The Professional Practice of Nursing Administration

Lillian M. Simms, Ph.D., R.N., F.A.A.N.
Associate Professor
School of Nursing
The University of Michigan
Ann Arbor, MI

Sylvia A. Price, Ph.D., R.N.
Professor
College of Nursing
University of Tennessee
Memphis, TN

Naomi E. Ervin, Ph.D., R.N.
Clinical Assistant Professor
College of Nursing
University of Illinois at Chicago
Chicago, IL

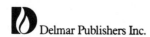 Delmar Publishers Inc.

I(T)P™

NOTICE TO THE READER

Cover design by: Geoffrey Deihl

Delmar Staff
Senior Acquisitions Editor: William Burgower
Project Editor: Melissa Conan
Production Coordinator: Mary Ellen Black
Art/Design Coordinator: Mary Siener
Assistant Editor: Debra Flis

COPYRIGHT © 1994
BY DELMAR PUBLISHERS INC.
The trademark ITP is used under license.
For information, address
Delmar Publishers Inc.
3 Columbia Circle, Box 15015
Albany, NY 12212-5015

Printed in the United States of America
Published simultaneously in Canada
by Nelson Canada,
a division of The Thomson Corporation

10   9   8   7   6   5   4   3   2   1   XX   00   99   98   97   96   95   94

Library of Congress Cataloging-in-Publication Data

Simms, Lillian M. (Lillian Miller)
   The professional practice of nursing administration / Lillian M.
Simms, Sylvia A. Price, Naomi E. Ervin. — 2nd ed.
    p.   cm.
Includes bibliographical references and index.
ISBN 0-8273-4965-3
1. Nursing services—Administration.   I. Price, Sylvia
Anderson.   II. Ervin, Naomi E.   III. Title.
[DNLM: 1. Administrative Personnel.   2. Nurse
Administrators.   WY   105 S592p   1993]
RT89.S58   1993
362.1'73'068—dc20
DNLM/DLC
for Library of Congress   93-12005
                                                CIP

To all professional nurses around the world who seek to understand how to accomplish their work wherever they practice

CONTRIBUTORS

Yvonne M. Abdoo, Ph.D., R.N.
Assistant Professor
Division of Nursing and Health Systems
The University of Michigan
School of Nursing
Ann Arbor, MI

Kathryn Barnoud, M.S.N., R.N.
Nurse Consultant
Memphis, TN

Eunice A. Bell, Ph.D., R.N., C.N.A.A.
Director of Clinical Education
Memorial Medical Center
Savannah, GA

Judith A. Bernhardt, M.S., R.N.
Senior Health Care Consultant
Pitts Management Associates, Inc.
Baton Rouge, LA

Catherine Buchanan, Ph.D., R.N.
Medical-Legal Consultant
Bloomfield Hills, MI

Peter I. Buerhaus, Ph.D., R.N.
Assistant Professor, Health Policy and Management
Harvard University
School of Public Health
Department of Health Policy and Management
Boston, MA

Sandra R. Byers, Ph.D., R.N., C.N.A.A.
Director, Health Policy
The Ohio Hospital Association
Columbus, OH

Harriet Van Ess Coeling, Ph.D., R.N.
Associate Professor
Kent State University
School of Nursing
Kent, OH

Betty Sue Cox, M.S.N., R.N.
Director, Cardiovascular Services
Baptist Memorial Hospital
Memphis, TN

Deborah Sweeney Hooser, M.S.N.A., R.N., C.N.A.
Nurse Manager, Cardiovascular Surgery
Heart Transplant Unit
Memphis, TN

Marjorie Mullin Jackson, M.S., B.A., R.N.
Associate Professor Emeritae
The University of Michigan
School of Nursing
Ann Arbor, MI

Paula R. Jaco, M.S.N., R.N.
Associate Administrator of Patient Care Services
Crawford Memorial Hospital
Van Buren, Arkansas

Marylane Wade Koch, M.S.N., R.N., C.N.A.A., C.P.H.Q.
Vice President, Alternative Care Services
Methodist Health Systems
Memphis, TN

Joanne L. Lound, M.H.S.A., C.P.A., F.H.F.M.A.
Assistant to the Vice Provost for Medical Affairs
The University of Michigan
Ann Arbor, MI

Charlotte McDaniel, Ph.D., M.Ed., B.S.N., B.A., R.N.
Assistant Professor, School of Nursing and
Associate, The Center for Medical Ethics
University of Pittsburgh Medical Center
Pittsburgh, PA

Mary L. McHugh, Ph.D., R.N.
Director, Nursing Research & Development
St. Francis Regional Medical Center
Wichita, KS

Richard W. Redman, Ph.D., R.N.
Associate Professor and
Director, Division of Nursing and Health Systems
The University of Michigan
School of Nursing
Ann Arbor, MI

Contents

Foreword   xv

Preface   xvii

Introduction   xix

**PART I   A Framework for the Practice of
             Nursing Administration**   1

Chapter 1   **Integrated Professional Nursing
             Administration in Multiple Settings**   2

Chapter 2   **Nursing Theories and Conceptual Models**   13

Chapter 3   **Evolving Theories of Management**   30
             Sylvia A. Price and Paula R. Jaco

Chapter 4   **Through the Looking Glass: Making Sense
             of Organizations**   46

Chapter 5   **The Person in the Role of Nurse Executive**   61

**PART II   The Context of Nursing
             Administration Practice**   79

Chapter 6   **Creating the Environment for Professional
             Practice**   80

Chapter 7   **Blending Clinical Practice with
             Organizational Design**   90

Chapter 8   **Receptivity to Innovation**   104

Chapter 9   **Organizational Culture**   120
             Harriet V.E. Coeling

Chapter 10   **Operationalizing Professional Nursing**   137

PART III   **Current and Emerging Challenges**   **145**

Chapter 11   **Current and Emerging Practice Settings**   **146**

Chapter 12   **Developing Human Potential**   **162**

Chapter 13   **Managing Fiscal Resources**   **173**
                  Joanne L. Lound

Chapter 14   **Conflict Management in Personal and**
                  Professional Life   **185**

Chapter 15   **Leadership in Care of Older People**   **203**

PART IV   **Facilitating Professional Nursing Practice** **221**

Chapter 16   **Ethical Decision Making and**
                  Moral Judgments   **222**
                  Charlotte McDaniel

Chapter 17   **Personal and Group Empowerment**   **231**
                  Lillian M. Simms

Chapter 18   **Strategic Planning**   **248**
                  Eunice A. Bell

Chapter 19   **Integrated Quality Management**   **257**
                  Marylane Wade–Koch

Chapter 20   **Advancing Nursing Research in a**
                  Professional Practice Climate   **270**

PART V   **Managing Resources**   **279**

Chapter 21   **Mobilizing Existing Resources**   **280**

Chapter 22   **Facilities Planning**   **295**
                  Judith A. Bernhardt

Chapter 23   **Nurse Staffing and Scheduling**   **310**
                  Yvonne M. Abdoo

Chapter 24   **Building Effective Work Groups**   **327**
                  Sandra R. Byers and Lillian M. Simms

Chapter 25   **Human Productivity**   **339**

PART VI   **Communication**   **351**

Chapter 26   **Effective Communication**   **352**

Chapter 27   **Mentorship and Networking**   **365**
                  Catherine Buchanan

Chapter 28   **From Enabling to Assistive Technology**   379

Chapter 29   **Enhancing Productivity Through Computerized Information Systems**   392
Mary L. McHugh

Chapter 30   **Collective Action—Labor Relations**   411
Richard W. Redman

PART VII   **Moving Beyond the Ordinary**   421

Chapter 31   **Quality in Health Care Environments**   422
Naomi E. Ervin

Chapter 32   **Marketing Nursing and Nursing Services**   435
Sylvia A. Price

Chapter 33   **Nursing Economics and Politics in a Global Economy**   449
Peter I. Buerhaus

Chapter 34   **Humor in Administration/The Comedy of Management**   460
Marjorie M. Jackson

Chapter 35   **The Nursing Administration Imperative: Integrating Practice, Education, and Research**   476

APPENDIX   489

Situations for case study   489

A   **Implementation of a change process**   489

B   **Gainsharing as an innovative approach**   489
Deborah Hooser

C   **Problem-oriented recording**   490

D   **Community/rural hospital nursing system**   491

E   **Urban hospital nursing system**   492

F   **Sharing of services as a cost-effective measure**   492

G   **Operationalizing professional nursing**   493

H   **Introducing quality assurance in a nursing home**   494

I   **Marketing a product line**   494
Betty Sue Cox

J   **Introduction of bedside terminals**   497
Kathryn Barnoud

FOREWORD

Foreword

A seminal work for the future of nursing administration! This book is a contribution to the literature that even outdistances the first edition. It harbors a completely new look at nursing administration, providing for the changes that will continue to challenge the nurse executive.

Simms, Price, and Ervin define a new cutting edge for nursing administration, offering a novel menu of the key elements of nursing administration. The proposed conceptual model addresses every practice setting, synthesizing the clinical, research, management, and teaching/learning knowledge into the position of nurse executive. It is the first nursing administration text to emphasize the teaching/learning role of the nurse executive; this revised book proposes new learning behaviors and the development of creative learning environments as the responsibility of the nurse executive. This new emphasis on creative teaching/learning is fostered through the examples of the authors, who change formats to meet the purpose of various chapters in the book.

The "seeds" sown in this seminal work are the product of intense interdisciplinary search and study as well as the scholarly research of the authors. Sources quoted from outside nursing bring the latest in thought from business and organizational fields about the future needs of organized work.

Establishing "an environment for creativity" and "flexible work groups" are popular catch words that the authors have operationalized for today's world. Discussion includes the efficient use of resources, the greatest of which is people and their innate abilities to think and create.

The future of health care lies in a global effort to provide for the welfare of all peoples. Soon it will extend also to those living in space. This book defines the organization and functioning of health care, DEFINING, not just addressing, the cutting edge of leadership for the provision of health care for all.

The authors offer this text for the second level of professional practice, that of nursing administration. It is recommended both for the practicing nurse in any setting and for graduate study. I feel its seeds need to be introduced at the baccalaureate level so that beginning practicing nurses will have a conceptual model of practice to serve them immediately and into the next century. We now expect of the new professional nurse that s/he manage a group of patients, an area of care, without acknowledging that we have not prepared her/him for this responsibility. The new professional nurse is not the dewy-eyed, naive 21-year-old that one remembers from the past, but a mature professional, probably over 35 years of age, with a wealth of life's experiences brought to nursing. S/he is capable of comprehending this new knowledge, and needs it for safe practice in today's complex health care world.

Barbara Fuszard, Ph.D., R.N., F.A.A.N.

Preface

The great diversity in approaches to nursing management or administration has led to confusion as to what this field encompasses. Because of this diversity, a comprehensive synthesis of ideas is needed about nursing administration. This revised edition of *The Professional Practice of Nursing Administration* presents a synthesis of key elements of nursing administration that can be used now and into the twenty-first century. For too long, nurses have argued about naming the first level of differentiated nursing practice with little attention to the second level. This book addresses the second level of practice, the professional practice of nursing administration. The title of nurse executive can no longer be reserved for corporate level nurses who manage health service systems and other health-related enterprises. Every professional nurse needs executive skills, and executive roles include existing nursing titles and those yet to be introduced.

Nurse executives are responsible and accountable for clinical practice, education, management, and research in ambulatory, acute, community health, home health, and long-term health care settings. A proposed conceptual model for professional nursing administrative practice emphasizes the integration of clinical, research, management, and teaching/learning knowledge in all these settings. Because the role of the nurse executive as a teacher/learner has been largely unrecognized, the revised book addresses the need for learning new behaviors in creative learning environments that maximize human potential and places major emphasis on the learning facilitative role of the nurse executive.

The revised book is comprehensive, research-based, and scholarly: an essential text for practicing clinicians, managers, researchers, and educators. This revised edition marks the first integrated approach to professional nursing practice that will appeal to students, practitioners, and other health care professionals. The revision updates all chapters, reflects changing thought, and includes essential content that has emerged since the first edition. Human development and lifelong learning permeate the book and provide the background for understanding the people-to-people skills essential for living and working in new-age participatory environments.

The book is designed for masters and doctoral students, upper division undergraduate students in nursing, and registered nurses in BSN completion programs in the United States and around the world. It is an appropriate resource for students and professional nursing practitioners at all levels in a variety of health care settings, including ambulatory, acute, community health, long-term, and home care. For example, clinical nurse specialists in line or staff positions, case managers, care coordinators, research project directors, entrepreneurs, nurse educators, nurse administrators, and health care professionals at all levels, as well as those who aspire to a career at the senior executive management level, will find this book a valuable resource.

Throughout the book, diversity is emphasized by variation in learning activities. Food for thought and study questions appear in several chapters as appropriate. Selected case studies are provided in the Appendix. Because the authors seek to stimulate new thoughts, previous objectives have been replaced by Chapter Highlights at the beginning of each chapter. The book blends ideas from the business and organizational fields with nursing, bringing a unique synthesis of relevant content. The authors have also built on their unique professional experiences in nursing to bring theory and practice together.

Special acknowledgement is given to Richard J. Simms, Sr., who provided extensive assistance with the design of illustrations throughout the text. The authors would also like to acknowledge Beverly G. Ware, Dr.P.H., and Barbara Fuszard, Ph.D., R.N., F.A.A.N., for their critique of the manuscript.

Lillian M. Simms
Sylvia A. Price
Naomi E. Ervin

Introduction _____

The computer has changed the way we think about our work, our organizations and the way we practice our profession. What were considered effective and efficient organizations in the past are now costly dinosaurs. New organizational structures are like cobwebs that can be built anywhere. To function in the new age, nurse executives must have an understanding of the knowledge and skills necessary to function in ever-changing organizations. Nursing administration is practiced everywhere and globalization of health care will soon be transformed to interplanetary health care. Practicing in the global community demands that individual professionals take personal responsibility for lifelong learning.

This book is not written as a traditional nursing administration text but, rather, as a book that will appeal to any nurse practicing in any setting and wishing to acquire an understanding of administrative knowledge and skills. If the computer has changed the way we think about working and communicating with each other, the realization that people can learn over the life span has changed the way we look at human resources and the development of effective work skills. Major emphasis has been placed, therefore, on human development and personal responsibility for quality care delivery. A unique chapter on leadership in care of older people is included as one relevant change in our society today. To understand aging and caring over the life span is to understand growth and development of the professional self.

The work of nursing is cast in a new light, moving past the factory models of the past. Work can be exciting, and nowhere is there work more exciting than nursing care that can be delivered in a wide variety of settings. The authors break loose from the traditional vision of past specialties of community health, medical-surgical, parent-child nursing and others to recognize that modern nursing administration can be practiced anywhere care must be delivered: in the home, in the neighborhood, in the military, in acute care hospitals, long-term care facilities, walk-in centers, in the bush country of Africa, in rural areas, in sports arenas, and anywhere else imaginable. Our practice is not defined by the traditional divisions but rather by a vision of community that encompasses wherever humans live.

Chapters are organized in groups according to major themes that could pertain to any organizational structure. Learning activities are not consistent for each chapter. They vary by chapter and appear as appropriate study questions, food for thought, occasional case studies, and activities immersed within the chapter. This is deliberate, as nursing texts have been overrun with objectives and fixed "Thou shalt learn this" approaches. We want this book to be interesting and readable, to be read in its entirety or to be relished in chapters, or even pages, that have particular individual relevance. We want readers to gain new ideas about themselves and how they can view the changing world of work.

Major emphasis is also placed on the importance of personal learning and the creation of learning environments, regardless of organizational setting. A unique approach to participatory action research is included as one way to create a relevant research environment. Facilitating participation in decision making and research is perceived as a key component of personal and group empowerment in any setting. This idea propels the meaning of integrated nursing administration to the real world of practice. Research is part of the nurse executive and not the role preserved for occasional visitors seeking research projects of their own interest.

In essence, the book is delivered in sections that are relevant anywhere on earth or in space. In Part I, the reader will move through a trajectory of a new vision of integrated practice, relevant clinical and management theories, a new look at organizations, and a soul-searching discussion of the nurse executive as a person. Part II presents a view of the context of nursing administrative practice with heavy emphasis on blending clinical practice with organizational design. The importance of organizational and unit culture as important to the business of operationalizing nursing and creating learning environments responsive to innovation makes this part vital. Part III presents current and emerging challenges with emphasis on the development of human potential; managing fiscal resources and conflict lead into the chapter on care of older people as the most striking health care responsibilities of our time.

Part IV addresses the facilitation of professional nursing administration practice in any setting. Ethical decision making, empowerment, strategic planning, quality management, and nursing research are all portrayed as essential knowledge areas for the practicing nurse executive. Part V places major emphasis on building and managing resources in any setting. Resources include facilities, people, and productivity abilities not usually addressed in administrative texts. Maximizing the creativity of workers in a non-zero sum-based power environment is encouraged through continual learning and functioning in flexible work groups. The communication chapters in Part VI have been expanded to include assistive technology as knowledge, skills and equipment for nurse executives and consumers, and computerized information systems. Collective action-labor relations is also a new addition in this text that extends the discussion of effective work groups to a total organizational environment.

The last part, number VII, is truly unique. Building on the concept of quality in any environment, the section covers marketing nursing services through entrepreneurship and nursing economics and politics in a global economy. An unusual chapter on humor and comedy in management is considered essential content for any nurse executive and part of the personal development of executive skills. The book closes with reaffirmation of the earlier imperative in the first edition. Clinical practice, teaching/learning, research, and management must be integrated in the nurse executive role. For too long we have created great division in our profession by preparing special elites, the most recent being the nurse researcher. The authors believe we must bring these components together in one new revolutionary role, the nurse executive. Nursing research sits on shelves of numerous places, unused in practice because it is not seen as being relevant to practice. The clinical nurse manager must be one and the same with the researcher and teacher/learner if we are to bring wholeness to our work.

This book is bold and not to be read by the faint hearted. We are proposing a totally new direction in nursing administration but one we believe will become the hallmark of professional nursing schools around the world. If we truly want to take our place in the "Health for All" agenda of the World Health Organization, we must take drastic steps in preparing our professionals so that we give them the tools they need to practice anywhere and that we develop nursing administration curricula that will appeal to diverse students with various backgrounds that could enrich our work.

PART I

A Framework for the Practice of Nursing Administration

CHAPTER 1

Integrated Professional Nursing Administration in Multiple Settings

---

Highlights

- Emergence of the nurse executive
- Professions and professionalism
- Nursing practice
- Professional practice disciplines
- Integrated professional nursing administration

The purpose of this chapter is to present a conceptual framework for integrated professional nursing practice. Since the 1985 edition of this book, nursing administration has advanced rapidly. Modern professional nursing has become nursing administration and deliberations on the fit of administration with clinical nursing are beginning to cease. Professional nursing practice combines care provision and care coordination in the mature integrated discipline of nursing administration and the title of nurse administrator has changed to nurse executive in most progressive settings.

The title of nurse executive can no longer be reserved for corporate-level nurses who manage health service systems and other health-related enterprises. Every professional nurse needs executive skills (Sovie, 1987). All professional nurses must be able to work with multiple groups. All professional nurses must develop team-building skills and knowledge essential to engage in participative management. Executive roles include head nurses, supervisors, coordinators, directors, chiefs, clinicians, managers, faculty members who manage courses, principal investigators and students, deans, vice presidents, presidents, and chief nurse executives under whatever title yet to be introduced. This does not mean there will not be senior nurse executives. These roles will change dramatically, however, and we can expect to see more visionary Nightingales and Walds who are unafraid to put theory and action together and who are unafraid to explore the development of new theories to nurture quality patient care.

Florence Nightingale was an extraordinary person and the first nurse executive to appreciate the importance of linking care provision and care management (Simms, 1991). Modern nursing and hospital administration emerged from her work and she was never content to provide only nursing care without tackling the physicians and the environment to improve patient care. In addition to advancing the cause of medical reform, she helped to pioneer the revolutionary notion that phenomena could be objectively measured and subjected to mathematical analysis. Although unaware of modern research methods, she fully understood the importance of collecting and analyzing data.

According to Cohen (1984), Nightingale not only instituted sanitary reforms in the hospitals at Scutari in 1854, she recognized the importance of medical statistics as a tool for improving medical care in military and civilian hospitals. She systematized the chaotic record-keeping practices and developed graphical representations of statistics. She invented polar-area charts, in which the statistic being represented is proportional to the area of a wedge in a circular diagram. These charts, called "coxcombs" in her writings, were used to dramatize the number of preventable deaths in the Crimean campaign. Her statistical charts and diagrams became an important part of the Royal Commission Report, a document that was widely distributed in Parliament, the government, and the army and had an important effect on the improvement of environmental conditions in hospitals.

Nightingale (Cohen, 1984) had little interest in the germ theory of disease and its implications for the treatment of contagious diseases. However, she was ahead of the times in her clinical efforts to improve ventilation, heating, sewage disposal, water supply, and kitchens. It is interesting to note that in modern times, we have again returned to environmental factors in disease prevention. And the major cause of death, as Nightingale noted, is still "diarrhea," which is related to poor sewage disposal, inadequate water supply, and malnutrition (Michigan League for Nursing, 1990). It is important to note that Nightingale managed patient care and the environment while at the same time she paid strong attention to physicians and government policy makers, recognizing their influence on her freedom to practice.

Lillian Wald also was a superb nurse executive (Kalisch and Kalisch, 1986). Wald was a public health nurse who graduated from New York Hospital School of Nursing in 1891. Unhappy with her scant nursing knowledge, she enrolled in Medical School at Woman's Medical College in New York. She used her nursing and entrepreneurial business skills to establish a nurses' settlement house in one of the slum sections of the Lower East Side. By 1909, the East Side Settlement moved to Henry Street and became the Henry Street Settlement. This very creative business included first-aid homes in densely populated sections of the city, small surgical offices for dressings, and a small obstetrical service. The Henry Street Settlement grew in size from two nurses living on the top floor of a tenement house to a highly organized social enterprise with many departments. Wald and her staff provided care for inner city people and much of her care focused on that of immigrant women and children who could neither read nor write the English language. The world has the same needy populations today, and the need for nurse executives who can combine clinical and management skills is greater than ever.

In 1977, the World Health Organization (WHO) set a global objective "the attainment of Health for All citizens of the world by the year 2000" and in 1978, primary health care was introduced in Alma-Ata as the primary strategy to achieving this goal (Kiereini, 1989). Although progress has been made, many barriers exist — perhaps the most important being the disease orientation of most health professionals, including nurses, and the relative incompetence among all health professionals to effectively develop and manage new health care systems that can meet current and emerging needs.

Maglacas (1988) forcefully states that nursing's choice for the twenty-first century is simple. We can participate in "health care for a few" or "health for all." This demands an integrated managerial process for national health development, stressing the concept of broad-based planning for health and development rather than for health services alone. It also places great emphasis on policy formulation, on the political and social processes in planning, and on strong links among clinical knowledge, planning, and management. Furthermore, says Maglacas, this implicitly requires reorientation of national health systems so that each system develops an appropriate structure for primary care. This has tremendous implications for the nursing profession wherein the struggle is still underway to keep at least 150 specialties alive and well in spite of tremendous overlap of services and competition for students. The artificial barriers that exist between nursing administration, community health, and medical-surgical nursing need to be taken down. The Berlin Wall came down, why not the walls within nursing?

In many countries of the world, there is an oversupply, underuse, and unemployment of various categories of health personnel, physicians and dentists in particular. There is a tremendous shortage of nurses offering care. Health promotion as nursing's focus must go beyond responsibility for merely delivering medical care services. Nurses should be running nursing and health services around the world, not participating only in illness services. Holleran (1988) supports the need for appropriate nursing care in institutions as well. In any case, nurses must be better prepared to influence the quality of care provided in home, community, or institutional settings.

Influence on health care must take place in the home, the workplace, and wherever humans abide. To accelerate the delivery of essential health services to the people of the world, particularly underserved populations, the transformation of the nursing profession is critical and professional nurses must assume roles as leaders and active participants in these changes. All professional nurses must master the skills of visionary and strategic thinking to have an impact on the institutional and political forces that control health development (O'Hara-Devereaux, 1989).

Nursing services constitute a core function of health care delivery systems, and nurse executives conduct and control clinical nursing practice. As health care delivery systems change and as professional roles are redefined, effective nursing leadership is essential. Nurses participate in policy and decision making, assume responsibility for managing nursing service and related activities, and work cooperatively with professionals from other health disciplines to ensure that quality client-centered care is administered. The acquisition and allocation of human and physical resources required to meet the goals of clinical care are facilitated by the nurse executive. For example, nurse executives generally influence the largest proportion of the budgets of hospitals and other health care institutions and make major decisions affecting the quality of patient care.

Because the health care industry is a human services endeavor, nurse executives must have a theoretical grounding in the behavioral sciences. It is also essential that they both acquire knowledge and understanding of administrative theory and are aware of changing concepts in the field. This knowledge will enable nurse executives to develop a conceptual framework for their nursing administrative practice in regional, national, and global environments.

DEFINITION OF A PROFESSION AND PROFESSIONALISM

Nursing is an emerging *profession* and a *professional practice discipline*. One must have comprehensive understanding of both terms to promote the highest level of nursing administrative practice. Many writers have discussed the history, development, definition, and application of the concept of a profession (Etzioni, 1969; Schein, 1972; Kelly, 1981; Simms, 1991). Although these writers exhibit considerable diversity, there is consensus on the basic premise that *professionalism* involves autonomy, mastery of a body of knowledge, and a community of colleagues. The following are essential criteria of a *profession*:

1. Provides practical services that are vital to human and social welfare
2. Possesses a specialized body of knowledge and skills
3. Educates its practitioners in institutions of higher education
4. Attracts people who emphasize service over personal gain or self-interest and recognize their occupation as a long-term commitment
5. Formulates and controls its own policies and activities and has practitioners who function relatively autonomously in the performance of functions and activities

6. Has a code of ethics that is usually enforced by colleagues or through licensure examinations

7. Has a professional association that promotes and ensures quality of practice

It should be noted that profession is a social concept. The authority for nursing is based on a social contract that is derived from a complex social base. Donabedian (1961) states:

There is a "social contract" between society and the professions. Under its terms, society grants the professions authority over functions vital to itself and permits them considerable autonomy in the conduct of their own affairs. In return, the professions are expected to act responsibly, always mindful of the public trust. Self-regulation to assure quality in performance is at the heart of this relationship. It is the authentic hallmark of a mature profession. (p. xiii)

Although there is some agreement as to what constitutes a professional nurse, much variation in opinion remains. One area of diversity involves the length and type of educational preparation necessary to qualify for the status of professional nurse. Another issue is whether nursing is really an occupation, rather than a profession, such as medicine, theology, and law. Writers who present this issue acknowledge that some nurses now perform expanded roles and functions, whereas others lack the educational basis for such a practice. Therefore, it is often difficult to distinguish among associate-degree, diploma, and baccalaureate-prepared nurses.

Nurses provide services in a variety of settings and assume more responsibility and accountability for the consequences of their decisions than in the past. This extension of nursing practice also involves increased collaboration with physicians and other health practitioners in the performance of their respective roles in the provision of health services. In collaborative practice, nurses emphasize psychosocial aspects of health care, coordination of patient care services, and advocacy of patient rights (Simms, Dalston and Roberts, 1984).

As an emerging profession, nursing is recognizing the need to formulate a theoretical base for its practice and to articulate that base to others. Research is evolving in the clinical areas to test nursing theories and related theories on which the practice of nursing is based. Similarly, research in the practice of nursing administration provides an empirical knowledge base for the various functions and responsibilities associated with nursing administration. Nursing must initiate and promote research to support the organizational restructuring of the delivery of nursing services, to define nurses' roles and responsibilities in interdisciplinary endeavors, and to provide a data base for a systematic evaluation of the impact of nursing.

Professional roles and functions of nursing are being reexamined and redesigned. The professional role of the practitioner of nursing has been expanded, leading to a repatterning of nursing education and emphasis on lifelong learning and career commitment to nursing. This trend has further emphasized the need for nurses who are creative and possess competencies to function in a collegial relationship with other health care professionals.

NURSING PRACTICE

Nursing is concerned with human health and well-being. It involves the delivery of humanistic care to people to promote and maintain health, prevent illness, cure illness and restore health, and coordinate health care services to improve continuity of care.

Discussing the nature of nursing, Virginia Henderson (1961) states:

The unique function of the nurse is to assist the individual, sick or well, in the performance of those activities contributing to health or his recovery (or to peaceful death) that he would perform unaided if he had the necessary strength, will, or knowledge. And to do this in such a way as to help him gain independence as rapidly as possible. This aspect of her work, this part of her function, she initiates and controls; of this she is master. In addition she helps the patient carry out the therapeutic plan as initiated by the physician. She also, as a member of a medical team, helps other members, as they in turn help her, to plan and carry out the total program whether it be for the improvement of health, or the recovery from illness, or support in death. (p. 42)

The American Nurses Association Congress for Nursing Practice has proposed a definition that attempts to differentiate between professional and vocational nursing:

The practice of nursing means the performance for compensation of professional services requiring substantial specialized knowledge of the biological, physical, behavioral, psychological, and sociological sciences and of nursing theory as the basis of assessment, diagnosis, planning, intervention, and evaluating the promotion and maintenance of health, the casefinding and management of illness, injury, or infirmity, the restoration of optimum function, or the achievement of a dignified death. Nursing practice influences but is not limited to administration, teaching, counseling, supervision, delegation, and evaluation of practice and execution of the medications and treatments prescribed by any person authorized by state law to prescribe. Each registered nurse is directly accountable and responsible to the consumer for the quality of nursing care rendered.

The practice of practical (vocational) nursing means the performance for compensation of technical services requiring basic knowledge of the biological, physical, behavioral, psychological, and sociological sciences and of nursing procedures. These services are performed under the supervision of a registered nurse and utilize standardized procedures leading to predictable outcomes in the observation and care of the ill, injured, and infirm, in the maintenance of health, in action to safeguard life and health, and in the administration of medications and treatments prescribed by any person authorized by state law to prescribe. (ANA, 1980, p. 6)

Schlotfeldt (1981) emphasizes that nurses should search for a conceptual focus and definition of their profession that permit inclusion of phenomena related to human beings' seeking optimal health. She believes that a definition is needed that will help to establish nursing as a profession whose practitioners are responsible for the general health of human beings. Thus, her definition is, "Nursing is assessing and enhancing the general health status, health assets, and health potentials of human beings" (p. 298). This definition is unambiguous; focuses on nursing practice, education, and research; and conveys nurses' knowledge, practice, and scope of accountability. Because it does not encroach on the responsibilities of other helping professionals, it is conceptually appropriate and politically acceptable. Schlotfeldt emphasizes that nursing will become a recognized, learned profession and that nurses will provide essential services that will enhance the health and well-being of our society.

The nursing profession makes significant contributions to the evolution of a health-oriented system of care. Nursing practice has been health-oriented for over half of a century because of its focus on individuals as persons and on the family as the necessary unit of service (ANA Social Policy Statement, 1980).

PROFESSIONAL PRACTICE DISCIPLINES

Both the legal responsibility and the scope of nursing practice are regulated by the nursing practice acts of each state. For example, according to the State of Michigan Public Health Code, House Bill No. 4070 (1978), the practice of nursing is "the systematic application of substantial specialized knowledge and skill derived from the biological, physical, and behavioral sciences to the care, treatment, counsel, and health teaching of individuals who are experiencing changes in the normal health processes or who require assistance in the maintenance of health and the prevention or management of illness, injury, or disability." This definition is appropriate for a professional practice discipline such as nursing. It conveys that nursing emphasizes human health and well-being, which are the concerns of nurses and determine the essential nature of nursing.

Lysaught (1981) reports that the National Commission for the Study of Nursing and Nursing Education presents an interactive model of nursing practice that envisages three dynamic continua that operate in close relationship to one another and, taken together, explain the entire domain of needs for nursing and expertise (see Figure 1.1). One axis classifies the set of nursing behaviors ranging from the initial assessment of client condition through intervention, instruction, and assessment of outcomes and results. The second axis classifies patient condition: well, unwell, or acutely unwell. The commission emphasizes that the "concept of maintaining wellness and limiting illness is as much a part of the full practice of nursing—or medicine—as is the treatment of acute illness." The third axis depicts the environmental setting (e.g., institution, outpatient setting, clinic, home, or community). This axis contains areas for the enactment of nursing behaviors classified, for simplicity, in two categories: episodic care, which includes curative and restorative care; and distributive care, which is geared toward health maintenance and disease prevention and takes place with increasing frequency in community and emergent care settings.

In determining proper role functions in accordance with client needs and in relationship to selecting the optimum environment for care, Lysaught's interactive model focuses on whether the nurses' role is independent or interdependent. This conceptual framework suggests no single focus for nursing practice; it argues for nursing as a variety of specific capacities, rather than a group of simple skills, and for a relocation of the patient and his or her needs to an elemental position in the decision-making process related to intervention and care. This model argues for nursing as a profession—not just nurses as individuals—to be prepared for health intervention in a kaleidoscope of situations. There is room for a variety of concentrations and specializations, both horizontally, across the range of client care needs (from acute cardiac care

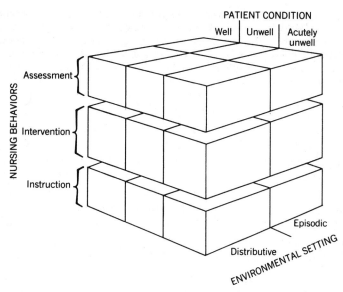

Figure 1.1 Interactive model of an emergent, full profession of nursing. Episodic care is that domain of nursing practice that is essentially curative and restorative, generally treating ill patients, and most frequently provided in a hospital setting or other inpatient facility. Distributive care is that domain of nursing practice that is essentially designed for health maintenance and disease prevention, generally continuous in nature, seldom acute, and increasingly provided in community or emergent care settings. (From Lysaught, J. P. (1981). *Action in Affirmation: Toward an Unambiguous Profession of Nursing.* New York: McGraw-Hill. Reprinted by permission.)

through a mild illness) and vertically, within a nursing practice (from staff nurse to master clinician).

This conceptual scheme also argues for variation in the educational patterning of preparatory and advanced studies to ensure the education of the variety as well as the number of nurses needed to implement a full range of client services. It provides for a commitment and career perspective that includes mobility and increments in responsibility, authority, and recognition. Furthermore, it provides for the integration of management skills that are so essential for the care coordination and action responsibilities of the modern nurse executive.

Donaldson and Crowley (1978) distinguish between academic and professional disciplines. The purpose of academic disciplines is to know (and, for some, to apply that knowledge); therefore, they develop descriptive theories. Because the professional disciplines have an added component of service to people, their theories are both descriptive and prescriptive in nature. Whereas academic disciplines involve basic and applied research, professional disciplines also involve clinical research. Donaldson and Crowley (1978) caution that:

The discipline, which is a body of knowledge, must not be confused with its associated practice realm, which embodies the processes of conducting research, giving service, and educating. Furthermore, some members of the profession must engage in enquiry that is not immediately applicable to current clinical practice. As a branch of knowledge, the discipline embodies more than the science of nursing and requires researchers who employ a variety of approaches from nursing's perspective. (p. 119)

Nurse researchers, clinicians, and educators use information from many disciplines and must understand or conduct research in these fields outside nursing.

Professional practice disciplines such as nursing, medicine, and dentistry are defined by the application of knowledge in relation to the health of clients. Although clinical practice is a major thrust of nursing, other components of professional practice must be considered, including research, education, and management. The four components, therefore, of integrated professional nursing administration are *(1)* clinical practice (application of knowledge), *(2)* research (development of knowledge), *(3)* education (learning and transmission of knowledge), and *(4)* management (care coordination and utilization of knowledge), as shown in Figure 1.2. These components

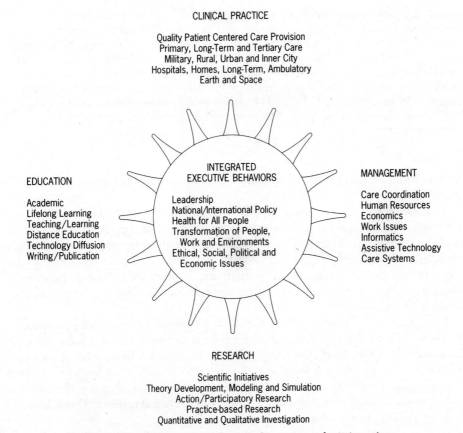

Figure 1.2 Integrated professional nursing administration.

need to be articulated and coordinated toward the full attainment of a professional practice discipline. The education component influences policy formation by administration, which in turn nurtures research-based clinical practice. Nurse administrators are responsible for nursing practice, research, and education as they relate to professional nursing within an institution.

Administrative support provides the environment and structure in which nursing practice can occur. The majority of nurses are employed by health care institutions, and their clinical practice must interface with administrative philosophy and policy. The amount of control that nurses have over their own practice is related to many factors in this employer-employee relationship. The following chapters cover innovative administrative approaches and factors that influence nursing practice on both conceptual and pragmatic levels. A nurse executive must consider both conceptual and pragmatic levels to construct a supportive and growth-producing environment for professional nursing practice.

Summary

For nursing administration to be a recognized professional practice discipline, nursing must do more than formulate a theoretical basis for its practice. Nursing theories and models provide a conceptual framework for the implementation of nursing practice. Management theories and models provide a framework for putting action into nursing practice. The next chapter examines selected nursing theories and models.

STUDY QUESTIONS

1. Formulate a definition of nursing administration.
2. What are the distinguishing characteristics that differentiate professional and vocational nursing?
3. According to the National Commission for the Study of Nursing and Nursing Education's interactive model, there is no single focus for nursing practice. Explain.
4. Why is the field of nursing administration considered a professional practice discipline rather than an academic one? Explain.
5. Describe the four components of professional nursing administrative practice.
6. Compare Nightingale and Wald with modern nurse entrepreneurs.

References

American Nurses Association. (1980). *Nursing: A social policy statement.* Kansas City, MO: American Nurses Association.

American Nurses Association. (1981). *The nursing practice act: Suggested state legislation.* Kansas City, MO: American Nurses Association.

Cohen, I. B. (1984). Florence Nightingale, *Scientific American, 250*(3), 128–137.

Donabedian, A. (1976). Foreword. In M. Phaneuf, *The nursing audit and self-regulation in nursing practice* (2nd ed.). New York: Appleton-Century-Crofts.

Donaldson, S., & Crowley, D. (1978). The discipline of nursing, *Nursing Outlook, 26*(2), 113–120.

Etzioni, A. (Ed.). (1969). *The semi-professions and their organization.* New York: The Free Press.

Henderson, V. (1961). *Basic principles of nursing care.* London: International Council of Nurses.

Holleran, C. (1988). Nursing beyond national boundaries: the 21st century, *Nursing Outlook, 36*(2), 72–75.

Kalisch, P. A., & Kalisch, B. J. (1986). *The advance of American nursing* (2nd ed.). Boston: Little, Brown.

Kelly, L. (1981). *Dimensions of professional nursing* (4th ed.). New York: Macmillan.

Kiereini, E. M. (1989, May 26–27). *Health policy: Barriers and means of achieving health for all by the year 2000.* Paper presented at the conference on Nursing Leadership: Using Research for Policy Making in Primary Health Care. Yonsei University: Seoul, Korea.

Lysaught, J. P. (1981). *Action in affirmation: Toward an unambiguous profession of nursing.* New York: McGraw-Hill.

Maglacas, A. M. (1988). Health for all: Nursing's role, *Nursing Outlook, 36*(2), 66–71.

Michigan League for Nursing. (1990). Nurses desperately needed in the developing world, *Nursing Focus, 7*(3), 5,9.

O'Hara-Devereaux, M. (1989, May 26–27). *Leadership development: Key to effectiveness at the policy level.* Paper presented at the conference on Nursing Leadership: Using Research for Policy Making in Primary Health Care. Yonsei University: Seoul, Korea.

Schein, E. H. (1972). *Professional education.* New York: McGraw-Hill.

Schlodtfeldt, R. (1981). Nursing in the future, *Nursing Outlook, 29*(5), 295–301.

Simms, L. M., Dalston, J. W., & Roberts, P. W. (1984). Collaborative practice: Myth or reality, *Hospital and Health Services Administration, 29*(6), 36–48.

Simms, L. M. (1991). The professional practice of nursing administration: Integrated nursing practice, *Journal of Nursing Administration, 21*(5), 37–46.

Sovie, M. D. (1987). Exceptional executive leadership shapes nursing's future, *Nursing Economics, 5*(1), 13–20.

State of Michigan, 79th Legislature. Enrolled House Bill No. 4070. (1978) *Michigan Public Health Code.*

CHAPTER 2

Nursing Theories and Conceptual Models

Highlights

- Theories
- Orem's self-care theory
- Roy adaptation model
- King's general systems theory
- Levine's conceptual model for nursing
- Implications for nursing administrative practice

The purpose of this chapter is to introduce the concept of theory and its relationship to nursing administrative practice. Nursing theories and models provide the conceptual framework for patient-centered nursing practice. In a practice discipline such as nursing, conceptual frameworks are necessary in directing the thinking of scholars, in the development of theories, and in guiding the observation of practitioners as the processes of assessment and intervention are implemented. This chapter focuses on nursing theories that are patient centered with patients considered to be bio-psycho-social beings and partners in the care delivery process.

THEORIES

A theory consists of a set of interconnected propositions designed to describe, explain, and predict an event or phenomenon. Chinn and Kramer (1991) envision a theory as a systematic abstraction of reality intended to serve some purpose. A systematic abstraction is defined as an organization pattern underlying the creation and design of theory as well as the notion that theory is not reality itself. Chinn & Kramer imply that what is systematized is also abstract; that is, it is a representation of reality, not reality itself. Approaches to theory development are themselves organized and patterned or systematic. The systematization of abstractions requires rigorous thought and action. The words and symbols that comprise a theory are labels associated with an object, property, or event in the real world. For example, the word "computer" represents an abstraction that denotes a real object. A theory consists of words (such as the label "computer") that represent abstractions, such as the mental image of a computer, that denote reality, such as the object "computer." Words and other symbols enable theories to be communicated and understood.

Hage (1972) states that concepts that refer to classes or categories of phenomena may be called nonvariable. Such concepts are observed in typologies in which classes are clearly defined, based on the presence or absence of the property of interest, for example, a nurse or a patient. General variables are concepts used to order phenomena according to some property or concepts that refer to dimensions of phenomena, for example, degree of anxiety or level of mobility. Hage stresses that concepts that vary over a continuum should be used more frequently than nonvariables in conceptualization and theory construction. Generally, variables are not restricted to time and place and lend themselves to more subtle description and classification than do nonvariable concepts.

In general, theories are constructed either deductively or inductively. In deductive theory construction, the concepts under study proceed from general to specific. Thus, deductive theory construction begins with general axioms and propositions. Deductive theories are developed through a logical process that relates concepts in general statements so that increasingly specific statements can be deducted from them.

The process of inductive theory construction proceeds from the specifics of empirical situations to generalizations about the data. This approach is best illustrated in the grounded theory of Glaser and Strauss (1967). This process involves sequential formulation, testing, and redevelopment of propositions until a theory is generated that is integrated, consistent with the data, and in a clear form, operationalized for later testing in quantitative research.

Simms (1981) in referring to the theory of Glaser and Strauss, cites four states in the constant comparative method they used in formulating the grounded theory approach:

(1) Comparing incidents applicable to each category, (2) integrating categories and their properties, (3) delineating the theory, and (4) writing the theory. The elements of theory that are generated by comparative analysis are the conceptual categories, their conceptual properties, and generalized relations among the categories and their properties.
To evaluate propositions and refine categories and their properties, relevant qualitative data are drawn from field and documentary sources. Principles underlying theoretical or purposive sampling guide the selection of comparison groups . . . The active search for relevant data continues until critical variables and their interrelationships have been saturated and no new relationships emerge that suggest more information be collected.
After the conceptual categories and properties are established and interrelationships evaluated, the researcher uses the information to formulate a theory. Each element is used to create an

explanation for the problem or phenomena under study, as well as questions for further research. The generation of theory must be viewed as a process. Concepts and propositions emerge gradually, and the ultimate generation of theory is dependent upon the data collected throughout the study. (pp. 356–357)

Theory formulation in the discipline of nursing provides a guide for professional nursing practice. Some nurse theoreticians use the deductive process with selected concepts from fields such as sociology, psychology, and physiology. They begin with general concepts and use these as parameters for analyzing specific nursing situations. Other theoreticians use the inductive approach to theory building in nursing, Wald and Leonard (1964) speculate that theorists begin with practical nursing experience and develop concepts that they feel will fit.

In their classic, yet contemporary article, Dickoff, James, and Wiedenbach (1968) describe the relationship of inductive theory to practice. They emphasize that a theory is neither a useless fairy tale nor a picture of the real. As such, the various kinds of theories can be grouped into four levels: *(1)* factor-isolating theory; *(2)* factor-relating, or situation-depicting, theory; *(3)* situation-relating, or predictive, theory; relationships; and *(4)* situation-producing, or perspective, theory. In this classification, each higher level presupposes the existence of theories at the lower level. Dickoff et al. (1968) state that a "situation is depicted in terms of actors already isolated; predictive or promoting theories conceive relationships between depictable situations; and situation-producing theories prescribe in terms of available predictive and promoting theories, and use depicting theories in the characterization of goal-content" (p. 420).

The *factor-isolating* theory, or naming, must be considered first because all scientific theory begins with the naming of factors. The essential function of naming is to facilitate reference to and communication about the factor associated with the name. This theoretical activity is called classifying or the introduction of technical terminology. To neglect factor-isolating theory is particularly detrimental when a theory is self-consciously being developed for the first time, as in nursing.

After factors are identified, they should be observed in relationships. The level of theory is *situation–depicting* in that it relates the factors that have been identified. Theories that depict or provide conceptions of interrelations among factors, as opposed to among situations, are correlations: the presence or absence or range of variation between two factors. Correlations do not imply causation or reference to time sequence; the two factors simply coexist.

Theories classified in the third level, are *situation–relating*. Factors are related in such a way that predictions can be made, because predictive theory can state relationships only between such situations as are depictable, which is dependent on what factors have been identified. Casual relationships must show the qualities of priority and direction among variables. For example, if A causes B, one must show that A precedes B, that when A occurs, so does B; that when A increases, B increases; and that when A decreases, B decreases. Therefore, situations may be connected causally.

The highest level of theory is *situation-producing* theory. This level exceeds predictive theory by stating not only that A causes B but also how to bring about A or how to facilitate A's production of B.

Dickoff et al. (1968) contend that to have an impact on practice, nursing theory must be at the highest level: situation-producing theory. Nurses confronted with a variety of complex situations must have a prescription for action. This prescription is made as a result of situation-producing theory.

Newman (1979) emphasizes that for a theory to have direct application, it must meet the following criteria:

1. The focus is on human beings.
2. The purpose is understanding the patterns of the life processes that relate to health.
3. A total elaboration of the theory contains an action component that facilitates health.

These criteria are consistent with the current conceptual models of nursing that include prescriptive-level theory.

MODELS

The relationship between variables may be depicted by a model. Hardy (1974) states that an investigator may formalize a theory, identify its postulates, identify or derive its propositions, and then decide that the problem of relationships is best represented by a model. A model is a simplified representation of a theory, certain complex events, structures, or systems. It is a conceptual representation of a reality situation.

Conceptual models provide a framework that directs the work of scholars in the formulation of theories. Differences among the various conceptual models of nursing are apparent in terms of emphasis, underlying assumptions, definition of health and illness, and designation of the goal of nursing.

The following nursing theories and conceptual models illustrate these differences. The objective of this discussion is to familiarize the nurse executive with selected nursing models and theories that are currently being implemented in nursing practice. It is important that nurse executives be knowledgeable about differences in emphasis so that they may adapt these models to interface with the philosophy of nursing practice within the context of their organizational (practice) setting. These models offer guidelines for nursing practice.

CONCEPTUAL MODELS AND THEORIES OF NURSING PRACTICE

Orem's Self-Care Theory

Dorothea Orem's (1991) general theory of nursing is a descriptive explanation of the human foundations of nursing and of nursing actions. She emphasizes that nursing is a response of human groups to one recurring type of incapacity for action to which human beings are subject, that is, the incapacity to care for oneself or one's dependents is limited because of the health or health care needs of the care recipient.

From the nursing perspective, human beings are viewed as needing continuous self-maintenance and self-regulation through a type of action termed "self-care." Self-care is care that is performed by oneself for oneself when this individual has reached a state of maturity that enables one to take consistent, controlled, effective, and purposeful action. Self-care involves the practice of activities that people initiate and perform on their own behalf in maintaining life, health, and well-being.

Her major concepts include *(1)* self-care; *(2)* self-care agent or provider of self-care; *(3)* dependent-care agent or provider of infant care, child care, or dependent adult care; *(4)* the agent who is the person taking action; *(5)* the nursing agency refers to the provision of nursing to individuals and families requiring that nurses have specialized abilities that enable them to provide care; and *(6)* the nursing system refers in a general way to all the actions and interactions of nurses and patients in nursing practice situations.

Orem's general theory of nursing is referred to as the self-care deficit theory of nursing because it explains the relationship between the action capabilities of individuals and their demands for self-care or the care demands of children or adults who are their dependents. Deficit is the relationship between the action that individuals take (action demanded) and the action capabilities of individuals for self-care or dependent care. It is important to note that deficit should be interpreted as a relationship, not a human disorder. However, these self-care deficits may be associated with the presence or human functional or structural disorders.

The essence of Orem's model is on the individuals' self-care needs and their capabilities for meeting these needs. She stresses that self-care has purpose. It is action that has pattern and sequence when it is effectively performed, contributes to human structural integrity, human functioning, and human development. The purposes attained through self-care actions are referred to as self-care requisites. Orem describes three types of self-care requisites:

1. Universal self-care requisites are common to all human beings during all stages of the life cycle, adjusted to age, developmental state, and environmental and other factors. They are associated with life processes, with the maintenance of the integrity of human structure and functioning, and general well-being.
2. Developmental self-care requisites are associated with human developmental processes; conditions and events occurring during various stages of the life cycle (e.g., prematurity and pregnancy); and events that can adversely affect development.
3. Health-deviation self-care requisites are associated with genetic and constitutional defects and human structural and functional deviations and with their effects, and with medical diagnostic and treatment measures. (p. 125)

Universal self-care requisites are universally required by all human beings. These eight requisites include the:

1. Maintenance of sufficient intake of air.
2. Maintenance of sufficient intake of water.
3. Maintenance of sufficient intake of food.
4. Provision of care associated with elimination process and excrements.
5. Maintenance of a balance between activity and rest.
6. Maintenance of a balance between solitude and social interaction.
7. Prevention of hazards to human life, human functioning, and human well-being.

8. Promotion of human development within social groups in accord with human potential, known human limitations, and the human desire to be normal. (p. 126)

Orem stresses that self-care related to the need for normalcy may be directed toward the promotion of integrated human functioning or the protection and care of the body. It is important to note that when individuals perform sets of actions for meeting these requisites, they are enhancing their health and well-being.

Development self-care requisites are sets of actions that must be performed to prevent developmental disorders and promote development in accord with human potential. Orem separates developmental disorders into the following two categories:

1. Bringing about, and the maintenance of, living conditions that support life processes and promote the process of development that refers to human progress toward higher levels of the organization of human structures and toward maturation during:
   a. The intrauterine stages of life and the process of birth
   b. The neonatal stage of life when *(1)* born at term or prematurely and *(2)* born with normal birth weight or low birth weight
   c. Infancy
   d. The developmental stages of childhood, including adolescence and entry into adulthood
   e. The developmental stages of adulthood
   f. Pregnancy in either childhood or adulthood
2. Provision of care associated with effects of conditions that can adversely affect human development.
   Subtype 2.1: Provision of care to prevent the occurrence of deleterious effects of conditions.
   Subtype 2.2: Provision of care to mitigate or overcome existent deleterious effects of such conditions. Conditions include such things as:
   a. Educational depreciation
   b. Problems of social adaptation
   c. Failures of healthy individuation
   d. Loss of relatives, friends, associates
   e. Loss of possessions, loss of occupational security. (p. 131)

Health-deviation self-care requisites exist for persons who are ill or injured; who have specific forms of pathology, including defects and disabilities; and who are under medical diagnosis and treatment. Obvious changes in *(1)* human structure, such as edematous extremities or tumors, *(2)* physical functioning, such as dyspnea or joint immobility, and *(3)* habits of daily living (e.g., sudden mood changes, loss of interest in life) focus a person's attention on him- or herself. When a change in health status results in total or almost total dependence on others for the needs to sustain life or well-being, the person moves from the position of self-care agent to that of patient, or receiver of care. The role of nursing focuses on assisting the individual, family, or significant others to meet universal self-care demands or develop new methods of providing self-care.

Orem states that when these three types of requisites are effectively met, they are productive of human and environmental conditions that support life processes, maintain human structures and functioning within a normal range, support development, prevent injury and pathology, contribute to the cure and regulation of pathological processes, and promote general well-being. The essence of this concept is that effectively meeting universal and developmental self-care requisites in well individuals relates to primary prevention of disease and ill health.

A related concept to self-care requisites is therapeutic self-care demand. This refers to the actions needed to meet the three types of requisites (universal, developmental, and health-deviation) that determine the therapeutic self-care demands of patients. The calculation of these demands requires antecedent knowledge of such areas as human structure and functioning, human growth and development, family and occupational life, and preventive health care.

Another major concept is the self-care agency, which Orem defines as qualities ascribed to individuals that refer to the complex acquired abilities necessary for the performance of self-care at a therapeutic level. These self-care actions at the therapeutic level are: *(1)* supportive of life processes; *(2)* remedial or curative when related to disease processes; and *(3)* conducive to personal development and maturation. It is important to note that adequacy of self-care agency is measured by comparing number and types of self-care actions that individuals can engage in with the number and types of actions that are required to meet the existing or projected therapeutic self-care demand. The term "self-care deficit" is the relationship between the self-care agency and the therapeutic self-care demands of individuals in which capabilities for self-care, due to existent limitations, do not meet some or all of the components of the therapeutic self-care demands.

In implementing Orem's model in nursing practice, the major emphases of the nursing assessment are the individual's self-care requisites, self-care agency or capabilities, and the influencing components related to the self-care agency. On the principle that nurses, patients, or both can act to meet patients' care requisites, three variations of basic nursing systems are recognized. These are *(1)* wholly compensatory, *(2)* partly compensatory, and *(3)* supportive-educative (see Figure 2.1). The nursing system is formed by the nurse's selection and use of methods of assisting patients and prescribes particular roles for the nurse and the patient.

The criterion measure for determining the need for a wholly compensatory nursing system exists when the patient is unable to engage in those self-care actions requiring self-directed and controlled ambulation and manipulative movement. These patients cannot or should not engage in any form of deliberate action. In the partly compensatory, the nurse and the patient perform care measures or other actions involving manipulative tasks or ambulation. It is intended for situations in which the patient can perform some, but not all of, the care measures required. In the supportive-educative system a patient can or should learn to perform the required self-care measure but cannot do so without assistance.

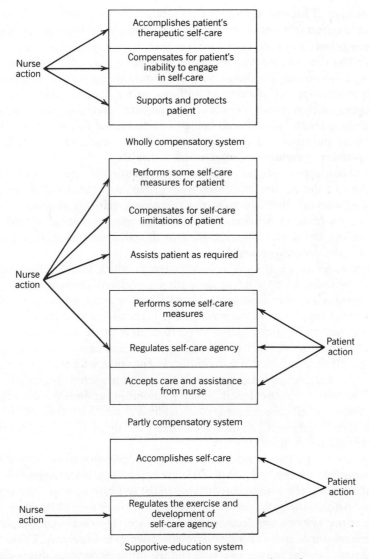

Figure 2.1 Basic nursing systems. (From Orem, D. E. (1991). *Nursing: Concepts of Practice*, 4th Edition. (p. 288) St. Louis: Mosby-Year Book. Adapted by permission.)

The family, community, and environment are important components considered in self-care actions, but the primary focus is on the patient. The outcome measures for evaluating nursing care are used to determine whether the patient's self-care requisites are met, and if the patient can achieve self-care management and does perform therapeutic self-care measures on an ongoing basis. The goal of nursing action is to involve the patient in his or her own self-care activities whenever possible.

Roy Adaptation Model

Sister Callista Roy's (1976, 1989) adaptation model of nursing practice can be viewed primarily as a systems model even though it also contains interactionist levels of analysis. The person is a bio-psycho-social being who, to be understood, has parts or elements linked together in such a way that force on the linkages can be increased or decreased. Roy emphasizes that increased force, or tension, occurs because of strains within the system or from the environment that impinges on the system. The units of analysis of the nursing system are the system of the person and his or her interaction with the environment, whereas mode of nursing intervention involves the manipulation of parts of the system or the environment.

Roy has identified that the person has four subsystems: *(1)* physiological needs, *(2)* self-concept, *(3)* role function, and *(4)* interdependence (Roy, 1976, p. 14). The self-concept and role function systems are envisioned as developing in an interactionist framework. This interaction process is one of the elements to be assessed with the system. Roy stresses that one of the nurse's primary tools in manipulating elements of the system or the environment is one's interaction with the patient.

In Roy's model, an assumption is a statement accepted as true without proof. These assumptions may be explicitly stated or implied with the discussion of the model, and are based on the model's approach to the concept of person and to the process of adaptation. The following are the basic assumptions of the Roy adaptation model:

1. The person is a bio-psycho-social being.
    The nature of the person includes a biologic component (such as anatomy and physiology) along with psychological and social components. The behavior of the individual is related to the behavior of others on a group level. Methods of analysis of the person must come from the biological, psychological, and sciences, and the person must be viewed from those perspectives as a unified whole.

2. The person is in constant interaction with a changing environment. Daily experience with such things as vicissitudes of the weather, or traffic conditions, supports this assumption. The person confronts physical, social, and psychological changes in the environment and is continually interacting with these.

3. To cope with a changing world, the person uses both innate and acquired mechanisms (biological, psychological, and social in origin). These acquired mechanisms are used to cope with the world (an example of this is dressing to suit the weather). Other mechanisms are innate (natural reaction of thirst in response to water loss through perspiration).

4. Health and illness are one inevitable dimension of a person's life. Each person is subject to the laws of health and illness. This dimension is one aspect of the total life experience.

5. To respond positively to environmental changes, the person must adapt. A changing environment demands a positive response, which is hopefully adaptive.

6. Adaptation is a function of the stimulus a person is exposed to and his or her adaptation level.

The person's adaptation level is determined by three classes of stimuli: *(1)* focal stimuli, which are stimuli immediately confronting the person; *(2)* contextual stimuli (all other stimuli present); and *(3)* residual stimuli (such as beliefs, attitudes, or traits, which have an indeterminate effect on the present situation).

7. The person's adaptation level is such that it comprises a zone indicating the range of stimulation that will lead to positive response. If the stimulus is within the zone the person responds positively; whereas, if the stimulus is outside the zone, the person cannot make a positive response.

8. The person is conceptualized as having four modes of adaptation:

   a. Person adapts according to his or her *physiological needs* (adaptation to temperature).

   b. Person's *self-concept* is determined by interactions with others (outside stimuli cause the person to adapt according to his or her self-concept).

   c. *Role function* is the performance of duties based on given positions within society (the way one performs these duties is constantly responsive to outside stimulation).

   d. *Interdependence relations*. In relations with others, the person adapts according to a system of interdependence, which involves ways of seeking help, attention, and affection. (Roy, 1989, pp. 106–108)

Roy emphasizes that the elements of a practice-oriented model imply values and include goal patency, source of difficulty, and intervention. The model implies values that, taken together, point to the desirability of the model's goal content. The basic values behind the goal can be summarized as follows:

1. Nursing's concern with the person as a total being in the areas of health and illness is a socially significant activity.

2. The nursing goal of supporting and promoting patient adaptation is important for patient welfare.

3. Promoting the process of adaptation is assumed to conserve patient energy; thus, nursing makes an important contribution to the overall goal of the health team by making energy available for the healing process.

4. Nursing is unique because it focuses on the patient as a person adapting to those stimuli present as a result of his or her position on the health-illness continuum. (Roy, 1989, p. 109)

The Roy adaptation model states that the goal of nursing is the person's adaptation in the four adaptive models previously described. Roy emphasizes that all nursing activity will be aimed at promoting the person's adaptation in physiological needs, self-concept, role function, and relations of interdependence during health and illness. The criterion used for judging when the goal has been reached is generally any positive response made by the recipient to the stimuli present that frees energy for responses to other stimuli. This is applied to each specific nursing intervention for which a specific goal of adaptation has been set.

Roy envisions the person as an adaptive system receiving stimuli from the environment inside and outside of its zone of adaptation. The recipient of nursing is the person in the dimension of his or her life related to health and illness. For example, the patient may be ill, or at risk of illness and in need of preventive services. The person may be adapting positively or not. It is important to emphasize that if the patient is adapting, the nursing goal is to maintain that response.

The newest element of this model is the source of difficulty that is described as the originating point of deviations from the desired state or condition. A need is described as a requirement in the individual that stimulates a response to maintain integrity. Roy implies that as internal and external environments change, the level of satiety for any need changes, and when this satiety changes, a deficit or excess is created. This deficit or excess then triggers the appropriate adaptive mode. Coping mechanisms whose activity is aimed at integrity are with each of the adaptive modes. The manifestations of this activity are the adaptive or ineffective behaviors. The source of difficulty is the coping activity that is inadequate to maintain integrity in the event of a need deficit or excess.

Intervention includes both focus and mode. This intervention focus involves the kind of problems found when deviations from the desired state occur that describe the kinds of disturbances that are to be prevented or treated. Each adaptive mode is related to underlying needs. For example, the physiological adaptive mode is related to the need for physiological integrity (such as exercise and rest, nutrition and elimination, fluid and electrolytes). The intervention mode is the means of preventing or treating the problems identified in the intervention focus; that is, it is the action that can be used to change the course of events toward the desired end product. It is what the nurse can do to promote patient adaptation. According to Roy's model, the nurse acts as an external regulatory force to modify stimuli affecting adaptation either by increasing, decreasing, or maintaining stimulation. This takes place within the nursing process, a problem-solving approach to diagnosing patient problems and to planning, carrying out, and evaluating patient care.

Roy's theory development is explanatory and an example of situation producing because it explains how the nurse can encourage adaptation through the manipulation of stimuli. The nurse must be able to consider each client as an individual, assess his or her needs, and act, accordingly. The model encourages the nurse to become more proficient in the total assessment of the patient through observation, interviews, and the performance of a variety of nursing care activities. An understanding of Roy's four adaptive modes for responding to change enables the nurse to bring a broad perspective to the planning and evaluating of nursing care based on individual client needs.

King's General Systems Theory

Imogene King's (1981) theory of nursing is based on the concept that patients and nurses are personal systems that coexist with other personal and group systems, as well as society as a whole. It is based on general systems theory as introduced by von Bertalanffy (1956) as a "complex of elements standing in interaction." He noted that general systems theory is a general science of "wholeness . . . in itself purely formal but applicable to the various empirical sciences" (p. 37). The distinguishing characteristics of systems include goals, structure, functions, resources, and decision making. Individuals are influenced by their interactions with both the internal and external environment and they, in turn, influence the environment. Three dynamic interacting systems comprise King's theory. These are *(1)* personal systems (individuals); *(2)* interpersonal systems (dyads, triads, and small and large groups); and *(3)* social systems (family, school, industry, social organizations, and health care delivery systems) (King, 1981).

King stresses that the goal of her conceptual system of nursing is health. Nurses help individuals attain and maintain their health, and if some disturbance occurs such as an illness or disability, nurses' actions are goal directed to assist the individual in regaining health or to help the individual live with a chronic disease or disability. Therefore, health is a dynamic state of an individual in which change is constant and an ongoing process.

King states that perception is a comprehensive concept in personal systems. This varies from one individual to another because each human being has different backgrounds of such things as knowledge, skills, abilities, needs, values, and goals. These perceptions of nurses and patients influence their interactions. Perception along with communication provide a channel for relaying information from one person to another. Self, growth and development, learning, body image, time, and space are concepts that also relate to individuals as personal systems.

A comprehensive concept in interpersonal systems is interaction. King emphasizes that knowledge of interaction is essential for nurses to understand a fundamental process for gathering information about human beings, and that purposeful interactions lead to transactions. Communication, transactions, role, and stress are related concepts. King notes that knowledge of the concepts identified in personal systems is also used to understand interactions.

Organization is a comprehensive concept in social systems because knowledge of organization is essential for nurses to understand the variety of social systems with which individuals grow and develop. Related concepts are power, authority, status, decision making, and control. King further states that all the concepts from personal and interpersonal systems provide knowledge for use within the social system.

In King's theory, concepts of the general systems framework are applied in nursing through the interaction-transaction process model. This model is defined as a "dynamic interpersonal process in which nurse and patient are viewed as a system with each affecting the behavior of the other and both being influenced by the factors within the situation" (Daubenemire & King, 1973, p. 513).

King's conceptual framework is a system of processes, which includes those of perception, communication, purposeful interactions, information, and decision making. She defined nursing as a "process of action, reaction, and interaction whereby nurse and client share information about their perceptions in a nursing situation. Through purposeful communication they identify specific goals, problems or concerns. They explore means to achieve a goal and agree to means to the goal" (1981, p. 2).

Nursing is described as a process of human interactions between nurse and patient in which each perceives the other and the situation. By means of communication, they mutually explore and set goals and agree on means to achieve those goals. The consequences or outcomes of the attained goal is also proposed. The basic premise of the theory is the interrelationship that exists between the nurse and the patient through action, interaction, and transaction for the purpose of achieving mutual goal attainment.

Levine's Conceptual Model For Nursing: The Four Conservation Principles

Myra Levine's theory (1973, 1989) of nursing is based on the concept of "wholeness" of the individual and the need to provide total patient care, from which she derives four conservation principles that serve as the basis for her nursing model. She emphasizes that the unity, integrity, the oneness, and the wholeness of human experience are universal.

Levine's theory (1973) reflects her definition of nursing in which she makes the assumptions that nursing is a human interaction, a discipline rooted in the dependency of people and their relationship with other people, and is based on intervention that supports or promotes the person's adjustment (pp. 1–3). She envisions nursing as holistic, individualized to meet each person's needs, and supporting adaptation. Therefore, the components of her theory are:

1. The patient is in the predicament of illness.
2. The nurse must recognize the patient's holistic response, which indicates the nature of the adaptation to illness.
3. The nurse who participates actively in every patient's environment must recognize the organismic response of the patient, make an intervention in the patient's environment, and evaluate the intervention as therapeutic or supportive. (Levine, 1973, p. 13)

Levine makes the assumptions that the nurse-patient interaction is determined by *(1)* the conditions in which the patient enters the health care setting, *(2)* the functions of the nurse in the situation, and *(3)* the responsibilities of the nurse in the situation. The theory implies that the nurse is able to make judgments that will promote or support the patient's adaptation to the situation based on knowledge. The nurse also is expected to possess the skills necessary to implement these interventions. Levine refers to the environmental setting of the nurse-patient interaction as the hospital.

Supporting her holistic beliefs, Levine views a person holistically as requiring four elements to be in a state of health. These are *(1)* structural integrity, *(2)* personal integrity, *(3)* social integrity, and *(4)* energy to be in state of health. If any one of these elements is disrupted or changed, the person is in a state of altered health. Health and disease are patterns of adaptive change and, they are never static entities. Nursing interventions are based on the conservation of these four elements. Levine defines conservation as the "keeping-together" function that should be the major guideline of all nursing interventions where it occurs. The purpose of conservation is to maintain the unity and integrity of the patient. The four conservation principles are:

1. Conservation of energy of the individual.
   Energy is eminently identifiable, measurable and manageable. For example, changes in the energy of heat production in the individual provide signals as to how effectively his or her body is functioning. Pulse rate, respiratory rate,

measurement of blood gases are energy measures. Energy conservation is an empirical activity of nursing care.

2. Conservation of structural integrity of the individual.
   This conservation principle is concerned with healing. Individuals are taught to have confidence in the ability of bodies to heal, that is, to restore wholeness and continuity after injury or illness, and to return to their pristine state. Healing is the defense of wholeness and is also a consequence of an effective immune system. Nurses have empirical awareness of the necessity to defend the structural integrity of individuals (such as proper positioning to prevent subluxations and other skeletal deformities or preventing pressure areas where decubiti might occur).

3. Conservation of personal integrity of the individual.
   The conservation of personal integrity implies that the sense of "self" is much more than a physical experience of the whole body, although it is a part of that awareness. The defense of self is reaching into the person. Everyone seeks to defend his or her identity as self. Even in those instances where the relationship with others is intimate and close—between parent and child, husband and wife—only by analogy is it known that our experience of selfhood is somehow an expression of personal identity. Nothing threatens that pride of self more than vulnerability of dependence. It is impossible for one individual to surrender his or her privacy to another, no matter how much the individual must depend on the good offices of the caregiver. It is much more difficult to articulate the anxiety created by a threat to self—to share it with another individual. The emphasis over the years on extracting psycho-social information about patients neglects the inevitable guarding of the privacy that cherishes self. It is possible that the use of private information as a component of the nursing care plan may be more damaging to the personal integrity of the individual than respecting a desire to withhold information. It may be that the most generous psycho-social approach would be to limit the recording of confidences to only those generalizations that actually make a difference in the choice of treatment plans. Individuals must participate freely in decisions that affect them.

4. The conservation of social integrity of the individual.
   This concept refers to the acknowledgement of the individual within the context of his or her social environment. Selfhood needs definition beyond the individual and this is the message of the conservation of social integrity. Individuals define themselves by their relationships (an identity places one in a family, a community, a cultural heritage, a religious belief, a socioeconomic slot, an educational background, a vocational choice). Coping refers to the way in which the individual responds to given social instant. Coping patterns are judged by the social acceptance of the behavior that is manifested. For example, coping patterns are categorized as everyday responses that have proved to be adequate and acceptable for the individual in the past. (Levine, 1989, pp. 331–336)

Levine emphasizes that the conservation principles do not operate singly and in isolation from each other. "They are joined within the individual as a cascade of life events, churning and changing as the environmental challenge is confronted and resolved in each individual's unique way" (p. 336). The nurse as caregiver becomes part of the environment bringing his or her own cascading repertoire of skill, knowledge, and compassion. She believes it is a shared enterprise and each participant is rewarded.

Similar to Orem's conceptual framework, Levine's nursing theory focuses on the individual (patient). The nurse is concerned with the patient's family and significant others as they influence the patient's progress. Levine's theory depicts nursing as an independent practice profession. Because her focus is on the hospital-based practice arena, Levine does not consider the collaborative relationship of nursing within the total health care setting. However, nurses in acute care settings could use this model. For example, the theory emphasizes the patient's dependency (illness) states with limited participation in planning his or her care. In such settings, the nurse has the major responsibility for assessing the patient's ability to participate in his or her own care, which is in contrast to Orem's self-care deficit theory model.

IMPLICATIONS FOR NURSING ADMINISTRATIVE PRACTICE

Meleis (1985) emphasizes that "Theory helps to identify the focus, means, and the goals of practice" (p. 31). Nursing administration must facilitate the implementation of patient-centered theoretical models for nursing practice. The nurse executive is the catalyst for instituting the use of nursing theoretical models that inspire, challenge, and influence clinical nursing practice within the organization.

Nurse executives and their staffs could select a conceptual model or framework of nursing that is congruent with the institutional and nursing division's philosophy, mission, structure, and goals, or they could develop a model for practice based on unit data collected in a grounded theory approach. Building a conceptual model for practice can be an important part of developing a shared vision. A prerequisite to the implementation of the model is the revision or development of guidelines and standards of nursing practice. Process and outcome quality measures of nursing care will need to be identified to reflect the concepts and terminology of the model. Other critical factors include preparation for implementing the model, available resources (technological, human, financial), and analysis and evaluation of the model in clinical nursing practice.

Summary

Nursing is attempting to formulate a theoretical basis for its practice. Many nurse scholars have advanced postulates, theories, and conceptual frameworks as a mechanism to achieve this goal. Orem focuses on the individuals' self-care needs and their capabilities of meeting these needs. Her belief is that self-care has a purpose because it emphasizes action that has pattern and sequence when it is effectively performed that contributes to human structural integrity, human functioning, and human development. Nursing actions are directed toward enhancing the self-care ability and therapeutic self-care ability of individuals. Roy's adaptation model of nursing practice can be perceived primarily as a systems model. The units of analysis are the person and his or her interaction with the environment, whereas mode of nursing intervention involves the manipulation of parts of the system or the environment. Roy espouses that nursing is an interpersonal process that is initiated by the individual's maladaption to change in the environment. The goal of nursing is to assess the adaptation level and intervene to promote positive adaptation and integrity. Similar to Roy, King's theory of nursing depicts a systems approach depicting patients and nurses as personal systems with other personal and group systems within the confines of society as a whole. King implies that through a systems approach by means of communication, nurses and patients will mutually explore and set goals and agree on means to achieve those goals, and the outcomes attained will become evident. Levine emphasizes the conservation principles of energy, structural integrity, and personal and social integrity. The goal of nursing is the wholeness of the individual that occurs by conservation in four areas when adaptive needs are manifested. She stresses an important point: that individuals (patients) must participate freely in decisions that affect them.

Chapter 3 addresses the major concepts and theories of management that are applicable to nursing administrative practice.

STUDY QUESTIONS

1. Formulate a definition of theory.

2. List the conditions under which you would use the constant comparative theory approach as depicted by Glaser and Strauss. Describe how you would formulate a grounded theory for a specific hypothetical situation.

3. What are the major differences between an inductive and a deductive theory?

4. Explain the rationale for the statement by Dickoff and James that the highest level of theory building is situation-producing theory. Why must nursing theory be at this level?

5. Formulate a definition of a model.

6. Distinguish among Orem's, Roy's, King's, and Levine's conceptual models of nursing practice.

7. Select from among the preceding nursing conceptual models the one that would be most applicable to incorporate patient-centered nursing practice within your health care organization. What are the implications for nursing administration in the application of the model to nursing practice?

References

Chin, P., & Kramer, M. K. (1991). *Theory and nursing: A systematic approach* (3rd ed.). St. Louis: Mosby Year Book.

Daubenmire, M., & King, I. M. (1973). Nursing process models: A systems approach, *Nursing Outlook, 21*(8), 512–517.

Dickoff, J., James, P., & Weidenback, E. (1968). Theory in a practice discipline—Part I, *Nursing Research, 17*(5), 415–434.

Dickoff, J., James, P., & Weidenback, E. (1968). Theory in a practice discipline—Part II, *Nursing Research, 17*(6), 545–554.

Glaser, B., & Strauss, A. (1967). *The discovery of grounded theory.* Chicago: Aldine.

Hage, F. (1972). *Techniques and problems in theory construction in sociology.* New York: Wiley.

Hardy, M. (1974). Theories: Components, development, evaluation, *Nursing Research, 23*(2), 100–107.

King, I. M. (1981). *A theory for nursing.* New York: Wiley.

Levine, M. (1973). *Theory development in nursing* (2nd ed.). Philadelphia: F. A. Davis.

Levine, M. (1989). The conservation principles of nursing: Twenty years later. In J. Riehl-Sisca, *Conceptual models for nursing practice* (3rd ed.). (pp. 325–337). Norwalk, CT.: Appleton & Lange.

Meleis, A. (1985). *Theoretical nursing: Development & progress.* Philadelphia: Lippincott.

Newman, M. (1979). *Theory development in nursing.* Philadelphia: F. A. Davis.

Orem, D. (1991). *Nursing: Concepts of practice* (4th ed.). St. Louis: Mosby Year Book.

Roy, C. (1976). *Introduction to nursing: An adaptation model.* Englewood Cliffs, NJ: Prentice-Hall.

Roy, C. (1989). The Roy adaptation model. In J. Riehl-Sisca, *Conceptual models for nursing practice* (3rd ed.). (pp. 105–114). Norwalk, CT.: Appleton & Lange.

Simms, L. (1981). The grounded theory approach to nursing research, *Nursing Research, 20*(6), 356–359.

von Bertalanffy, L. (1968). *General systems theory.* New York: Braziller.

Wald, F., & Leonard, R. (1964). Towards theory development of nursing practice theory, *Nursing Research, 13*(4), 309–313.

CHAPTER 3
Evolving Theories of Management

Sylvia A. Price
Paula R. Jaco

Highlights

- **Classical writers**
- **Bureaucratic model**
- **General systems theory**
- **Contingency management movement**
- **Theory X and theory Y**
- **Theory Z and theory F**

The purpose of this chapter is to trace the development of management theories and their application to nursing administrative practice. Because nurse executives are responsible and accountable for clinical nursing practice, education, and research in a variety of health care settings, they must be knowledgeable about management theories. The following discussion of the major management approaches will familiarize nurse executives with pertinent concepts and principles in the field. Relevant humanistic organizational theories will be presented in Chapter 4. This knowledge will enhance the incorporation of specific concepts into nursing administrative practice.

This chapter addresses the concepts of administration and management. "Administration" is a process of effectively and efficiently coordinating both human and material resources toward the accomplishment of the organization's goals. Robbins (1980) emphasizes it as the universal process of efficiently getting activities completed with and through other people. Many believe the practice of managing is an art, whereas the organized knowledge fundamental to this practice is a science. These are not mutually exclusive and the science underlying management is still evolving and imprecise.

The term "management" is often perceived as primarily for profit-making enterprise, often with negative implications. Others envision administration as more readily acceptable in both profit and not-for-profit organizations. The perceived dissimilarity between the two terms is insignificant. Our view is that the terms are synonymous. Florence Nightingale organized the first nursing services as they are still conceived today. Her work established the principles of nursing administration, and it is interesting to note that she used the terms administration and management interchangeably.

The administrative process also refers to the planning, organizing, leading, and evaluating that occur to accomplish organizational goals. Goals are an essential activity that must be directed toward some end or accomplishment. Although Nightingale sometimes described the science of administration as "the driest, most technical, and the most difficult . . ." (Cope, 1958, p. 28), she recognized that the health of each individual and a nation's well-being depended on proper management of patient care by nurses at the bedside, in communities, and in organizations (Henry, Woods, & Nagelkerk, 1990). Administrators must not only be effective, but efficient in achieving the goals within the scope of limited resources.

Administrators may be viewed negatively, especially by their subordinates. Administration often refers to powerful individuals who are in situations where conflict is frequently evident. Others see administrators as only those in corporate or top level administrative positions with luxurious offices, chauffeured limousines, private jets, and exorbitant salaries and benefits. In today's society, however, an administrator's role varies with the setting but regardless of position, title, or level, it is an extremely challenging one. This role involves critical decisions that affect such variables as production, performance, and morale that, in turn, significantly influence corporate culture.

Early in this century, the study and formulation of theories of modern management began. Over the years, several administrative or management theories have developed, such as classical, behavioral, management science, general systems, and contingency approaches. Concepts from all of these approaches have been incorporated into the field of nursing administration.

CLASSICAL WRITERS

The classical theory of management emphasizes the functions of a manager. The classical writers focus on prescriptive management theory: on how managers should perform their functions. According to this approach, the function of management is to discover the "one best way" to perform manual tasks. This approach is based on the classical economic theory that human beings are basically motivated by a desire for economic betterment. The classical theorists identify three components of the management process: planning, organizing, and controlling. This approach consists of scientific management, or the management of work, and classical organizational theory, or the management of organization.

One of the major contributors to the field of scientific management is Frederick W. Taylor (1911) who was a mechanical engineer at the Midvale Steel plant in Pennsylvania. In 1911, he published *The Principles of Scientific Management.* This work, along with studies conducted before and after its publication, established Taylor as the father of scientific management. He focused on making management a science rather than an individualistic approach that was based primarily on experience. In it, he defines guidelines for improving production efficiency. At the turn of the century, business was expanding and new products were being developed, but labor was in short supply. To offset these labor shortages, two solutions were available: either substitute capital for labor or use labor more efficiently. Taylor theorized that the cause of industrial conflict was the inefficient use of scarce resources. His work concentrated on the observation of the worker's performance as he performed his task. He observed the phenomenon of "that men were," which means that men were producing far less than their capacities would permit. Taylor's principal interest was to increase production efficiency to reduce costs and increase profits and worker earnings through their higher productivity. The inducement was economic reform. The solution to increases in productivity was more efficient work performance. His premise was that workers had to be shown a better organized, more methodological way to work.

Taylor's philosophy and work techniques are still being implemented today. Industries produce products on an extensive scale within a specified time frame and base worker compensation on individual productivity. Taylor's four principles of scientific management are *(1)* develop a science for each man's work, *(2)* select and train workers scientifically, *(3)* accomplish work objectives through the cooperation of management and labor, and *(4)* divide responsibility more equitably between managers and workers.

A colleague of Taylor's at the steel plant was a young engineer named Henry L. Gantt who was concerned with improving worker efficiency at the shop-floor level. He also recognized the human element of production work. Gantt developed a chart (called the Gantt chart) that compares the relationship between work planned and work completed on one axis and time elapsed on the other. This facilitates the administrative functions of planning, controlling, and evaluation by establishing designated outcome points.

Taylor's efforts inspired others to continue his work. Frank and Lillian Gilbreth, a husband-and-wife team, conducted time and motion studies. Lillian Gilbreth was an industrial psychologist who received her doctorate in that field in 1915. She raised 12 children and was depicted in the book and movie *Cheaper by the Dozen.* The Gilbreths directed their efforts toward work arrangements, eliminating unnecessary hand and body motions, and designing the proper tools for optimizing work performance. Frank Gilbreth worked as an apprentice bricklayer and observed the work of the skilled bricklayers. He was convinced that many of the body movements could be combined or eliminated so that the procedure would be simplified and production increased. He also emphasized that when applying principles of scientific management, one must consider the workers and understand their personalities and needs. The Gilbreths concluded that it is not the monotony of work that results in worker dissatisfaction but, rather, management's lack of interest in the worker.

Contemporary with the work of Taylor is that of Henri Fayol, who worked as the managing director of a large coal-mining company in France. This experience provided Fayol with the background for his impressions about the managerial process. He sought to discover principles of management that determine the "soundness and good working order" of the firm. His ideas were first committed to writing in 1916 when Fayol contributed to the bulletin of a French industrial association. A more comprehensive statement of these ideas did not appear until 1929 with the publication of his book entitled *General and Industrial Management*. However, no English translation was widely available in the United States until 1949. Fayol was also concerned with principles of organization and the functions of an administrator. He defines administration as consisting of the functions of planning, organizing, commanding, coordinating, and controlling.

Fayol developed 14 management principles to guide the thinking of managers in resolving concrete problems and to direct the design, creation, and maintenance of an organizational structure. These principles are:

1. *Division of Work*
   Specialization of labor is the natural means by which institutions and societies have progressed and developed. This results in increased productivity through reduction of job elements expected of each worker.

2. *Authority and Responsibility*
   These terms are highly abstract and difficult to define. Fayol defines authority as the right to give orders and the power to exact obedience, which is balanced by responsibility for performing necessary functions. He distinguishes authority as official (holding an office) and personal (derives from the office holder's own personality, experience, etc.). The ultimate check on authority has to be the integrity and moral courage of the administrator.

3. *Discipline*
   There should be obedience to agreements reached between parties in the firm. Clear statements of agreements are necessary.
   Discipline is a result of the ability of leadership. Fayol emphasizes that discipline requires good supervisors at all levels.

4. *Unity of Command*
   Fayol believed that the existence of dual command (two supervisors, one subordinate) causes severe breakdowns in authority and discipline. Employees should receive orders from only one superior. He believed that recognition and observance of this principle would eliminate the causes of interdepartmental and interpersonal conflict arising from jurisdictional issues.

5. *Unity of Direction*
   Each group of activities having the same purpose should operate under one head and one plan. It derives from a sound organizational structure that is

departmentalized in an appropriate manner. This principle refers to the structure of the organization.

6. *Subordination of Individual Interest to General Interest*
   The whole is greater than the sum of its parts or the overall objectives that the group seeks to achieve take precedence over the objectives of the individual.

7. *Remuneration of Personnel*
   Remuneration of workers and managers for services rendered should be based on a systematic attempt to reward well-directed effort. Fayol discusses advantages and disadvantages of compensation plans, day rate, piece rate, and profit-sharing plans.

8. *Centralization*
   There is one central point in the organization that exercises control of all parts. Centralization refers to the degree to which the importance of the subordinates' role is reduced. The degree of centralization should be related to the character of the manager, reliability of subordinates, and conditions of the business.

9. *Scalar Chain*
   A graded chain of authority from top to bottom must exist through which all communications flow. The scalar chain implements the unity-of-command principle and centralization provides for the orderly transmission of information.

10. *Order*
    Even as the material instruments of business must be arranged logically and neatly, so must the human instruments. A manager must determine the exact nature and content of each job and demonstrate its relationship to both the end product and other jobs. Interrelationships appear in the form of an organizational chart.

11. *Equity*
    The enforcement of established rules must be tempered by a sense of kindliness and justice. Fayol believed that employees respond to equitable treatment by carrying out their duties in a sense of loyalty and devotion.

12. *Stability and Tenure of Personnel*
    Fayol observes that prosperous firms usually have a stable group of managerial personnel. Top management should implement practices that encourage the long-term commitment of employees, particularly of managers, to the firm.

13. *Initiative*
    Employees must be encouraged to think through and implement a plan of action. Fayol believed that the opportunity to exercise initiative is a powerful motivator. The only limits on personal initiative should be the authority relationship defined by the scalar chain and the employee's sense of discipline.

14. *Esprit de Corps*
    There should be a unity of effort through harmony of interests. This principle stresses the need for teamwork and the maintenance of interpersonal relationships.

Over the years, Fayol's principles have been discussed and criticized in management literature, especially those principles concerning centralization, scalar chain of authority, and order. Fayol's principles do not focus on degree or specificity. He emphasizes that the balance of the 14 principles and the moral character of the manager determines the ultimate outcome of management.

BUREAUCRATIC MODEL

Max Weber (1952), a German sociologist, studied man, his work environment, and productivity. His primary concern was the bureaucratic structure and how this affected productivity. Weber described the bureaucratic organization as a highly structured, formalized, and impersonal organization.

Weber viewed this bureaucratic organizational design as the most efficient model that could be used for complex organizations. Rational-legal authority is the major management premise evident in bureaucratic structures. Rational-legal authority is defined as the "right to exercise authority based on position." Legal authority facilitates depersonalization and promotes legal obligation and obedience to the established order. In the case of legal authority, it extends to the people exercising the authority of the office under it only by virtue of the formal legality of their commands within the scope of the authority vested in that office.

It must be emphasized that the rational-legal authority is based on the position within the organization. When this authority evolves into an organized administrative staff, it takes the form of a bureaucratic structure. Within this organizational structure, each member of the administration occupies a position where there is *(1)* a specific delineation of power and compensation in the form of a fixed salary, *(2)* the various positions are organized in a hierarchy of authority, *(3)* fitness for office is determined by technical competence, and *(4)* the organization is governed by rules and regulations. Power is in the position or office, not in the individual, and proper respect is due because of the position. There is an assigned division of labor so that each task performed by employees is systematically established and legitimitized as an official duty.

Weber's analysis tends to be descriptive (what he saw and how it should be interpreted), whereas Taylor ascribes to a prescriptive approach (how it must be done). The preceding dimensions are present in varying degrees, resulting in a highly mechanical model. Weber's discussion of bureaucracy is an example of a closed-technical system. The emphasis of this model is on the internal workings of the organization, with little attention given to environmental factors. In this highly impersonal approach, Weber views individuals as "officials" without personality or individual variations.

As a complex organization, the hospital is seen as a bureaucracy as previously described. The typical characteristics are *(1)* a hierarchical structure, with each managerial member responsible for subordinates' actions and decisions; *(2)* clear division of labor; *(3)* control by rules and regulations, so that official decisions and actions are uniform, anticipated, and stable; *(4)* impersonal relationships, so control over individuals and activities in the organization can be efficiently established; and *(5)* career mobility.

Organizations dominated by professionals often do not fit the traditional Weber-ian bureaucratic model. For example, nursing professionals, who are employed in a bureaucratic setting, procure a relatively standard body of knowledge on which they are examined and licensed. Their education evolves outside of the organization, and staff nurses are hired for their basic level of skill. Their practice is regulated through an official board of nurse examiners. Nurses define an appropriate code of ethics for practice affecting both patients and nurses. Thus, professional authority is granted because of nursing's unique body of knowledge. The professional organization, the American Nurses Association (ANA) is the group that develops standards of prac-tice. Control of the professional nursing practice in the hospital is through stan-dards delineated by a variety of accrediting or regulatory agencies external to the organization.

The command model (a few at the top giving orders and a great many at the lower level obeying them) remained the norm for nearly 100 years. Drucker (1988) states that this model was never static, as its longevity might suggest. The first university-trained engineer in manufacturing industry was hired in Germany in 1867 and within 5 years, he had built a research department. Other specialities followed, and by 1914, the typical functions of a manufacturer included such areas as manufacturing, sales and finance and accounting, and later, human resources.

It is interesting to note that at this time, another important management-directed development occurred, which was the application of management to manual work in the form of training. Drucker emphasizes that during World War I, large numbers of totally unskilled, preindustrial people had to be made productive workers in a very short time. To meet this demand, businesses in the United States and the United Kingdom began to apply Taylor's scientific management principles to the systematic training of blue-collar workers on a large scale. They analyzed tasks into individual, unskilled operations that could be learned rather quickly. These operations were further developed during WWII, and the training aspect was implemented by the Japanese and, 20 years later, by the South Koreans, who made it the foundation for their countries' remarkable development.

HUMAN RELATIONS AND BEHAVIORAL SCIENCE APPROACHES

Behavioral scientists have challenged some established classical theories, especially the assumption that human beings are basically economically motivated. In the 1940s and early 1950s, the first branch of the behavioral school used a human relations approach and the second branch, begun in the 1950s, used a behavioral science approach.

The human relations approach modifies the premises of the classical theorists to take into account differences in individual behavior and the influence of the work group on the individual. The movement began when a group of researchers headed by Elton Mayo from Harvard University were requested to conduct studies at the Chi-cago Hawthorne plant of Western Electric. The purpose of the studies was to deter-mine the relationship between employee productivity and physical working condi-tions. Illumination, temperature, and other working conditions were selected as representative features of the physical environment. Experiments were conducted to determine the effects of illumination changes on productivity. The conclusions were that working conditions, fatigue, and pay were secondary factors in productivity aspects. Major factors were the human aspects, such as the presence of a friendly, nonauthoritarian supervisor and increased participation in decision making. The Hawthorne studies found that employee productivity improved when people were noticed and that when they received a lot of attention, they produced more and had a higher morale. The results of these studies indicated that social variables were more important than physical variables in affecting production.

Both the human relations writers and the behavioral science workers examine the underlying determinants, types, characteristics, and roles of work groups. The behavioral science approach to the study of management is defined as "the study of observable and verifiable human behavior in organizations, using scientific procedures. It is largely inductive and problem centered, focusing on the issue of human behavior, and drawing from any relevant literature, especially in psychology, sociology and anthropology" (Filley, House, & Kerr, 1976, p. 8).

The behavioral science approach added to the earlier body of knowledge, because the behavioral scholars provided a means to test the earlier theories. Donnelly, Gibson, and Ivancevich (1975) state that advocates of the behavioral science approach were concerned that both practitioners and scholars had accepted without scientific validation so much of the management theory that preceded them. Through the work of the behavioral scientists, some aspects of the early theories have been modified, whereas others have withstood the test of scientific validations. Classical writers overemphasize the technical and structural components of management, whereas the human relationists exaggerate the psychological aspects.

MANAGEMENT SCIENCE APPROACHES

The proponents of the management science approach attempt to apply scientific knowledge to the solution of large-scale management problems in all types of organizations. Management science can be considered an extension of scientific management. The primary emphasis of this approach is on the establishment of normative models of organizational behavior for maximizing efficiency. This approach is also referred to as management science, operations research, or decision science and is related to industrial engineering and mathematic economics.

Although attempts have been made to distinguish between operations research and management science, it is very difficult to do. Several writers emphasize that the term "management science" is broader than the term "operations research" because it encompasses such fields as mathematical economics and the behavioral sciences and is also closely related to the physical sciences and engineering. Operations research is operationally oriented, whereas management science is directed toward the establishment of a broad theory. There is also a close relationship between management science and industrial engineering. Both disciplines are concerned with the same problems and often use similar techniques.

Kast and Rosenzweig (1985) emphasize that although management science and operations research represent a loose conglomeration of interests and approaches, there are several key concepts that permeate the field:

1. Emphasis on scientific method
2. Systematic approach to problem solving
3. Mathematical model building
4. Quantification and utilization of mathematical and statistical procedures
5. Concern with economic-technical rather than psychological aspects
6. Utilization of computers as tools
7. Emphasis on the systems approach
8. Seeking rational decisions under varying degrees of uncertainty
9. Orientation toward normative rather than descriptive models. (p. 90)

GENERAL SYSTEMS THEORY

The development of general systems theory has provided a basis for the understanding and integration of scientific knowledge from a variety of specialized fields. Kast and Rosenzweig (1985) define a system as "an organized, unitary whole composed of two or more interdependent parts, components, or subsystems and delineated by identifiable boundaries from its environment suprasystem" (p. 103).

When one applies the definition and key concepts of general systems theory to organizations, it is imperative also to define the structure and characteristics associated with that particular organization. The information obtained from this dissecting process provides a basic understanding of the organization in terms of its functional and operational capabilities.

The key general systems theory concepts that are common to all systems are as follows:

1. A system is more than the sum of its parts; it must be viewed as a whole.
2. A system has boundaries that separate it from its environment.
3. Systems have subsystems and are also part of a suprasystem; they are hierarchical.

Systems can be further identified as open or closed. Open system organizations interact with their external environment, whereas closed system organizations exist within their own environment. The key concepts associated with open and closed systems are depicted in Table 3.1.

Organizations can be considered in terms of an open system model. The internal functioning of an organization must be congruent with the demands of organizational tasks, technology, external environment, and the needs of its members if the organization is effective.

The view of an organization as an open system suggests a different and more challenging role for the nurse executive than his or her role would be in a closed system. The open system interacts with its environment and moves toward a steady state while maintaining capacity for work flow and energy transformation. Management must deal with external uncertainties and ambiguities and be flexible to adapt to new and changing requirements. For example, the hospital organization receives input from its external environment in the form of personnel, financial and material re-

TABLE 3.1 Comparison of Open and Closed Systems Models in General Systems Theory

Open System	Closed System
Exchanges information, energy, or material with its environment	Does not interact with its environment
Receives inputs from its environment	Does not receive inputs from its environment
Does not experience entropy if the inputs from the environment are as great as the energy the systems use plus the energy and materials used in the operations of the system	Subject to entropy due to lack of inputs being received from their environment; this results in the failure of the entire system
Exchanges information, energy, or material with its environment	Does not interact with its environment
Dynamic equilibrium is achieved when there is a balance or steady state; open systems have a greater potential to remain in a dynamic equilibrium through their ability to allow the inflow of materials, energy, and information	Dynamic equilibrium can be achieved in closed systems for a period of time until the lack of available resources, such as materials, energy, and information are depleted
The feedback of information required to maintain a steady state may come from inside or outside the system	The feedback of information required to maintain dynamic equilibrium may come only from inside the system
Tends toward increased elaboration, differentiation, and a higher level of organization	Tends toward entropy and disorganization
Equifinality is a process used by open systems to achieve desired results; established expected outcomes may be accomplished in a variety of ways, using assorted inputs	The cause and effect relationship is the common process associated with closed systems; regimentation and specified sequencing result in the designed or expected outcomes

From Kast, F., & J. Rosenzweig. (1985). *Organization and management: A systems and contingency approach* (p. 107). New York: McGraw-Hill. Adapted by permission.

sources, and information. These inputs facilitate the accomplishment of outcomes expected of health care organizations. In addition, employee participation is reinforced and rewarded for achieving organizational goals.

An early systems theorist was Chester Barnard, who in 1938 wrote *The Functions of the Executive*, based on his years of experience as president of the New Jersey Bell Telephone Company. He focuses on the psychosocial aspects of organization and management. Barnard (1938) considers the organization a social system in his definition of a formal organization as "a system of consciously coordinated activities or forces of two or more persons" (p. 73). He defines the functions of the executive in a formal organization as the following: *(1)* the maintenance of organizational communication through a scheme of organization coupled with loyal, responsible, and capable people; *(2)* the securing of essential services from individuals in the organization; and *(3)* the formulation and definition of purpose.

Katz and Kahn (1978) conceptualize the role of the executive or manager as one of a number of organizational subsystems. Such subsystems operate together to meet needs and accomplish necessary tasks. They identify maintenance structures that function to maintain stability and predictability in the organization. The purpose of such structures is to preserve a steady state of equilibrium. Such structures may result in a tendency toward organizational rigidity, the preservation of the status quo in absolute terms, or they may necessitate mediation between task demands and human needs to keep the structures in operation. Such mechanisms for maintaining stability seek to formalize, or institutionalize, all aspects of organizational behavior.

The boundary structures of procurement of materials and personnel and product disposal involve transactional exchanges with the environment. These mechanisms concern acquiring control of sources of supply and creating an organizational image.

Adaptive structure concerns the survival of the organization. Both the maintenance and adaptive structures move in the direction of preserving constancy and predictability in the conditions of organizational life. Katz and Kahn (1978) emphasize that the adaptive function can focus either on attaining control over external forces and maintaining predictability in the operations of the organization or on achieving internal modifications of organizational structures to meet the needs of a changing world.

The managerial subsystem cuts across all the operating structures of production, maintenance, environmental support, and adaptation. The managerial system is the controlling, or decision-making, aspect of the organization. The authors further state that "the complexity of organizational structures implies that the functions of management are also complex. Three basic management functions can be distinguished: *(1)* the coordination of substructures, *(2)* the resolution of conflicts between hierarchical levels, and *(3)* the coordination of external requirements with organizational resources and needs" (p. 91).

The goals, resources, and outcomes as well as technical, adaptive, psychosocial, and managerial subsystems, are all essential elements of the overall organizational structure within a general systems model framework. For example, because they were concerned with developing management principles and improving production efficiency, classical management theorists focused on the structural and managerial subsystems. The human relations and behavioral science approaches, on the other hand, emphasized the psychosocial aspects, differences in individual behavior, and the influence of the work group on the individual. The contemporary systems approach envisions the organization interacting with all of its subsystems and the external environment.

CONTINGENCY MANAGEMENT MOVEMENT

Investigators who examine the functioning of organizations in relation to the needs of their members, the internal environment, and the external forces impinging upon the organization emphasize the contingency approach to management. The contingency management perspective involves understanding the interrelationships of systems and subsystems within an organization as well as the dynamics occurring between the organization and its environment.

Contingency theory originated in the late 1950s when Woodward (1958), a British researcher, attempted to determine whether the principles espoused by the scientific management theorists had any relationship to business success. She studied 100 British manufacturing firms, measuring success in relation to productivity, market standing, reputation of the firm in the community, and rate of supervisory turnover. Woodward measured the relationship between organizational structure and success, but no consistent pattern emerged. She examined the firms according to production techniques and complexity. Woodward's findings implied that different technologies imposed varying demands on individuals and organizations that had to be met through an appropriate organizational structure. This study questioned the classical theorists "one best way" approach as organizational technology was contingent on the appropriate organizational structure.

Robbins (1980) points out that the contingency movement began by identifying common characteristics that might exist in a variety of situations, creating the potential to qualify a theory to the specifics of a situation. If one cannot say, "If X, then Y," possibly one can say, "If X, then Y, but only under the conditions specified in Z."

The contingency or situational approach emphasizes the ability of the organization to adapt based on the behavioral aspects of its members, circumstances or situations, and internal and external forces that are evolving in both the organization and its environment. Additionally, attempts are made to identify or predict patterns of behavior based on certain configurations of variables. The evaluation of the success of the organization is determined by the ability to achieve the goals or outcomes of the organization under its distinctive circumstances.

Compared with the systems approach, contingency views of organizations emphasize more specific characteristics and patterns of interrelationships among subsystems. Some theorists make no distinction between open systems and contingency theory. Others emphasize that the purpose of the contingency approach is to specify functional relationships between independent environmental and dependent management variables.

Three components of the contingency approach are the environment, management concepts, and techniques. The relationship between each of these components contributes to the functional understanding and operation of an organization using contingency theory. For example, management concepts and techniques may be classified as *(1)* process variables, including planning, organizing, directing, commanding, and evaluating; *(2)* quantitative variables such as decision making, linear programming, and operations research models; *(3)* behavioral variables, including learning, behavior modification, motivation, and group dynamics; and *(4)* systems variables, including general systems theory, systems design, and management information systems. The contingency approach is designed to relate the environment to these various management concepts and techniques.

THEORY X AND THEORY Y

Douglas McGregor (1960) believes that the vertical division of labor proposed by the classical management theorists is based on a set of negative assumptions many managers have about their employees. He has suggested that organizations can achieve their goals more effectively if they address the human needs of organizational members and utilize their potential. What McGregor calls theory X is based on traditional autocratic assumptions about people, whereas theory Y is founded on behaviorally based assumptions about people. Most management actions flow directly from the particular theory of human behavior that individual managers espouse.

Theory X refers to an autocratic approach to managing. It assumes that most people dislike work and will try to avoid it if at all possible. Because of this dislike of work, most people must be coerced, controlled, and threatened with punishment to get them to put forth adequate effort toward the achievement of the organization's goals. According to this theory, people have little ambition and avoid responsibility. The average human being prefers to be directed, lacks responsibility, has little ambition, and wants security above all.

In contrast, theory Y implies a humanistic and supportive approach to the management of people. It assumes that people are not inherently lazy and indolent but that they may become so as a result of experience. According to this theory, the average human being leans, under proper conditions, not only to accept but to seek responsibility. Avoidance of responsibility, lack of ambition, and emphasis on security are generally consequences of experience, not inherent human characteristics. Commitment to the organization's objectives is a function of the rewards' association with their achievement. They have potential along with imagination, ingenuity, and creativity that can be applied to their work situation.

McGregor argues that the conventional management approach ignored the facts about people because these managers adhere to theory X and follow an outmoded set of assumptions about their employees. McGregor contends that most people are close to the theory Y assumptions. The theory X manager will have a predisposition to develop autocratic or paternalistic approaches. These managers should change to a whole new theory of working with people: theory Y.

THEORY Z AND THEORY F

Advocates of theory Z suggest that involved workers are the key to increased productivity. With the interest in quality management in relation to Japanese theory Z management, the question arises whether such participatory management techniques will be adapted by American organizations.

William Ouchi (1982) proposes that American managers learn to create some of the family-like, or industrial-clan, qualities that come more naturally to Japanese organizations. He contends that the Japanese quality edge is the result of a management style based on trust, subtlety, and worker involvement. Trust and subtlety (such as fewer explicit rules because the common culture communicates the ground rules, more discussion and sharing of information, focus on the group, the team, rather than individuals) improve productivity through effective coordination. The assumption is that if workers' ideas are heard, the result is a satisfied, motivated, and productive work force. Consensus, participative decision making, lifetime employment, establishment of a particular kind of bond between supervisors and their employees (e.g., supervisors often regard their employees' problems as their own), and a commitment to organizational goals are the facets of this approach.

One expression of the consensual aspect in a theory Z management approach is the quality circle. The quality circle was developed in Japan as a useful method of achieving high quality, improved productivity, and increased employee morale. Quality circles are disciplined operations. It is imperative that the staff be knowledgeable regarding concept of theory Z. Quality circle educational programs must be a part of the implementation plan.

A typical ad hoc quality circle consists of four to ten employees who volunteer or are assigned to that circle. Each circle's employees, representing all managerial levels, form a working group in which everyone's work is related. Workers meet together regularly, usually for a designated time period, identify a problem or problems, and collect data on the nature of the problem. At the conclusion of this designated time period, members analyze the data, develop and implement solutions, and evaluate results. If this process is successful, a solution is identified and implemented. Once these solutions are implemented, the circle must monitor the outcome. The results are compared with the goals to determine the extent to which the identified problem was corrected. If the goal was not achieved, the circle analyzes why. The circle formulates another solution and plan for implementation. A formal report of the circle's activities is presented to the appropriate group within the organization.

Michael Jablow, an American who founded an electronics marketing firm in Tokyo, finds that negative factors now play a far more important role inside Japanese companies than the humanistic principles stressed by Ouchi. Jablow has come up with his own, somewhat unconventional, theory, Theory F (Kotkin & Kishimoto, 1986). Because promotion systems tied to seniority and most large corporations set retirements at age 55, the Japanese executive has at best only 15 years to gain power and position. He also knows that if he fails, there are hordes of often more technically qualified young executives "bucking" for the same position. According to Jablow, advocates of theory Z don't talk about how the system actually works. It is actually fear that moves those managers and there is no tolerance for failure. In theory F, the penalty for failure is out, finished; it is the powerful motivating force. Jablow states that executives who reach the top in Japanese companies are those who succeed at every step in their career paths. If they fail, there are no second chances. Jablow states that the choice for an executive who fails is a "one-way ticket to oblivion" in a remote subsidiary or early retirement.

Those critical of theory Z emphasize that firms in Japan do not consistently show the conditions Ouchi selects as representative of familylike organizations. Managers may be more autocratic, organizations more bureaucratic, career paths more specialized, and employment less stable than may appear. It has not been demonstrated that satisfaction or belongingness causes increased productivity or that theory Z organizations are more successful than non-theory Z organizations.

However, the proponents of a theory Z organization emphasize that the participative process is one of the mechanisms that provides for the dissemination of information and values within the organization. Consensual decision making provides the direct benefits of information and value sharing and, at the same time, openly signals the commitment of organizations to those values.

Summary

Classical management theory focuses on the structure of formal organization, the process of management, productivity, and the functions of the manager. The human relations and behavioral science approaches modify the premises of the classical theorists examining the underlying types, characteristics, and roles of the work group. The

proponents of the management science approach attempted to apply scientific knowledge and mathematical modeling of systems to the solution of management problems in organizations.

Systems concepts provide the conceptual framework for understanding organizations. General systems theory includes concepts related to the understanding and integration of knowledge from a variety of disciplines. Systems theorists generally view an organization as an open system interacting with its environment. The contingency approach to management emphasizes that there should be a congruence between the organization and its environment and among its various subsystems.

McGregor's theories X and Y have helped clarify direction for the field of organization behavior toward a more humanitarian approach. The philosophy of a theory Z Japanese management approach is that the organization can significantly benefit from a management style based on trust and on workers' involvement in discussions that affect them and their product. Theory F implies that it is actually fear that moves managers in Japanese management; that is, there is no tolerance for failure within the system.

Drucker (1988) eloquently states that "Management is about human beings. Its task is to make people capable of joint performance, to make their strengths effective and their weaknesses irrelevant. That is what organization is all about, and it is the reason that management is the critical determining factor" (p. 75). The nurse executive should select a management theory or model that is compatible with the required work and purpose of the organization. These models provide a framework for evaluating the outcomes of both nursing administrative and clinical practice. Chapter 4 addresses the nature of organizations as people-centered workplaces.

STUDY QUESTIONS

1. What is the major premise of the classical theory of management, the human relations and behavioral science approach, and the management science approach?

2. Describe the contributions of the following individuals to their respective management approaches: Taylor, Fayol, the Gilbreths, Weber, Mayo, and Barnard.

3. Which of Fayol's management principles have influenced nursing administration? Explain.

4. Discuss the emergence of the systems approach in the study of organizations.

5. What is the difference between an open and a closed system?

6. How is the systems approach applicable to management practices in nursing administration?

7. What is meant by a contingency view of an organization?

8. What assumptions do theory X managers and theory Y managers make about people?

9. Compare and contrast theory Z and theory F.

10. Select a problem in nursing administrative practice that can be reduced or eliminated by utilizing the theory Z management approach.

References

Barnard, C. (1938). *The functions of an executive.* Cambridge, MA: Harvard University Press.

Cope, Z. (1958). *Florence Nightingale and the doctors.* London: Museum Press.

Donnelly, J., Gibson, J., & Ivancevich, J. (1975). *Fundamentals of Management.* Dallas: Business Publications, Inc.

Drucker, P. (1988). Management and the world's work, *Harvard Business Review, 66*(5), 65–76.

Fayol, F. W. (1949). *General and industrial management.* London: Sir Isaac Pitman & Sons.

Filley, A., House, R., & Kerr, S. (1976). *Managerial process and organizational behavior.* Glenview, IL: Scott, Foresman.

Henry, B., Woods, S., & Nagelker, J. (1990). Nightingale's perspective on nursing administration, *Nursing & Health Care, 11*(4), 201–206.

Kast, F., & Rosenzweig, J. (1985). *Organization and management: A contingency approach* (4th ed.). New York: McGraw-Hill.

Katz, D., & Kahn, R. (1978). *The social psychology of organizations.* New York: Wiley.

Kotkin, J., & Kishimoto, Y. (1986). "Theory F". *Inc., 8*(4), 53–60.

McGregor, D. (1960). *The human side of enterprise.* New York: McGraw-Hill.

Ouchi, W. (1982). *Theory Z.* Reading, MA: Addison-Wesley.

Robbins, S. (1980). *The administrative process.* (2nd ed.). Englewood Cliffs, NJ: Prentice-Hall.

Taylor, F. W. (1911). *The principles of scientific management.* New York: WW Norton.

Weber, M. (1952). The essentials of bureaucratic organization: An ideal-type construction. In R. K. Merton et al. (Eds.) *A Reader in Bureaucracy* pp. 18–27. Glencoe, IL: The Free Press.

Woodward, J. (1958). *Management and technology.* London: Her Majesty's Stationary Office.

CHAPTER 4

Through the Looking Glass: Making Sense of Organizations

The proliferation of complex organizations has made almost every human activity a collective one. We are born, raised and educated in organizations. We work in them and rely on them for goods and services. Many of us will grow old and die in organizations. (Bolman and Deal, 1991, p. 5)

Highlights

- **Perspectives on organizations**
- **The human side of clinical administration**
- **Participatory approaches to organizational design**
- **The learning window**
- **The nurse executive role in learning organizations**
- **Professional associations**
- **Managing boundaries**

There is a great need for professional nursing administration to reorganize its services, practice settings and educational policies if nurse executives are to be able to function in current and emerging environments. Attention to the development of the "self" must be seen as a vital and integral part of continuing learning experiences, AND attention to persons in groups is equally vital. Most nursing administration texts are written about managers to describe the hierarchy of managers and the span of control of managers. Very little attention is paid to the work of the organization or workers. Organizational theorists have tended to focus on either public or private organizations, whereas all organizations have similarities. Nurse theorists have tended to focus on theories of nursing without any understanding of organizations. This chapter seeks to provide a way of looking at health care organizations as composed of autonomous, yet tightly coupled groups with various interacting networks. It assumes a different theme, that every nurse is an executive and every nurse executive is a worker in multiple organizations. It also assumes that traditional organizational theories no longer explain modern organizations, which are now viewed as networks or linkage points of distinctive competencies or areas of specialization on a global scale (Schneider, 1991).

Most traditional organizational charts are pecking orders for managers with the front line workers perceived to be off the page somewhere. Health care organizations have been the ultimate of pecking orders with the physician always at the top in capital letters. To understand the concept of organization, let us for the moment assume that organization refers to Webster's dictionary definition: "the unification and harmonizing of the elements of work for a defined purpose." Organizations exist in nature, and may or may not have buildings as we know them. The ants have their nests, the bees their hives, and the wolves their caves for extended families. Organizations provide environments for work in which humans can struggle to provide for food, shelter, clothing, and tools for survival. In rural cultures, work seems closely tied to subsistence — less so in urban communities and especially health care organizations where work is linked with professional behavior. All in all, the understanding of work is essential to the understanding of workers in organizations. The neurosurgeon operating in a modern hospital, the nurse executive coordinating care in various settings, the potato picker in the field are all working.

PERSPECTIVES ON ORGANIZATIONS

Bolman and Deal (1991) have consolidated the major schools of organization thought into four perspectives or frames to characterize the major vantage points. They define frames as both windows on the world and lenses to bring the world into focus. Every manager, consultant, or policymaker, they say, uses a personal frame or image to make judgments and determine how to get work done. They describe four major frames. The structural frame emphasizes the importance of formal roles and relationships. Commonly depicted by organizational charts, structures are created to fit an organization's environment and technology. The human resource frame is based on the premise that organizations are inhabited by human beings with skills, needs, feelings, and prejudices. The political frame views organizations as arenas in which different interest groups compete for power and scarce resources. Conflict abounds during this competition. Bargaining, negotiation, coercion, and compromise are everyday organizational activities. In the symbolic frame, organizations are viewed as tribes, theater, or carnivals. In this view, say Bolman and Deal (1991), organizations are cultures that are propelled more by rituals, ceremonies, stories, heroes, and myths than by rules, policies, and managerial authority. Organizations are theater in this frame. This is especially true in health care delivery settings where health professionals play numerous roles in various parts of the organization many times on the same day.

Our goal is to break the gap between managers and workers, to realize that managers are workers and workers are managers and that other perspectives or frames must be brought into account if nurse executives are to understand the multiple environments in which they practice. Nurse executives no longer practice in settings but rather in systems of care that now have extended boundaries in other countries and soon, on other planets. A change in position descriptions and role relations via restructuring is no longer adequate for developing optimal work environments for clinical practice and patient care delivery. We propose the following windows as essential to understanding the various ways nurse executives could look at organizations (Figure 4.1). Figure 4.2 graphically portrays the interacting systems in clinical organizations.

WINDOW	PERCEPTION OF VIEWER
Personal	Personal perception of place(s) where and how work is accomplished in organizations; innovation and resource discovery are possible; organizations viewed by some as chaos and others as places for creativity.
Structural	Organizational charts depicting formal roles and relationships; boxes and lines cloud vision of potential; rule by policies and managerial authority; some see boxes; others see only information links between boxes; others see only local and global networks.
Political	Arenas in which different groups compete for power and resources. Bargaining, negotiation, coercion and "dog eat dog" are everyday activities.
Symbolic	Public or private cultures that are orchestrated by rituals, ceremonies, stories, heroes, rumors, and myths. History, tradition, and celebrations are important. Different theater playing in different units.
Systems	Combined clinical management approaches to care delivery. Solutions are chosen from multiple alternatives. Commonly described as a tool for selection of actions based on competing resources and benefits.
Geographic	Spheres of influence with flexible boundaries that separate an organizational system from its environment; boundaries also delineate the parts and processes within the system. Maps would make a better organizational picture.
Work	Socio-technical systems with emphasis on machine and human productivity and interdependence; elements of flow and play; accomplishment of meaningful work outcomes; interaction with clients.
Play	Least recognized window. In childhood, our play is our work; adults search for ways to make work joyful and exciting; personal and work activities in synchrony; stress and monotony-breaking activities.

Figure 4.1 *(Continued on next page)*

Clinical	Community of competent and trusted human and health care resources for the treatment of physical and mental discomforts; comfort, safety, and machine care available; a healing site; a health education center or central place either to be cured or learn how to cope with discomfort. Birth to death scenarios—daily scripts of health to illness to death phenomena and travel through diverse health care delivery settings.
Learning	Perception of organizations as learning environments with all workers sharing learning and power.
Professional	Perception of health care organizations as a stage for health professionals, professional practice considered the major role in everyday life; self-disciplined clinical professional groups.
Associations	View of organizations as professional associations; cause of major conflict in organizations where professional organizations are bargaining units also provide arenas for managers and workers to meet on common ground to discuss topics of mutual interest in a nonthreatening environment.
Laboratories	Houses of research for clinical research with animal and human research in separate sections of adjacent or separate buildings.
Knowledge	Information-based enterprises composed largely of knowledge and service specialists who direct and discipline their own performance or are managed by others; offer knowledge-based services.
Symphony	An orchestra wherein all the players (workers) are specialists and the chief executive knows how to make good music and knows something about each instrument but does not pretend to be an expert in each specialty.

Figure 4.1 Through the looking glass: Windows on clinical organizations. (A synthesis of ideas by author Simms drawn from Drucker, 1988; Csikszentmihalyi, 1990; Bolman and Deal, 1991; and Schneider, 1991).

THE HUMAN SIDE OF CLINICAL ADMINISTRATION

Veninga (1982) made a sincere attempt to bring in the human element in organizations, but most of his writings still remain fixated on the idea of formal arrangements with administrators telling subordinates what to do and how to do it. The formal structure of departments and divisions creates fixed environments for the accomplishment of work. The grouping of work segments and the levels of management are paramount. Managers are much more interested in their span of control than the knowledge level of individual workers or their ability to figure out how to do their own work. Simms, Dalston, and Roberts noted in 1984 that a persistent reluctance to differentiate work assignments among nurses remains the crucial barrier to differentiated practice. All nurses are mistakenly considered to have the same capabilities by most practicing nurse executives.

Veninga (1982) further noted that the personal and social relations not established by formal authority constitute the informal social system of work groups, with the

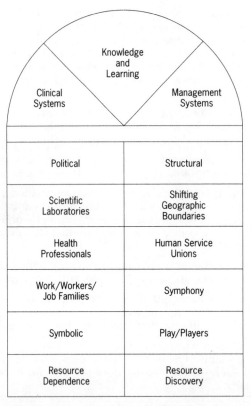

Figure 4.2 Interacting windows in the clinical organization.

political structure creating the environment for goal setting, distribution of authority, and setting the stage for power to affect and control resources. Without organizations, there are no leaders and followers and no opportunity for followers to be leaders. Political leadership can be defined only in terms of and to the extent of realization of purposeful substantive change in the conditions of peoples' lives.

Do nurse executives make any difference in meeting peoples' needs? The financial structure, although comprising humans in Veninga's model, is of paramount importance. The bottom line, what you have now, and what profits you expect to make are all important. The fiscal means that enable you to live in this organization seem more important than what resources might be discovered through creative thought and creative learning environments.

Idour (1980) described the need for health organizations to be a total community effort (Figure 4.3). The community or society is not only a unit of organization, according to Idour, it is also a unit of living, interdependent individuals. The nurse executive must be able to work with other members of society — professional and lay — to design organizational models of care delivery that meet client/customer needs and priorities. Idour further noted that illnesses that prevail are increasingly of a

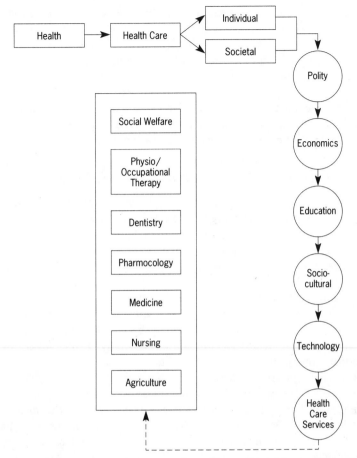

Figure 4.3 "Health"—A total community effort of health professionals and services. (From Idour, M. (1980). *The Social Concept and the Relevancy of Nursing Curricula* (p. 22). Unpublished manuscript. Adapted by permission.)

chronic nature requiring community boundary changes beyond traditional health institutions. Strauss, Fagerhaugh, Suczek, and Wiener (1985) also noted that the work of physicians, nurses, and associated technicians has been radically altered today by a prevalence of chronic illnesses. They bring a sociological perspective to hospital work describing machine, safety, comfort, sentiment, articulation, and patient work as important in analyzing the sociology of work.

Patient involvement in collaborative practice is one factor rarely mentioned. With consumer interest in health care and self-care, it is important to have patient representation on various joint practice activities. Patients could be involved in discharge planning. The effectiveness of planning could therefore be measured in terms of patient compliance with health regimens as prescribed by care-givers. There are several reasons for supporting patient representation on discharge planning teams.

Currently, consumers are interested in disease prevention, health promotion, and self-care. Patient involvement is a rapidly emerging part of hospital-based educational programs. Nationally, concern exists about increased health care costs and the decreased financial support. Individuals want more control of their own health; they want to assume responsibility for present and potential health care needs. More patients seek involvement in the decision-making process regarding their own care. They reject the role of passive recipients with decisions made by physicians and nurses without patient input. In the future, patient involvement will become increasingly important and should be a part of evaluation procedures.

PARTICIPATORY APPROACHES TO ORGANIZATIONAL DESIGN

Although recent attention has been focused on the introduction of shared governance in nursing, little attention has been given to participatory action research methods in redesigning clinical work groups in nursing. Shared governance, described as a philosophy, model, or structure in which nurses have explicit and legitimized control over nursing practice, has become the new "buzz" word for transformation without empirical underpinnings (Perry, 1991). Furthermore, early literature on shared governance suggested governance be shared at the nursing department general policy level. Only recently has the importance of shared governance at the nursing unit level been emphasized so that staff nurses can be actively involved in the day-to-day clinical decision-making process (Kramer, 1990; Porter-O'Grady, 1989; Wake, 1990). Most of the supporting literature is anecdotal and only one study by Ludemann and Brown (1989) linked participatory management with shared governance. No studies have examined the impact of nursing work redesign on patient outcomes.

Several authors have linked participatory management to the human relations theorists such as Likert, McGregor, and Argyris (Perry, 1991), but there has been no theoretical development of how participatory management relates to shared governance. Weick (1979) clarified the importance of each individual worker actively participating in the formation and maintenance of an organization. Although Weick has been influential in describing the process of organizing, a process that comes about by the active involvement of each individual worker, he has not delineated a theoretical framework for his emphasis on the worker, as contrasted with the usual organizational emphasis on the manager. This focus on interactions between rank-and-file workers is often referred to as a "bottom-up" or action approach as compared with the traditional "top-down" approach.

However, bottom-up approaches with clear pathways to redesigning clinical work and practice patterns in nursing do not exist. Quite divergent definitions of primary nursing, case management, team nursing, functional nursing, total patient care, and integrated nursing exist in the literature and in practice. Even though current literature supports increasing interest in collaborative practice in health care (Simms et al., 1984), little attention has been given to meaningful interdisciplinary and intradisciplinary flexible work groups. Unnecessary duplication of effort exists across health care disciplines and between professional and technical nurses. With the exception of the Planetree Model for training patients to be partners in care (Martin, Hunt,

Hughes-Stone, & Conrad, 1990), patient involvement in care planning efforts is rarely discussed.

IMPACT ON THE ORGANIZATIONAL DESIGN OF CARE DELIVERY SYSTEMS

The Patient Intensity for Nursing Index study using Division of Nursing definitions suggests that only one-third of nursing time is spent in direct clinical care (Prescott, Phillips, Ryan, & Thompson, 1991). Other work-sampling studies reported by these authors confirmed this finding. The majority of time (over 50 percent) is spent in combined indirect care or unit management activities. Reducing inefficiencies in information flow and charting routines and reassigning aspects of unit management could save approximately 48 min per nurse per shift. Staff nurses have little creative personal time and only spend about 14 percent in activities such as meals, breaks, personal phone calls, or socializing with co-workers. The Prescott et al. (1991) research supports *(1)* the redesign of work and work groups through restructuring the role of the registered nurse, *(2)* developing assistive nursing personnel, and *(3)* implementing labor-saving assistive technologies.

During the past decade, revolutionary changes have involved every aspect of health care in this country. Extensive basic medical research has yielded an expanding array of diagnostic and monitoring equipment. Life support systems permit surgeons to remove, repair, or replace components of the body as never before in the history of the human race. The manned space programs have yielded a tremendous amount of knowledge related to physiology and communication systems. Major advancements in robotics and the development of assistive technology are dramatically changing patient education and rehabilitation for self-care. As nurses are the principal care givers in various health care delivery settings, it is essential to take a new look at the nature of the work of nursing and propose innovative models for nursing practice that take into account emerging labor-saving assistive technologies as well as rapidly changing health care needs. In essence, nurses must change the way do their clinical work and how they spend their time in clinical practice. Nurse executives must develop new organizational models for care delivery that reflect changing thought about organizations.

THE LEARNING WINDOW

The importance of work group culture and worker learning is beginning to be recognized as important in organizational analyses and technology transfer. One aspect of culture is a group's readiness to change. Receptivity to innovation may be the critical factor in orchestrating change and learning to use technology. Schein (1984) notes that excessive stability may prevent innovation unless large numbers of people are redistributed or replaced or the organizational culture is changed and the workers become involved in decision making.

Changing technology and work environments have created a new potential for worker learning as well as a need for better approaches to the learning process. In fact, Deutsch (1989) has proposed a new norm that it is okay to spend time learning at work. A key point stressed by various researchers is the need for effective organizations to strive consciously toward a participatory work environment to best utilize technology and human resources. Worker learning and the shaping of the work environment are important aspects of human growth and development, especially in the face of rapid technological change. Crisis conditions have accented the need for worker learning in anticipation of changed work environments. The key role of new technology cannot be overstated; it is revolutionary and "the greatest challenge for those involved in worker learning efforts will continue to be to devise ways to move from the narrow and technical to broader issues of worker knowledge, active involvement, and an ever-expanding base of learning how to learn in an on-going process" (Deutsch, 1989, p. 251). Deutsch further suggests a model for expanded learning that increasingly goes from workplace specific issues to larger matters of the work situation depicting a fluid process for everyday learning.

Brown and Duguid (1989) suggest that learning is not the process of amassing data and working is not a series of unenlightening lower level routines but rather both are closely interrelated sense-making, reflective, culture-bound activities. They see human learning as the bottleneck through which innovation must pass. Conversely, innovation is becoming the learning burden of those whose working practices are constantly being changed. Brown and Duguid (1989) further suggest that working, learning, and innovation are related processes and if innovation can be developed out of or in relation to workplace learning, the bottleneck of human learning and burden may be avoided. The authors suggest that the activity of small groups and individuals can lead to insightful learning and this learning is potentially innovative at the organization level. Thus, the small group around the coffee pot, the drinking fountain, or the lunch room should not be assumed to be wasting time. In these small informal groups, real working knowledge about real working practices is commonly exchanged and developed. The lack of personal time at work for staff nurses noted earlier by Prescott et al. (1991) must be viewed as detrimental to creative thinking and interaction in the workplace.

Achieving goals of workplace democracy and freedom to take personal time depends on informed, growing, and self-confident individuals and groups within a supportive work group culture. Brown (1985) and Elden (1981) have shown how workplace participatory research can be viewed as a colearning process where researchers and workers share in some or all stages of work research. Increased learning through participative empowerment processes can make a fundamental contribution to organizational outcomes as confident workers are competent workers. Kornbluh and Greene (1989) propose a learning consciousness in an organization model that focuses on four areas:

- developing learning enabler roles for managers and workers
- developing work organizations as learning milieu
- developing meaningful participatory processes
- developing a work climate committed to learning.

The way work is organized affects the quantity and quality of worker learning; dull, repetitive, fragmented work does not produce a positive learning milieu.

Workers can be deeply involved in processes of research related to their work situations. Elden (1981, 1983) and Brown (1985) have done empirical and analytical work on this issue and have developed the concept of workers and researchers as colearners.

Within the framework of ranges of human needs, McClusky (1974) proposed a theory of margin, postulating that people are constantly engaged in a struggle to maintain a margin of energy and power. Margin is a function of the relationship of load to power. Load refers to the self and the social demands a person must meet to maintain a minimal level of autonomy. Power is made up of the resources, abilities, possessions, positions, allies, and so on, that a person can command to cope with load. Margin can be increased by reducing load or increasing power. Margin can be decreased by increasing load or reducing power. The crucial element is the surplus, or margin, of power in excess of load. This margin confers autonomy on individuals, gives them an opportunity to exercise a range of options, and enables them to achieve growth and development. A major force in the achievement of this outcome is learning, which will assist in creating margins of power for the maintenance of well-being and continuing growth toward self-fulfillment.

Kornbluh, Pipan, and Schurman (1987) also related empowerment to learning and defined empowerment learning as unlimited energy in an organization. Human learning is considered an organizational asset, and in transformed organizations, human learning and problem-solving abilities are viewed as vitally important resources in empowering people—a continuous source of energy. Their thesis questions the zero-sum conception of power in command and control organizations that assumes that power is a finite commodity in which some may gain only if others lose. In turn, a radically different approach is proposed—a non-zero-sum model of power in which the total amount of power is always expanding. This situation is believed to occur in a learning environment. Learning is not a process of receiving verbal information. At the workplace, learning is the process of continually expanding coherence, collaboration, and innovation within a particular community of practice (Brown & Duguid, 1989). The creation of a learning environment empowers workers to use their intellectual abilities to individual development and work-group advantage. In this model, every worker is respected and every worker exerts control over performance and quality of work and life variables. Worker participation and learning environments go hand in hand, and work redesign should be regarded as a continuous process, not a goal.

THE NURSE EXECUTIVE ROLE IN LEARNING ORGANIZATIONS

The need for creativity in the role of the nurse executive has never been greater. Middle managers are frequently threatened by an educative, participative work environment, even though a climate of sharing information is fundamental to professional nursing practice. With the shift to consumer locus of control and demands for high quality patient-centered care, the head nurse as the front line nurse executive is extremely important in creating work environments in which integrated professional practice can occur. The classical view of the manager as the organizer, coordinator, planner, and controller becomes less important in organizations that support participatory management. Mintzberg (1990) suggests that effective management incorporates a balance of cerebral and insightful aspects. He further suggests that the effective manager's role involves interpersonal, informational, and decisional activities. The manager's effectiveness is significantly influenced by insight into the nature of the work.

The learning enabler facilitator role needs to be learned by managers (Kornbluh & Greene, 1989). A very different role compared with traditional management roles, the facilitator role involves performing the function of enabler of learning and constantly creating the conditions for learning. Learning in groups has enormous potential, as described by Hirschhorn (1988), in studying training and learning needs of workers in the new computer-based work organization. Drucker (1988) supports the notion of participatory management because the work force has changed with the introduction of the better educated knowledge worker. This suggests that the manager's primary task is to support joint performance by nurturing common goals, common values, the right structure and ongoing training, and development needed to perform and respond to change. Much of the redesign literature has focused on factors related to redesigning the work of staff nurses. Flarey (1991) asserts that first-line managerial roles must change as well. The role of the first-line manager must take on new dimensions to facilitate quality patient care and patient care provider outcomes.

Failure of unit nurse executives to use professional nurses congruent with their education and expertise is perceived by many nurse leaders to be contributing to the continuing nursing shortage. Prescott et al. (1991), however, debunk arguments of nursing shortage and make a strong case for the idea of inadequate professional nursing practice. Based on work sampling studies about how nurses spend their time, they conclude that hospitals use nurses inappropriately in two ways: nurses do the work of other departments and clinical decision-making authority of nurses is severely limited in many hospitals. Both result in too little professional nursing practice and inappropriate use of nurses' time.

In general, too much emphasis has been placed on limited organizational variables and too little emphasis has been placed on workplace and learning variables. The concept of work excitement, first introduced in a publication by Simms, Erbin-Roesemann, Darga, and Coeling (1990), has tremendous potential for affecting nursing practice. This research supports Pressler and Fitzpatrick (1988), who believe that patient behavior in response to nursing action is of considerable importance for nursing practice. If one considers behavior to be part of nursing action, then the link between work excitement and nursing practice is an important issue to explore. Behavior of health care providers is thought to significantly influence patient clinical outcomes (Knaus, Draper, Wagner, & Zimmerman, 1986). Specifically, if work excitement behaviors are found to be linked to positive outcomes for patients, improvement in quality care could be the end product. If nursing is, indeed, losing the best and brightest potential and current nurses to other professions, creative thinking must be used to halt this progression. Without expert clinicians, the profession will not exist because the social mandate for nursing includes direct care for individual consumers and groups.

The recent shift to a consumer/customer locus of control, emphasis on clinical outcomes in health care, and the increasing availability of various personal assistive technologies mandate different approaches to nursing practice. Decisions regarding changes in staff numbers have generally been determined by management with little opportunity for staff nurse involvement or consumer input. Job redesign solutions have seldom included workers' input. In the future, worker/management/consumer participatory discussion will be essential to decision making about technological change and will be a fundamental component of organizational learning processes.

THE PROFESSIONAL ASSOCIATIONS

A basic element of any profession is the formal organization of professional associations—for example, the American Nurses Association (ANA), the National League for Nursing (NLN), the American Medical Association (AMA), and so forth. Such groups are highly visible phenomena in society and give credibility to participant members as legitimate professionals (Hegyvary, Duxbury, Hall, Krueger, Lindeman, Scott, & Scott, 1987). Professional associations play a vital role in activities of professional life and offer a common ground for discussion and dealing with political issues of conflict among managers and workers who cannot regularly meet in fruitful conversation in the regular world of work. However, they should not be viewed as the equivalent of care delivery organizations. They have very different missions and goals. Professional associations offer wonderful opportunities to learn negotiation, bargaining, and sound management skills in a relatively friendly environment and this is one of the major reasons why nurse executives at all levels should encourage active participation in professional organizations.

MANAGING BOUNDARIES

How boundaries are managed and how that relates to levels of differentiation and integration necessary for effective functioning within organizations has become an issue of paramount importance for nurse executives at all levels. Schneider (1991) provides a meaningful perspective on the concept in her recent discussion of boundaries as both defined and flexible. Boundaries separate a system from its environment and delineate the various parts and processes within that system. As systems develop, they require increased differentiation and integration.

In family systems, managing the boundaries between members is considered important. In organizations, the management of boundaries between and among job families is equally important. Relatedness is forced through concern for patients and quality patient care. Job-family fighting may be a symptom of threatened individual or particular family autonomy. For example, the infighting between nurses, physicians, and social workers over responsibilities for patient care reflect the relatively low autonomy of nonmedical health workers. Descriptions of hospitals as medical care facilities rather than health care facilities further denies the existence of nonmedical health professionals.

The boundary issues present at the group level also exist between groups within organizations and between organizations and their environments (Schneider, 1991). The extent of external control greatly influences boundary management. During reorganizations and work redesign, boundaries are redrawn and redefined. The renegotiation of boundaries is frequently marked by anxiety and a scramble for power among group members. The resolution of boundaries should be dynamic and continuously changing and should restore the necessary requirements for interdependence and interaction. The role of the nurse executive is to manage the boundary between what is outside to preserve the integrity of groups (nursing and non-nursing job families) and the internal coherence of the system.

Boundary problems between professional roles and tasks can create continuing problems with tensions especially pronounced between nurses and physicians. Overlapping services create blurred boundaries that require negotiation for staffing, responsibility, and accountability. Other hostilities are created by ideological boundaries of a community-oriented vs. medical-model approach to care (Schneider, 1991). Competing camps vie for reimbursement of overlapping services. Professional boundaries are jealously guarded and without the National Institutes of Health (NIH) and the Joint Commission for Accreditation of Healthcare Organizations (JCAHO), mandates for attention to patient outcomes, it is likely that patients would have stayed forever at the bottom of the hierarchy with the least to say about their treatment.

Summary

The way clinical organizations are viewed is extremely important and everything in this chapter is essential content for those nurse executives considering organizational innovation at any level. Basic to understanding the chapter theme, it seems important to believe that: *(1)* boundaries are necessary and need to be established for appropriate levels of differentiation and integration and *(2)* autonomy for individual workers is essential to self-development. Boundaries cannot be managed without autonomy of individuals and groups. Allowing projects to develop outside established organizational structures and policies provides the rationale for "skunkworks," which are loosely coupled with the parent structure but not strays, by any means.

In other words, says Schneider (1991), organizations need appropriate levels of differentiation and integration with boundaries established within that are firm yet flexible. Firm but flexible boundaries enable interpersonal intimacy, group cooperation, and organizational interdependence. An effective nurse executive must define and redefine flexible work groups within the central organization while negotiating and planning with networking groups. Today, organizations are viewed as networks, as linkage points of distinctive competencies or specialties on a global scale that require greater and greater efforts at integration without losing differentiation (Ghoshal & Bartlett, 1990). Differences between internal and external stakeholders have become less clear; for example, organizational members such as staff nurses have become customers as well. The nurse executive at all levels must be conscious of unit, organizational, and external boundaries. The process of managing flexible boundaries can be learned and is essential during birth, innovation, work redesign, and creation of new departments and businesses.

Bolman and Deal (1991) suggest that reframing or changing your organization is a four-dimensional process (human, structural, political, and symbolic frames) with major investment in training. We suggest that nurse executives in clinical organizations give attention to all the windows described in Figures 4.1 and 4.2 and that an environment of total learning replace simple training activities. Peter Drucker (1988) talks about the coming of the new organization with the hospital, the university, and the symphony orchestra serving as models. It will bear little resemblance to the factory models of the past. Nursing divisions with numerous levels of managers have been and continue to be structured as factory models. In the coming organizations, health care delivery businesses will be knowledge-based organizations composed largely of specialists who direct their performance through organized feedback from colleagues, customers, and headquarters. Computer technology will make information, formerly considered only for managers, available to everyone who needs it. Successful information-based organizations will have no middle management at all. Senior executives will function more like orchestra conductors. Decentralization into autonomous units with flexible task forces will be essential. Physicians and nurse executives will function collaboratively with health services administrators in a variety of new practice patterns and work groups. What will you see when you look through the looking glass at your organization?

References

Bolman, L. G., & Deal, T. E. (1991). *Reframing organizations*. San Francisco: Jossey-Bass.

Brown, J. S., & Duguid, P. (1989). *Learning & improvisation: Local sources of global innovation*. Unpublished manuscript, University of Michigan, Ann Arbor.

Brown, L. D. (1985). People-centered development and participatory research, *Harvard Education Review, 55*(1), 69–75.

Csikszentmihalyi, M. (1990). *Flow—The psychology of optimal experience*. New York: Harper & Row.

Deutsch, S. (1989). Worker learning in the context of changing technology and work environment. In H. Leymann & H. Kornbluh (Eds.). *Socialization and Learning at Work* (pp. 237–255). Brookfield, VT: Gower Publishing Co.

Drucker, P. F. (1988). The coming of the new organization, *Harvard Business Review, 88*(1), 45–53.

Elden, M. (1981). Sharing the research work: Participative research and its role demand. In P. Reason & J. Rowan (Eds.). *Human Inquiry*. New York: John Wiley.

Elden, M. (1983). Democratization and participative research in developing local theory, *Journal of Occupational Behavior, 4*(1), 21–33.

Flarey, D. L. (1991). Redesigning management roles, *Journal of Nursing Administration, 21*(2), 40–45.

Ghoshal, S., & Bartlett, C. A. (1990). The multinational corporation as an interorganization network, *Academy of Management Review, 15*(4), 603–625.

Hegyvary, S. T., Duxbury, M. L., Hall, R. H., Krueger, J. C., Lindeman, C. A., Scott, J. M., & Scott, W. R. (1987). *The evolution of nursing professional organizations.* Kansas City, MO: American Academy of Nursing.

Hirschhorn, L. (1988). Psychodynamics of the workplace. In *The Workplace Within* (pp. 1–15). Cambridge, MA: MIT Press.

Idour, M. G. (1980). *The social context and the relevancy of nursing curricula.* Unpublished thesis. Massey University, New Zealand.

Kornbluh, H., Pipan, R., & Schurman, S. J. (1987). Empowerment learning and control in workplaces: A curricular view, *Zeitschrift Fur Sozialisationsforschung Und Erziehungssoziologie (ZSE) J. Jahrgang/Heft 7*(4), 253–268.

Kornbluh, H., & Greene, R. T. (1989). Learning, empowerment and participative processes. In H. Leymann & H. Kornbluh (Eds.). *Socialization and Learning at Work* (pp. 256–274). Brookfield, VT: Gower Publishing Co.

Knaus, W., Draper, E., Wagner, D., & Zimmerman, J. (1986). An evaluation of outcomes from intensive care in major medical centers, *Annals of Internal Medicine, 104*(4), 410–418.

Kramer, M. (1990). The magnet hospitals: Excellence revisited, *Journal of Nursing Administration, 20*(9), 35–44.

Ludemann, R. S., & Brown, C. (1989). Staff perceptions of shared governance, *Nursing Administrative Quarterly, 13*(4), 49–56.

Martin, D., Hunt, J. R., Hughes-Stone, M., & Conrad, D. A. (1990). The planetree model project: An example of the patient as partner, *Hospital & Health Services Administration, 35*(4), 591–601.

McClusky, H. Y. (1974). Education for aging: The scope of the field and perspectives for the future. In S. M. Grabowski & W. D. Mason (Eds.). *Education for Aging.* Syracuse, NY: ERIC.

Mintzberg, H. (1990). The manager's job: Folklore and fact, *Harvard Business Review, 68*(2), 163–172.

Perry, B. (1991). *Shared governance in nursing: A review and critique of the literature.* Unpublished manuscript. University of Michigan, Ann Arbor.

Porter-O'Grady, T. (1989). Shared governance: Reality of sham? *American Journal of Nursing, 89,* 350–351.

Prescott, P. A., Phillips, C. Y., Ryan, J. W., & Thompson, K. O. (1991). Changing how nurses spend their time, *IMAGE: Journal of Nursing Scholarship, 23*(1), 23–28.

Pressler, J., & Fitzpatrick, J. (1988). Contribution of Rosemary Ellis to knowledge development for nursing, *IMAGE: Journal of Nursing Scholarship, 20*(1), 28–30.

Schein, E. L. (1984). Coming to a new awareness of organizational culture, *Sloan Management Review, 25*(2), 3–16.

Schneider S. C. (1991). Managing boundaries in organizations. In M. K. deVries (Ed.). *Organizations on the Couch* (pp. 169–190). San Francisco: Jossey-Bass.

Simms, L. M., Dalston, J. W., & Roberts, P. W. (1984). Collaborative practice: Myth or reality, *Hospital and Health Services Administration, 29*(6), 36–48.

Simms, L. M., Erbin-Roesemann, M., Darga, A., & Coeling, H. (1990). Breaking the burnout barrier: Resurrecting work excitement in nursing, *Nursing Economic$, 8*(3), 177–186.

Strauss, A., Fagerhaugh, S., Suczek, B., & Wiener, C. (1985). *Social organization of medical work.* Chicago: The University of Chicago Press.

Veninga, R. L. (1982). *The human side of health administration.* Englewood Cliffs, NJ: Prentice-Hall, Inc.

Wake, M. M. (1990). Nursing care delivery systems: Status and vision, *Journal of Nursing Administration, 20*(5), 47–51.

Weick, K. E. (1979). *The social psychology of organizing.* Reading, MA: Addison-Wesley.

CHAPTER 5

The Person in the Role of Nurse Executive

Highlights

- **The nurse executive as a leader**
- **Maslow, McClusky, and the nurse executive**
- **Leadership styles and excellence in administration**
- **Personal attributes of successful nurse executives**
- **Personal support systems**
- **Time and chance**

The purpose of this chapter is to emphasize the person in the role of nurse executive by focusing on the importance of personal attributes and leadership skills. It is a myth that only those who cannot practice, teach, and those who cannot teach, administrate. True administrators are leaders who love the challenge and hard work of creating a climate in which professional nursing practice can occur. They are catalysts not only for their own activities but for those of others. Contrary to the beliefs of many nurses, the excellent nursing administrator must possess the highest level of ability and the greatest personal skills. Such leaders are not bound by thinking about what cannot be done. Rather, they see the same puzzles others see, but they envision different ways of putting them together.

There is a leadership crisis in nursing and a critical shortage of executives with the political, psychological, and social management skills needed to cope with today's changing world (Kulbok, 1982; Simms, 1991). Nurses are unprepared or unwilling to assume leadership roles. Women are not socialized to assume leadership roles, nor do existing nursing programs really address the need to prepare nursing leaders who are effective administrators. Chaska (1978) spoke of the nursing profession as being in a "mist" of conflicting views about professionalism and professional practice. In 1990, Chaska confirmed that nursing is in the midst of advancing change with multiple evidence of turning points in the profession.

The hospital is the primary area of employment for nurses, with the majority of all nurses employed in a hospital setting (Spitzer, 1981, p. 21). Hospitals are big business, and most nurse executives are not prepared to function within a complex corporate structure. It may be possible that much of the burnout experienced by nurses at all levels is due to the inability of nurses in leadership roles to function in complex corporate structures.

Regardless of the setting for practice—whether hospital community health agency or long-term care setting—nurse executives must know how to compete effectively in a businesslike world. Spitzer (1981) suggests that they should:

1. Reverse the tendency toward isolationism and communicate with others outside of nursing as well as within nursing.
2. Expand teamwork skills.
3. Understand management concepts and organizational goals.
4. Promote an organizational structure and environment that encourage involvement of staff nurses at all levels rather than the practice of creating and maintaining "Queen Bees." (p. 24)

The prevalence of the queen bee syndrome interferes with the advancement of professional nursing in any institutional setting.

The "Queen Bee" syndrome has been identified by Halsey (1978) as certain antifeminist behaviors of women who successfully secure positions in management and other traditionally male-dominated career worlds. Queen bees in nursing administration positions are not an advantage to nursing. These individuals have a desire to work independently of other nurses, identify with people outside nursing, align tenaciously with the institution, and have little interest in making changes that would benefit nursing. They seek to preserve their own images, demand personal loyalty, and have a strong need to run the entire show at the expense of other competent women. They are high achievers and excellent in their area of interest, but they are not leaders.

Early directors of nursing, called superintendents, did run the whole show in hospitals but not necessarily at the expense of other nurses. Erickson (1980) describes the nursing superintendent as the forerunner of modern hospital and nurse executives. These early directors were responsible for nursing service and education. They were expected to have technical knowledge as well as executive ability. Financial knowledge and training in every detail of work were essential skills. Some of these early directors may well have been queen bees, but it is unlikely that they separated themselves from the rest of nursing because they lived in the hospital and directed and knew the nursing staff extremely well.

THE NURSE EXECUTIVE AS A LEADER

Nurse executives cannot create a climate for professional practice unless they are leaders as well as managers. Administration can be carried out by nonnurses, but true leadership in a professional practice setting must be manifested by a nurse with leadership skills. The work of nurse executives differs from that of other hospital administrators in that nursing involves professionals, or what Drucker (1980) calls "knowledge workers." The productivity of knowledge workers requires that people be assigned where there is potential for results and not where knowledge and skill cannot produce results. The utilization of nursing resources according to level of education, experience, and strengths is of critical importance today for all nurses in administrative posts.

There are no known ways of training great leaders, and the preparation of leaders in nursing has become the challenge of this decade for schools of nursing. Most deans and program directors will claim to be preparing leaders, but the fact remains that true leaders simply are not emerging from nursing graduate programs.

According to Zaleznik (1981), managers and leaders differ fundamentally in their world views, perceptions, and personal characteristics:

- Attitudes toward goals: managers tend to adapt impersonal attitudes toward goals; leaders adapt personal and active attitudes toward goals.
- Conception of work: managers act to limit choices as they seek the accomplishment of specific tasks through predetermined combinations of people and ideas; leaders work to develop fresh approaches to long-standing problems and to open issues for new options.
- Relation with others: managers prefer to work with people, avoid solitary activity, and relate to people according to the roles they play; leaders are more empathetic and are concerned with the effects that events and decisions have on participants.
- Sense of self: managers are once-born personalities and belong to the institutional environment; leaders tend to be twice-born personalities and separate from their environment; they may work in organizations but never belong to them.

Managers develop through socialization, and leaders develop through personal mastery. For a leader, self-esteem does not depend solely on positive attachments and real rewards. Leaders cannot be bought by the institution. They have visions and dreams that managers may never see. As nursing seeks to become recognized as a profession, it is increasingly important to have visionaries in leadership roles to find new answers to old, unresolved questions.

Who, then, are leaders? Lundberg (1982) says that leaders are people who:

- Know where they are going.
- Know how to get there.
- Have courage and persistence.

- Can be believed.
- Can be trusted not to sell their cause for personal advantage.
- Make missions important, exciting, and possible.
- Make subordinates feel that their roles in the mission are important.
- Make others feel capable of performing their roles.

Managers, says Drucker (1980), are paid to enable people to do the work for which they are paid. Nurse executives do not earn their pay if they do not create a professional practice climate in which nurses can do their work. Leaders make a difference in the lives of those who work for them and with them. In fact, according to Veninga (1982), one of the most important executive functions is the teaching responsibility. Instructing staff in how to carry out assignments is an important part of work accomplishment.

MASLOW, McCLUSKY, AND THE NURSE EXECUTIVE

The able nurse executive is not only self-motivated but is also able to create an environment in which others are motivated. To motivate others requires a strong self-concept and a high place on the ladder of Maslow's hierarchy of needs (1962). In other words, the able executive is one who has reached or is approaching the stage of self-actualization. New style organizations demand leaders who are interested in the development of others, not just their own personal success. Such leadership involves self-development and a true sense of knowing oneself intellectually, bodily, emotionally, and spiritually (Kinsman, 1986).

Maslow's theory of motivation can be applied to almost every aspect of human life, but it has special significance for those who lead and guide others. Maslow's theory provides a basis for the higher needs of psychological growth. People are initially motivated by basic physiological needs. As those needs are satisfied, the individual moves toward the level of higher needs and becomes motivated by them. This is the heart of Maslow's theory. Most previous studies assumed that needs could be isolated and studied separately. Maslow considered the individual as an integrated whole. The identification of needs for growth, development, and utilization of potential are an important part of self-actualization. Maslow has described this need as the "desire to become more and more what one is, to become everything that one is capable of becoming" (1962).

Figure 5.1 depicts Maslow's hierarchy of needs. Maslow's hierarchy has been applied to patient needs. It also has significant application for the nurse as a person. Nurse executives as nurse persons and leaders of other nurse persons have a special need to reach the level of self-actualization. Nurse persons are described by Simms and Lindberg (1978) as fully functioning individuals who are comfortable with using the self as well as technical skills in professional practice. This implies the need for growth and development of the nurse as a person.

Self-actualization is the desire for self-fulfillment, to make actual all one's potentialities. Maslow related potential to the concept of growth, and by growth, he meant the constant development of talents, capacities, creativity, wisdom, and character. To play a role satisfactorily, a person must have a self-concept that fits the role.

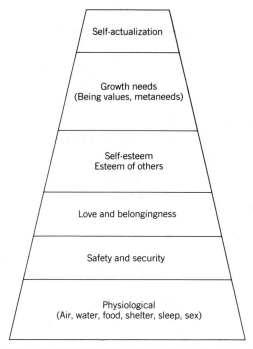

Figure 5.1 Maslow's hierarchy of needs.

Howard McClusky (1974) of the University of Michigan, delineated educational needs for older people, ranging from survival through maintenance to growth and beyond. The McClusky conceptual framework is readily adaptable to the growth and development of nurse executives and provides a companion schema to Maslow's hierarchy. Within the framework of ranges of needs, McClusky proposed a theory of margin. According to this theory, people are constantly engaged in a struggle to maintain a margin of energy and power.

"Margin" is a function of the relationship of "load" to "power." "Load" refers to the self and the social demands a person must meet to maintain a minimal level of autonomy. "Power" is made up of the resources, abilities, possessions, positions, allies, and so on, that a person can command to cope with load. Margin can be increased by reducing load or increasing power. Margin can be decreased by increasing load or reducing power.

The crucial element in this scheme is the surplus, or margin of power in excess of load. This margin confers autonomy on individuals, gives them an opportunity to exercise a range of options, and enables them to achieve growth and development. A major force in the achievement of this outcome is education that will assist in creating margins of power for the maintenance of well-being and continuing growth toward self-fulfillment.

Figure 5.2 demonstrates the scope of needs in McClusky's hierarchy, ranging from coping needs to transcendence. The first level "coping needs," refers to the need for

---

TRANSCENDENCE NEEDS
Self actualization
Comprehensive, individualized learning

INFLUENCE NEEDS
Civic and political organization
Education for leadership, community action and problem solving

CONTRIBUTIVE NEEDS
Societal contribution
In-service leadership
Community awareness

EXPRESSIVE NEEDS
Physical education
Liberal education
Hobbies and personal interests

COPING NEEDS
Physical well-being
Social adjustment
Psychological health

Figure 5.2 Categories of educational needs. (From McClusky, H. (1974), in Grabowski & Mason (eds.) *Education for the Aging.* Syracuse, NY: ERIC Clearinghouse. Adapted by permission.)

---

basic education for survival and self-sufficiency. The second category, "expressive needs," is based on the premise that people have a need to engage in activities for the sake of the activity itself. The human personality is capable of a wide range of expression beyond habitual routines. Talents and interests flower if properly cultivated.

Category 3, "contributive needs," refers to the assumption that all people have a need to give to others and society, a desire to be of service. "Influence needs" comprises category 4. People must exert influence on the circumstances of living and the world about them. Applied to nursing, the right kind of education and utilization of experience can greatly enhance the nurse executive's power base and ability to influence others. McClusky's category 5, the need for "transcendence," matches Maslow's level of self-actualization. Although McClusky envisioned transcendence as uniquely relevant to the later years, it is also pertinent to the nurse executive who must move beyond self in motivating others. One rarely reaches this level early in life. By definition, achieving the highest level of one's existence is a feature of the later years.

Figure 5.3 depicts an adaptation of the McClusky hierarchy of education in terms of the developing administrator. A great educator, Howard McClusky believed that education is not an option but, rather, an indispensable means of existence. For the fully functioning professional person, lifelong learning is mandatory.

Many nurses rebel at the possibility of becoming an executive. They are bound up in the care functions and feel that unless they personally deliver hands-on care, they have somehow abandoned the profession. They fail to see that influencing others to deliver quality care can have greater impact on the quality of care than any individual effort could.

HIGH SELF-ESTEEM

Regard for needs of others; international perspective on health for all
Able to follow others as well as to lead
Visionary executive leadership in a variety of roles
Not threatened by competition; able to take risks
Active in professional nursing and health organizations

OWN LEADERSHIP STYLE

Builds on own uniqueness
Established lifelong learning pattern
Motivates self and others
Integrates management activities in everyday activities regardless of role

SELF-ESTEEM

Recognizes self as a fully functioning nurse executive
Additional education and specific interests
Personal anchors and supports in place
Self-directed learning

LOVE AND BELONGINGNESS

Comfortable in clinical world
Middle management skills in line or staff positions
Head nurse, clinical manager or clinical specialist roles
Graduate education at either the master's or doctoral level

SAFETY AND SECURITY

Beginning work experience
Comfortable with clinical knowledge
Little if any risk taking
Increased involvement in professional nursing organizations

PHYSIOLOGICAL

Basic education in nursing
Beginning involvement in professional nursing organizations
Beginning recognition of interest in professional career

Figure 5.3 The developing nurse executive.

What, then, is the able executive like? What characterizes the Ruth Freemans, the Lillian Walds, the Florence Nightingales? To begin with, they all conveyed a sense of togetherness—wholeness, confidence, wisdom. They were teachers, rational thinkers, dreamers, and independents. They did not seek to emulate others' leadership styles. They had their own. In true Maslovian fashion, they moved up the ladder to strong self-concept and self-actualization. They were the sum total of their individual lives, educations, genes, and experiences. Nurse executives should be leaders; if they are not leaders, they should not administrate.

LEADERSHIP STYLES AND EXCELLENCE IN ADMINISTRATION

The leadership literature is voluminous, and yet no theorist has been able to fully describe the "perfect 10," the effective leader-administrator who is a self-actualized person who can lead common people to do uncommon things in a productive fashion. Robbins (1980) discusses three basic approaches to explaining effective leaders:

1. Trait studies are designed to find universal personality traits that leaders have to a greater degree than nonleaders.
2. Behavioral research is undertaken to explain leadership in terms of behavior.
3. Contingency models are constructed to explain situational variables as well as leadership traits and behavior.

Research efforts to isolate traits have resulted in inconsistent conclusions. The major central idea that has emerged is that intelligence, extroversion, self-assurance, and empathy tend to be related to achieving and maintaining a leadership position. Leadership style traits can be identified, however (Moloney, 1979). Although requisite traits are inconsistent, the following traditional and emerging leadership styles can be observed in practice:

1. Autocratic leader: demonstrates aggressive dominance; commands and expects others to follow.
2. Participative leader: includes followers in decision making; assumes followers can be motivated to self-direction, self-actualization, and creative performance.
3. Laissez-faire leader: permits group members to have freedom to function and set goals independently of the leader.
4. Instrumental leader: exhibits rational rather than supportive behavior; plans, directs, organizes, controls, and coordinates the activities of followers.
5. "Great man" leader: behavior based on the belief that people can learn leadership from studying the examples of the lives of great men.
6. Teacher-learner leader: an emerging model based on the belief that leading is learning and good management is teaching. (Veninga, 1982; Adams, 1986)

The two most popular behavioral studies to date have been conducted by Kerr, Schriesheim, Murphy, and Stogdill (1974) at Ohio State University and Kahn and Katz (1969) at the University of Michigan. These studies identified two dimensions of leadership behavior: *(1)* initiating structure and *(2)* consideration. Initiating structure refers to the extent to which a leader defines and structures his or her role and those of subordinates. Consideration refers to the interpersonal relationships variable. Blake, Mouton, and Tapper (1981) addressed two concerns: *(1)* production of results and *(2)* concern for personnel as people. None of the three approaches addressed the social situations in which leaders must act.

For example, the social situation varies according to the characteristics of the group, the nature of group tasks, and the particular circumstances relevant to a given leadership position. Hershey and Blanchard, cited in Moloney (1979), studied the relationship of the psychological, or person, dimension to the sociological, or role, dimension in specific situations. Their work has added to the leadership literature in terms of self-understanding, group tasks, the concept of group behavior, individual behavior within a group, and the importance of interpersonal relationships within a given situation.

The work of Blake et al. (1981) is particularly useful for nurse executives as they attempt to understand and develop their own leadership style and ability to work with groups in a given situation. Figure 5.4 depicts 81 positions categorizing the relation-

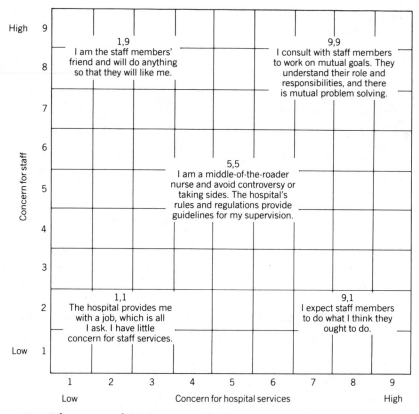

Figure 5.4 The nurse administrator grid. (From R. R. Blake, J. S. Mouton & M. Tapper. (1981). *Grid Approaches for Managerial Leadership in Nursing* (p. 2). St. Louis: Mosby. Used with permission.)

ship between the nurse manager and the nursing staff. Position 9.9 is considered excellence and connotes an administrator who is moving to the ultimate in mature, meaningful relationships.

Other leadership research produced the contingency models, with *(1)* the autocratic-democratic continuum, *(2)* the Fiedler, and *(3)* the path-goal models becoming the best known (Robbins, 1980). The autocratic-democratic model depicts two extreme positions on either end of a continuum, with many positions between. The contingency approach suggests that neither the democratic nor the autocratic extreme is effective in all situations.

The Fiedler (1967) model suggests three contingency dimensions:

1. Leader-member relations: how well liked, respected, and trusted the leader is
2. Task structure: the procedural nature of job assignments
3. Position power: the degree to which the leader has influence over power variables

The basic premise of Fiedler's theory is that the performance of a group is contingent on the style of the leader and how favorable the situation is for the leader. Robert House (1971), of the University of Toronto, has proposed a contingency path-goal model of leadership that integrates the expectancy model of motivation with the structure and consideration research developed by Kahn and Katz (1969). The model describes the leader as being responsible for "increasing the number and kinds of personal payoffs to the subordinates for work-goal attainment and making paths to these payoffs easier to travel" (House & Mitchell, 1974). The path-goal model proposes that the scope of the job and the characteristics of the subordinates moderate the relationship between a leader's behavior and subordinates' performance and satisfaction.

In applying path-goal theory to nursing, the leader uses skills in structuring and consideration to increase worker motivation (Calkin, 1980). The leader initiates structure by defining his or her own role and the roles of subordinates toward goal achievement. Volunteers need a high level of direction, staff nurses less, and clinical nurse specialists very little. The leadership skill lies in knowing how to balance structure and consideration with the particular situation.

All nurse executives should be leaders; if they are not, they should develop the capability or be replaced. The morale and motivation of staff nurses are highly dependent on the leadership skills of the nurse executive and on the work climate.

PERSONAL ATTRIBUTES OF SUCCESSFUL NURSE EXECUTIVES

Donna Diers (1979) aptly discussed the personal attributes of successful nurse executives as the softer aspects of leadership—those characteristics that do not fall conveniently into boxes in a diagram. They are intangible traits that are not easily researched, for example:

- Vision
- Political skills
- Creativity

- Charisma
- Knowledge of other peoples' motivations and pressures
- Ability to read the dynamics of a situation

It is not enough to be able to plan, organize, set goals, and achieve goals. One must be able to dream—to envision the future. Says Diers, "A vision serves as an energy source, a star to guide us, a hook on which to hang dreams of glory. Goals, on the other hand, are achievable end points, termini to measure progress. A good vision will outlive any leader; it gives one a legacy" (p. 7).

Often people in leadership roles get so involved with their work that they never step back to see if they are on target. They do not take the time to assess their personal and professional goals or their strengths and weaknesses. Moon (1981) suggests that professional nurse executives must pursue excellence in themselves to improve the quality of life in their institutions. This means developing and maintaining their knowledge base, keeping up to date, sharing knowledge with colleagues, and taking time to "smell the flowers."

Successful executives in nursing must have goals and dreams and ideas and a love of their work. Benjamin Mays (1980), at the White House Conference on Aging, expressed his views on professional administration in the following statement:

It must be borne in mind that the tragedy in life doesn't lie in not reaching your goal. The tragedy lies in having no goal to reach. It isn't a calamity to die with dreams unfulfilled, but it is a calamity not to dream. It is not a disaster to be unable to capture your ideal, but it is a disaster to have no ideal to capture. It is not a disgrace not to reach the stars, but it is a disgrace to have no stars to reach for. Not failure, but low aim, is sin. (p. 7)

Of the possible personal attributes that nurse executives need, courage, conviction, and creativity are the most important. One's survival as a nurse executive depends on these three attributes.

Courage

A nurse executive with courage has the mental or moral strength to venture, persevere, and withstand danger, fear, or difficulty. Courage implies a firmness of mind and will in the face of difficulty and a determination to achieve one's ends. Courage is synonymous with mettle, spirit, resolution, and tenacity.

One may not ordinarily think of the nurse executive as courageous, but he or she assuredly should be. It takes courage to make changes that need to be made, even though those changes are unpopular and little appreciated. It is very risky to move into uncharted water. For example, establishing a unification model between nursing service and nursing education in an environment of alienation and distrust can be very stressful. The nurse executive attempting to establish such a model must be prepared to withstand personal and professional criticism. Many barriers must be broken down and many friendships established before the two groups can collaborate within a total nursing community.

Courage may also be required to establish meaningful joint practice modalities ranging from integrated charting to true collaborative care planning and implementation. Nurse executives must listen to all the arguments against joint practice and still persevere toward establishing a feasible institutional or unit model. They must be prepared to face the wrath of nurses and physicians alike who are unwilling to collaborate in a professional, meaningful way.

Nurse executives must be willing to meet one to one, in small groups or in large groups—whatever it takes to nurture discussion and identify opposition. Allowing one's ideas to be thoroughly challenged and questioned enables one to verify those ideas and to remain in one's goal without becoming known as a stubborn tyrant. Stubbornness is not to be confused with courage, for stubbornness implies a closed mind, one that is not willing to test out new ideas.

It takes courage to work in the midst of negative criticism. It takes courage to meet with opponents and try to achieve a meeting of the minds. It also takes courage to face the opposition and maintain presence of mind and dignity without becoming pompous or resorting to shallow thinking. It takes courage to swim daily with the sharks as well as the friendly dolphins. It takes courage to maintain composure and not show one's wounds, though some may be deep. Above all, it takes courage to remain dry eyed, even when angered to frustration and tears (Cousteau, 1981).

Conviction

A conviction is a strong persuasion and belief, an opinion held with complete assurance despite opposing arguments, a belief stronger than an impression and less strong than positive knowledge. One cannot have courage without convictions, and one cannot have convictions without strong inner discipline and high ideals. One who has conviction about nursing ideals is willing to attempt to convert others to the same way of thinking and to establish goals that are meaningful to nursing and the institution.

With conviction comes the ability to communicate one's opinion. Not only does one have an opinion, but one is also able to communicate that opinion orally and in writing. A lot is written about communication in the nursing literature, but little is written about having something to communicate. The nurse executive must communicate from a base of knowledge and experience that reflects understanding of the issues under discussion.

The nurse executive with conviction is a nagger, one who keeps needling away at others to move toward goals of worth: when others believe an idea has been dropped, they soon realize they are being bombarded from another quarter. Executives with courage and conviction bring about change and desired internalization of ideas in others without force. They bring about such results by planting the seeds of a desired change and then rigorously making sure the seeds grow and multiply.

Creativity

A distinctly human quality, creativity is not any one thing, but contains the common elements of all creative thought: divergent thinking, flexibility, fluency, and originality. Creativity is the highest order of conceptualization and problem solving. By definition, to create is to evolve something from one's own thought. True innovation must come from within. Innovating means not succumbing to the fallacy that there is not enough time to be creative. It comes from a can-do, rather than a cannot-do, philosophy.

Creativity sets the excellent executive, the true leader, apart from the minimum-level performer. Anyone can be taught the four maxims of management: planning, organizing, implementing, and evaluating. One can learn to memorize the rules of delegation and time management and still not have anything to delegate or any reason to save time.

Successful nurse executives are creative problem solvers. To be creative, they must free themselves from their own premature judgment. They must allow themselves time for theorizing and hypothesizing. Many creative people recognize that they give intermittent attention to problems of interest; that is, they are aware of incubation periods when much subconscious activity may be occurring. It is important, therefore, to develop an increased awareness of the problems to which one would like to direct attention. Functioning creatively, one can combine intuition and scientific principles to achieve superlative problem solving. Such functioning is the highest level of professional skill. Creativity is truly the art of seeing what everyone else is seeing but thinking what no one else has thought.

The essential problem for teachers of the professions is the difficulty of providing a transition from academic experience to work experience. Many educators struggle over how to teach administrators the qualities of a leader. Epstein (1982) discusses the "missing factor" in the teaching: leadership skills and the need for leadership are packaged together for students without the opportunity to make creative inferences. The competency-based movement in education threatens to shroud further the development of creative leaders. There is a difference between competence and the full functioning of excellence in the practice of administration.

The excellent executive is a leader who is creative. Creativity can be recognized only if it is observable by others. The outcomes of creativity are recognized in the results of one's labors, either as accomplished, recognizable feats or as changed behavior of fellow workers.

The creative leader is in fact an effective teacher, one who influences the thinking and behavior of others. The creative leader is one who can take advantage of teachable moments and seize opportunities for infiltrating the minds of others. Such a leader is also well able to take advantage of optimal "learning movements" in which vision and understanding of complex problems occur.

The highest level of creativity requires the ability to conceptualize, the ability to lift any idea or problem from the mundane to a level of abstraction so that it may be treated and studied in an innovative manner. In building a conceptual framework for nursing administration, one uses concepts from nursing, basic sciences, and behavioral sciences. Concepts can serve as powerful organizational tools for thinking, and the sorting and matching of concepts is a practical skill of creativity. Consider, for example, the conceptualization of a new organizational structure. Organizational charts are usually complex concepts developed first in one human brain, transmitted to others by a teaching-learning exercise, and completed on paper only when firmly understood by all concerned. Creativity, then, produces the paths to achievement of those dreams, visions, and goals.

PERSONAL SUPPORT SYSTEMS

There is more to life than work. Work time is measured in terms of work-related objectives, and personal time is measured in terms of satisfaction, emotional gain, quality of relationships, and fulfillment or service to others (Douglass & Douglass, 1980). Personal goals and objectives are part of the whole human picture of the nurse executive. They constitute an essential dimension of self-actualized, fully functioning leaders with the capability for mature relationships.

Other management literature suggests that personal life goals cannot be left out of performance plans (Levinson & La Monica, 1980). Management by objective and performance appraisal processes as typically practiced may be self-defeating if attention is not given to personal life goals and their relevance to organizational objectives. Workers whose personal and work lives are in flow are significantly happier, more creative, and more satisfied (Csikszentmihalyi, 1990).

Whatever supports are important to the individual must be identified and nurtured. Who are those individuals or groups whom one can laugh with and love? Who supports and understands one? What serves as a release for confusion and frustration? Where are the quiet and restful corners at home where comfort and solace are assured? What hobbies and activities produce the greatest sense of optimism and positive thinking? Pets, for example, can be the most significant others an executive can have, and their value should not be underestimated.

Humor in all settings leads to greater sensibility and an appreciation of the temper of other people. It is a social lubricant and a human connection (Bennett, 1981). The ability to see humor in various situations is a means of releasing the energy accompanying excessive tension. A sense of humor is both a personal attribute and a personal support system. Humor is a powerful weapon that can help establish trust and fellowship at work, at home, and in group interactions. Jackson (1980) proposed the use of humor as a deliberate nursing technique, "Laughing with someone enfolds him/her within a network of human love, understanding, and support" (p. 12).

The phenomenon of burnout deserves special attention and is more fully addressed later in this book. Burnout is not unique to executives, but they are prime victims of what is known to the military as battle fatigue. Maslach (1976) aptly describes burnout as a "syndrome of emotional exhaustion and cynicism that frequently occurs among people who do 'people' work—who spend considerable time in close encounters." Nurse executives need to recognize that burnout can happen to them and that steps should be taken to mitigate its occurrence. Personal support systems become extremely important in providing channels through which individuals can tune off their work role and its demands. Female executives, especially, must see their families as support systems rather than handicaps. Too often, children of working women are perceived as interferences with productivity rather than as assets.

TIME AND CHANCE

The self-actualized, fully functioning nurse executive has mastered time management, for time management is really self-management. McCarthy (1981) emphasizes that one cannot really manage time. To be a good self-manager, one must have a positive professional self-image and enough initiative to change oneself. McCarthy stated that there are five degrees of initiative, ranging from waiting to be told what to do to acting on one's own.

To determine personal and career goals, one must conduct a formal time analysis. Douglass and Douglass (1980) suggest that most people have about 2 hours a day to do various personal things. They suggest that executives should determine how they currently spend their time in eight broad areas and then decide how they would like to spend their time. Douglass and Douglass propose that the things people value most can be divided into these eight categories: career, family, social life, financial stability, health, personal development, spiritual development, and leisure. To achieve a satisfying, fulfilling life, one must control one's life and decide how one will spend one's time in these areas. Every day, each person has a new 24 hours to unfold and to spend and a chance to write a new page of one's life.

The focus of this chapter has been the person. Within the conceptual framework, time can be seen as a personal resource that enhances one's power to cope with the demand, or load, of one's job. As discussed early in this chapter, the surplus of power—the margin—enables individuals to be autonomous. Time is perhaps the single resource over which the individual can maintain a large degree of control. Powerless executives are "can't" people, "never have enough time" people. Lack of time is an excuse for all manner of uncompleted tasks.

The fully functioning nurse executive maintains a margin of power and energy through time management and timing. Time and chance are linked, and time is perceived as opportunity. In administration, one has seconds, minutes, days, seasons, and years to accomplish one's goals. Many conferences and books address the issue of time management. None provides a formula that works unless the individual sees time as an energy and power resource.

Summary

Personal attributes and leadership skills are crucial to the role of the nurse executive. Personal attributes, personal support systems, and learned administrative behaviors combine with management skills to produce a competent leader-administrator. Knowing one's strengths and weaknesses, building on one's educational and work experiences, and the uniqueness of one's life experiences and leadership capabilities are essential components of a satisfying, rewarding experience in administration. The work of Maslow and McClusky in developmental psychology is a useful conceptual framework for the development of the self-actualized, transcended leader-administrator capable of creating a climate of motivation and productivity for others.

SELF-DEVELOPMENTAL ACTIVITIES

1. Explore Maslow's concept of self-actualization and McClusky's concept of transcendence in terms of your own development. Where do you perceive yourself on the ladder?

2. Relate the concepts of courage, conviction, and creativity to a situation in your practice. To what extent does your personal administrative style influence the operationalization of these concepts?

3. Update your curriculum vitae every 6 months.

4. Examine the concept of personal support systems as it applies to you.

5. Regularly develop a personal and professional performance plan.

6. Assign yourself new learning activities based on weaknesses identified in your self-assessment and CV update.

References

Adams, J. D. (Ed.). (1986). *Transforming leadership.* Alexandria, VA: Miles River Press.

Bennett, A. C. (1981). It's no joke — healthcare exec needs a sense of humor, *Modern Health Care, 11*(8), 146, 150.

Blake, R. R., Mouton, J. S., & Tapper, M. (1981). *Grid approaches for managerial leadership in nursing.* St. Louis: Mosby.

Calkin, J. D. (1980). Using management literature to enhance new leadership roles, *Journal of Nursing Administration, 10*(4), 24–29.

Chaska, N. L. (1978). *The nursing profession.* New York: McGraw-Hill.

Chaska, N. L. (1990). *The nursing profession.* New York: McGraw-Hill.

Cousteau, V. (1981). How to swim with sharks: A primer, *American Journal of Nursing, 81*(10), 1960.

Csikszentmihalyi, M. (1990). *Flow. The psychology of optimal experience.* New York: Harper & Row.

Diers, D. (1979). Lessons on leadership, *Image, 11*(3), 3–7.

Douglass, M. E., & Douglass, D. N. (1980). *Manage your time, manage your work, manage yourself.* New York: AMACOM.

Drucker, P. F. (1980). *Managing in turbulent times.* New York: Harper & Row.

Epstein, C. (1982). *The nurse leader: Philosophy and practice.* Reston, VA: Reston.

Erickson, E. H. (1980). The nursing service director, 1880–1980, *Journal of Nursing Administration, 10*(4), 6–13.

Fiedler, F. E. (1967). *A theory of leadership effectiveness.* New York: McGraw-Hill.

Halsey, S. (1978). The queen bee syndrome. In M. E. Hardy & M. E. Conway (Eds.). *Role Theory: Perspectives for Health Care Professionals.* New York: Appleton-Century-Crofts.

House, R. J. (1971). A path goal theory of leader effectiveness, *Administration Science Quarterly, 16*(3), 321–328.

House, R. J., & Mitchell, T. R. (1974). Path-goal theory of leadership, *Journal of Contemporary Business, 3*(4), 81–97.

Jackson, M. M. (1980). The nurse who laughs, lasts: The comic spirit in nursing, *The Michigan Nurse, 53*(4), 12–14.

Kahn, R., & Katz, D. (1969). Leadership practices in relation to productivity and morale. D. Cartwright & A. Zauder (Eds.). *Group Dynamics: Research and Theory* (2nd ed.). Elmsford, NY: Row Paterson.

Kerr, S., Schriesheim, C. A., Murphy, C. J., & Stogdill, R. M. (1974). Toward a contingency theory of leadership based upon the consideration and structural literature, *Organizational Behavior and Human Performance, 12*(1), 62–82.

Kinsman, F. (1986). Leadership from alongside. In J. D. Adams (Ed.). *Transforming Leadership* (pp. 19–38). Alexandria, VA: Miles River Press.

Kulbok, P. (1982). Role diversity of nursing administrators, *Nursing and Health Care, 3*(4), 199–203.

Levinson, H., & La Monica, E. L. (1980). Management by whose objectives? *Journal of Nursing Administration, 10*(9), 22–30.

Lundberg, L. B. (1982). What is leadership? *Journal of Nursing Administration, 12*(5), 32–33.

Maslach, C. (1976). Burn-out, *Human Behavior, 5*(9), 16–22.

Maslow, A. H. (1962). *Toward a psychology of being.* New York: Van Nostrand.

Mays, B. (1980). *Report from the White House Conference on Aging, no. 2.*

McCarthy, M. J. (1981). Managing your own time: The most important management task, *Journal of Nursing of Administration, 11*(11,12), 61–65.

McClusky, H. Y. (1974). Education for aging: The scope of the field and perspectives for the future. In S. M. Grabowski & W. D. Mason (Eds.). *Education for the Aging.* Syracuse, NY: ERIC Clearinghouse.

Moloney, M. M. (1979). *Leadership in nursing.* St. Louis: Mosby.

Moon, D. J. (1981). Professionalism: A commitment to excellence, *Nursing Homes, 30*(2), 2–4.

Robbins, S. P. (1980). *The administrative process* (2nd ed.). Englewood Cliffs, NJ: Prentice-Hall.

Simms, L., & Lindberg, J. (1978). *The nurse person.* New York: Harper & Row.

Simms, L. M. (1991). The professional practice of nursing administration: Integrated nursing practice, *Journal of Nursing Administration, 21*(5), 39–46.

Spitzer, R. (1981). The nurse in the corporate world, *Supervisor Nurse, 12*(4), 21–24.

Veninga, R. L. (1982). *The Human Side of Health Administration.* Englewood Cliffs, NJ: Prentice-Hall.

Zaleznik, A. (1981). Managers and leaders: Are they different? *Journal of Nursing Administration, 11*(7), 25–31.

PART II

The Context of Nursing Administration Practice

CHAPTER 6

Creating the Environment for Professional Practice

Highlights
- Environment of the nurse executive
- Concept of environment
- Authority of the nurse executive
- Using the environment model
- Fiscal implications

The purpose of this chapter is to discuss the concept of and a model for the environment for professional nursing practice. The term "environment" is commonly used in the literature on organizations to mean the conditions and structures outside an organization. Areas of the external environment that are important for organizations are technological, legal, political, economic, demographic, ecological, and cultural (Hall, 1977). The term "internal environment" is used in this chapter to refer to conditions and characteristics within an organization. The internal environment for nursing practice may be viewed for the purposes of this discussion as all organizational elements, both tangible and intangible. Tangible elements include, for example, the physical plant, equipment, and staff. Examples of intangible elements include communication patterns, philosophy of the agency, values, and leadership styles.

The climate of the organization is also an important aspect of the internal environment and is classified in this chapter as an intangible element of the internal environment. Climate is defined as "the psychological atmosphere that results from and surrounds the operation of the structure" (Jones, 1981, p. 160). Organizational climate is the quality of the total organizational environment that is a result of the interaction of the formal organizational policies, the personality factors, and the stress created when individual and organizational goals are integrated. The climate of an organization is considered an important factor because it serves as a link between such variables as policies and organizational structure and such end result variables as satisfaction and turnover (McMahon, Ivancevich, & Matteson, 1977).

The specific aspects of an environment for nursing practice will vary with different settings, regional customs, and institutional history. However, the general concepts and frameworks presented herein may be adapted to fit a particular situation. Because the external environment also influences nursing practice, certain aspects are explored in later chapters.

THE ENVIRONMENT AND THE NURSE EXECUTIVE

The environment created by the nursing department serves as the foundation of the four components of professional nursing: clinical practice, administration, education, and research. Although all four components may not exist simultaneously in each practice setting, the established environment can ease the introduction of additional components at different points in time.

Unfortunately, the environment created by a nursing department does not constitute the total environment in which nursing is practiced. Some aspects of the total institutional or societal environment will no doubt have more impact on the nursing staff at times than does the nursing environment. If these other aspects are negative, nursing practice may stagnate even with a well-planned basis for the nursing environment. On the other hand, the nursing-created environment may cushion the impact of some aspects of the broader environment. For example, if a nursing shortage forces an institution to hire additional, less skilled staff, aspects of the nursing environment, such as job description, appropriate practice policies, and orientation, could reduce the impact on the overall quality of nursing care.

There are numerous other reasons for the nurse executive to provide leadership in creating the environment for nursing practice. For example, in a survey of nurses, lack of administrative support was found to be the main reason that nurses left practice in Oregon (Three new studies, 1981). The chief conclusion of another study of nurse shortages was that nurses leave nursing primarily because of the working conditions tolerated or promoted by administration (Wandelt, Pierce, & Widdowson, 1981). In the Oregon study, complaints from nurses included statements about nursing directors who did not support good nursing practice. In another report, the American Nurses Association Commission on Nursing Services stated that a serious factor in the nursing shortage was the amount of time that nurses spend performing non-nursing functions (Culprit in shortage, 1981).

Although these study findings cannot be generalized to all nursing service settings, their conclusions direct nurse executives to examine the organization in which they practice for factors and situations that may contribute to a less than adequate environment for nursing practice. Such an evaluation should include examination of both the nursing service and the overall institutional environments. To carry out this examination systematically, the nurse executives should have a conceptual framework. The proposed framework that follows may be used both to examine a current situation and to plan an environment that promotes nursing practice.

The Concept of Environment

Conceptual approaches to environment have been identified in the fields of business and organizational behavior. As mentioned previously, most of these approaches are geared to the environment external to the organization. The organizational universe model represents one approach that does include both the internal and the external environment. This model can provide a basis for "looking through the whole to those structures and processes that need to be monitored before change can be managed effectively" (Jones, 1981, p. 155).

The organizational universe model (Figure 6.1) has values as the core of any human organization. The set of values is reflected in the philosophy that defines the purpose for which the organization was established and the reason for its existence. Goals may be viewed as articulated values or operational statements of the organization's values. The next layer of the model depicts the structure, which consists of the systems needed to carry out the goals. The climate component of the model is "the psychological atmosphere that results from and surrounds the operation of the structure; consequently, it is both a result of and a determinant of the behavior of individuals and groups within the structure" (Jones, 1981, p. 160). The outermost ring of the model depicts the many aspects of the external environment, or milieu, with which an organization must interact to accomplish its goals.

For the purpose of analyzing and designing an internal environment for nursing practice, the health organization-environment model (Figure 6.2) is presented. This model arbitrarily separates the internal environment into tangible and intangible aspects. Both types of aspects are viewed as having structure, process, and outcome components, which are primarily used in models for quality assurance.

In a quality assurance model, the structure components are the human, physical, and financial resources needed to provide care. Structure includes the number, distribution, and qualifications of personnel, as well as the equipment, the physical facility, and the organizational structure of the health care facility. The process components involve the activities of health care providers in their management of patients. Outcomes are the end results of care for the patient (Donabedian, 1969).

In the model for the health organization-environment, the process and outcome components are not the same as those of a quality assurance model. The process components in the environment are those activities carried out to implement the goals and objectives of the organization, for example, patient care conferences, decision-

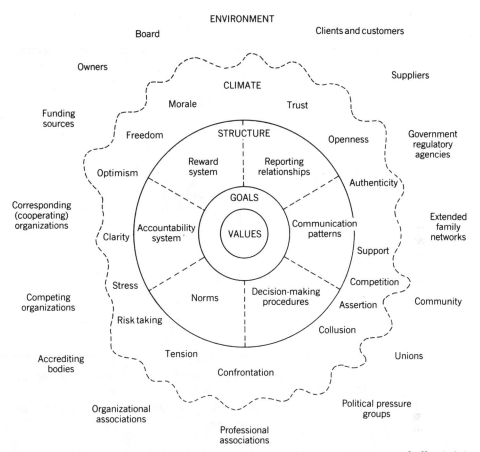

Figure 6.1 The organizational universe. (From J. E. Jones, & J. W. Pfieffer (eds.). (1981). *The 1981 Annual Handbook for Group Facilitators* (p. 162). San Diego: University Associates. Used by permission.)

making procedures, and communication procedures. The outcome components are the aspects of the environment that result from the processes, for example, staff satisfaction, staff turnover, and achievement of objectives.

In quality assurance, structure, process, and outcome are interrelated, but the relationships are not clear, especially the direct relationships of specific processes to specific patient outcomes (Given, Given, & Simoni, 1979). Donabedian (1980) classifies structure and outcome as indirectly related to assessing the quality of care. He states that structure can indicate only general tendencies. As a measure of the quality of care, structure is limited also because of insufficient knowledge about the relationships between structure and performance. Donabedian maintains that the use of outcome is likewise an indirect approach for assessing quality: "When changes in health status are observed, there must not only be a prior basis for assuming a possible relationship to

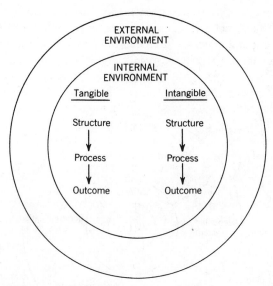

Figure 6.2 Health organization-environment model.

antecedent care; further ascertainment is also often needed, at least to show the absence of other factors that might explain the findings, preferably together with the presence of the kind of care that can explain them" (Donabedian, 1980, p. 83).

Similar arguments can be raised about the relationship of structure, process, and outcome components in the internal environment as a basis for nursing practice. Many unanswered questions exist about the relationships between, for example, a specific organizational structure and outcomes in terms of efficiency, effectiveness, staff satisfaction, and numerous other variables. Given these complexities, the nurse executive is responsible for and faced with the challenges of leading the nursing department and thus maintaining or developing the environment in which nursing is practiced. Before the use of the health organization-environment model is discussed, some of the elements required for the nurse executive to create the environment for nursing practice are considered.

The Authority of the Nurse Executive

Basic to beginning the process of creating the environment for nursing practice is the nurse executive's authority to institute changes within the department of nursing. The concept of authority, as part of the organizational structure, is the expectation that someone should exert control and direction over others (Dalton, Barnes, & Zaleznik, 1968). Although the nurse executive may possess both professional and positional authority, such authority will, no doubt, have limits. However, the limits of the authority may not become an issue until a conflict arises. Many conflicts arise when changes in the nursing department result in required changes in other departments. For example, when the staff nurse position is changed to exclude certain housekeeping tasks, the housekeeping department or unit management must incorporate these tasks. In such situations, interdepartmental conflict may be minimized with thoughtful planning and effective interdepartmental communication.

To institute change, the nurse executive requires at least three key elements: administrative support, budgetary control, and authority to approve nursing practice components. In all nursing practice settings, other aspects of authority and support are also important, for example, support of the nursing staff and authority to make personnel changes. The support of the medical staff may play a crucial role in some areas where changes affect the functioning of or interaction with physicians, for instance, the type of documentation used for nursing care.

Administrative support should not be interpreted to mean that the agency or institution administrator agrees with all decisions made by the nurse executive. The nurse executive does, however, require administrative backing for well-planned projects that are pivotal for creating the environment for nursing. For example, the organizational structure of the nursing department is one of the most important components of an environment that promotes and supports professional nursing practice. If the nurse executive does not have both the authority and administrative support to implement, within approved resources, the organizational structure, her authority to implement the other environmental components may certainly be very limited.

A second important element for the nurse executive is budgetary control. Basically, this means that the nursing department is allocated a budget and the nurse executive is responsible for specific allocation approval and monitoring expenditures. This range of authority allows the nurse executive to make many personnel changes as well as to initiate new programs within budgetary allocations.

The third element important for the nurse executive is the authority to approve nursing practice components, such as standards, policies, job descriptions, and performance evaluation mechanisms. This authority is closely related to that for making changes in general but is much more crucial to the actual practice of nursing. The lack of nursing control in this area may mean that the nurse executive position is ineffective or merely a figurehead for the real source of control in medicine or the institutional administration.

If a key element of authority is lacking or unclear, the nurse executive should begin the environment development process with discussion and clarification of these issues. When contemplating a change of position, the nurse executive is in a better situation to negotiate for specific authority. However, experience and the development of administrative skills also contribute greatly to a favorable outcome for the nurse executive in requesting and obtaining authority for creating the environment for nursing practice.

USING THE ENVIRONMENT MODEL

To use the health organization-environment model, the nurse executive must begin with an assessment of the current situation, including data collection and the identification of problems. Because an assessment of every component of the environment is not practical, the process should begin with those aspects of the department that are considered priorities, and the other aspects should be incorporated into the long-term plan for the nursing department.

How does the nurse executive know which components are priorities? Several approaches may be used to identify priorities:

- Survey of the nursing staff
- Survey of the nursing staff and selected others in the organization
- Study conducted by an in-house committee or individual
- Study conducted by an outside consultant
- Combination of approaches

Attempts to study or survey broadly for all possible components results in frustration in the typical institution. However, a well-designed study of a few key areas could result in a valid basis for recommendations for creating the environment for nursing practice. A beginning point for looking at the current environment could be the assessment of the formal systems of the organizational structure: reporting relationships, communication patterns, decision-making procedures, norms, accountability system, and reward system (Jones, 1981). The area or areas that appear to be troublesome should be assessed in more depth, but a few key questions to the staff about each area could be included in a survey.

The environment model provides a systematic approach to environment development as well as to a study or series of studies of the nursing department (see Figure 6.2). Table 6.1 depicts some of the structure, process, and outcome components of the internal organization environment and provides a compilation of the major items defined in this chapter as part of the environment for nursing practice. Components have been arbitrarily placed in a category, but they may be arranged differently without harming the concept.

TABLE 6.1 Internal Environment Components

Structure Components	Process Components	Outcome Components
Department organizational structure	Patient care documentation system	Staff satisfaction
Philosophy statement	Nursing care plans or nursing orders	Acceptable staff turnover rate
Policies		Achievement of objectives
Procedures (nursing practice guidelines)	Patient care criteria and standards	Achievement of patient care criteria and standards
Nursing assignment patterns	Management objectives and work plans	Staff morale
Staff numbers and mix	Decision-making patterns	Trust
Job descriptions	Clinical judgments	Support
Qualifications of all nursing staff		Tension
Performance criteria		Level of stress
Compensation system that reflects qualifications, responsibilities, and clinical competence		Openness
		Degree of risk taking

Several of the components are explained in depth in other chapters, and the reader should refer to those sources for definitions, conceptual frameworks, and discussion. For purposes of example, a component from each category is discussed briefly here.

As structure components, nursing policies provide guidelines for the staff. Policies should free the nursing staff from the burden of making routine, decisions, while not restraining the practice of professional nursing. Because policies reflect the philosophy and mission of the nursing department, they are a reflection, in turn, of the organization goals and mission (Alexander, 1978). In creating an environment conducive to nursing practice, policies should be congruent with statements such as the American Nurses Association (ANA) Code for Nurses, the ANA Standards of Nursing Practice, the state nursing practice act, the ANA Standards for Nursing Services, standards of accrediting bodies, and requirements of regulatory agencies (American Nurses' Association, 1979). Precisely what policies should be developed and how they should be stated are decisions to be made by appropriate nursing staff with nursing administrative approval.

Nursing care plans are process components that provide for continuity of nursing care and constitute one mechanism of professional accountability. Care plans should be written so as to become a permanent part of patients' records. The contents should be individualized for each patient, even if standardized nursing care plans are used for some patient populations. Among other characteristics, a system for planning patients' care should aim for economical use of the nurse's time, be readily accessible to all staff, incorporate standards of care, and emphasize nursing care. In addition, the staffing of the supportive environment should be sufficient to allow enough time for care planning.

An example of an outcome component of the environment model is staff satisfaction. Although many variables affect satisfaction, several of these variables for nurses are within the nursing department and may be influenced by the nurse executive. The National Commission on Nursing cited evidence to support this: "Although they are accountable for nursing care, nurses at all levels often have insufficient decision-making authority in management of patient care and in other areas of the environment in which nurses practice." Furthermore, staff nurses reported that the nursing administrator's position and influence in the institution were important factors in their job satisfaction (National Commission on Nursing, 1981, p. 9).

FISCAL IMPLICATIONS

The nurse executive must always be mindful of the costs associated with any change. Frequently, fiscal constraints more or less dictate the form and content of such environmental components as the nursing assignment pattern. As nursing services have implemented primary nursing, for example, obtaining the initial budget for a larger registered nurse staff has been delayed or has resulted in implementation by phasing in various units.

Fiscal constraints may totally prevent the implementation of some aspect considered critical for nursing practice. Although a carefully prepared plan will not eliminate the fiscal problems, they may be minimized if planning is done on a long-term basis. In addition, alternative methods for arriving at the same outcome should be considered in the planning process. Fiscal planning is not easy to accomplish, because the nurse executive frequently must find methods of expressing quality factors in quantitative terms (Alexander, 1978). Chapter 13, on fiscal management, offers some assistance with this administrative responsibility.

Summary

The internal environment of a health care organization consists of the conditions and characteristics within the organization. The health organization-environment model is one approach the nurse executive can use in assessing, planning, and implementing the environment in which nurses will practice. According to this model, the internal environment is composed of tangible and intangible elements. The categories of structure, process, and outcome can be used to classify the components of an organization. The authority to make changes, control the budget, and approve nursing practice components is necessary for the effective performance of a nurse executive undertaking the establishment of an environment for nursing practice.

STUDY QUESTIONS

1. What do you consider the two most important structure, process, and outcome components in the nursing practice environment?

2. What are some other components that could be added to each list?

3. Develop a model other than the health organization-environment model that could be used for assessing and planning the environment for nursing practice.

References

Alexander, E. L. (1978). *Nursing administration in the hospital health care system* (2nd ed.). St. Louis: Mosby.

American Nurses Association (1979). Characteristics of a professional climate of administration and practice in a nursing department. In *Roles, Responsibilities and Qualifications of Nurse Administrators.* Kansas City, MO: Author.

Culprit in shortage is misuse of RNs, says commission, *American Journal of Nursing, 81*(2), 264, 274.

Dalton, G. W., Barnes, L. B., & Zaleznik, A. (1968). *The distribution of authority in formal organizations.* Boston: Harvard University Division of Research, Graduate School of Business Administration.

Donabedian, A. (1969). *A guide to medical care administration* (vol. 2). *Medical care appraisal: Quality and utilization.* New York: American Public Health Association.

Donabedian, A. (1980). *The definition of quality and approaches to its assessment* (vol. 1). Ann Arbor, MI: Health Administration Press.

Given, B., Given, C. W., & Simoni, L. E. (1979). Relationships of process of care to patient outcomes, *Nursing Research, 28*(2), 85–93.

Hall, R. H. (1977). *Organizations: Structure and process* (2nd ed.). Englewood Cliffs, NJ: Prentice-Hall.

Jones, J. E. (1981). The organizational universe. In J. E. Jones & J. W. Pfeiffer (Eds.). *The 1981 Annual Handbook for Group Facilitators*. San Diego: University Associates.

McMahon, J. T., Ivancevich, J. M., & Matteson, M. T. (1977). A comparative analysis of the relationship between organizational climate and job satisfaction of medical technologies, *American Journal of Medical Technology, 43*(1), 15–19.

National Commission on Nursing. (1981). *Initial report and preliminary recommendations.* Chicago: Hospital Research and Educational Trust.

Three new studies seek reasons for RN shortage. (1981). *American Journal of Nursing, 81*(2), 264, 273, 292.

Wandelt, M. A., Pierce, P. M., & Widdowson, R. R. (1981). Why nurses leave nursing and what can be done about it, *American Journal of Nursing, 81*(1), 72–77.

CHAPTER 7

Blending Clinical Practice with Organizational Design

Highlights

- **Organizational design and context for practice**
- **Nature of committees**
- **Span of control**
- **Authority relationships**
- **Models of organizational structures**

Scientific and technological advances have significantly influenced the pattern of delivery of health care services. The majority of these health services are delivered within an organizational environment. Health care organizations orchestrate human and technological resources to create an environment in which care delivery can occur.

The focus of this chapter is to analyze various patterns of relationships associated with design or structure of health care organizations as they relate to the context for nursing administrative practice. It further identifies concepts that apply to analyzing, developing, or restructuring a nursing department or division. As selected designs of organizations are identified, it will become evident that, for a health care organization, a structure—the formal relationships among individuals in various positions—combines a set of variables involving technology, tasks, and human resources that will enable the organization to accomplish its purpose, mission, and goals. Nurse executives and other health care professionals must be knowledgeable about organization design. They must be able to recognize the most appropriate organizational design, the criteria for its selection, and how the organizational structure influences the behavior of individuals and groups.

FIT BETWEEN ORGANIZATIONAL DESIGN AND CONTEXT FOR PRACTICE

Organizations are composed of people performing tasks within formal or informal organizational networks. Whenever individuals join in a common effort, organizations should be employed to obtain effective and productive results. The interrelated conditions in which professional nursing administrative practice occurs, comprise the organization design of nursing divisions. The goal of organizational design is to identify the specific structures and processes that best accommodate the types of individuals and nature of the work to be performed in a given organization.

Leatt, Shortell, and Kimberly (1988) state that when a new organization is formed a new design will be created. This is an ongoing process where the design needs will change as the organization changes. Ideas about the appropriate design should be derived from the organization's mission and strategic plan.

Organizational design is the way in which authority, responsibility and information networks are blended within an organization. Organizational elements can be designed to include departments or division into sections or units, determination of the number of management levels, locus of decision making, accessibility of information, and the physical facility.

Mintzberg (1981) asserts that "a great many problems in organizational design stem from the assumption that organizations are all alike: mere collections of component parts to which elements of structure can be added and deleted at will, a sort of organizational bazaar" (p. 103). Whereas, the opposite assumption is that effective organizations achieve coherence among their component parts; that is, one part cannot be changed without considering the consequences to all the others. To design effective organizations, managers need to determine the most effective structure for the set of units that constitutes the organization as a whole.

PURPOSE AND PHILOSOPHY

An essential step in determining the appropriate organizational structure is understanding the purpose, philosophy, goals, and objectives of the organization, which should be congruent with the parent organization's mission. It is important to design a structure that is congruent with the institution's purpose and philosophy. It is also important to know the major organizational product(s).

The philosophy within a nursing division is made up of the beliefs and values that directly influence the professional practice of nursing within the health care setting.

The philosophy should incorporate the theory of nursing that is reflected in the practice of nursing. The basic purposes of the nursing division are to provide meaningful work environments and quality nursing care to the client. The process of developing or redesigning purpose, philosophy, and objectives in the nursing division should be reflective of the overall institution's purpose and philosophy statements. Because most nursing divisions have written statements of philosophy and purpose, the task is usually to redesign them rather than to develop original statements.

A philosophy may be evaluated for usefulness and thoroughness using various criteria. The following criteria are suggested for general applicability:

1. Reference is made to the purpose of the nursing service.
2. Terminology can be understood by nurses, clients, and others.
3. The philosophy is concise.
4. Statements of beliefs and values are included.

The purpose of the division of nursing is its reason for existing. The philosophy of the division of nursing is developed as a statement of the values and beliefs that underlie the way in which the purpose is achieved. Cantor (1973) states that "thoughtfully prepared statements of purpose, philosophy, and objectives based on reality, understood and used by those responsible for implementation, can promote efficiency and effectiveness in the operation of institutions, departments, and programs. Statements lacking these qualities are merely collections of words" (p. 25).

SHARED GOVERNANCE

An innovative approach to implementing philosophy, purpose, and goal statements that provides structure and accountability for nursing practice is to design an organizational model that may be supported by a framework of bylaws. These bylaws should incorporate elements such as the name, purpose, and mission of the organization, nursing staff membership, appointments to staff, nursing council structure, and the organization and coordination of clinical services. Bylaws are used to operationalize professional nursing practice models such as shared governance.

Poster-O'Grady (1986) indicates that shared governance models are not participatory management models. They are an accountability-based governance system for professional employees. Authority, control, and autonomy occur in the organization based on specifically defined areas of accountability that arise according to need and location for best expression. All issues related to practice are dealt with by the practitioner, with the manager having no legitimate role in that specified clinical decisional framework. It is important to note that the manager's role is to facilitate, integrate, and coordinate the system and resources required for its maintenance and growth.

Structure is devised from the center of the shared governance work environment rather than from the hierarchical periphery. Authority is established in specified processes rather than in individuals. Porter-O'Grady states "from these functions and placements of accountability, the professional organization takes form. In nursing, the major service components generally involve practice, quality, education, peer process, or governance. Within these five functional characteristics, most operational processes unfold" (p. 283). Therefore, the goal of a shared governance model is to determine the base of accountability for each of the major components and to devise appropriate structures.

NATURE OF COMMITTEES

Within nursing divisions or departments, there are usually formal or informal mechanisms for allocating functions. To accomplish customary functions, nursing organizations often create committees. Functions are identified, and a structure of committees is evolved to fulfill these functions. Committees are a necessary and integral part of organizational life. It is important to emphasize that committees must arise out of a need and be established for a specific purpose. The function and nature of the committee should be stated in the bylaws or rules of the organization.

Some examples of committee purposes in a division of nursing are to revise policies and procedures, to make recommendations about improving the quality of nursing care, and to formulate new projects or programs. Some committees engage in managerial functions such as developing or revising policies and procedures. Certain committees are vested with the authority to make decisions, whereas others make recommendations but do not have the authority to implement decisions.

A committee may be designated as having either line or staff authority. If the authority vested in the committee involves decision making affecting subordinates responsible to it or organizational policies, it is a plural executive — a line committee. If its authority relationship to the nurse executive or chief executive officer is advisory, then it is a staff committee.

Committees are also classified as formal or informal. Formal committees, which are part of the organizational structure, with designated functions and responsibilities, are usually referred to as standing committees. Informal committees are organized without specific delegation of authority. The purpose of informal committees may vary; for example, they may be organized for group discussion or for problem solving on a particular issue.

Committees that are established for a specific purpose and for a specified time period are called ad hoc committees. When the committee's work is completed, it is disbanded. Task forces are also formed to accomplish a particular purpose; thus, the term "task force" is often used instead of committee. A task force may be a work group of standing committees or a separate group that is given a specific work assignment.

Because professionals need to participate in the decision-making process, health care administrators should design a committee structure that allows such participation. Some administrators do this reluctantly. Leavitt and Lipman-Blumen (1980) view such reluctance as part of a direct management style. They imply that the direct types of people tend to do it themselves, organize and compete to win regardless of what the "it" happens to be. These administrators often see committees as a necessary evil. That is, they believe that committees exist to keep people content but that they are burdensome and unproductive. Administrators who use a direct management style insist that most of the work done by committees could be accomplished more efficiently by top management, provided that the organizational climate permits this.

Other administrators value committees because they feel that shared decision making cannot be achieved through a direct, authoritative approach. Leavitt and Lipman-Blumen (1980) refer to this as a relational management style. Administrators who use a relational style tend to help, support, and back up other people — often getting enjoyment from contributing to the success of others or from a sense of belonging. In contrast to the direct management style administrators, these relational style individuals envision committee work as a valuable end in itself because through it, people learn to work with each other, come to understand the challenges of the organization, and complement one another's creativity in making the enterprise as effective as possible.

The cost of committee meetings in relation to time is usually very significant. Several variables that affect committee outcomes are length of meetings due to excessive deliberation, travel time required by members, and cost of personnel time in terms of salaries. It is essential that when a decision is made to form a committee, consideration should be given as to whether a group decision is necessary or whether an individual decision would be as appropriate. The question arises as to whether the benefits of a committee are worth its cost, especially, when the emphasis in many organizations is on cost containment. Often these benefits, such as increased morale and satisfaction or the experience of teamwork, are difficult to measure. Committees do function effectively when costs are justified, authority for decision-making responsibility is defined, the scope of the subject matter is considered, members are representative of the interests they serve, and sufficient resources are allocated.

ORGANIZATIONAL STRUCTURE

Structure enables the organization to achieve its purposes, goals, and objectives. Organizations have activities that must be performed. The grouping together of activities and responsibilities of a specialized nature through a formalized mechanism is a widely accepted management practice. This type of structure is founded on the functional basis of departmentalization. For example, in a hospital, nurses are generally placed within the nursing division and pharmacists within the pharmacy division. Organizational structure is more than a group of boxes or lines on an organizational chart or table; it delineates the formal relationships of individuals in the various positions within an organization. An organizational chart is a graphic representation of the departmentalization process that shows the functional and reporting relationships and depicts the downward flow of authority and responsibility and the upward flow of accountability.

The organizational chart serves useful purposes such as orienting new staff and depicting formal relationships within the division of nursing and other departments. In a visual sense, the chart maps the entire operation of the organization. It is necessary to reevaluate and update organizational charts frequently to reflect changes in the enterprise.

These organizational charts have several limitations. The executive-level position on the chart is not synonymous with high status within the organization. Status is affected by factors other than position that include the authority, power, and influence vested in the position. For example, the vice president of nursing may be on the same level as other division heads, even though he or she may have more functions and responsibilities for influencing the budget than do the others.

When one analyzes an organization, it is important to examine the various systems that exist to get the task accomplished to maintain the organization. One must also consider the processes or procedures that have been developed to coordinate the work to be done. To conceptualize how the organization functions, it is imperative that one know the recruitment practices, the method of selecting individuals for positions, the reporting relationships, and the informational network.

SPAN OF CONTROL

The number of subordinates who report directly and are supervised by any one manager is referred to as the span of control of management. There is a limit to the number of individuals a manager can supervise that is dependent on the impact of several underlying factors. Koontz and Weihrich (1990) identify the following factors that influence the number and frequency of contacts the manager has with subordinates and therefore affects the span of control: *(1)* the better the training of subordinates, the less required of their manager's time and also less contact with them is necessary; *(2)* clarity of delegation authority—identifying the work tasks and clearly defining authority enables the subordinate to perform the task with a minimum of the manager's time and attention; *(3)* clarity of plans provides a framework of operations to guide the subordinates, which necessitates fewer contacts with managers; *(4)* use of objective standards enables the manager to delegate in confidence and reduce unnecessary control-centered relationships; *(5)* rate of change refers to stability in policies so that subordinates have guides to thinking and do not have to appeal for policy decisions and direction; *(6)* communication techniques—ability to communicate plans and directions clearly and concisely tends to increase a manager's span; *(7)* amount of personal contact needed—allowance is given for cases where the subject matter demands personal contact; *(8)* variation by organization level is that the size of the most effective span varies by organizational level; *(9)* other factors include *(a)* managerial competence: a competent manager can effectively supervise more people than one who does not have these attributes; and *(b)* complexity of task: simple tasks may allow for a wider span than tasks that are more complex.

As reflected in an organizational chart, a wide span of control usually has two to four levels and is referred to as a flat, or horizontal, organizational structure. A narrow span of control has many levels and is referred to as a tall structure.

AUTHORITY RELATIONSHIPS

Concepts of line and staff authority are frequently ill defined, referring to functions or authority relationships. Early classical administrative writers made a distinction between line and staff authority. They defined managers with line authority as exercising direct responsibility for accomplishing organizational objectives with staff authority as supporting the line in the achievement of those objectives. However, the difficulty of separating these two concepts in modern complex organizations makes this distinction obsolete. The empirical data regarding the proper use of staff are often confusing. As long as organizations continue to use line and staff authority, conflict seems inevitable.

Line and Staff Authority

The concept of line authority is clear when it is designated that a superior exercises direct control over a subordinate; such a structure consists of a direct vertical relationship and reflects the Fayol scalar principle. This principle is applicable to this concept in that the clearer the line of authority from the executive-level management position to the subordinate position, the responsibility for decision making and communication will be more effective (See chapter 3). Line functions are those that have direct impact on the achievement of the organization's objectives.

Staff authority is advisory and does not entail the authority to enact policy decisions. Staff personnel assist line officers in implementing their managerial activities. An important distinction is that line and staff are differentiated by their authority relationships, not by departmental functions. Thus, personnel activities at X Home Health Care Agency may be considered staff, whereas at Home Health Care Agency Y, placement of personnel may be a line function. In a staff relationship, the clinical nurse specialist (CNS) or advanced nurse practitioner has responsibilities and functions that are advisory. This individual is not in a command position; the line superior makes decisions and issues directives that are developed in consultation with the CNS or advanced nurse practitioner.

Functional Authority

Functional authority is the right delegated to an individual or department to control specified practices, processes, or policies within an organization outside one's own areas of command. Functional authority is a type of formal authority that enables specialists in a given set of activities (i.e., finance or personnel) to enforce directives within a clearly defined scope of authority. This authority can be regarded as a small section, or piece, of the authority of the line superior. For example, the personnel director in hospital X may give staff ratio advice to the assistant vice president for nursing (staff authority), supervise his or her own personnel (line authority), and determine specific personnel procedures for the management staff with his or her own specialist authority (functional authority).

Functional authority can be dysfunctional within an organization. It may cause overlapping relationships and increase the possibility of conflict between departments. However, Robbins (1980) emphasizes that in large organizations "such authority can increase efficiency, because of specialization of skills and also improved coordination when those responsible for a particular activity have commensurate authority to ensure its attainment" (p. 228).

Chain of Command

Figure 7.1 shows the organizational chart of the division of nursing within a large community hospital. It indicates authority relationships by identifying the chains of command, which are the supervisor-subordinate relationships starting at the top level of the organization. The chain of command establishes an authority hierarchy in

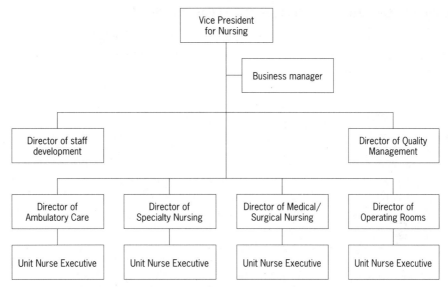

Figure 7.1 Division of nursing organizational chart.

which formal communication evolves along this chain. (The chain, as illustrated in Figure 7.1, is senior nurse executive——middle level executive——unit nurse executive.)

Delegation of Authority

The delegation process involves responsibility, authority, and accountability. This process is vital to an organization because it enables superiors to pass authority downward to subordinate managers, giving them certain rights as well as prescribing limits within which they must operate. Administrative personnel are authorized to make certain decisions and to direct the staff under their jurisdiction. They are also accountable for the results. When an activity is delegated to subordinates, the supervisory personnel retain responsibility for it. Subordinates are responsible to the individual who delegated the task to them. Therefore, delegation includes assigning an activity to subordinates, granting them the authority necessary for it to be fulfilled, and acceptance by subordinates of responsibility and accountability for satisfactory performance of the activity.

An interesting question arises as to whether responsibility can be delegated. Classical administrative theorists note that because the delegator is held responsible for the action of the delegatees, responsibility cannot be delegated. Robbins (1980) recognizes two forms of responsibility: operating and ultimate responsibilities. Administrators give out operating responsibility but retain ultimate responsibility. Robbins states that an administrator is ultimately responsible for the actions of subordinates to whom he or she has given operating responsibility. It is imperative that the administrator delegate operating responsibility equal to the delegated authority. Ultimate responsibility can never be delegated.

MODELS OF ORGANIZATIONAL STRUCTURES

The concepts of centralization and decentralization are related to delegation of authority. The degree of delegation of responsibility, power, and authority to the lower levels in an organization is used to classify the organization as centralized or decentralized.

Decentralized Organizational Structure

Decentralization reflects a particular philosophy of organization and management. In a decentralized structure, decision making, responsibility, authority, and accountability are incorporated at the operational, or practitioner, level of the organization. The concept of decentralization emphasizes the importance of human relationships within an enterprise. It requires careful selection of which decisions will be made at the operational level and which will be decided at the executive level. Decentralization entails granting subordinates authority to make decisions, determining which decisions will be made at the operational level, and enacting policies to guide decision making. Dale (1952) formulated some objective criteria that can be useful in determining the extent of decentralization. He implies that the degree of decentralization is greater when:

1. More decisions are made lower down the management hierarchy.
2. More important decisions are made lower down the management hierarchy.
3. More functions affected by decisions are made at lower levels.
4. Less checking is required on decisions. (p. 118)

In a decentralized nursing service, professional nurse practitioners participate in the management of services to their patients/clients and in decisions that affect their nursing practice. The decisions are usually made by individuals with the clinical expertise to provide quality nursing care. In this structure, managers at the first and middle levels are involved in decisions regarding the implementation of programs, because staff are more knowledgeable than upper level managers about the details of day-to-day operations and are able to implement those decisions. This expanded responsibility has encouraged the development of self-managed teams. Self-managed teams are also referred to as cross-functional teams, high performance or super teams (Dumaine, 1990). These self-managed teams perform functions such as determining schedules, hiring and firing authority, ordering supplies and equipment, and developing productivity and quality standards.

At the operational level, nurse managers have greater authority than in a centralized structure and are held accountable for operations at this level. Their participation in the decision-making process provides a high degree of congruence with organizational goals and objectives.

Decentralization generally increases motivation and satisfaction of staff at the middle- and first-management levels. The advantages of decentralization are job enrichment because there is more effective utilization of managerial skills, greater potential for innovation and creativity in fulfilling the responsibilities of the position, more autonomy encouraged in decision making, and an increase in overall satisfaction.

Limitations of decentralization are based on such contingency factors as the size of the organization. Size is a critical determinant of decentralization. An organization may not be large enough to warrant decentralization, as it may not be feasible or cost effective to have autonomous units within the agency. Senior executive-level administrators may not desire decentralization, because they may not want to relinquish authority to subordinates who do not have the managerial abilities and motivations to make effective decisions. Division managers may identify with one unit to the point of developing favoritism toward it; this may result in competition among units to the extent that is detrimental to the overall objectives of the enterprise. In addition, fragmentation may occur due to problems of control and nonuniform policies.

Centralized Organizational Structure

Centralization implies a tightly controlled communication network, uniformity of policy and action in decision making, identification of power and authority with position, and controlling authority over financial resources, planning, and the mandating of changes of direction or programs for the organization. It is usually advantageous to centralize those activities or functions within an enterprise that interacts with the overall environment. For example, financial, governmental, and labor relations activities are often centralized to standardize procedures to maintain continuity within the organization.

The disadvantages of centralization are due to the investiture of decision-making authority at the executive level, which often results in the delay of implementation at the operational, or practitioner, level. Innovative thinking and creativity tends to be stifled, and changes imposed from the top often become subverted and do not get implemented.

Matrix Organization

Matrix management has become increasingly popular in recent years. Matrix organizations were initially developed in the aerospace industry, where the focus was on products and markets as well as on technology.

The matrix organization superimposes a project or program management directly over a functional, hierarchical organizational structure. This allows for maintenance of the day-to-day operations and implementation of new projects or programs within an enterprise. The single most characteristic element of the matrix organization is a dual authority, or chain of command, in that both the heads of the functional areas and the project (product-line) managers have authority over those working in the matrix unit. Within this dual authority structure, responsibilities are assigned to functional departments oriented toward specialized resources.

Three critical management roles are distinguishable in a matrix structure: the top leader; the matrix bosses, or managers, who share subordinates; and the two-boss managers. Lawrence, Kolodny, and Davis (1977) state that the matrix approach requires a strong, unified command at the top executive level to ensure a balance of power at the next level. The role of the top executive involves three unique aspects: power balancing, managing the decision, and standard setting.

First, the top executive has authority over, or controls, both of the organization's command structures: administrative and technical. The existence of dual pressures requires balanced decision making that considers both structures to establish and sustain a reasonable balance of power between the two sectors. The second aspect of the role relates to the necessary condition for an effective matrix; that is, a very high volume of information must be processed and focused for use in making key decisions. This requires that authority and responsibility for decision making be shared. Third, the top executive sets the standards of performance. This aspect is vital to the allocation of financial and human resources. Unless the top executive has high expectations for the organization, it is unlikely that the matrix organization will respond to the environmental pressure for resource deployment.

The matrix manager holds a middle management position and shares many of the decisions such as tasks, assignments, and performance evaluations with product-line, business, or other functional managers. In contrast to the situation in a traditional pyramidal organization, no individual manager in a matrix organization is autonomous or controls his or her own destiny. Rather, each manager has unit objectives that are partially determined by the resource demands of projects and businesses.

The most challenging aspect of the matrix organization is the often-conflicting demands of the two-boss managers. Conflicts may arise between the demands of the manager's functional position and those of the project team. Such conflicts emanate from multiple demands from above and beyond a manager's immediate command. The manager must heed the competing demands, make trade-offs, and manage the conflicts that cannot be resolved. Such situations can create anxiety and stress from above, but it is important to emphasize that two-boss managers must also be responsible for their subordinates. This role need not be shared. Any skillful politician knows that alternative sources of power increase one's flexibility, which is the key to successful performance as a two-boss manager.

Matrix organizations are a challenge to manage. Because personnel in the matrix have two bosses, conflicts within the system are inevitable. To cope with such conflicts, managers must develop a high level of interpersonal skills and a willingness to take risks. They must rely on their own personal qualities and the ability to persuade through their own knowledge and expertise.

Hospitals have been classified as matrix organizations because of their hierarchical coordination through departmentalization and their formal chain of command and horizontal coordination across departments through patient care teams. Each team has a leader and members representing technical, social, and service departments. In the nursing model, the professional nurse, a nurse manager, is responsible for coordinating patient care. Johnson and Tingey (1976) emphasize that the structure of the patient care teams should not be confused with the more traditional structure of nursing teams. In the traditional structure, the team is composed of aides, orderlies, and other related personnel who report administratively to the nurse manager. In the matrix structure, the team includes personnel from other departments, and the team members do not report to the nurse administratively, the nurse's function is primarily coordination and communication rather than direct supervision. An example of a nursing matrix model is depicted in Figure 7.2.

NURSING MATRIX MODEL

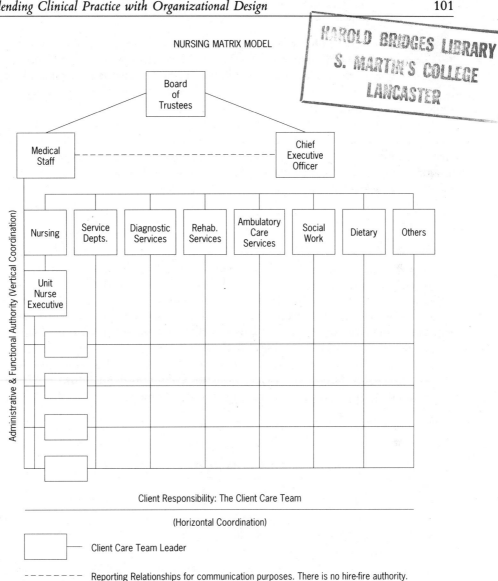

Figure 7.2 Nursing matrix model. (From Johnson, G., & S. Tingey. (1979). Matrix organization: Blueprint of nursing care organization for the 80s. *Hospital & Health Services Administration, 21*(1), p. 33. Adapted by permission.)

Bartlett and Ghoshal (1990) stress that most successful organizations are those whose top executives recognize the need to manage the new environmental and competitive demands by emphasizing less on the quest for an ideal structure and more on developing the abilities and performance of individual managers. One senior executive stated "The challenge is not so much to build a matrix structure as it is to create a matrix in the minds of our managers." Bartlett and Ghoshal emphasize that "developing a matrix of flexible perspectives and relationships within each manager's mind, however, achieves an entirely different result. It lets individuals make the judgments and negotiate the trade-offs that drive the organization toward a shared strategic objective" (p. 145).

Because the matrix organization focuses on a specific product line or products, it is able to generate information and mobilize resources needed to respond quickly to changes. The matrix structure should be implemented when an organization has unique problems in a market area or requires increased specialization associated with the technological requirements of the environment.

Summary

Organizational design facilitates the accomplishment of the work of nursing and structure accommodates the types of individuals and nature of the work to be performed within a given system. The organizational structure should be designed to be congruent with the institution's philosophy, purpose, goals, and objectives. To ensure such congruity, the executive must understand the types of authority relationships and the models of organizational structure that best apply to the enterprise. Nurse executives must be knowledgeable about organizational designs and their effect on human behavior.

THOUGHT PROVOKING QUESTIONS

1. Why is it important that nurse executives be knowledgeable about the organizational design process?
2. Why are philosophy, purpose, and objectives necessary for a division of nursing?
3. Describe the concept of shared governance.
4. Describe the factors to be considered when planning for and implementing a committee structure within a division of nursing.
5. What problems exist in relation to the traditional line, staff, and functional authority relationships?
6. Illustrate in a chart the distinguishing characteristics such as the nature of decision making, communication patterns, and delegation of authority of the centralized, decentralized, and matrix structures.

References

Bartlett, C., & Ghosal, S. (1990). Matrix management: Not a structure, a frame of mind, *Harvard Business Review, 68*(4), 138–145.

Cantor, M. (1973). Philosophy, purpose and objectives: Why do we have them? *Journal of Nursing Administration, 3*(4), 21–25.

Dale, E. (1952). *Planning and developing the company organization structure.* Research Report 20, New York: American Management Association.

Dumain, D. (1990). Who needs a boss? *Fortune, 121*(10), 52–60.

Johnson, G., & Tingey, S. (1976). Matrix organization: Blueprint of nursing care organization for the 80s, *Hospitals & Health Services Administration, 21*(1), 27–39.

Koontz, H., & Weihrich, H. (1990). *Essentials of management* (5th ed.). New York: McGraw-Hill.

Lawrence, P., Kolodny, H., & Davis, S. (1977). The human side of matrix, *Organizational Dynamics, 6*(1), 43–61.

Leatt, P., Shortell, S., & Kimberly, J. (1988). Organization design. In S. Shortell, A. Kaluzny et al. (Eds.). *Health Care Management: A Text in Organization Theory and Behavior* (2nd ed.). Albany, NY: Delmar Publishers Inc.

Leavitt, H., & Lipman-Blumen, J. (1980). A case for the rational manager. *Organizational Dynamics, 9*(1), 27–41.

Mintzberg, H. (1981). Organization design: Fashion or fit? *Harvard Business Review, 59*(1), 103–116.

Porter-O'Grady, T. (1986). Shared governance and new organizational models, *Nursing Economics, 5*(6), 281–286.

Robbins, S. (1980). *The administrative process* (2nd ed.). Englewood Cliffs, NJ: Prentice-Hall.

CHAPTER 8

Receptivity To Innovation

Highlights

- **Change and innovation theories and models**
- **Participatory action research**
- **Stages of change**
- **Strategies for change**
- **Resistance to change**

Innovation is often perceived as threatening because it usually is accompanied by change while individuals tend to seek stability within their internal or external environment. The field of nursing administration is continually undergoing change. Changes in the health care delivery system, in science and technology, and in government regulations have made a significant impact on the practice of professional nursing administrative practice. Nurse executives at every level within the organization must facilitate receptivity to change and innovation. In addition, they are often responsible for planning, initiating, and implementing innovation within a division of nursing by converting new ideas or thoughts into action. Change and innovation are closely related concepts. In our society, change is inevitable and innovation is a necessary component of our culture.

Drucker (1985) indicates that innovations may spring from a "flash of genius." However, most innovations, especially the successful ones, result from a conscious, purposeful search for innovation opportunities that are found in only a few situations. He suggests that every organization needs strategies for innovation. These include *(1)* Be the firstest with the mostest. Be first in the market and be first to improve a product or cut its price or both, which discourages prospective competitors; *(2)* Be the second with the mostest strategy. Let someone else establish the market. Be able to satisfy markets with narrow needs and specific capabilities. Provide excellent products for narrow market segments, that is, big purchases with narrow needs. Offer few features; *(3)* Use the niche strategy. Locate a finite market and establish yourself so that it is not worthwhile for others to enter because the market cannot be expanded; *(4)* Make the product your carrier. Develope one product to carry another. An example would be computer software programs that can only be used with a certain brand of computer.

Pearson (1988) also asserts that successful innovations require the following key components: "*(1)* a champion who believes that the new idea is really critical and who will keep pushing ahead, no matter what the roadblocks; *(2)* a sponsor who is high up enough in the organization to marshal its resources — people, money, and time; *(3)* a mix of bright, creative minds (to get ideas) and experienced operators (to keep things practical); *(4)* a process that moves ideas through the system quickly so that they get top-level endorsement, resources, and perspective early in the game — not in the bottom of the ninth inning" (p. 101).

Nurse executives at all organizational levels must be committed and personally involved in the processes of change and innovation. Leaders and members of successful organizations generally set demanding goals for themselves, are more innovative, take more risks, and change at a more accelerated rate. Change has a dominant role within any organizational enterprise. The survival of health care organizations within our society is largely dependent on their responding appropriately to the forces of change. These forces include such things as science and technological innovations, the knowledge explosion, and social changes. Managing change is a critical element of the nurse executive role. Nurse executives need and use their skills in orchestrating change. Therefore, they must be knowledgeable about the theoretical basis of the change process, understand the reasons for resistance to change, and pursue opportunities for innovation.

CHANGE AND INNOVATION THEORIES AND MODELS

Lewin's Force Field Theory

One of the major influences in the early development of change theory was Kurt Lewin (1951), a social scientist. He managed situations where tensions and conflicts were evident by focusing on the cooperative humane element within the situations and by devising ways of managing and improving them. He was a founder of the group dynamics movement; he established the first organization devoted to research on group dynamics in 1945.

Lewin described the phenomenon of force field theory as a state in which equilibrium is maintained in an organization by the existence of both *driving* and *restraining* forces. Organizations may be experiencing equilibrium with forces pushing for change, while at the same time, there are forces resisting change to maintain the status quo. For change to occur, the driving forces increase as a result in some movement. These driving forces tend to facilitate change because they push individuals in the desired direction. However, this alteration may also increase resistance by adding strength to the restraining forces. An effective approach might be to reduce or eliminate the restraining forces, thus reaching a new level of equilibrium.

Lewin described changing as a three-step process by *(1)* unfreezing the existing equilibrium or present level. It is in this stage that motivation for change occurs. The group must first make a diagnosis of the problem. Active participation in the identification of the problem and generation of alternate solutions helps to modify attitudes; *(2)* change itself. The emphasis is on moving to a new level of equilibrium in which participants agree that the status quo is not gratifying to them. The actual change or moving requires that new responses be developed based on collected information; *(3)* refreezing or stabilizing the change. The involved individual(s) in this stage integrate new concepts into their own value system that are congruent with the individual's existing self-concept and values. Reinforcement of the new behavior is essential to a successful implementation of the change.

Planned change theory can be envisioned from various perspectives that have their foundations in the Lewinian approach. Changes that are conscious, deliberate, and intended, at least on the part of one or more agents of change, are planned changes. The process of planned change involves a change agent, a client system, and a collaboration to resolve the clients' problems.

Lippitt's Theory

Lippitt (1973) expanded Lewin's theory to a seven-phase planned-change model. His focus was on what the change agent must do, rather than on the evolution of the change. However, he did emphasize the importance of participation of members of the target system. Problem identification, communication, and rapport building are key aspects of the change process. The phases of the model include:

1. Diagnosis of the problem. This is an important step. Involve key individuals in data collection, analysis, and problem identification.

2. Assessment of the motivation and capacity to change. The success of any change program is based on accurate assessment of the potential for change in individuals, groups, and the environment. Awareness of the need to change must be translated into a desire to change and also requires a readiness and capacity to change. Assess factors such as the availability of resources (human, financial, and physical), organizational climate, structure and function of the organization, timeliness, and the credibility of those initiating the change.

3. Assessment of the change agent's motivation and resources. It is important that the initiator of change clearly assess his or her role in a particular situation. The change agent may be external or internal to the client system. Whether to have an external or internal change agent is dependent on the identified problem and the environmental conditions in which the change occurs. The external change agent must have credentials and expertise and must gain acceptance with the client system. The internal change agent can usually determine the organizational climate, readiness of the participants to change, and the power bases of key individuals in the organization. A combination of both an external and internal change agent may also be effective.

4. Selection of progressive change objectives. Formulate an action plan, strategies for the change, and establish criteria for evaluation with key individuals participating. The change is usually implemented for a trial period, evaluated, and modified.

5. Identification of the appropriate role(s) for the change agent. The change agent can act as an expert, consultant, facilitator, coordinator, leader, or a combination of these roles. It is important that whichever role(s) is (are) designated, the participants involved understand the expected outcomes.

6. Maintenance of the change. Emphasis on this phase is on the communication process with continuous feedback on progress to all those involved in the change process.

7. Termination of the helping relationship. The change agent gradually withdraws from the situation, allowing the client system to maintain or operationalize the change.

There are limitations to the planned change approach to organizational change. For example, how effective or realistic is the planned change model in today's complex, changing environment? Because health care organizations deal with a high degree of uncertainty, is it realistic to assume that change is conscious, deliberate, and intended as depicted in the planned change model? Can individuals change their behavior if they do not anticipate that this change will give direction and meaning to their work within the organization?

Nurse executives who manage innovative organizations must condition themselves to look for change and innovative opportunities within their organization. They must search for clues on ways to change without disruption. Change must be seen as a challenge, not a threat. Drucker (1990) emphasizes that one should refocus and change the organization when one is successful. Put your efforts into successes, improve the area of success, and change them. He stresses that innovative organizations systematically look both outside and inside for clues to innovative opportunities.

Another way of examining innovation is to focus on personal characteristics of the individuals involved. Rogers (1983) reviewed studies and used summative techniques to identify personality and demographic characteristics associated with innovativeness. The following discussion illustrates his diffusion of innovation theory.

Rogers' Diffusion of Innovation Theory

Rogers envisioned the change process as having antecedents that included both the background of individuals involved in the change and the environment where the change occurred. His five-phase innovation-decision model is a mental process that describes *(1)* how an individual (or other decision-making unit) passes from first knowledge of an innovation, *(2)* forming an attitude toward it, *(3)* making a decision to adopt or reject it, *(4)* implementing the new idea, and, *(5)* confirming the decision (p. 20). He emphasizes the reversible nature of change because participants may initially adopt a proposal or at a later date *discontinue* it; whereas, the reverse may occur, that is, initially reject the proposal but adopt it at a later date.

Rogers conceptualizes the following five-step process to the diffusion of innovation:

1. Knowledge occurs when the individual (or other decision-making unit) is exposed to the innovation and begins to understand how it functions.

2. Persuasion occurs when the individual (or other decision-making unit) forms a favorable (or unfavorable) attitude toward the innovation.

3. Decision occurs when the individual (or other decision-making unit) participates in activities that lead to a choice to adopt or reject the innovation.

4. Implementation occurs when the individual (or other decision-making unit) operationalizes the innovation and reinvention or alterations may occur.

5. Confirmation occurs when the individual (or other decision-making unit) seeks reinforcement that the decision was correct. If there are conflicting messages about the innovation, the original decision may be reversed.

Rogers emphasizes that two important components to a successful change process are that key individuals and policymakers must not only be interested in the innovation but committed to making it happen.

Tornatzky, Eveland, and Fleischer (1990) assert that individual characteristics of innovators do seem to make some difference. In any given setting in which innovation-related activities occur, the personal attributes of participants may be equal to or more important than the group or organizational factors. They state that "no matter what pains are taken to provide the right decision-making processes or reward system, and no matter how pressing and persuasive the external economic environment is, if rigid and timid people are employed in jobs that are key to fostering an innovation process, it will likely fail" (p. 35). However, they note that the best and brightest people do not guarantee success. In many cases, the promise of desirable individual characteristics of participants may be "smothered" by organizational or environmental context.

There are also limits to the use of individual characteristics in relation to making a difference in innovating systems. Certain individual characteristics such as sex or personality tend to be difficult to change. The authors state that the only practical way to use this information is through the selection of participants, which is difficult to do, because we usually have a workforce to start with and rarely have freedom to select at will.

Organization Development Model

A contemporary approach to the management of change and the development of human resources in organizations has become known as organization development (OD). Davis and Newstrom (1985) emphasize that OD is an intervention strategy that uses group process to analyze the characteristics and features of the organization to focus on change. French and Bell (1978) assert that OD is a long-range effort to improve an organization's problem-solving and renewal process, particularly through participation in collaborative decision making. They stress that special emphasis must be directed toward the culture of the formal work teams by a change agent, or catalyst, and the use of the theory and technology of applied behavior science, including action research, are essential to the process.

OD is an intervention strategy that uses the group process to achieve planned change by concentrating on the organization's culture. It is based on the assumption that change involves a systematic diagnosis of the total organization, the development of a strategic plan for improvement, and the mobilization of resources to carry out the effort. Changing beliefs, attitudes, values, and structures will be necessary for the organization to grow as well as to survive.

There were two major reasons that OD became an important tool in organizations. First, the reward structure on the job did not provide adequate reinforcement for conventional training programs and it often failed to carry over in the job (Ehrenberg, 1983). Second, technological advances and the acceleration of change requires flexibility in organizations. OD can encourage the organization to foster and respond to change by opening channels of communication, increasing the amount and accuracy of information, and building trust and rapport through a process of group problem solving at all levels of the organization.

In OD, the emphasis is on the total system and the creation of a climate that fosters learning, creativity, and innovation opportunities that permeate the total enterprise. Change agents, either internal or external, function to stimulate and coordinate change within the group. The experiential learning techniques used include training, role playing, problem solving, discussion groups, and lectures. It is important to note that with regard to the methodologies used, emphasis is placed on gaining competence in dealing with interpersonal relationships. Goals often are concerned with developing skills in areas such as communication processes and decision making. The value system includes an integration of individual needs and management goals, enhanced learning opportunities, and encouragement of more open human relationships.

Davis and Newstrom (1985) describe an action research approach used in OD:

- Initial diagnosis. A decision by management to use and support OD is followed by selection of a change agent or consultant. This individual meets with top management to outline a process to examine the nature of the organization's problems and, subsequently, to develop the series of OD approaches.

- Data collection. Surveys or interviews may be undertaken to determine organizational climate and existing and potential managerial problems. The consultant usually meets with specified work groups within the organization to develop information. Questions to be addressed include: What conditions contribute to or interfere with your job effectiveness? What would you most like to change in the way you function in the organization? What would you most like to change in the way the organization functions?

- Data feedback and confrontation. Small groups are selected to analyze the data collected. Areas of disagreement are mediated and priorities for change established.

- Action planning and problem solving. Groups use the data analysis and report to develop specific recommendations for change. The discussion focuses on issues in their department, group, or activity. Plans are specific, including specifying who is responsible, and deadlines for completion of action taken.

- Team building. During the entire period of group meetings, the consultant encourages the groups to examine how they work together. The consultant helps them to value open communication and trust as prerequisites for improved group functioning. Team building may be encouraged further by having individual managers and their subordinates work together as a team in OD sessions.
- Intergroup development. After development of small-group teams, there may be development among larger groups comprising several teams from all levels of the organization.
- Evaluation and follow-up. The consultant helps the organization evaluate the result of the OD efforts and develops additional programs in areas where additional results are needed.

OD appears to be a beneficial organizational intervention. Its focus is on a behavioral approach to problem solving within the total organization. OD is time consuming and costly. Factors such as invasion of privacy and psychological harm must be considered in some of the methods used. The potential for contribution for redesigning work groups to yield productive teams is critical to a successful OD approach.

PARTICIPATORY ACTION RESEARCH

Participatory action research provides a legitimate model for creating a learning environment that focuses on maximizing the individual's potential. Brown (1985) believes that using people-centered development and participatory research is a means for maximizing human resource development. Participatory action research asks adults to be interdependent participants and co-learners rather than dependent and researcher controlled. The researchers learn skills for general problem solving such as managing meetings, collecting information, organizing work, or planning activities. The control of learning in participatory action research can seldom be predicted or planned in detail across projects and is participant-learner dependent rather than researcher-teacher controlled. It is a way to promote people-centered development in various systems that encourage local empowerment (Simms, 1991). This is especially appropriate for nurse executives at all levels as they seek to transform nursing work environments and redesign work groups and organizational downsizing, especially in relation to reduction in the workforce.

Examples of successful-action research studies have been described in the labor and occupational studies literature. Kornbluh, Pipan, and Schurman (1987) have reported positive findings on empowerment learning and control in workplaces in industry. Israel, Schurman, and House (1989) have a highly credible record in involving workers as researchers and using action research methods in their study of occupation stress.

ORGANIZATIONAL BEHAVIOR MODEL

Organizational behavior emphasizes the nature of individuals and organizations. It is the study of how individuals perform within an organization. The key elements include individuals, structure, technology, and the environment in which the enterprise operates. The role of management is to provide a climate in which organizations function effectively. A major tenet of the organizational behavior approach is understanding of both individual and group behavior. Understanding of this behavior is a complex process. Nadler and Tushman (1980) stress that organizational behavior must be managed in spite of this complexity. Ultimately, the organization's work is accomplished through people, individually or collectively, on their own or in collaboration with technology. They believe that the management of organizational behavior is central to the management task. This task involves the capacity to *understand* the behavior of individuals, groups, and organizations to *predict* what behavioral responses will be elicited by managerial actions and, finally, to use this understanding and these predictions to achieve control.

Nadler and Tushman have developed a congruence model of organizational behavior that reflects the basic systems concepts and characteristics (see chapter 3). This model specifies four critical inputs: *(1)* the environment of all factors outside the organization being examined including such areas as markets, suppliers, governmental and regulatory bodies, labor unions, and competitors; *(2)* organization's resources referred to as a range of different assets to which it has access—employees, technology, capital, and information. One concerns the relative quality of those resources or value in light of the environment; *(3)* the organization's history is important because there is growing evidence that the way organizations function today is influenced by past events; and *(4)* a fourth derivative input, strategy, including the issue of matching the organization's resources to its environment or making the fundamental decision of "What business are we in?" Strategy is a critical input because it determines the work to be performed by the organization and it defines desired organizational outputs.

The major outputs are what the organization produces, how it performs, and how effective it is. One needs not only to be concerned about system's basic output—the product—but to think about other outputs that contribute to organizational performance. When evaluating organizational performance three factors to consider are *(1)* goal attainment, or how well the organization meets its objectives; *(2)* resource utilization, or how well the organization makes use of available resources; and *(3)* adaptability, or whether the organization continues to have a favorable position vis-a-vis its environment. In other words, whether it is capable of changing and adapting to its environmental changes.

The last element is the transformation process. Given an environment, a set of resources, and history, the question is "How do I take a strategy and implement it to produce effective performance in the organization, in the group/unit, and among individual employees?" Their model is based on how well components fit together, that is, the congruence among the components; the effectiveness of this model is based on the quality of these "fits" or congruence. These component parts are the fundamental means for transforming energy and information from inputs into outputs.

As depicted in the Nadler-Tushman transformation model, organizations are composed of the following four major components:

1. **Task** is the basic or inherent work to be done by the organization and its subunits or the activity the organization is engaged in. Emphasis is on the specific work activities or function that need to be done and their inherent

characteristics. For example, analysis of the task would include a description of the basic work flow and function (knowledge or skills demanded by the work, kinds of rewards provided by the work). It is assumed that the reason for the organization's existence is to perform the work (task) consistent with strategy.

2. Individuals who perform organizational tasks. Identify the nature and characteristics of the organization's members (individual skills and knowledge, different needs or preferences that individuals have, perceptions or expectancies that they develop, other background factors that may influence individual behavior).

3. Formal organizational arrangements. These include the structures, methods, procedures that are explicitly and formally developed so that individuals will perform tasks consistent with organizational strategy. This activity encompasses a number of factors, including the way jobs are grouped together in units, internal structure of those units, and the coordination and control mechanisms used to link the units together. Other factors to consider are job descriptions, and the work environment which characterizes the immediate environment where work is done, and the organization's formal systems for attracting, placing, developing, and evaluating human resources.

4. Informal organization. Informal arrangements are usually implicit and unwritten but may influence behavior as they include the structures, processes, and arrangements that emerge from within the organization. These adaptations may either aid or hinder the organization's performance. (pp. 43–45) (See Figure 8.1.)

The steps in the problem-analysis process of the model are *(1)* to identify symptoms and list data indicating possible existence of problems; and *(2)* to specify inputs by identifying the system and determine the nature of its environment, resources, and history. Identify critical aspects of strategy. Then, identify outputs by indicating data that define the nature of outputs at various levels (individual, group/unit, organizational). This specification should include desired outputs (from strategy) and actual outputs being obtained.

Problems are then identified by indicating areas where there are significant and meaningful differences between desired and actual outputs. To the extent possible, identify penalties; that is, specific costs (actual and opportunity costs) associated with each problem. The basic components of the organization are described in relation to the basic nature of each of the four components with emphasis on their critical factors.

Assess congruence (fits). Conduct analyses to determine relative congruence among organizational components. Generate, identify, and analyze causes to fit with specific problems. Identify action steps and indicate the possible actions to deal with problem causes.

This congruence model and the problem-analysis process are tools for structuring and dealing with the reality of the complexities of organizational life. It must be noted that there is no one best way of handling a particular situation. Nadler and Tushman emphasize that the model and process could assist the manager in making a number of decisions and evaluating the consequences of them.

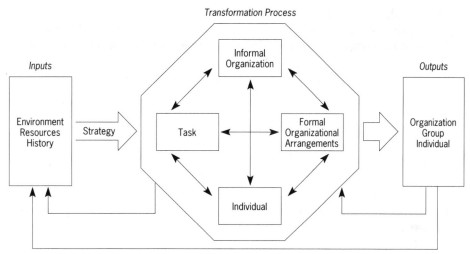

Transformation Process

Inputs

Informal
Organization

Outputs

Environment
Resources
History

Strategy

Task

Formal
Organizational
Arrangements

Organization
Group
Individual

Individual

Feedback

Figure 8.1 A congruence model for organizational analysis. From Nadler, D., & M. Tushman. (1980). A model for diagnosing organizational behavior. Reprinted, by permission of the publisher, from *Organizational Dynamics, 9*(4), p. 47 (Autumn 1980 © 1980). American Management Association, New York. All rights reserved.)

THE 10 STAGES OF CHANGE

Perlman and Takacs (1990) imply that organizations rarely deal consciously or constructively with the human emotions associated with organizational change. Yet, these are the resources and energy from within individuals that are necessary to help accomplish change. They emphasize that to cope with and work through the changes that affect the organization, members must deal with the emotional processes of letting the past die and of experiencing depression. The model presented by Kuebler-Ross in her book, *On Death and Dying*, is useful in dealing with a major aspect of change: grief. Although she deals with death and dying on an individual level, the stages she presents are compatible with those encountered in organizational change. Perlman and Takacs added five phases to Kuebler-Ross's original five to more fully explain the problems associated with change.

The purpose of the model is to enable practitioners to face some of the more personal and emotional issues that change produces, and to offer tools that will assist them in making conscious choices about dealing with change in the organization.

Phase Equilibrium

1. High energy level. State of emotional and intellectual balance. Professional and personal goals are in harmony.
   Intervention: Inform employees of any change in the environment that will have impact on status quo.

2. Denial. Energy is drained by the defense mechanism of rationalizing or denying of the reality of the change. Employees experience negative changes in physical health, emotional balance, logical thinking patterns, and normal behavior patterns.

   Intervention: Employ active listening skills; for example, be emphatic, use reflective listening techniques. Focus on impact of the change.

3. Anger. Energy used to ward off and actively resist the change by blaming others. Frustration, anger become visible.

   Intervention: Recognize symptoms, legitimize employee feelings, focus on positive aspects of change.

   Active listening, problem-solving skills needed by managers.

4. Bargaining. Energy used in an attempt to eliminate the change. Talk is about "if only." Others try to mediate the problem. Bargains can compromise the needed change.

   Intervention: Explore ways of achieving desired changes through conflict management techniques.

5. Chaos. Diffused energy, feeling of powerlessness, sense of insecurity.

   Intervention: Quiet time for reflection and listening. Recognition of being in state of flux.

6. Depression. No energy left to produce results. Self-pity, remembering past, expressions of sorrow, and feeling nothingness and emptiness.

   Intervention: Provide necessary information in a timely fashion. Allow sorrow and pain to be expressed openly.

7. Resignation. Energy expended in passively accepting change. Lack of enthusiasm.

   Intervention: Hold employees accountable for their own behavior, but allow them to move at their own pace.

8. Openness. Availability of renewed energy. Willingness to expend energy on what has been assigned to individual.

   Intervention: Patiently explain again in detail the desired change.

9. Readiness. Willingness to expend energy in exploring new events. Reunification of intellect and emotions begins.

   Intervention: Assume directive management style: assign tasks, monitor; provide direction/guide.

10. Reemergence. Rechanneled energy produces feelings of empowerment, employees become more proactive.

    Intervention: Mutual answering of questions; mutual understanding of role and identity. Employees will take action based on their own decisions.

The generators of change and recipients of change in an organization must work through the various stages to deal effectively with the emotional dimensions of change. If those involved work through the intellectual and emotional issues in each phase, Perlman and Takas indicate that the organization and its employees will become stronger and the change is more likely to be successful and lead to success.

STRATEGIES FOR CHANGE

Chinn and Benne (1976) propose a three-way classification of the strategies of change. *Empirical-rational* strategies of change are based on the assumptions that humans are guided by reason and follow their rational self-interest once it is disclosed to them. A change is proposed by some person or group that knows of a desirable solution. It is assumed that the individual or group will adopt the proposed change if it can be rationally justified and if it can be demonstrated that the individual or group will gain by the change.

The basic tenet of this strategy is that trust in the scientific method is the predominant motivator by which to change human behavior. Change agents using this model will use research methods to scientifically study the organization to determine the need for change, how it should be carried out, and whether the change, once initiated, has improved the effectiveness of the organization.

Elements of empirical-rational strategies include such areas as recruitment and retention. For example, personnel selection and replacement: there may be an incongruence between the people occupying positions and the job responsibilities. Improving performance requires the development of scientific testing of potentialities and attitudes. Use of applied research and linkage systems for diffusion of research results is another element in this model.

The objective of the *normative reeducative* strategies of change is to improve the problem-solving capabilities of a system. A problem-solving process must impact on both the human problems of the organization as well as the system's task requirements set by its goals of production and distribution. Problem-solving processes must be developed to deal with sociotechnical difficulties by converting them into identifiable problems and organizing the relevant processes of data collection, planning, intervention, testing of solutions, evaluation, feedback to results, and replanning. All of these processes are required in the solution of a problem. Intervention by outside agents is used extensively in implementing this approach to change.

The assumption of this model is focused on human motivation; individuals are motivated primarily by unsatisfied needs. Employees do not passively wait for an administrator to suggest changes. They are in the pursuit of realizing their potential and will initiate changes on their own, if possible.

The person is the basic unit of the social organization. Intervention methods are designed to assist people to discover themselves as "persons" and achieve commitment to continuing personal growth in their interrelationships. People must learn from their experiences if self-directed change is to be maintained and continued. The elements of normative-educative strategies imply that the emphasis is on the client system and involvement in programs of change and improvement. The role of the change agent is to implement the change by intervening mutually and collaboratively with the client system.

Power-coercive change strategies approaches to effecting change are based on the assumption that power is part of all social interaction. The differences among social interactions lie in the sources of power on which the strategies of change depend and the ways in which power is generated and applied in the processes of effecting change. The application of power results in a state wherein those with greater power alter the behaviors of those who have less power. The ingredients of power that power-coercive strategies use are the political and economic sanctions in the exercise of power. Political power carries with it legitimacy and the sanctions associated with those who break the law. Economic power exerts coercive influence over the decisions of individuals to whom it is applied.

The objective of power-coercive strategies of change is to increase political and economic power for the goals that the strategists of change have determined to be desirable. The elements of this model focus on the use of nonviolent strategies for indicating value conflicts and specifying the inequities in existing patterns. Sit-ins and other types of nonviolent demonstrations are also used. Political power is essential to achieving changes in institutional life; normative reeducative strategies must be combined with political coercion before and after the political action so that the public is adequately informed and accepts the changes in practice.

Beer, Eisenstate, and Spector (1990) state in a provocative article that although senior managers understand the necessity of change to cope with new competitive realities, they often underestimate what it takes to bring it about. They tend to assume that promulgating company-wide programs that include mission statements, "corporate culture" programs, training courses, quality circle programs, and new pay-for-performance systems will transform organizations and change employee behavior. In their study of organizational change at six large corporations, they found the opposite to be true: the major obstacle to revitalization is the idea that it comes about through company-wide change programs, especially when a corporate staff group such as human resources is the sponsor. They believe successful change efforts focus on the work itself, that is, by aligning employee roles, responsibilities, and relationships to address the organization's most important competitive task, or "task alignment." It is their belief that any approach to change starting at the periphery and moving steadily toward the corporate core is the most effective way to achieve enduring organizational change. Managing change involves process over specific content, recognizes organization as a unit-by-unit learning process rather than a series of programs, and acknowledges the payoffs that result from persistence over a long period of time are superior to quick fixes.

This change strategy could be applicable to health care organizations because of the need to make changes in providing programs that address issues in cost containment and involve consumers in their choice of health care options.

RESISTANCE TO CHANGE

A significant aspect of the change process involves an alteration in the status quo. Often when any change is proposed, resistance may surface. Organizational change efforts frequently encounter human resistance. Nurse executives must assess those individuals in the organization who are likely to resist the change initiative and attempt to ascertain their reasons for resisting. Individuals or groups can react very differently to change — from being apathetic to it, to aggressively opposing it, or to quickly adopting it, or sabotaging it. Nurse executives need to be aware of the most common reasons people resist organizational change. Kotter and Schlesinger (1979) present the following reasons:

- People think they will lose something of value because they focus on their own best interests and not those of the total organization.
- People misunderstand the change and its implications, and they perceive that it is likely to cost them more than they will gain.
- People assess the situation differently from those initiating the change and believe that greater costs than benefits will result from the change for themselves as well as for the organization.
- People have low tolerance for the change because they fear they will not be able to develop the new skills and behavior that are required of them.

Resistance to change may be caused by errors on the part of the change agent or consultant who may not communicate trust or may not understand the nature of the advocated change and its relevance to the client system. Resistance should be viewed constructively by change agents.

Rubin, Plovnick, and Fry (1974) point out that by resisting change, whether actively or passively, an organization is communicating a message—it is providing data. In a very real sense, an organization is telling us something about "who it is"—its major resources and limitations, its attitude toward outsiders and change, its important internal norms and values, and the nature of its relationship to other systems in the environment.

Zaltman and Pinson (cited in Zaltman and Duncan [1977]), state that resistance is not simply lack of acceptance or the reverse of acceptance of a proposed change. It may reflect clients' attitudes toward innovation itself. For example, when an innovation is incompatible with a particular norm, it may be accepted by one person as a symbol of defiance and rejected by another who fears social disapproval. An innovation may be a source of attraction to visionaries and a source of resistance to more conservative clients.

One of the most important sources of resistance to change is the perception that the change will be a threat to the power or influence of various parts of the organization. When two or more organizations merge, a difficult problem to overcome is the feeling on the part of the individual organizations that they are going to lose, or have diminished control, over decision making. Change should be presented in a way that minimizes the degree to which it is perceived as threatening. Members of the merged organizations must be informed about the need and consequences of the change. They must be active participants in the change process. Nurse executives and unit nurse managers need to assist their staff in accepting change by providing necessary information, emotional support, and an educational environment for upgrading skills.

The structure and climate within an organization can effect resistance to change. Individuals should be able to experience a need for change, accept the reality of change, and be committed to it. Finally, there must be a potential for change in the system and some control or influence over the anticipated change.

Summary

Receptivity to innovation can be envisioned from various perspectives. Innovation can be a flash of genius or changes that are conscious, deliberate, and intended — at least on the part of one or more agents of change. Lewin's theory of change involves three stages of change which are referred to as unfreezing, moving and refreezing. Lippitt expanded Lewin's theory to a seven-phase change-process model. Rogers model focuses on the innovation-decision process.

Proponents of an organizational behavior model believe that it is the management of organizational behavior that is central to the management task. Organizational development (OD) on the other hand, is an intervention strategy that uses group processes in an attempt to modify and/or change beliefs, attitudes, values, and structures for the organization to adapt and survive in our changing society. The participatory action research model is a way to promote people-centered development in systems that encourage local empowerment.

For change to succeed in an organization, whether through planned change, OD, the application of organizational behavior models, or by participatory action research, the individuals must be supportive of or agreeable to the change. Significant components of the nurse executive role include continually pursuing sources of opportunities for innovation and being a facilitator in providing a learning environment that enhances the change process. Organizations must constantly search for ways to innovate and change to survive in today's competitive marketplace.

References

Beer, M., Eisenstat, R., & Spector, B. (1990). Why change programs don't produce change, *Harvard Business Review, 68*(6), 158–166.

Brown, L. (1985). People-centered development and participatory research, *Harvard Education Review, 55*(1), 69–75.

Chin, R., & Benne, K. (1976). General strategies for effecting changes in human systems. In W. Bennis, K. Beene, & K. Corey (Eds.). *The Planning of Change* (3rd ed.) (pp. 22–45). New York: Holt, Rhinehart & Winston.

Davis, K., & Newstrom, J. (1985). *Human behavior at work: Organization behavior.* New York: McGraw-Hill.

Drucker, P. F. (1985). The discipline of innovation, *Harvard Business Review, 43*(3), 67–72.

Drucker, P. F. (1990). *Managing the nonprofit organization.* New York: Harper Collins.

Ehrenberg, L. (1983). How to ensure better transfer of learning, *Training and Development Journal, 2,* 81–83.

French, W., & Bell, C. (1978). *Organizational development* (2nd ed.). Englewood Cliffs, NJ: Prentice-Hall.

Israel, B., Schurman, S., & House, J. (1989). Action research on occupational stress: Involving workers as researchers, *International Journal of Health Services, 19,* 135–155.

Kornbluh, H., Pipan, R., & Schurman, S. (1987). Empowerment learning and control in workplaces: A curricular view, *Zeitschrift Fur Sozialisationsforschung Und Erziehungssoziologie (SZE) J. Jahrgang/Heft, 7*(4), 253–268.

Kotter, J., & Schlesinger, L. (1979). Choosing strategies for change, *Harvard Business Review, 57*(2), 106–114.

Kuebler-Ross, E. (1969). *On death and dying.* New York: MacMillan.

Lewin, K. (1951). *Field theory in social science: Selected theoretical papers.* New York: Harper & Brothers.

Lippitt, G. (1973). *Visualizing change: Model building and the change process.* Fairfax, VA: NTL Learning Resources Corporation, Inc.

Nadler, D., & Tushman, M. (1980). A model for diagnosing organizational behavior, *Organizational Dynamics, 9*(4), 35–51.

Pearson, A. (1988). Tough-minded ways to get innovative, *Harvard Business Review, 67*(3), 99–106.

Perlman, D., & Takas, G. (1990). The 10 stages of change, *Nursing Management, 21*(4), 33–38.

Rogers, M. (1983). *Diffusion of innovations* (3rd ed.). New York: The Free Press.

Rubin, I., Plovnick, M., & Fry, R. (1974). Initiating planned change in health care systems, *Journal of Applied Behavioral Science, 10*(1), 107–124.

Simms, L. (1991). The professional practice of nursing administration: Integrated nursing practice, *Journal of Nursing Administration, 21*(5), 37–46.

Tornatzky, L., Eveland, J., & Fleischer, M. (1990). Technological innovation as a process. In L. Tarnatzky & M. Fleischer (Eds.). *The processes of Technological Innovation* (pp. 27–50). Lexington, KY: Lexington Books.

Zaltman, G., & Duncan, R. (1977). *Strategies for planned change.* New York: Wiley.

CHAPTER 9

Organizational Culture

Harriet V. E. Coeling

Highlights

- **Definitions of organizational culture**
- **Corporate and subgroup cultures**
- **Sources of organizational culture**
- **Value of understanding organizational culture**
- **Changing organizational culture**
- **Ethics related to organizational culture**

The past decade has witnessed the sudden and widespread popularity of a concept called organizational culture. The purpose of this chapter is to present the concept of culture and its importance in nursing administration practice. The concept of culture, developed by the discipline of anthropology, was embraced by both management theorists and organizational practitioners in the 1980s (Smircich & Calás, 1987). Nurse executives today are increasingly concerned with the culture of their organizations. Several conditions in the late 1970s contributed to this interest in organizational culture.

One condition was the shift in thinking in the human sciences. For many decades positivistic science had predominated scientific fields (Smircich & Calás, 1987). An important goal of positivist science was control. It was believed that the process of positivistic science, involving construct validity and the measurement of dependent variables, would lead to findings that could be generalized. Scientists who used these processes were considered superior to scientists who sought understanding by looking at the creation of meaning within an organization and who did not seek generalizations.

In the late 1970s, however, management theorists began to value understanding, in addition to control, as a goal of management research. They began to study organizational culture in an attempt to understand what was happening as people interacted together within an organization. This new path of inquiry allowed them to ask radically different questions about the environments in which people worked. It allowed management theorists to study some of the more expressive aspects of organizational life. Part of this desire to find new ways to study organizations was a response to the realization that previous studies focusing on the measurement of variables in organizations had yielded few definitive findings (Starbuck, 1982). This shift in the goal of research has also occurred in the study of nursing management.

Another factor contributing to the study of organizational culture was the economic success of industry in Japan, along with increased foreign competition in steel, electronics, and other markets that the United States and Europe had dominated for years. The realization that other cultures did things differently, yet very successfully, prompted an openness to new ways of thinking and doing things among those who manage organizations. The loss of market share to other countries and the recent turbulence and instability of the U.S. economy, in which traditional management practices no longer seem to produce their usual results, prompted managers to grasp any concept that promised help. Organizational culture offered such help. As a concept, organizational culture can be studied at the corporate level, where it is referred to as corporate culture, or at the department or unit level, where it is called work group culture (Reimann & Wiener, 1988).

PERSPECTIVES ON ORGANIZATIONAL CULTURE

Because the study of organizational culture has been advanced by three different traditions, namely, anthropologists, management theorists, and organizational practitioners, the organizational culture literature represents diverse and often conflicting recommendations. It is important for nurse executives to recognize the basic assumptions from which recommended management strategies are derived. Sackmann (1989) provides a comparison of these three traditions, or sets of assumptions, which reflect different goals and offer different rewards.

The goal of the cultural anthropologist is to understand a group's behavior. Because anthropologists are interested in understanding human variation, their goal is to describe unique situations, rather than to establish universal laws. The product of such research is a description of a cultural pattern that enables the manager to better recognize how the group works. Anthropologists do not see culture as power, nor do they see culture as causing behavior; rather, culture is the situation in which behavior occurs.

The goal of the organizational theorist is to revitalize organizational theory and develop a better conceptualization of organizational life. This research, which increases our understanding of all organizational participants, facilitates the prediction of both worker and manager responses.

The goal of the organizational practitioner or manager is to guide and control what goes on in organizations. The practitioner desires to find managerial formulas for success. The practitioner seeks to "master" the organization to make it function more effectively. Managing culture is seen as a powerful activity that enhances organizational effectiveness and financial success. It should be noted, however, that this effectiveness is defined by those who hold power. It is effectiveness as seen from management's perspective, not necessarily the worker's perspective.

Each perspective has its limitations for the nurse executive. The weakness of the anthropologist's approach is that it is limited to describing. Mere descriptions of group behavior are generally not associated with increased corporate profitability or a better style of organizational life.

The theorist has somewhat the same weakness as that of the anthropologist. By using an understanding of culture to predict behavior, however, the theorist can guide the nurse executive by predicting what outcomes might flow from certain interventions. The theorist, however, recognizes that multiple factors play a role in any organizational outcome and makes no promises of success if a certain strategy is used.

The culture controlling perspective, which seeks to identify the excellent culture, is intuitively appealing to the nurse executive because it offers strategies for success through the effective exercise of cultural levers. However, it has several potential pitfalls that the nurse executive would do well to recognize (Sackmann, 1989). First, this perspective advocates cultural-value engineering where administrators hold the power to prescribe certain values the employee must accept. Not all of today's nurses may want to give this power to their employers; nor is giving such power necessarily consistent with nursing practice excellence. Clinical leaders thrive more in a supportive environment than in a controlling environment. Second, it is questionable whether human behavior can be controlled to the extent that all nurses can be made to accept certain values and to follow a given set of rigid organizational rules. Culture, based on survival strategy, is not easily manipulated. Enduring change must be based either on the organization's survival behaviors and the policies that give these behaviors form or on a changing environment that requires new strategies for survival (Taft, 1988a, 1988b). Third, research has not yet proved what is the "best" culture for a health care organization. Finally, the assumption often associated with this perspective, namely, that a "good" culture is stable and homogeneous, is problematic in that such a culture has a negative effect on innovation and adaptation and robs the practitioner of some degree of autonomy and creativity.

Sackmann (1989) notes that when the concept of culture is used by anthropologists, management theorists, or organizational practitioners, they are usually not aware of their different interests and expectations. Each group uses culture to meet its own needs. Although practitioners attempt to use culture to support managerial control, the discipline of anthropology warns against attempts to control a culture. Today, the efforts of the theorist and the practitioner seem to be merging. Barley, Meyer, and Gash (1988) note the movement is in the direction of the practitioner and suggest this is occurring because both theorists and practitioners are responding to an environment of declining productivity and competitiveness. Yet, it remains important for nurse executives to differentiate the goal of understanding a culture from the goal of controlling the culture. Schein (1985) highlights these differences by disputing any inevitable link between culture and effectiveness and encourages practitioners to be more cautious about management's ability to manipulate culture. Nurse executives can profit from his advice.

DEFINITIONS OF ORGANIZATIONAL CULTURE

Considering the variety of perspectives that address the concept of organizational culture, it is not surprising that there is an even greater variety of definitions of organizational culture. Anthropologists define culture broadly to include knowledge, beliefs, artifacts, values, and customs. This broad definition is reflected in descriptions of organizational culture as "the way we do things around here" (Deal & Kennedy, 1982). However, more specific definitions of organizational culture are also common in the literature.

One approach is cognitive in nature. It focuses on what goes on inside of people. It focuses on the values (basic assumptions about what is desirable to do) and beliefs (basic assumptions about how the world actually works) people share in common. Schein (1984) typifies this school of thought by defining organizational cultures as the pattern of basic assumptions that a given group has invented, discovered, or developed in learning to survive by coping with its problems of external adaptation and internal integration, and that has worked well enough to be considered valid and, hence, should be taught to new members as the correct way to perceive, think, and feel regarding these problems. Quinn (1988), too, defines culture as the underlying assumptions and values present in the organization. This cognitive approach focuses on culture as a set of values.

In contrast, other writers take a more behavioral approach toward defining organizational culture. They focus on what organizational members actually do. They study behavioral norms, behavioral rules, and what the organizational member is expected to do. Van Maanen and Barley (1985) characterize this line of thought. They define organizational culture as a set of solutions devised by a group of people to meet specific problems posed by the situations they face in common. This behavioral approach describes culture as a set of norms.

Many writers approach culture as including both basic values and behavioral norms and emphasize that culture is an integrated whole. Hall (1990) describes a culture as a group of people who interact in a specific environment, recognize common behavioral norms and values, have relatively similar beliefs, and use a common language. Pettigrew (1979) notes that culture may be defined as an amalgam of beliefs, ideologies, language, ritual and myth. Meyerson and Martin (1987) also study organizational cultures as patterns of behaviors, values, and meanings.

It should be noted that all culture scholars emphasize that culture emerges as a response to situations faced by the group members. Over time, these responses become entrenched in group behavior. These responses can be seen clearly in health care organizations that have existed for many years. Culture provides its members with a sense of unity and helps make their lives predictable.

Both groups also recognize that although culture is passed on to new members, it is done so in an informal manner. Work group rules are seldom if ever written down or presented formally to newcomers; they are inferred from what members say and do. Pfeffer (1981) comments that the crucial feature that distinguishes culture from other management phenomena is that culture is conveyed to its participants through the expression of sentiments, beliefs, and attitudes. Denison (1990) notes that culture is a form of internal control. Thus, culture stands in contrast to externally controlled, power-dependent activities, such as clearly stated goals, consciously derived strategies, carefully drawn organizational charts, codified policies and procedures, and consistently applied sanctions. Culture is what nursing has often called the informal organization. An organization's culture may or may not coincide with the formal management activities or it may do so to a greater or lesser extent.

RELATIONSHIP BETWEEN CORPORATE AND SUBGROUP CULTURES

As has been noted, culture was originally studied by anthropologists. Their focus was on ethnic and national cultures. When management scholars began to investigate culture, they brought the study of culture to the organizational level. Early on, the culture of the organization was studied at the corporate level. The culture was identified by observing the norms and values of members of top management. It was assumed that the culture at the corporate level penetrated down to all levels of the organization. Peters and Waterman (1982) suggested that well-run companies have a unitary culture, that is, one common culture shared by both workers and management. Hence, the terms organizational culture and corporate culture became almost synonymous.

As the study of organizational culture progressed, however, the belief that well-run companies have only a unitary culture was questioned. Van Maanen and Barley (1985) recognized that even the best run companies have a variety of cultures. Subsequent research has identified subcultures at the department level, the occupational level, and the work group level.

Although Deal and Kennedy (1982) focused on the unitary culture of each company, they did suggest that most companies are actually a mix of different cultures. They described the cultures of different departments by proposing that within companies the marketing department may reflect the "tough guy" culture, sales and manufacturing are often characterized by working and playing hard, research and development frequently typify the "bet-your-company" culture, and the accounting department tends to be more process-oriented in nature. Rousseau (1978) studied departments within an electronics firm and a radio station and found cultural differences among departments in the same organization.

Cultural differences among different occupational groups have also been identified. Gregory (1983) described differing occupational cultures between computer scientists and software engineers in a Silicon Valley corporation. The computer scientists were interested in the academic aspects of computers and enjoyed writing papers about what they did, whereas the software engineers were interested in building things and enjoyed producing a useful product. Bullis (1990) found differing occupational cultures in the U.S. Forest Service among the biologists, whose goal was to manage ecosystems; the foresters, who concentrated on managing resources for people; and the engineers, who focused on managing the forest to preserve the timber resources. Coeling & Wilcox (1991) identify cultural differences among different health care professionals within a hospital. Physicians focus on maintaining life above all else, nurses emphasize individualizing patient care, and respiratory therapists strive to get oxygen into the cells.

Research also supports the existence of culture at the work group level. Short and Ferratt (1984) reported differing types of work group cultures in industry, and Coeling and Wilcox (1988) described different nursing unit cultures within the same hospital. Cultural differences between shifts on nursing units has also been observed.

Schein (1985) recommends that culture be viewed as a property of any independently defined stable social unit. If one can demonstrate that a given set of people have shared a significant number of important experiences in the process of solving external and internal problems, one can assume that such common experiences have led them, over time, to a shared view of the world. Recognizing that different groups within a health care agency will have different cultures is important for the nurse executive to help groups work together to meet the needs of the client.

Culture researchers are currently studying how the culture at one organizational level compares with that at another level. Coeling and Wilcox (1988) looked at two nursing unit work group cultures in a health care organization. They found that group A emphasized teamwork and a sense of family, whereas group B focused on innovation and moving ahead professionally. A year later, Mullins (1989) studied the corporate level culture of that same organization. A comparison of the two studies suggests that the corporate values identified were general and broad in scope. Important organizational values included innovation, teamwork, and a feeling of family. Although both nursing units valued these cultural elements of innovation, teamwork, and a feeling of family, the groups differed in the emphasis given to the various behaviors. Group A was relatively less concerned with innovation and more inclined to emphasize teamwork and a sense of family than was group B. In contrast, group B spent a considerable amount of the time innovating and much less time promoting teamwork and a sense of family. Although the culture of the work groups did not conflict with corporate level cultural elements, the emphasis given to different behaviors varied between the groups within the organization. Bullis (1990) questioned whether a change in the organizational mission of the U.S. Forest Service would lead to a more common culture. She found that when the meaning of the mission statement diverged from the foresters' professional values, the foresters held to their professional values rather than adopting the values of their employing agency. Morley and Shockley-Zalabak (1991) studied the degree to which corporate culture penetrates down the hierarchy. They found that the organizational founders perceived the corporate culture to be much stronger than did other levels of organizational members. Other recent studies also describe the existence of subcultures among workers in organizations (Friedman, 1989; Jones, 1990; McMillan, 1989; Nickerson, 1990).

SOURCES OF ORGANIZATIONAL CULTURE

A variety of factors contribute to the formation and continual shaping of a culture. These factors include group leaders, group members, the internal environment, and the external environment. A consideration of the variety of factors that impact on the culture reveals the difficulty of changing the culture by changing only one of these factors. It is the wise nurse executive who, in attempting to change a culture, takes into consideration all the forces that affect the culture.

Early studies of organizational culture focused on the corporate level of culture. Early theories about the source of culture gave considerable attention to the influence of the organizational founder on the current culture (Morley & Shockley-Zalabak, 1991; Schein, 1983). Because the founders have considerable influence on the organization, their values, goals, and preferences often become those of the organization, and their approaches to matching a particular technology with a market opportunity prevail.

Another source of culture, where applicable, is the institution that founded the organization. This may be especially true in health care institutions, which often are founded by an established community or a religious organization. In such cases, the values of these founding groups impact on the nature of the culture because the purpose of the facility is to further the goals of the founding organization.

Although administrators have considerable power over members, they do not have total power. Workers bring to the organization their own values, goals, and customary behaviors. Over time, workers' norms are incorporated into the group culture. This is especially likely to occur when a large number of new employees who have similar values join the group at the same time. This might occur in nursing when several new graduates from the same school join a unit together.

If there is an acceptable fit between the new member and the group, the new member will reflect the values of the group. If, however, the new member's values and norms are dissimilar from the group, the new member will have to choose whether to adopt the norms and values of the group, remain an outsider, or leave the group. Groups differ in the extent to which they are willing to tolerate members whose behaviors deviate from that of the group's culture. Nursing units can often predict whether a new nurse will fit in with the unit after the new nurse has worked only a few days.

Various internal forces also influence the shape of the culture. One force is that of the technology of the work. In a health care setting, a group whose primary focus is to improve the client's physiological functioning may develop a different culture than a group whose focus is to assist the client with interpersonal processes. Also the acuity of the client determines the culture. Many nurses today are reporting changes in their culture that they attribute to the increased acuity of their clients.

Another force is critical incidents that have occurred within the history of the group. A strike that occurred 10 years ago may still determine how people interact and who talks to whom. Unusual behaviors reinforced by the leaders and talked about by the members also shape the culture. For example, when one or two nurses are positively reinforced for taking initiative in an emergency situation and performing "medical" functions to save a client's life, the behavior may quickly become a group norm.

Physical facilities impact on group culture. The furniture provided will affect the formality of the atmosphere, which can, in turn, affect how group members interact with each other and do their work. The layout of the nursing station and client rooms may determine how closely co-workers interact to help each other, socialize with each other, and criticize each other.

Conditions in the external environment also influence a group's culture. If the organization is to successfully function in a given community, the value system of the surrounding community will have to be incorporated into that of the organization. The economic environment of the surrounding community is also very powerful in shaping a group's culture. If money is scarce and the community is unwilling and/or unable to purchase the hospital's services, the organization will have to adapt their services to what the client will buy.

THE VALUE OF UNDERSTANDING ORGANIZATIONAL CULTURE

Understanding organizational culture is important to nursing management theorists. The goal of the management theorist is to find new, more effective ways to study organizations. A culture study can serve as a necessary, prequantitative description for researchers interested in devising quantitative measures. A culture study can be used in conjunction with a quantitative study to help interpret or place in context results from a statistical analysis of an organization. An organizational culture approach can also provide both a managerial and a nonmanagerial (worker) account of sense making in a particular organization by describing organizational life in all its fullness and thus enhance understanding of the work context. As Pacanowsky and O'Donnell-Trujillo (1982) note, a culture study may even have the capacity to reject theories by noting whether or not predictions are borne out in real life. In short, organizational culture research has theory-generative, theory-contextualizing, and theory-testing functions for the nursing management researcher.

Understanding organizational culture also has practical benefits for employees. This understanding is useful for nurses who are looking for a new position, being oriented to a new position, or seeking to change an aspect of his/her organizational culture. If nurses both know the essential cultural elements for a given group and are aware of their preferences regarding each of these elements, then during the interview, they can inquire about the typical behaviors and values of the group and thereby decide if they would be compatible with this group. Furthermore, if new orientees understand how groups may differ in their responses to a situation, orientees will know what to watch for and what to ask about to learn about the job. This knowledge can help new members understand why things happen the way they do. Also knowing how to assess a group's culture will guide the nurse who wants to change the group. Being aware of the established way of doing things will help nurses appreciate the impact a change would have on the group and develop some tentative plans for the best way to bring about the change on the unit.

In the same manner, an understanding of organizational culture is beneficial to nurse executives and management consultants for hiring, orienting, integrating a new technology, decreasing conflict, predicting a competitor's next move, and merging groups. An understanding of the culture, along with the ability to determine the preferred culture of a potential employee, will assist the interviewer in determining whether a prospective employee would be a good match for the group. Early identification of an incompatible match can prevent premature resignation and the financial loss associated with such an event. A conscious awareness of the group culture can also assist in orienting a new employee. The faster new members learn the culture, the more quickly they will be productive for the organization. Knowledge of the culture also helps integrate a new technology. If the technology, such as a new piece of equipment or information processing system, supports the group culture, one can expect the innovation to be quickly adapted by the group. If the innovation conflicts with the culture, it will probably be resisted. Sathe (1985, p. 383) has developed the following formula to predict resistance to culture change:

Resistance to culture change = Magnitude of the   × Strength of prevailing
                               change in the content   culture, i.e., strong versus
                               of the culture, i.e.,   weak culture
                               radical versus
                               incremental change
                               in the culture's
                               content

Altering the innovation so that it is compatible with the culture can facilitate its acceptance (Coeling & Wilcox, 1990; Pondy and Huff, 1985). Understanding culture can also help alleviate one source of group conflict. Sometimes, some nurses on a unit attempt to develop and/or sustain one cultural pattern, whereas other nurses support a different response to the problem at hand. Bringing these differences to conscious awareness will enable the nurses to make more conscious choices regarding the resolution of the conflict. Also an appreciation of the dominant culture of a competitor can be useful in anticipating future moves and competitive responses (Reimann & Wiener, 1988). Finally, an awareness of organizational culture is beneficial when merging units within a hospital or when merging two hospitals. Conflict, rather than acceptance, can be expected when groups merge and one of the two cultures expects or attempts to dominate the other. A conscious awareness of the cultural differences can enable the two groups to work together.

THE POSSIBILITY OF CHANGING ORGANIZATIONAL CULTURE

Organizational practitioners, such as nurse executives, are under intense pressure to bring about organizational change. In today's environment, where there is tremendous pressure on managers and managerial consultants to find new ways to increase productivity and assure organizational survival, changing culture has been billed as the new solution on the horizon. Early studies of organizational culture suggest that having the right culture is the key to organizational success (Deal & Kennedy, 1982; Peters & Waterman, 1982).

However, nurse executives are wise to be cautious and resist rushing forward to try to change a culture. Although there is considerable agreement on the value of understanding organizational culture, there is no consensus on the value of changing the culture. Scholars coming from the anthropological tradition are slow to encourage culture change. They argue there is currently little evidence to support the belief that one culture is better than another (Hall, 1990; Leininger, 1985; Lessem, 1990). They ask not whether any culture is good, but rather what the culture is good for; that is, what does it accomplish for the group and does this correspond to the group's goal?

Others who have studied organizational culture in depth, theorists and practitioners alike, have also questioned the effectiveness of using organizational culture as a means of control for organizational survival. Ray (1986) describes how the concept of culture has become the latest strategy of organizational control but questions its effectiveness for increasing organizational success. Frost (1985) writes that organizational culture as a "quick fix" is passe. Schein (1985) advises that we do not assume culture can be manipulated like other matters under the control of managers. He adds that culture controls the manager more than the manager controls culture. By definition, innovation will not be congruent with the current culture. The motivation for change does not come from the power of the manager, but rather it comes from the fact that some incongruity (culture change) may be needed for continued survival. Kilmann, Saxton, and Serpa (1986) also warn about the promise of culture as being a quick single remedy to a complex problem. They add that it is virtually impossible to improve the functioning of a complex organization by any quick fix, no matter how appealing this is. Sathe (1985) notes that companies seen as having excellent cultures developed these cultures in their formative years while they were still small in size. The easiest time for the nurse executive to influence the culture is when the group is in its formative years.

As Schein (1985) notes, to label a change as "culture change" enhances the drama of what is happening so it may have some motivational value, but it does not make the change occur any faster. Another value of a nurse executive calling a change a culture change is the recognition that people are changing from preexisting values and behaviors that are firmly entrenched, closely interrelated, and intricately embedded in a culture to new adaptive values and behaviors. Because culture consists of the firmly entrenched, and often unconscious, values and behaviors that have been in place for a long time, it is to be expected that culture will be much harder to change than the formal management processes and tools, which are the surface manifestations of culture and are not as deeply embedded in one's value system. Culture can be changed and, in fact, is always changing in a slow evolutionary manner as the environment changes. But it is unrealistic to expect culture to change quickly, especially if the change involves basic values, unless many of the factors that facilitate the change are already in place. Denison (1990) writes that culture changes occur more readily in response to an outside threat, a change in leadership, or a high turnover of personnel. He adds that cultures have tremendous inertia, and the larger the organization, the greater the inertia.

To answer the question of how easily an established organizational culture can be changed, it is important for the nurse executive to define clearly what she/he means by culture. As noted above, culture can refer to everything, to values, and/or to specific behaviors. Both Schein (1985) and Sathe (1985) note that it is possible to change behavioral norms without changing values and beliefs. Although some correlation between values and behavior has been observed, this link has not been found to be nearly as strong as is sometimes assumed (Wicker, 1969). Culture change that involves a change in specific behaviors is much easier than culture change involving underlying values and beliefs. The nurse executive must remember that change involving internalization of new values and beliefs occurs at a deeper, more lasting level but takes more effort than a change in a specific behavior.

Factors that facilitate culture change include clear goals, organizational reward systems, a desire by participants to change, and a flexible work group environment. Clear goals are necessary to make explicit the desired change and enable the participants to see what they and their clients are gaining from the change. Early signaling and the use of symbols by leaders warn the members of upcoming changes and allow some early testing of responses. Wilkins and Patterson (1985) recommend the formulation of a plan to avoid costly mistakes related to change by asking the following questions:

1. Where do we need to be going strategically as a group?
2. Where are we now as a culture?
3. What are the gaps between where we are and where we should be?
4. What is our plan of action to close those gaps?

A thorough assessment and a clear plan of action involving participants at all levels of the organization are essential for successful culture change.

A reward system that supports the culture change is also critical. Culture change is an attempt to alter firmly entrenched values and behaviors. This often involves the loss of rewards associated with former behaviors. Hence, the reward for the new behavior must be great enough to compensate for the incurred loss. That it is easier to reinforce changes in behavior than changes in values suggests to the nurse executive that an initial focus on changing behaviors, rather than values, may be the most productive approach. Reinforced behaviors will eventually change values.

Support by staff nurses can be encouraged by prompting them to question their own values, by pointing out the conditions in the environment that necessitate changed behavior, and by changing behavior one step at a time. Brown (1985) recommends the use of participatory research for changes involving values, ideologies, and possible conflicts with power holders. Participatory research is a way to promote people-centered development in political and economic systems that encourage local empowerment. This is especially relevant as nurse executives seek to transform the work environment by attempting to change cultural values. Participatory research involves having participants identify and analyze the problem as they see it and clarify a common vision for the future. The cultural assessment tools described in the following section, which assist nurses to identify both current and preferred culture, are especially suitable for this process. Weick (1979) emphasizes the importance of slow, evolutionary change, which enables employees to adjust to changes in small bits and to experience one small change before determining the most appropriate next step.

Under certain conditions, a strong culture can inhibit change. Change can be difficult when a given culture has existed intact for a long period of time and the members of the culture have no desire to change. Del Bueno (1990) notes nurse turnover may be desirable and necessary to allow changes essential for an organization's survival.

ASSESSING ORGANIZATIONAL CULTURE

Early studies of organizational culture used the traditional anthropological method of analysis, namely, participant observation and questioning. The goal was to understand organizational life. Just as the anthropologist is interested in the workways, folk tales, and ritual practices of a culture, so also these early organizational culture scholars were interested in the workways, folk tales, and ritual practices of an organization. Pacanowsky and O'Donnell-Trujillo (1983) suggest workways that reflect the culture include courtesies, pleasantries, sociabilities, and privacies. Stories that are important to listen to include personal stories, collegial stories, and corporate stories. They recommend personal, communication, task, social, and organizational rituals be considered when doing a cultural assessment. Sathe (1985) has contributed to this assessment process by describing a systematic procedure for deciphering the culture by making inferences from such data.

Although observation and questioning provide the richest information regarding a given culture, they do require substantial time and skill on the part of the person who seeks to analyze that culture. In an attempt to assist the manager or worker who is relatively untrained in assessing a culture and who has a limited amount of time to assess a group's culture, several culture scholars have developed either specific categories of behaviors and values to investigate or tools designed to assess organizational culture.

Schein (1985) lists five categories of behaviors and values that provide important descriptors of an organization's culture: *(1)* the organization's relationship to its environment; *(2)* the nature of reality, truth, time, and space; *(3)* the nature of human nature; *(4)* the nature of human activity; and *(5)* the nature of human relationships. These content areas are based on the categories developed by the anthropologists Kluckhohn and Strodtbeck (1961) to study culture at any level. Wilkins (1983) provides guidelines for understanding the group's assumptions about the nature of work, its means, its ends, and its rewards, as well as the interests that are served by work and the equitability with which people are treated.

Several nurses have contributed categories and samples of questions that can be used to better understand the culture of health care organizations. Del Bueno and Freund (1986) identify the need to consider health professionals' deportment, status symbols and reward systems, environment and ambiance, communication patterns, meeting rules, rites, rituals, ceremonies, sacred cows, and subcultures. Hughes (1990) draws on the work of Dandridge, Mitroff, and Joyce (1980) to discuss material symbols, behavioral symbols, verbal symbols, structural characteristics, and historical characteristics of health care settings.

Several researchers have developed survey tools to assist in assessing culture. One early tool that can be used to describe a culture is the Work Environment Scale by Moos and Insel (1974). This tool, which provides a numerical score on the three dimensions of relationships, personal growth, and system maintenance and change, was developed to describe the social climate of a work place. Halpin and Croft devised the Organizational Climate Description Questionnaire (Halpin, 1966). This tool was later modified by Duxbury, Henly, and Armstrong (1982) for use in a neonatal intensive care unit. These tools were developed before organizational culture became a popular topic in the literature. Although these tools purport to describe climate, the questions are similar to those on more recently developed tools designed to assess organizational culture.

The concept of organizational climate came into vogue before the concept of organizational culture. The organizational climate is an assessment of the atmosphere of the organization. It is perceived by workers and is described by a worker's attitude and emotions toward the workplace. Ott (1989) defines organizational climate as an amalgamation of feeling tones, or a transient organizational mood. Putnam and Cheney (1983) note that climate has typically been measured through individual perceptions while being used to describe a characteristic of an organization. They discuss this conceptual slippage associated with the term "climate" and offer the term "culture" as a broader concept that includes all aspects of a group, not merely the member's emotional reactions to the group. Denison (1990) argues that the debate over organizational culture and climate is in many ways a classic example of methodological differences obscuring a basic substantive similarity. He notes that the argument is not so much what to study as how to study it. Climate researchers have traditionally used questionnaires, whereas culture researchers began by using qualitative methods. Thus, many of the topics considered in climate scales are the same as those considered in cultural assessments. Culture consists of values and behaviors, however, not someone's emotional reaction toward these values and behaviors.

Another early survey tool, used primarily to assess organizational cultures in multinational organizations, is that of Hofstede (1980). Although Hofstede uses this survey to describe what he calls culture, many of the questions were derived from an attitude survey questionnaire. Hofstede's tool provides a numerical score on the four dimensions of power distance, uncertainty avoidance, individualism-collectivism, and masculinity-femininity.

A more recently developed tool is the Kilmann-Saxton Culture-Gap Survey (1991). This survey provides a numerical score on the dimensions of task support, social relationships, task innovation, and personal freedom. It assesses both current and desired work group norms. Differences between the actual and desired norms are referred to as "Culture-Gaps." Identifying these gaps can motivate nurses to change their culture.

Cameron (Quinn, 1988) has developed a tool to assess corporate culture. It provides a score on six dimensions of corporate culture. These dimensions include the organization's dominant characteristics, leader, glue, climate, criteria of success, and management style. The nurse executive can use the scores on these dimensions to describe the nursing culture in terms of its internal/external orientation and its flexibility/control orientation.

Coeling (Coeling, Simms, & Erbin-Roesemann, 1991) has designed a tool specifically to assess the culture of a nursing unit. This Nursing Unit Cultural Assessment Tool (NUCAT) is broad in scope. It assesses a variety of behaviors that, through a series of qualitative and quantitative studies, have been found both to be important to practicing nurses and to differ between nursing units. All items on the tool assess different elements of culture and, hence, vary independently. This allows the tool to assess a unit culture in its fullness and gives a broad description of life on the unit.

However, this variety and breadth preclude its being divided into different dimensions with scores for each dimension. It is intended to be used as an initial scanning tool. It can be followed by tools, such as those listed previously, which will provide a more definitive measure of a certain element if the need arises. Because it assesses the group's typical behavior and the individual's preferred behavior, it, too, can be used to identify unit behaviors that might be producing group conflict and/or to identify work penetration points at which innovations can be introduced.

ETHICS RELATED TO ORGANIZATIONAL CULTURE

Although assessing a group's culture can have great value, there are also some dangers associated with a cultural assessment. One danger is that the assessment may be inaccurate. Because culture is really a wholistic concept, a description of a pattern, one can never "measure" it in its full complexity. The best one can do is measure discrete elements of it as research variables and then attempt to describe the pattern these variables portray. Another danger is that conscious awareness of the culture might prompt a change to meet a specific standard when this change is not in the group's best interest (De Lisi, 1990). This phenomenon occurred as Americans gained world power and then tried to impose the American culture on natives in other lands and even on native Americans.

It has also been questioned whether administrators have the right to change the behaviors and values and beliefs of employees. Perhaps it is more important to build on individual cultural values in shaping the character of an organization or work group. The nurse executive is encouraged to recognize that a culturally diverse work group is a strong and productive work group. Drake and Drake (1988) recommend that cultural values represent the views of employees as well as the views of managers. Nurse executives should encourage input from throughout the organization regarding appropriate values and practices for the culture.

Summary

Organizational culture has become a major focus of management studies. It emphasizes the importance of understanding people, individually and collectively, to facilitate organizational success. Because it is a broad concept and one that derives from a variety of traditions, it is important for the nurse executive and the nurse researcher to clarify their working definition of culture and their basic assumptions and goals regarding culture. An understanding of culture can facilitate organizational hiring, orientation, technological and work process changes, and mergers. Hasty attempts by the nurse executives to change the culture are ill-advised. Rather the current culture should be assessed and predictions made about what aspects of the culture should be changed and what supports should be in place before the changes begin.

References

Barley, S. R., Meyer, G. W., & Gash, D. C. (1988). Cultures of culture: Academics, practitioners and the pragmatics of normative control, *Administrative Science Quarterly, 33,* 24–60

Brown, L. D. (1985). People-centered development and participatory research, *Harvard Educational Review, 55*(1), 69–75.

Bullis, C. (1990). *Organizational transformation through values: A comparison of unitary and pluralist perspectives.* Paper presented at the Annual Convention of the International Communication Association, Dublin, Ireland.

Coeling, H. V., Simms, L., & Erbin-Roesemann, M. (1991). *Identification of relevant cultural norms in nursing unit work groups.* Paper presented at the Midwest Nursing Research Society, Oklahoma City, OK.

Coeling, H. V., & Wilcox, J. R. (1988). Understanding organizational culture: A key to management decision-making, *Journal of Nursing Administration, 18*(11), 16–24.

Coeling, H. V., & Wilcox, J. R. (1990). Using organizational culture to facilitate the change process, *American Nephrology Nurses' Association Journal, 17,* 231–236.

Coeling, H. V., & Wilcox, J. R. (1991). Professional recognition and high-quality patient care through collaboration: Two sides of the same coin, *Focus On Critical Care, 18,* 230–237.

Dandridge, T. C., Mitroff, I., & Joyce, W. F. (1980). Organizational symbolism: A topic to expand organizational analysis, *Academy of Management Review, 5*(1), 77–82.

Deal, T. E., & Kennedy, A. A. (1982). *Corporate cultures.* Reading, MA: Addison-Wesley.

del Bueno, D. J. (1990). Warning: Retention may be dangerous to your organization's health, *Nursing Economic$, 8,* 239–243.

del Bueno, D. J., & Freund, C. M. (1986). *Power & politics in nursing administration: A casebook.* Owings Mills, MD: National Health Publishing.

De Lisi, P. S. (1990). Lessons from the steel axe: Culture, technology, and organizational change, *Sloan Management Review, 32*(1), 83–93.

Denison, D. R. (1990). *Corporate culture and organizational effectiveness.* New York: Wiley.

Drake, B. H., & Drake, E. (1988). Ethical and legal aspects of managing corporate cultures, *California Management Review, 30*(2), 107–123.

Duxbury, M. L., Henly, G. A., & Armstrong, G. D. (1982). Measurement of the nurse organizational climate on neonatal intensive care units, *Nursing Research, 31*(2), 83–87.

Friedman, R. A. (1989). Interaction norms as carriers of organizational culture, *Journal of Contemporary Ethnography, 18*(1), 3–29.

Frost, P. J. (1985). Does organizational culture have a future? In P. J. Frost, L. F. Moore, M. R. Louis, C. C. Lundberg, & J. Martin (Eds.). *Organizational Culture* (pp. 379–380). Beverly Hills: Sage.

Gregory, K. L. (1983). Native-view paradigms: Multiple culture and culture conflicts in organizations, *Administrative Science Quarterly, 28,* 359–376.

Hall, P. (1990). *A cultural basis for cultural equality.* Paper presented at the Annual Convention of the International Communication Association, Dublin, Ireland.

Halpin, A. W. (1966). *Theory and research in administration.* New York: Macmillan.

Hofstede, G. (1980). *Culture's consequences: International differences in work-related values.* Beverly Hills: Sage.

Hughes, L. (1990). Assessing organizational culture: Strategies for the external consultant, *Nursing Forum, 25*(1), 15–19.

Jones, M. O. (1990). A folklore approach to emotions in work, *American Behavioral Scientist, 33,* 278–286.

Kilmann, R. H., & Saxton, M. J. (1991). *Kilmann-Saxton Culture-Gap Survey.* Tuxedo, NY: XICOM and Organizational Design Consultants.

Kilmann, R. H., Saxton, M. J., & Serpa, R. (1986). Issues in understanding and changing culture. *California Management Review, 28*(2), 87–94.

Kluckhohn, F. R., & Strodtbeck, F. L. (1961). *Variations in value orientations.* Evanston, IL: Row, Peterson and Company.

Leininger, M. M. (1985). Ethnography and ethnonursing: Models and modes of qualitative data analysis. In M. M. Leininger (Ed.). *Qualitative Research Methods in Nursing* (pp. 33–71). New York: Grune & Stratton.

Lessem, R. (1990). *Managing corporate culture.* Brookfield, VT: Gower.

McMillan, J. J. (1989). Symbolic emancipation in the organization: A case of shifting power, *Communication Yearbook, 13,* 203–214.

Meyerson, D., & Martin, J. (1987). Cultural change: An integration of three different views, *Journal of Management Studies, 24*(6), 623–647.

Moos, R. H., & Insel, P. N. (1974). *Work environment scale.* Palo Alto, CA: Consulting Psychologist Press.

Morley, D. D., & Shockley-Zalabak, P. (1991). An examination of the influence of organizational founders' value, *Management Communication Quarterly, 4,* 422–449.

Mullins, D. G. (1989). Messages of values inculcation in a hospital organization. (Doctoral dissertation, Bowling Green State University, 1989). *Dissertation Abstracts International, 50,* 10A.

Nickerson, B. E. (1990). Antagonism at work, *American Behavioral Scientist, 33,* 308–317.

Ott, J. S. (1989). *The organizational culture perspective.* Chicago: The Dorsey Press.

Pacanowsky, M. E., & O'Donnell-Trujillo, N. (1982). Communication and organizational cultures, *The Western Journal of Speech Communication, 46,* 115–130.

Pacanowsky, M. E., & O'Donnell-Trujillo, N. (1983). Organizational communication as cultural performance, *Communication Monographs, 50,* 126–147.

Peters, T. J., & Waterman, R. H., Jr. (1982). *In search of excellence.* New York: Harper & Row.

Pettigrew, A. M. (1979). On studying organizational cultures, *Administrative Science Quarterly, 24,* 570–581.

Pfeffer, J. (1981). Management as symbolic action: The creation and maintenance of organizational paradigms. In L. L. Cummings & B. M. Staw (Eds.). *Research in Organizational Behavior* (vol. 3, pp. 1–52). Greenwich CT: JAI Press.

Pondy, L. R., & Huff, A. S. (1985). Achieving routine in organizational change, *Journal of Management, 11,* 103–116.

Putnam, L. L., & Cheney, G. (1983). *A critical review of research traditions in organizational communication.* Paper presented at the Annual Convention of the International Communication Association, Dallas, TX.

Quinn, R. E. (1988). *Beyond rational management.* San Francisco: Jossey-Bass.

Ray, C. A. (1986). Corporate culture: The last frontier of control, *Journal of Management Studies, 23,* 287–297.

Reimann, B. C., & Wiener, Y. (1988). Corporate culture: Avoiding the elitist trap, *Business Horizons, 31,* 36–44.

Rousseau, D. M. (1978). Characteristics of departments, positions, and individuals: Contexts for attitudes and behavior, *Administrative Science Quarterly, 23,* 521–538.

Sackmann, S. A. (1989). Managing organizational cultures: Dreams and possibilities, *Communication Yearbook, 13,* 114–148.

Sathe, V. (1985). *Culture and related corporate realities.* Homewood, IL: Richard D. Irwin.

Schein, E. H. (1983). The role of the founder in creating organizational culture, *Organizational Dynamics, 12*(Summer), 13–28.

Schein, E. H. (1984). Coming to a new awareness of organizational culture, *Sloan Management Review, 25*(2), 3–16.

Schein, E. H. (1985). *Organizational culture and leadership.* San Francisco: Jossey-Bass.

Short, L. E., & Ferratt, T. W. (1984). Work unit culture: Strategic starting point in building organizational change, *Management Review, 73*(8), 15–19.

Smircich, L., & Calás, M. B. (1987). Organizational culture: A critical assessment. In F. M. Jablin (Ed.). *Handbook of Organizational Communication* (pp. 228–263). Newbury Park, CA: Sage.

Starbuck, W. H. (1982). Congealing oil: Inventing ideologies to justify acting ideologies out, *Journal of Management Studies, 19*(1), 3–27.

Taft, S. H. (1988a). *Cultural pluralism in professional organizations: Processes of transition and change.* Unpublished manuscript.

Taft, S. H. (1988b). Professional cultures of medicine, nursing and health care administration: A study in internal integration in a changing organization. (Doctoral dissertation, Case Western Reserve University, 1988). *Dissertation Abstracts International, 49,* 04B.

Van Maanen, J., & Barley, S. R. (1985). Cultural organization: Fragments of a theory. In P. J. Frost, L. F. Moore, M. R. Louis, C. C. Lundberg, & J. Martin (Eds.). *Organizational Culture* (pp. 31–53). Beverly Hills: Sage.

Weick, K. E. (1979). *The social psychology of organizing.* Reading, MA: Addison-Wesley.

Wicker, A. W. (1969). Attitudes versus actions: The relationship of verbal and overt behavioral responses to attitude objects, *Journal of Social Issues, 25*(4), 41–78.

Wilkins, A. L. (1983). The culture audit: A tool for understanding organizations, *Organizational Dynamics, 12*(2), 24–38.

Wilkins, A. L., & Patterson, K. J. (1985). You can't get there from here: What will make culture-change projects fail. In R. H. Kilmann, M. J. Saxton, R. Serpa, & Associates (Eds.). *Gaining Control of the Corporate Culture* (pp. 262–291). San Francisco: Jossey-Bass.

CHAPTER 10

Operationalizing Professional Nursing

Highlights

- Model of nursing administration
- Prerequisites for operationalizing professional nursing
- Model for operationalizing professional nursing
- Use of the model
- Fiscal implications

The purpose of this chapter is to discuss the major aspects of operationalizing professional nursing in a patient care setting. To operationalize professional nursing, staff must be prepared to carry out assigned responsibilities. In any patient care setting, nursing has assigned tasks or functions as part of its responsibilities. In many settings, however, the functions that are considered within the realm of the professional nurse, for example, patient assessment, patient teaching, and developing nursing care plans, are carried out inconsistently or not at all. Although nursing leaders frequently decry these facts, little study has been undertaken to discover why these situations exist. Indeed, one could make a strong case for the argument that nurses themselves are not clear about what functions are expected of them. Because nursing is an emerging profession, not all functions are yet unequivocally identified. To make professional nursing operational, the nurse executive must make many assumptions and decisions about nursing practice. The theories and models presented thus far are designed to assist the executive with these decisions about nursing practice. This chapter continues this approach by presenting a model for the use of theories or conceptual frameworks.

MODEL OF NURSING ADMINISTRATION

Models are derived from speculation about what processes could have produced the observed results (Lave & March, 1975). Models assist us in gaining understanding of complex relationships (Robbins, 1991). Models of various aspects of nursing provide the nurse executive with frameworks for approaching problem identification and solution. Models may be useful when the nurse executive communicates with institutional administrators and members of other disciplines. As any nurse executive knows who has attempted to communicate the essence of professional nursing practice to a nonnursing audience, models are useful tools for communicating concepts without the need for a great amount of verbal detail.

The model of the role of the nurse executive represented in Figure 10.1 depicts the relationships among key components for the nurse executive. In this model, the nurse executive is viewed as the fulcrum between nursing practice and administration of the health care facility. In mechanics, the fulcrum is the support or point of support on which a lever turns in raising or moving something. A fulcrum is also a means of exerting influence or pressure (Webster's, 1984). The model is also meant to depict the role of the nurse executive in providing a balance between nursing practice and administration.

Each end of the lever—nursing practice and facility administration—has legitimate organizational functions and authority. If one end out-weighs the other, conflict and loss of productivity may occur. In keeping a balance between the two ends of the lever, the nurse executive performs many functions, including:

- Communication linkage between nursing and administration
- Interpreter of nursing practice to administration
- Interpreter of administrative policy and decisions to nursing staff
- Arbitrator between nursing practice and health care facility interests
- Negotiator for necessary nursing resources
- Advocate for increased understanding between nursing practice and administration

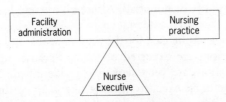

Figure 10.1 Model of the role of the nurse executive.

This role of the nurse executive is a delicate balancing act that may not always be satisfying but is almost always challenging. This model of the role of the nurse executive is the basis on which the nurse executive operationalizes professional nursing.

PROFESSIONAL NURSING

In this text, nursing has been presented as an emerging profession and a professional practice discipline. The model presented in Chapter 1 has four components of professional nursing practice: clinical practice, research, education, and management. In this chapter, the clinical component, application of knowledge, is the primary focus, because the nursing staff in most health care institutions have this realm as their primary responsibility. The nurse executive spends a great deal of time on matters of structure and process, for example, policy, procedures, planning, that lead to the application of nursing in the patient care setting.

Although disagreement exists about the need for nurse executives to retain clinical skills, the need for current theoretical clinical knowledge is obvious. For a nursing division to progress to professional nursing practice, some nurses in the environment must possess advanced clinical skills and knowledge, as well as understanding of and commitment to professional nursing. In some institutions, the nurse executive may be one of a few nurses with a degree.

To support the professionalization of nursing in a specific institution, the nurse executive needs a pragmatic understanding of what professional nursing means, not just an intellectual understanding of the concepts. If the nurse executive has practiced clinical nursing in a professional environment, it is a great advantage when introducing changes necessary to move toward professional nursing practice.

PREREQUISITES FOR OPERATIONALIZING PROFESSIONAL NURSING

Chapter 6 discussed the authority base of the nurse executive in relation to creating the environment for nursing practice. Those elements—administrative support, budgetary control, and authority to approve nursing practice components—also provide the foundation for operationalizing professional nursing. Perhaps the process could occur without the presence of all three elements; perhaps others are needed in some settings. The nurse executive must evaluate the particular situation to determine which specific elements in what combination are central to the authority to institute changes and control nursing.

One type of authority valuable to the nurse executive within the nursing division has been labeled "colleague authority." This type of authority derives from professional and management accomplishments that are recognized by the nursing staff (Marylander, 1974). The nurse executive's clinical knowledge and competence may have been the basis for promotion, but without administrative skills, these are inadequate for operationalizing professional nursing. As pointed out previously, nurses have indicated in numerous studies that lack of administrative leadership and support contributed to their leaving nursing practice.

Another prerequisite for operationalizing professional nursing is the presence on the staff of professional nurses, not only to serve as role models, but also to work closely with the staff in implementation of the professional nursing model. Without a cadre of professionally competent and confident nurses, the nurse executive is not likely to successfully implement all aspects of a professional model. Because the implementation of a model may require several years, the nurse executive does not have the time or all the skills required for total implementation. Recruitment of qualified staff may be the top priority while planning is continued for implementing a professional nursing model.

The type of institution or agency is particularly important when evaluating the support of the medical staff for professional nursing. Chronic disease institutions and rehabilitation hospitals are likely to provide a favorable environment for professional nursing. Many small hospitals tend to be less formal and thus to minimize the differentiation between medicine and nursing, whereas large hospitals tend to empha- size rigid job descriptions and thus restricted definitions of the nurse's responsibilities. The university medical center, which is dominated by the medical presence, tends "to push nursing aside, thereby minimizing its capability to negotiate and to reoccupy its place when the doctor is gone" (Mauksch, 1972, pp. 220–221). In community nursing agencies, the physician is frequently not in the formal organizational struc- ture. Medical support for professional nursing may not be a prerequisite in all institu- tions, but opposition will certainly make the nurse executive's job difficult, if not impossible, in terms of operationalizing professional nursing.

MODEL FOR OPERATIONALIZING PROFESSIONAL NURSING

Because models assist one in gaining understanding of complex relationships, it is advantageous to have a model for the very complex process of operationalizing professional nursing. The steps for the development of any model are *(1)* facts are observed; *(2)* the facts are looked at as if they were the outcome of some unknown process (the model), and speculation is made about what processes might have pro- duced these outcomes; *(3)* other implications or predictions are deduced from the model; and *(4)* whether these implications are true is questioned, and new models are produced if necessary (Lave & March, 1975).

For the nurse executive, the facts observed are those that, taken together, define professional nursing. The process that might result in professional nursing in a particular institution or agency is not known precisely. Although nurse executives have operationalized professional nursing based on some research findings, much has been based primarily on assumptions and the executives' individual experiences. Be- cause the research base from nursing and other fields is inadequate as a basis for operationalizing professional nursing, any model is necessarily speculative and based on assumptions, that is, circumstances and situations that the executive supposes to be true. Given that any model will be imperfect at this point in the development of professional nursing, the following model is presented for use and revision as new information becomes available.

The model depicted in Figure 10.2 presents a basic relationship framework among the three elements for operationalizing professional nursing: foundations, derived constructs, and operationalized results. Foundations are those theories, conceptual

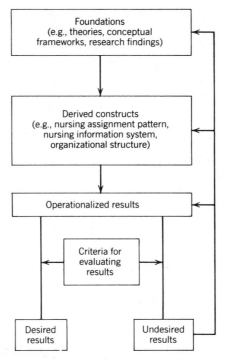

Figure 10.2 Model for operationalizing professional nursing.

frameworks, and research findings that are used as the bases for developing the elements in the environment for nursing, for example, theories of nursing, management theories, organizational theory, research findings about nurse performance, leadership theories, and values. Many nurse executives assume their positions with an understanding of and leanings toward various foundation components. In such instances, it is important for the nurse executive to be aware of bias before developing a plan for implementing professional nursing.

The derived constructs are the components of clinical practice and the environment most related to professional nursing. For example, if the foundation of a decentralized organizational structure is chosen, the nursing assignment pattern of primary nursing may be one derived construct related to decentralization. Operationalized results are those outcomes, from the derived constructs, that can be observed in terms of behavior. All of the results will not, of course, be those that were anticipated or desired, but with an imperfect model and incomplete data, revisions in the constructs are expected to be necessary. Perhaps a different foundation is required or a construct needs to be operationalized in an effective manner. All results require continuous evaluation and adjustments of the components when results are not adequate.

USE OF THE MODEL

Use of the model for operationalizing professional nursing presumes knowledge of theories and willingness to intellectually struggle with some ideas that are in various stages of development. Although theories in nursing and other fields may not be tested, they can provide guidance in areas of uncertainty. Some guidance is preferable to none or to using conflicting approaches. The major bases for professional nursing in a service agency are those used to develop the management and clinical practice components. One task of the nurse executive is to facilitate the incorporation of theoretical knowledge and research findings into the practice environment.

Some of the categories of theories and conceptual frameworks useful to the nurse executive in developing the organizational structure are organizational theory, management theory, leadership styles, communications, team building, and bureaucratic characteristics. These concepts are based on theory from psychology, sociology, and other fields. To understand these concepts, the nurse executive need not return to the study of the basic sciences, but at times, a review of a concept may be useful in attempting to operationalize some aspect of professional nursing.

Before developing or changing the organizational structure of a nursing service, the nurse executive must assess the structure of the total institution. Knowledge of theory and conceptual frameworks is also important for this assessment. Three types of organizational structures have been identified as centralized, decentralized, and matrix.

Although centralization and decentralization may be examined as separate organizational types, they may also be viewed as the ends of a continuum. Because decentralization implies the delegation of responsibility, authority, and decision making from higher management levels to lower levels of subordinates (Robbins, 1991), all large or complex organizations have some degree of decentralization. Determining the degree of decentralization within the organization gives the nurse executive major information from which to begin planning.

Obviously, the organizational structure of the nursing division must be compatible with that of the total organization. For example, in a highly centralized organization, a decentralized nursing division would probably create conflict and confusion for the nursing staff when interacting with other divisions. However, some aspects of responsibility, authority, and decision making could be decentralized, and must be, to attain a professional nursing model.

One approach for decentralizing decision making is based on the classes of decisions: those that can be predetermined and those that cannot be predetermined. Predetermined decisions generally concern measurable and objective physical phenomena. Nonpredetermined decisions involve humans and human values as well as "the assessment of situations in which information needs cannot be adequately anticipated or adequately filled" (Burlingame, 1971, p. 236). In a centralized organization, the pattern is to retain in a small group the responsibility for nonpredetermined decisions and to delegate only predetermined decision areas. In a decentralized organization, responsibility for decision making is assigned where the skills and competencies can reasonably be matched with required information. In a centralized organization, "the decision structure tends to be one where the decisions at the top are original and sensitive to human and social considerations; decisions at the bottom are more likely to be routine and insensitive to such considerations." In a decentralized organization, all types of decisions are made at all organizational levels, with only the extent and complexity of impact decreasing from top to lower levels (Burlingame, 1971, p. 236).

This analysis of decision making is not entirely applicable to the health care setting because all clinical decisions involve humans and human values. However, decision making can be centralized or decentralized. In deciding with other nurse managers what decision areas to decentralize, the nurse executive should maintain a high level of cognizance of what areas may result in conflict, and thus stress, for the nursing staff. For example, in some hospitals, if the head nurse had the authority to refuse patient admissions to the unit, the admissions office would find the situation unacceptable. Even without major organizational changes, many minor structural changes can result in a more effective and efficient nursing service. For example, hiring and disciplinary decisions can be made at the head nurse level instead of at the supervisor or director levels.

Another area in which the model for operationalizing professional nursing may be useful is in determining the nursing assignment pattern. Some common types of nursing assignment patterns are functional, team, and primary. In recent years, research has been completed comparing the effectiveness and efficiency of some nursing assignment patterns. Shukla (1982) postulates that primary nursing is more cost effective than team nursing when the nursing support system requires very little time of the registered nurse and the patients require highly skilled nursing care. Based on his conclusions from study results, probably a short-term acute care community hospital would not financially benefit from primary nursing. However, from other perspectives, for example, job satisfaction, quality of care, and patient satisfaction, primary nursing may still be desirable. Knowledge of theories and concepts can be used in the model as a basis for discussion in choosing a nursing assignment pattern.

Many decisions are made based on preference or subjective data. Although the use of the model for operationalizing professional nursing will not eliminate the use of subjective data by any means, it gives nurse executives an alternative approach for making changes in the nursing division. The strategies of change presented in Chapter 8 are foundations that could be used in the model as the basis of implementing a change within the division of nursing. The same change strategy may be used for several changes, or a different one may be more successful with different changes. The model for operationalizing professional nursing can be used to phase in various components or changes in the practice environment that the nurse executive has planned.

FISCAL IMPLICATIONS

All changes entail costs. Although most of the costs are in terms of personnel time, this is a costly item to a labor intensive organization such as a health organization. One costly pitfall to avoid is that of planning too extensively. At times, a nursing division may undertake a planning phase for a change or for introducing a new concept without a realistic level of commitment from staff or the health care organization administration. This is not to say that commitment must be in place before a change is discussed, but a core level of support for a concept will prevent wasted hours of planning something that will not be implemented.

A second costly pitfall is not planning enough for a change or for introducing a new concept. Although not every detail of a plan must be developed before implementation begins, the clear delegation of tasks and responsibilities will greatly facilitate efforts. Many good ideas are scrapped because of frustration during the implementation phase of a project. In addition, a poorly implemented concept is often not correctly implemented, thus leading to costly backtracking to attempt to work out problems. In some instances, the change or concept is dropped by staff as quickly as the implementation phase is completed. This can be a major cost to an institution if the change is critical to efficient functioning.

Although planning and the use of the model to operationalize professional nursing will not prevent costly errors, a more studied approach in nursing administration can lead to better organizational outcomes. If cost estimates are made for each change or concept to be introduced, the nurse executive also has more concrete data on which to make decisions.

Summary

The major prerequisites for operationalizing professional nursing are administrative support, budgetary control, and authority to approve nursing practice components. These factors provide the foundation on which the operationalizing process can occur. The major components of a model for operationalizing professional nursing are foundations, derived constructs, and operationalized results. These components must be individualized to each practice setting and compatible with the overall health care organization.

STUDY QUESTIONS

1. What are the two most important prerequisites for operationalizing professional nursing? Why?
2. Discuss one way in which a model for operationalizing professional nursing could be used.
3. List two specific theories that can be used in operationalizing professional nursing and discuss their application to a nursing division.

References

Burlingame, J. F. (1971). Information technology and decentralization. In P. P. Schoderbek (Ed.). *Management Systems* (2nd ed.). New York: Wiley.
Lave, C. A., & March, J. G. (1975). *An introduction to models in the social sciences.* New York: Harper & Row.
Marylander, S. (1974). The dual role of the director of nursing, *Hospitals, 48*(13), 119–120, 124.
Mauksch, H. O. (1972). Nursing: Churning for change. In H. E. Freeman, S. Levin, & L. G. Reeder, (Eds.). *Handbook of Medical Sociology* (2nd ed.). Englewood Cliffs, NJ: Prentice-Hall.
Robbins, S. P. (1991). *Management* (3rd ed.). Englewood Cliffs, NJ: Prentice-Hall.
Shukla, R. K. (1982). Primary or team nursing? Two conditions determine the choice, *Journal of Nursing Administration, 12*(11), 12–15.
Webster's II New Riverside University Dictionary. (1984). Boston: Houghton Mifflin.

PART III

Current and Emerging Challenges

CHAPTER 11

Current and Emerging Practice Settings

Highlights

- **Emerging practice settings**
- **Economic issues**
- **The global society**
- **Political issues**
- **Ethics and the nurse executive**

The purpose of this chapter is to discuss current and emerging practice settings for nurse executives and to address some specific current issues related to economics, society, politics, ethics, and health. The professional practice of nursing administration is carried out in a variety of settings where the opportunities for leadership at all levels of administration have never been greater. Nurses have always valued the whole person and from early times stressed the importance of the wellness-illness continuum. Patient-centered care and continuity of care are not new concepts in professional nursing; thus, the sudden awareness of these concepts by other health professionals is refreshing. Professional nursing administration is practiced in many settings — in fact, wherever professional nursing is part of health care delivery. These include ambulatory, acute, home, and long-term care settings. The nurse executive is also found in consultation agencies, schools of nursing, and various government positions at the policy-making level. The 1983 Institute of Medicine Report (1983) expands the list of practice settings to include health maintenance organizations, student health services, and complex physicians' offices.

EMERGING PRACTICE SETTINGS

Recent nurse executives have discovered entrepreneurship and are starting their own businesses (Norris, 1991). These businesses range from block nursing programs, nursing centers, contract supplemental staffing agencies, child care agencies, midwifery and womens health practices, and numerous variations of home health care practices. Hospices are a natural for nurses and uniquely packaged holistic models are sprouting everywhere.

Nurse executives are taking business skills seriously and are appreciating the need to diversify as in any successful professional business. The Block Nursing Program in St. Anthony Park in St. Paul, Minnesota, is an excellent example of a nurse-managed nursing service in a noninstitutional setting through nursing practice arrangements in communities (Jamieson, 1990). The Block Nursing Program is a creative at-home service delivery model for meeting the needs of older people.

On other fronts, nurses are serving on numerous health care agency boards. Nurses are cochairs with physicians in outcome research (AHCPR, 1991). Nurses are finding expanded opportunities in the military where leadership and management skills have for a long time been integrated with clinical expertise. Nurses are preparing for travel in space, recognizing that nurses with practice are needed wherever there are people (Czerwinski, 1987; Burge & Walker, 1992).

Significant levels of work excitement have been demonstrated among Navy Nurse Corps officers across a variety of settings and levels of responsibility (Savage, Simms, Williams, & Erbin-Roesemann, 1993). Practice patterns vary widely according to mission and available resources. Advanced leadership and management roles require superior administrative skill accomplished through education and experiences. Overall results indicated that Navy nurses are excited about the elements that are the essence of Navy nursing practice: variety, leadership and management experience, and the teaching/learning component were all found to contribute to overall work excitement.

After avoiding nursing homes for years, nurses are returning to nursing homes as researchers, nurse practitioners, and clinical nursing directors. The nursing home as a rehabilitation center is offering a challenging site for nurses who seek to integrate the components of the professional nurse executive. Faculty members forced to look for clinical placements beyond acute care settings are rediscovering the nursing home as a major practice setting. Despite the high prevalence of depression among older people, few controlled studies of depression have been reported from nursing home populations (Abraham, Neundorfer, & Currie, 1992).

For inpatient settings, the wide range of opportunity for administrative practice varies from the small rural hospital to the large multihospital system. In the small rural hospital under swing bed reimbursement regulations, patients will range from acute care to intermediate care to long-term care, depending on the needs of the community (Supplitt, 1982). Such a setting requires a nurse executive with different clinical knowledge than that of the nurse executive functioning at the corporate level in a multihospital system in a large urban area.

Nurses have a unique and difficult position in correctional systems. On one hand, they are health care providers whose focus is on health care services. On the other hand, they are corrections officers monitoring security and public safety. Nurse executives have key roles in developing and managing nursing services in correctional institutions.

On the national level, Davis and colleagues (Davis, Oakley, & Sochalski, 1982) stress the need for nurse executives to enlarge their role in health policy making by increasing their potential legislative expertise and activity. Until recently, nurses have relied on a small cadre of people to influence legislative policy development. To increase nursing's effectiveness in competing for scarce resources, the number of politically active nurse executives will have to increase. Political power can best be generated by the leadership in nursing. Nurse executives are in key leadership roles to affect policy issues at the local, state, and national levels.

In the United States, as well as internationally, the determinants of health are rooted in political, social, and economic realities (Morrow, 1982). Poverty and lack of education are the outstanding inhibitors for health in the developing countries. One should not be surprised that the same factors exist to a lesser degree in the United States. Of interest to nurse executives is the result of a World Health Organization analysis of the factors that were inhibiting improvement in the health status of the world's poor populations in the 1970s. This analysis shows that increasing resources for the health sector did not improve health status for the following reasons, among many:

1. Limited national resources were largely devoted to curative, urban, hospital-based services, which were inaccessible to the rural poor.
2. The greatest need for health care was for simple, preventive and promotive services that did not require highly trained personnel with sophisticated equipment.
3. The services required participation of the people.
4. Successful attainment of an integrated approach to health care required cooperation from other sectors, for example, agriculture, public works, education, and social welfare.

An analysis of factors that inhibit improvement of the health status of the poor population of the United States would probably reveal similar, if not the same, results. Nurse executives must be knowledgeable about the economic, social and political factors that affect health care and must work to change those factors for better health care for all.

Nursing in the United States is subject to all the economic, social, and political forces that shape and change any society. The current and emerging effects on nursing of several major issues are discussed in this chapter. In analyzing the reasons for the impact of these issues on nursing, a direction emerges for anticipatory actions to be taken.

ECONOMIC ISSUES

Over the past several years, our society has been bombarded with several major economic fluxes that have contributed to major shifts in thinking about how to finance health care or, more appropriately titled, sickness care. Inflation and high unemployment have had major effects on the cost and use of health care. The idea that health care costs must be brought under control has long been discussed but has had a greater number of advocates and been the target of more actions since the economy of the United States worsened during the 1980s and early 1990s.

Economic policy and strategy changes on the federal level affect nursing in very direct ways. One change that occurred in the early 1980s was a shift in federal spending from human resources to defense. In 1982 alone, a 25 percent cut was made in public health grants to the states (Davis, 1983). A second and related major change in federal policy was the shift to a prospective reimbursement system for hospital care. This major shift in federal funding of health care has brought about significant changes.

The change in federal funding for hospital care creates an unstable economic base for acute care hospitals. Because most nurses are employed in short-term, acute care hospitals, the unstable economic base, has affected the nursing component of hospitals. In some instances, decreased hospital revenue has brought a decrease in the size of the nursing staff. For some hospitals, this has increased stress on the nursing staff, because not all hospitals were adequately staffed before prospective reimbursement.

A decrease in nursing staff and shorter lengths of stay have resulted in less patient teaching. This is a crucial issue, because patients need more teaching, not less, if they are to be discharged as early as possible. The need for continuity of care is also apparent when looking at a prospective reimbursement system. Nurses have always demonstrated concern and interest in continuity of care, but health care agencies have not always been organized to allow or encourage a continuity of care system for patients. This need alone is reason enough for nurses to become much more oriented toward working together in different settings and toward developing models for health care delivery that emphasize principles of continuity of care.

An unstable economic base for acute care hospitals has resulted in their diversifying, that is, broadening their mix of products or services. This diversification is coming about because of the need for more income, because the demand for inpatient care is growing very slowly and hospitals are under pressure to contain and reduce their costs (Goldsmith, 1982). Thus, acute care hospitals are seeking ways to decrease their dependence on patient care revenue. A hospital with less dependence on patient-related revenue is on a sounder financial base because it does not have to cut services when major third-party payers withdraw support (Kernaghan, 1982). In the future, hospitals will face even more financial pressures as they experience an increase in the acuity level of patients while third-party payers will step up efforts to contain hospital costs (Goldsmith, 1982).

Some examples of diversification that hospitals have already undertaken include buying and operating apartment buildings; making other real estate investments; manufacturing hospital linens; leasing hospital space to nonhealth businesses, such as banks and fast food restaurants; and operating restaurants (Kernaghan, 1982). Although diversification into areas where the hospital lacks expertise is not recommended, there are numerous areas in which hospitals have not made use of the expertise on the staff, for example, expansion of ambulatory nutritional services for older people (Goldsmith, 1982). Diversification is a process in which the nurse executive should be involved in planning and developing areas for the expansion of nursing services. For example, classes for ambulatory patients and community members can provide nurses with creative practice opportunities as well as increase hospital revenue.

Home health care is an important area of diversification for hospitals and one in which nursing should play a major role. The importance of home health care for hospitals lies in the strategy of extending the hospital's sphere of influence to activities that may lead patients to seek hospital services in the future. "By linking both prehospital and posthospital services to the traditional inpatient services of a hospital, hospitals not only are meeting new community needs but also are securing control over their inpatient utilization by 'organizing' both entry and exit from the hospital" (Goldsmith, 1982, p. 70). In addition, hospitals will have difficulty internally financing capital needs, with cost-containment measures being implemented. As a result, hospitals are looking to less capital-intensive investments, such as home health care programs.

In developing home health care programs, the nurse executive should take the lead in part of the planning process. Nursing has the expertise to determine patient needs; to determine the type and mix of staff; and to hire, orient, and provide staff development for the home health care staff. Although a nurse executive who is knowledgeable in home health care should be hired to head the service, the nurse executive of an affiliated inpatient service should continue to support and be appropriately involved in planning activities.

Another major economic issue for nursing is that of third-party reimbursement for nursing services. In the late 1970s, nursing organizations began working to have state legislation introduced and passed to require health insurers to directly reimburse nurses for services provided. As of mid-1983, 14 states had passed laws mandating third-party reimbursement for registered nurses or specific nurse groups, such as nurse midwives, nurse practitioners, nurse anesthetists, and psychiatric nurse specialists (LaBar, 1983). With prospective reimbursement and pressure from the nursing profession for nursing services to be separated from room and board, third-party reimbursement for inpatient ambulatory and home nursing services is becoming a reality in all states.

What changes for nurse executives will occur with third-party reimbursement for nursing services? A greater knowledge of revenue forecasting, budgeting, and budget monitoring will be necessary as the fiscal systems become more complex. The nurse executive requires such knowledge, not to perform calculations, but to work with the financial management staff of the health care facility. Nursing has rarely been made accountable for delivering a specific amount of services, except perhaps in such agencies as visiting nurse associations. The ability to accurately predict revenue is still not well established for nursing services. In the future, this will become important to hospitals and other agencies that may have decreased revenue bases and shrinking patient numbers.

Understanding that nursing is a business as well as a professional practice has opened the doors to diversification. In former times, nurses have resisted business skills, particularly financial, hoping to achieve economic gains through bargaining units alone. The acquisition of management expertise along with a research passion has created unlimited possibilities for nursing businesses as intrepreneurships within existing health care systems and free-standing newly designed entrepreneurships.

Business language has entered nursing vocabulary and nursing schools are introducing components of a business plan in both leadership and clinical management courses. The cost consciousness of today's health care industry demands that nurses function as business people with skills in developing successful plans for building new product lines and expanding current nursing programs (Johnson, 1990; Vaiana, 1990). These new programs usually bring about new roles and new settings for practice.

THE GLOBAL SOCIETY

The shift to a global society has led to a massive change in thinking about "who does what" in health care. The old barriers between nurses and physicians are crumbling as the world moves towards the goal of "Health for All by the Year 2000." There is increasing interest by the public and by many health care providers to enact a universal access patient-centered health plan for the more than 60 million Americans who are now without insurance benefits (Weil, 1992). Grasping the concept of uninsured in America has led to a better understanding of the world populations who are without basic subsistence health care.

The "Health for All" agenda emerged in 1977 at the World Health Assembly (WHO). It was decided at that meeting that the main social target of governments and of WHO should be the attainment by all people of the world by the year 2000 a level of health that permits them to live socially and economically productive lives (Little, 1992). In 1978, the WHO and UNICEF adopted and published the now famous Declaration of Alma-Ata and further stated "An acceptable level for all the people of the world by the year 2000 can be attained through a fuller and better use of the world's resources, a considerable part of which is now spent on armaments and military conflicts" (Little, 1992). In 1981, the World Health Assembly unanimously adopted a "Global Strategy for All by the Year 2000."

Physicians in America are responding rapidly to the challenge. Rather than the oversupply of physicians predicted by Ginzberg (1981), the United States now faces a shortage of primary care physicians. Medical schools are changing curricula to emphasize preparation of the general practitioner who can serve in primary care and family practice. Nursing is in a unique position to respond to the challenge by restructuring educational programs in nursing schools. Management and clinical programs that can be blended are already in place awaiting the redesign that will be responsive to "Health for All."

Computerized information systems will allow nurses and physicians to collaborate in newly designed centers of care that can reach human beings from all walks of life and social levels. These are exciting times in nursing. National nursing organizations are working closely together and the relationship with the International Council of Nurses (ICN) is excellent. In the new age, however, nurses must work closely with physicians and other health care providers in flexible work groups with transdisciplinary patient-centered goals. The need for executive and primary care skills for nurses and physicians has never been greater.

POLITICAL ISSUES

In addition to the opposition that will come from physicians for expanded nursing roles in nursing practice acts, there may be attempts to introduce legislation to restrict the role of nurses so that physicians will have more opportunity to expand their roles into areas of health promotion and prevention. In one past difficult economic period, the Great Depression, the American Academy of Pediatrics promoted the expanded role of the physician in well-child supervision. In the Division of Child Hygiene of the Board of Health of the City of Newark, the number of physicians was doubled during this time period even though the effectiveness of nurses in reducing infant mortality had been demonstrated in that agency since 1913 (DeMaio, 1981).

The nurse executive must be alert and attuned to factors in the society and political environment that would result in inappropriate constriction of nursing practice. Being involved in the American Nurses Association and in specialty nursing organizations, such as the American Organization of Nurse Executives and multidisciplinary organizations, is one of the best avenues for receiving information about legislative and political issues.

The increase in the number of physician specialists may have some other long-term effects if the number of nurses is reduced in health care agencies. As pointed out in a study by Miller and Stokes (1978), the only health resource that has made an apparent difference in infant mortality and age-sex adjusted death rates was the increase in nurses per capita. As other health service resources increased, such as hospital facilities and physicians, either no effect occurred or mortality rates increased. Nursing needs to continue to conduct studies to document such relationships and to gain greater publicity of such studies. The nurse executive is continuously challenged to have such data to present when planning and decisions are to be made about use of resources within the health care agency.

Two other topics that are in the political arena are nurse-managed or community nursing centers and national health insurance. The concept of the community nursing center was introduced on the national level in the form of legislation that would allow the delivery of reimbursable nursing services to appropriate unserved or underserved populations. This mechanism would allow patient populations direct access to nursing services without the use of an intermediary, such as a physician. The centers would provide out-of-hospital services consistent with provisions of the state licensing authority. Although the idea of nurse-managed centers is not new, there were few operating in the United States in 1983 (Lang, 1983). The number of centers is increasing. Nurse executives are needed to assist in the development and operation of more community nursing centers, as well as to be active in the legislative process that will create part of the financial base on which the centers will operate. These new centers include sleep disorder, eating disorder, pain control, and birthing centers (Smith, 1988).

National health insurance has been discussed in the United States since at least the 1920s, but serious activity to adopt a national health insurance plan or system has been absent until recent years. Over a decade ago, several plans introduced in congress covered a variety of funding possibilities as well as benefits. However, there were criticisms of all plans that did not adequately address three major health care issues: distribution of health resources, quality of care, and cost control. What might be the effects on nursing and nursing services of a national health insurance plan? The nurse executive must become aware of the potential effects of a national health insurance plan on nursing service and become involved in forums to inform nurses about the advantages and disadvantages of such a plan.

American nurses have endorsed Nursing's Agenda For Health Care Reform (ANA, 1992), a unique plan for creating a health care system that assures access, quality, and services at affordable costs. The approach, now endorsed by most nursing organizations, calls for a restructured health care system that will focus on consumers and their health, with services to be delivered in familiar, convenient sites, such as schools, workplaces, and homes. The basic components of the restructured care system include:

A restructured health care system that enhances consumer access, fosters consumer responsibility for personal health and self-care, and facilitates utilization of the most cost-effective providers and therapeutic options.

A federally defined standard package of essential health care services available to all citizens and residents of the United States.

A phase-in of essential services especially for women and children.

Planned change to anticipate health service needs that correlate with changing national demographics.

Steps to reduce health care costs.

Case management for those with continuing health care needs.

Provisions for long-term care.

Insurance reforms to assure improved access to care.

Access to services assured by no payment at the point of service.

Establishment of public/private sector review.

Nursing is uniquely postured to participate fully in such a restructured health care system.

HEALTH PROMOTION AND DISEASE PREVENTION

Florence Nightingale established the importance for nursing of health promotion and disease prevention with her emphasis on the restoration and preservation of health and the prevention of disease. She identified that the basic principles inherent in nursing and health are the same (Chaska, 1990).

Today, the concepts of health promotion and disease prevention are equally, if not more, important, because many diseases and conditions result from life-style or behavior, for example, smoking, alcoholism, and malnutrition. To continue to extend the life span, science and health care must concentrate on how to facilitate life-style changes and prevent disability. This rationale is part of the basis for the increased interest in these areas of health care. However, the interest is not totally altruistic, being also related to the desires of health care agencies to increase their revenue levels and sources.

Although many programs and services are directed toward health promotion and disease prevention, these terms have not been clearly defined or consistently used. In general, the concept of health promotion is health care aimed at growth and improvement in well-being. Disease prevention is a separate concept and refers to health care provided to protect from or defend against disease (Brubaker, 1983).

Until recently, health promotion and disease prevention have been a small segment of the health care industry. However, current economic factors and price competition are directly affecting the development of services based on these concepts, primarily under ambulatory care. Gilbert (1983) defines ambulatory care facilities and organizations as those that provide home health care, outpatient rehabilitation and therapy, preventive health and fitness, hospice, diagnostic, and therapeutic services on an outpatient basis. The importance of the relationship between health promotion and ambulatory care is based partially on the following:

1. New technologies that increase the possibility of giving care on an outpatient basis;
2. Insurance coverage expanded to include ambulatory care;
3. Reimbursement based on cost efficiency and the resultant encouragement for hospitals to use less costly alternatives; and
4. Private entrepreneurs opening ambulatory care facilities. (Gilbert, 1983)

For the nurse executive, knowledge of the concepts of health promotion and disease prevention will become more important as increased emphasis is placed on developing new programs in these areas. Because these are areas of nursing expertise, nurses should be included in key positions in implementing the new and expanded programs of health promotion and disease prevention. Although there will be competition with nursing for positions in new programs, nurse executives can be prepared to present sound rationale for why nurses are best employed in many of the positions where one-to-one counseling and group guidance are provided, for example:

1. Nurses are knowledgeable about health and illness so they can make appropriate assessments and referrals of presumably well individuals.
2. Nurses use a comprehensive view of clients and thus can be more effective.
3. Nurses are cost effective because they can function in various phases of health promotion and disease prevention.

Although health promotion and disease prevention have been integral parts of nursing, practice environments have not always encouraged or allowed nurses to adequately include the concepts in their practice, except perhaps in public health nursing. Current practice settings, especially acute care settings, may not have the resources for or goal of implementing health promotion but could increase the content of disease prevention in the practice of nurses through small projects. For example, discharged patients with familiar histories of specific diseases could be given literature or referrals to appropriate counseling agencies, or an injury prevention program could be developed and implemented for both patients and employees. These examples also contribute to increasing the implementation of the concept of continuity of care, which should be a part of all nursing services.

CONTINUITY OF CARE

Continuity of care means that care is provided throughout time, from setting to setting and across the wellness-illness continuum. The concept of continuity of care also encompasses the goal of coordinated and uninterrupted services as well as comprehensive care, including health promotion, disease prevention, health maintenance, acute care, rehabilitation, custodial care, and terminal care. The major thrust of continuity of care is prevention, whether it is prevention of chronic disease through health promotion programs or prevention of rehospitalization (Bealty, 1980). Much of the earlier emphasis of continuity of care was on referral from the hospital to public health nursing or visiting nurses. The thrust is now included in the process of discharge planning that was mandated in 1972 Medicare and Medicaid amendments (Public Law 92-603) for hospitals, skilled nursing facilities, and home health agencies (Crittenden, 1983). Although discharge planning has been a component of quality nursing care and continuity of care, inpatient settings may still not be organized to consistently meet the patient's and family's needs on discharge. A renewed interest in continuity of care has resulted from several changes in society and the health care field.

A monumental increase in the number of older people has created what Somers (1983) describes as the geriatric imperative. This imperative has created new health care problems that demand health care policies that recognize prevention of disease and postponing or controlling chronic conditions. Maintaining quality of life in the later years is dependent on the availability of ambulatory, acute, and long-term care services.

The total number of community hospitals is expected to shrink from about 6,000 to 5,000, and of the remaining number, 55 to 60 percent are expected to join multiinstitutional arrangements (Somers, 1983). Multihospital arrangements can be horizontal models linking two or more hospitals or vertical models linking a hospital with one or more institutions of different levels, for example, a nursing home, health maintenance organization, hospice, or home care program.

Thus, the geriatric and cost-containment imperatives of the 1980s have greatly contributed to the new emphasis in hospital administration and the health care industry in general on functional independence rather than cure. Prevention of disease is emphasized at all ages, and patient education programs and departments have become part of many hospital-based human resources departments. In addition, there is common agreement among health professionals that public financing should be impartially distributed among diverse services rather than primarily to acute care. This will involve transfer of some resources from acute care to primary and long-term care.

The goal of functional independence, rather than cure, for patients demands a change in thinking on the part of health professionals. Continuity of care and discharge planning are processes, not end points. Both processes involve the patient and a team of individuals from various disciplines working together to facilitate the transition of the patient from one environment to another (McKeehan, 1981). These environments are usually hospitals, nursing homes, or the patient's home.

Because patient participation is a cardinal principle of continuity of care, the concept of self-care is fitting for incorporation into a nursing practice setting. By embracing the self-care framework, nursing is able to focus attention on assisting patients in self-care practices and on increasing self-care abilities through education. Orem (1991) stresses the importance of human agency and self-care agency. Human agency is the knowledge, power, or ability of a person to act, including cognitive knowledge, affective feelings, and psychomotor development. Self-care agency is the ability of a person to initiate and perform health activities for himself or herself in maintaining life, health, and well-being.

Levin (1981) has become one of the most outspoken proponents of self-care in this decade. Health professionals, according to Levin, are so rarely willing to trust people to make decisions about their own health that they have developed a negative view of people's roles in health. The health establishment has encouraged the growth of a "serviced society" in which health professionals seek to provide a service for every need and to stimulate a need for every service. Health services have emerged as an industry with values, operational styles, and plans for expansion like any other industry. A recent rise in public awareness of the limits of resources in health has added to the interest in self-care. Self-care is certainly part of continuity of care, wherein people function on their own behalf in health promotion and disease prevention in such roles as health maintenance, self-diagnosis, self-medication and self-treatment, and participation in professional care. These roles are carried out in collaboration with health professionals. Nursing services can contribute to the enhancement of self-care roles for patients as part of implementing the concept of continuity of care.

ETHICS AND THE NURSE EXECUTIVE

Nursing is in transition (National Commission on Nursing, 1982) and rapidly undergoing change. Technological advances, changing attitudes of patients and health care professionals, government regulations, and other internal and external pressures are creating changes that cannot be ignored within the profession. Computers, CAT scanners, and invasive techniques that require extensive medical care are coupled with nuclear energy possibilities to create an environment the world has never seen. The nuclear revolution is here, and the benefits for changing the work of the nurse are as dramatic as those of electricity in rural America.

Nursing will have time to be creative, time to evaluate ethical issues, time to consider the quality of life. Work in institutions will be done differently, and more people will be able to spend less time in acute care. More nursing time and expertise will be spent in home care, ambulatory care, health education, and health promotion.

Nurse executives will evolve a vision of nursing within a total health perspective. As technology has become increasingly advanced and as nursing has changed, ethical issues have been raised about life and death and the quality of life and death. Nurse executives also continue to face such ethical dilemmas as unethical behavior of professionals, withholding information from patients, and employee insubordination because of conscience. Rapid technological developments and financial constraints have made ethics a major concern of all health service administrators.

According to Westbury, "Ethics is the application of a person's values in decision situations. These values are derived from the individual's total life experience, including family upbringing, religious training, education, social contacts, employment experiences, and other influences" (1983, p. 7). Health care ethics are ethics applied to the health sciences. Health care ethics concern what is right or wrong or what ought to be done in a health science or care situation that requires a moral decision. Four areas are addressed by health care ethics: *(1)* clinical, *(2)* allocation of scarce resources, *(3)* human experimentation, and *(4)* health policy. The purpose of health care ethics is to provide approaches for systematically reasoning through an ethical dilemma that arises when moral claims conflict. A dilemma may be viewed as *(1)* a difficult problem that seems to have no satisfactory solution or *(2)* a situation involving a choice between equally undesirable alternatives (Westbury, 1983).

When is it appropriate to stop treating certain individuals as if we had a particular set of ethical and legal duties toward them? Veatch (1983) describes this dilemma as a debate over the "social system of death behavior." As health care settings become more sophisticated in stretching out the death process, nurses are faced with more and more patients whose hearts are beating but whose brains are dead. They are, in fact, cadavers. However, deciding to call a body dying or dead is essentially making a moral, legal, or political decision about how a body should be treated. There are important questions about shifting from acute curative care to comfort hospice care and where this care should be provided.

Nurse executives do now and will continue to serve on ethics and hospice committees wherein decisions are made about death and life. When is a fetus alive, and when is a body dead? There may be no single point at which death occurs. We may decide to remove organs for transplant when the brain is destroyed, read the will when the heart stops, and begin mourning at some other point (Veatch, 1983).

The issue of defining death is only one issue encountered in balancing knowledge from the sciences with ethical decision making. Although ethics will not provide instant solutions for complex moral-technical problems, ethics does provide frameworks for dealing with ethical dilemmas and issues (Benoliel, 1983).

DEALING WITH ETHICAL DILEMMAS

In dealing with ethical dilemmas or assisting nursing staff with them, the nurse executive can turn to some general sources of information and direction. The American Nurses Association Code for Nurses (1985) provides a basis for self-regulation in nursing. The requirements of the code can serve as one resource in dealing with questions of unethical behavior of registered nurses. The American Hospital Association Bill of Rights (1970) is not an ethical code but could provide useful information for discussions about ethical dilemmas. Other sources of direction may be found in the approaches suggested by Mamana (1983):

1. Peer review mechanisms using quality assurance committees;
2. Controls on health care technology by institutions, for example, the prohibition of heart transplants;
3. Hospital ethics committees to review new and existing technologies and their impact on humans;
4. Rationing system for resources controlled by federal or local health planning agencies.

Making decisions or choices of an ethical nature can be facilitated by using the following questions:

1. What has been learned or could be learned from the past that is relevant to this situation?
2. What do conscience and common sense demand in the present situation? In this dilemma, what makes sense for everyone involved?
3. What are the probable future consequences of each action? (Davis and Aroskar, 1983)

In addition to facilitating the discussion of these questions, the nurse executive should have knowledge of ethics so as to bring a broad base of thinking to the resolution of ethical dilemmas.

Some ethical dilemmas can be addressed before a crisis arises, for example, dealing with "do not resuscitate" orders. The nurse executive is in a key position to facilitate the establishment of a mechanism to resolve this kind of clinical dilemma. When a mechanism is in place, the nurse executive has the responsibility to monitor the effectiveness of the mechanism, for example, a committee, a panel of experts, or legal counsel. Another key responsibility of the nurse executive is to facilitate the establishment of a support system for nurses who deal with ethical dilemmas as daily routine. The support system may include such mechanisms as informal discussion groups led by a nurse ethicist or other knowledgeable professional, individual or group counseling provided by a mental health professional, and staff development programs and consultation provided by a clinical nursing specialist with knowledge of ethics.

Another mechanism to assist nursing staff in dealing with ethical dilemmas is the use of ethics rounds, in which the clinical aspects of a case study are the basis for an organized discussion of the ethical dilemma and possible solutions. Hypothetical cases, case histories, or cases under care may be used for ethics rounds. Because the purpose of ethics rounds is to reason through a case study ethically, the leader must be a knowledgeable nurse executive, clinical specialist, or someone from another field, such as philosophy or religion (Davis, 1982).

Whatever mechanisms are established for the nursing division to deal with ethical dilemmas, the nurse executive must demonstrate concern and caring for the nursing staff by listening to their concerns, working with them and others to solve the ethical dilemmas, and being an advocate for quality patient care.

Summary

In current and emerging practice settings, many economic, social, and political issues affect nursing. Major economic issues include federal economic policy, the economic base of acute care hospitals, and third-party reimbursement for nursing. Social issues include the structure of physician employment and the increase in the number of physicians. Political issues include constriction of nursing roles, decrease in the numbers of nursing staff, community nursing centers, and national health insurance.

Health promotion, disease prevention, and continuity of care have assumed new importance in health care due to price competition and economic factors. Nursing administration has key roles to play in planning and implementing services in all three of these areas.

Knowledge of ethics is essential for the nurse executive dealing with the four areas of health care ethics: *(1)* clinical, *(2)* allocation of scarce resources, *(3)* human experimentation, and *(4)* health policy. Mechanisms for dealing with ethical dilemmas and supporting staff include a decision process, informal discussion groups, counseling, staff development programs, consultation, and ethics rounds.

STUDY QUESTIONS

1. Describe some entrepreneurial settings in which nursing administration is and will be practiced.
2. Discuss the impact, actual or potential, on nursing of one economic, one social, and one political issue.
3. How do health promotion and disease prevention differ?
4. Define continuity of care.
5. Why is it important for a nurse executive to be knowledgeable about ethics?
6. How do currently legislated advance directives assist the nurse executive in ethical decision making?

References

Abraham, I., Neundorfer, M. M., & Currie, L. (1992). Effects of group interventions on cognition and depression in nursing home residents. *Nursing Research, 41*(4), 196–202.

Agency for Health Care Policy and Research (1991, May). *Outcomes of Health Care Services and Procedures.* (AHCPR #91-0004). Washington, DC: U.S. Government Printing Office.

American Hospital Association. (1970). *Patient's bill of rights.* Chicago: American Hospital Association.

American Nurses Association. (1985). *Code for nurses with interpretive statements.* Kansas City, MO: American Nurses Association.

Bealty, S. R. (Ed.). (1980). *Continuity of care: The hospital and the community.* New York: Grune & Stratton.

Benoliel, J. Q. (1983). Ethics in nursing practice and education. *Nursing Outlook, 31*(4), 210–215.

Brubaker, B. H. (1983). Health promotion: A linguistic analysis, *Advances in Nursing Science, 5*(3), 1–14.

Burge, J., & Walker, G. (1992, April 2–4). *Nursing and space life sciences: Preparing for living and working in space.* Third National Conference on Nursing and Space Life Sciences. Conference Curriculum. Huntsville, AL: College of Nursing.

Chaska, N. L. (1990). *The nursing profession: A time to speak.* New York: McGraw-Hill.

Crittenden, F. J. (1983). *Discharge planning for health care facilities.* Bowie, MD: Brady.

Czerwinski, B. (1987, June). Feminine hygiene in space. Sexuality and the menstrual cycle: Clinical and sociocultural implications. Seventh Conference of the Society for Menstrual Cycle Research. Ann Arbor: University of Michigan.

Davis, A. J. (1982). Helping staff address ethical dilemmas, *Journal of Nursing Administration, 12*(2), 9–13.

Davis, A. J., & Aroskar, M. A. (1983). *Ethical dilemmas and nursing practice* (2nd ed.). Norwalk, CT: Appleton-Century-Crofts.

Davis, C. K. (1983). Nursing and the health care debates, *Image: The Journal of Nursing Scholarship, 15*(3), 67.

Davis, C. K., Oakley, D., & Sochalski, J. A. (1982). Leadership for expanding nursing influence on health policy, *Journal of Nursing Administration, 12*(1), 15–21.

DeMaio, D. J. (1981). Health services for children: A descriptive analysis of an urban program. In L. H. Aiken (Ed.), *Health Policy and Nursing Practice.* Kansas City, MO: American Academy of Nursing.

Gilbert, R. N. (1983). Competition spurs ambulatory choice, *Hospitals, 57*(10), 67–68.

Ginzberg, E. (1981). The economics of health care and the future of nursing, *Journal of Nursing Administration, 11*(3), 28–32.

Goldsmith, J. (1982). Diversification: Broadening hospital services: What makes sense? *Hospitals, 56*(23), 68, 70–73.

Institute of Medicine. (1983). *Nursing and nursing education: Public policies and private actions.* Washington, DC: National Academy Press.

Jamieson, M. K. (1990). Block nursing: Practicing autonomous professional nursing in the community, *Nursing and Health Care, 11*(5), 250–253.

Johnson, J. E. (1990). Developing an effective business plan, *Nursing Economics, 8*(3), 152–154.

Kernaghan, S. G. (1982). Nontraditional revenue: Diversification for profit, *Hospitals, 56*(23), 75, 78–81.

LaBar, C. (1983). *Third-party reimbursement legislation for services of nurses: A report of changes in state health insurance laws.* Kansas City, MO: American Nurses Association.

Lang, N. M. (1983). Nurse-managed centers: Will they thrive? *American Journal of Nursing, 83*(9), 1290–1293.

Levin, L. S. (1981). Self-care in health: Potentials and pitfalls, *World Health Forum, 2*(2), 177–184.

Little, C. (1992). Health for all by the year 2000. Where is it now? *Nursing and Health Care, 13*(4), 198–201.

Mamana, J. P. (1983). Ethics and medical technology, *Michigan Hospitals, 19*(4), 11–13.

McKeehan, K. M. (1981). Conceptual framework for discharge planning. In K. M. McKeehan (Ed.). *Continuing Care.* St. Louis: Mosby.

Miller, M. K., & Stokes, C. S. (1978). Health status, health resources, and consolidated structural parameters: Implications for public health care policy, *Journal of Health and Social Behavior, 19*(3), 263–279.

Morrow, H. (1982). The fundamental influence of political, social, and economic factors on health and health care, *International Nursing Review, 29*(6), 183–186.

National Commission on Nursing. (1982). *Nursing in transition: Models for successful organizational change.* Chicago: American Hospital Association.

Norris, D. (1991). *How I became a nurse entrepreneur: Tales from 50 nurses in business.* Petaluma, CA: National Nurses in Business Association.

Nursing's Agenda for Health Care Reform. (1992). PR-3 220M 6/91. Kansas City, MO: American Nurses Association.

Orem, D. E. (1991). *Nursing: Concepts of practice* (4th ed.). New York: McGraw-Hill.

Savage, S., Simms, L. M., Williams, R., & Erbin-Roesemann, M. A. (1993). Discovering work excitement among navy nurses, *Nursing Economics, 11*(3), 153–161.

Smith, G. R. (1988). The evolution of alternative delivery systems: What will be nursing's role? *Nursing practice in the 21st century.* Kansas City, MO: American Nurses Foundation.

Somers, A. R. (1983). The geriatric imperative, *Hospitals, 59*(9), 77–81.

Supplitt, J. T. (1982). Swing beds, *Hospitals, 56*(22), 67–72.

Vaiana, D. A. (1990). Sample business plan: A laser section business plan, *Nursing Economics, 8*(3), 155–171.

Veatch, R. M. (1983). Definitions of life and death: Should there be a consistency? In M. W. Shaw & A. E. Doudera (Eds.), *Defining Human Life.* Ann Arbor, MI: Health Administration Press.

Weil, T. P. (1992). A universal access plan: A step toward national health insurance, *Hospital and Health Services Administration, 37*(1), 37–51.

Westbury, S. A. (1983). Ethics and hospital decision making, *Michigan Hospitals, 19*(4), 11–13.

CHAPTER 12

Developing Human Potential

Highlights

- **The power of education**
- **Changing behavior**
- **Motivation**
- **Humans becoming**
- **Developing leaders and followers**

The purpose of this chapter is to examine the concept of human potential and to present methodologies for creating an organizational climate in which that human potential can develop. Nowhere in the world of nursing is it more possible to influence the growth and development of other nurses than in nursing administration. The nurse executive creates an environment in which professional practice can flourish or deteriorate. This chapter focuses on human potential as an important concept in nursing administration. Inner-directed individuals who are highly self-motivated will produce the answers to the problems of productivity and dissatisfaction within nursing staff.

HUMAN POTENTIAL AND THE POWER OF EDUCATION

Nurses today want to be recognized as professionals. They want to be recognized for their contributions to patient care, and they want the right to control their professional practice within the limits of the law. Unquestionably, these rights always involve maximizing human potential. Human potential means all of one's potentialities: knowledge, talents, capacities, creativity, wisdom, character, and genetic makeup.

The acquisition of technical skill alone does not provide the necessary base for the independent thinking and action essential in today's nursing practice. Men and women have a great deal of unrealized potential, and helping staff discover that potential can be one of the most exhilarating experiences for the nurse executive.

The identification of needs for growth, development, and utilization of potential is an important part of Maslow's self-actualization. This concept was introduced in Chapter 5, "The Person in the Role of Nurse Executive." The fully functioning administrator encourages the development of human potential in self, peers, and subordinates. Optimal biopsychosocial functioning, so carefully nurtured in patients, needs also to be nurtured in oneself and one's fellow workers.

Howard McClusky (1974) had a passionate belief in the power of education to improve the condition of people's lives and to liberate them from the meanness of intolerance and self-interest. Lifelong learning and the fulfillment of growth needs are indeed powerful tools in enhancing human potential. Lifelong learning can help individuals become the persons they are best able to become. In most people, there is a large domain of unexpressed and underexpressed talent that could be developed through educative means.

McClusky (1974) further theorized that failure to internalize the learner role as a central feature of the self is a major restraint in the adult's achievement of his or her potential. Studying, learning, and intellectual adventure must become part of one's life in both work and social environments.

Striving to learn about employees and matching them with educational and work experiences can be one of the nurse executive's most stimulating and rewarding challenges. Because the power of education lies both in learning and in teaching abilities, the administrator needs to be a learner as well as a teacher. Satisfaction with work and assumption of responsibility for professional behavior flourish in an environment that fosters maximizing human potential through continued learning.

CHANGING BEHAVIOR

The role of the nurse executive as a teacher has been largely unrecognized. In fact, in their efforts to stay away from educational roles, many administrators may lose sight of the fact that most education occurs in noncredit or nonformal learning environments. Achieving one's maximum potential involves learning new behaviors. Many administrators spend a great deal of time teaching others how to perform assigned tasks rather than delegating the responsibility for those tasks. How much better it would be to teach individuals how to approach tasks so that they can grow and develop while unleashing their own creativity in resolving problems that contribute to the need for the assigned tasks. Understanding the logic and rationale behind various administrative strategies encourages the learner to have positive feelings toward the ongoing project; as a result, the learner is less likely to resent and thus negatively influence change.

Pritchard (1975) suggests that the individual who has been a successful teacher in nursing can also be successful in administration. The same fundamental principles apply to both areas. Administrative leadership inspires, encourages innovations, assists the nurse in the self-actualizing process, and promotes and facilitates excellent nursing practice. To teach is also to inspire, to encourage creative effort, and to foster the full potential of the individual. Both teaching and administration require the same basic principles for implementation: planning, organizing, leading, and evaluating.

Nurse executives may perceive themselves as preceptors or mentors. These roles are in essence teaching-learning roles. Within these roles, nurse executives can open new doors to the intellectual experiences that favor creativity and productivity. Staff nurses throughout the country have become increasingly critical of administration. Frequently, one criticizes and belittles what one does not understand. One administrative imperative is to plan to change behavior in the desired direction while recognizing the need to maximize staff potential that will allow everyone to move forward together. The importance of the teaching-learning responsibilities of the nurse executive has been supported in research by Pfoutz, Simms, and Price (1987).

MOTIVATION

Motivation is an internal force that incites a person to action; what motivates one person will not necessarily excite another. According to Herzberg's (Herzberg, Mausner, & Snyderman, 1959) research, rewards can be listed under two broad categories: hygienes, or extrinsic factors, and motivators, or intrinsic factors. The hygienes include:

1. Company policy and administration.
2. Supervision.
3. Relationships with supervision.
4. Work conditions.
5. Salary.
6. Relationship with peers.
7. Personal life.
8. Relationships with subordinates.
9. Status.
10. Security.

The motivators include:

1. Achievement.
2. Recognition.
3. Work itself.
4. Responsibility.
5. Advancement.
6. Growth.

If managers want to develop a highly motivated staff, says Herzberg, they should focus on the true initiators of action: the motivators, or intrinsic factors. These intrinsic factors are in keeping with the human need theory of Abraham Maslow (1962), which postulates that humans have the need to grow and develop beyond basic coping needs. A satisfied need does not motivate. If all basic and safety needs are met, one can move on to meeting belonging needs and so on up the ladder. Self-actualization needs are never fully met, and by definition, self-actualization is a self-perpetuating, ongoing, and never finished process.

The work of David McClelland (1961) must also be recognized as an important landmark in the field of motivation. He states that, to one degree or another, there are three basic human needs in all individuals:

- Achievement: the need to excel, to achieve in relation to a set of standards, to strive, to succeed
- Power: the need to make others behave in a way they would not have behaved otherwise
- Affiliation: the desire for friendly and close relationship

The nurse executive needs to recognize which needs are dominant in employees. To determine which needs are present, several approaches may be used. One tool is a questionnaire that incorporates questions about employee benefits, clinical career ladders, and promotion opportunities. Another approach could be part of the annual objective-setting process. Employees could be asked to write objectives related to goals they want to achieve in the coming year. Some of these objectives should be directed toward the employees' professional growth, for example, completing a B.S.N. to be eligible for promotion.

While some individuals are motivated by the need to exercise power, others are motivated by the need to achieve. The nurse executive's challenge is to find avenues for these needs to be met. There is also a strong need in staff nurses for affiliation. Some observers suggest this motivation as the major reason why many more young women than men enter nursing.

Expectancy theory suggests that the strength of a tendency to action in a certain way is dependent on the strength of an expectation that an act will be followed by an attractive outcome (Vroom, 1964; Robbins, 1980). Attractiveness, performance-reward linkage, and effort-performing linkage are the key variables in this approach to developing human potential. Attractiveness is determined by what one would like to have, such as a promotion or merit increase. Performance-reward linkage is the individual's perception that certain actions will lead to a desired reward. Effort-performing linkage is the perception that a desired reward, such as a raise, is worth the effort to achieve.

Expectancy theory also presupposes the importance of intrinsic factors. The theory holds that workers attempt to complete jobs they know can be accomplished and expend energy on those that will result in personal benefit. In the world of nursing, however, employees may not consider many activities, such as care plans and patient classification systems, to be meaningful activities; thus, the question arises as to how one chooses meaningful activities that also meet the goals of the nurse executive to provide excellent nursing care.

Deci's theory (Deci, 1975) highlights the concept of competence as a strong motivator. Elaborating on Herzberg's work, Deci describes intrinsic motives as informing those activities for which there is no apparent reward. Most people will actively look for stimulation in their work. When there is overstimulation, the individual withdraws and seeks another area of competence. Understimulation results in less than minimal competency. The skillful administrator seeks an environment balanced between overstimulation and understimulation.

Overstimulation can result from the occurrence of numerous clinical projects and changes at one time. Because staff need time to incorporate changes into their functioning, three or four changes attempted at the same time may result in very little lasting change. Also, staff may feel guilty if they neglect their usual tasks for innovative endeavors.

Understimulation can be the result of an environment of no changes or of rigidity. At times, staff require a period of time to become comfortable with changes, but this must not continue indefinitely. A situation of heavy work loads and understaffing can also result in understimulation because staff are forced to give up the challenging tasks — for example, patient teaching, patient care conferences, and committee work — to meet minimal patient needs.

Having staff involved in setting objectives can contribute to arriving at a balanced environment. However, staff may tend to overestimate the amount of work and underestimate the amount of time required to accomplish objectives. Trial and error are sometimes important learning tools as a group of staff struggle to put a new clinical concept into place.

Another useful concept in developing human potential is found in the classic work in operant conditioning conducted by B. F. Skinner (1953). The classic operant conditioning process is portrayed as:

Stimulus ⟶ response ⟶ consequences ⟶ future response to stimulation

Skinner's theory focuses on four variables: positive reinforcement, extinction, punishment, and avoidance learning. This theory provides guidelines for rewarding desirable behavior and for punishment as a negative reinforcer designed to stop negative behavior. The principles of reinforcement theory can be used to modify behavior in a desired direction. For example, consider the case of a nurse executive who wants to have the staff conduct group patient teaching sessions but none of the staff has enough confidence to volunteer. In such a situation, staff could be reinforced for learning and practicing skills that would lead to conducting group sessions.

Worker motivation appears to be a key factor influencing productivity and quality of employee performance. Gordon (1982) takes issue with motivation theorists who stress the responsibility of leaders and managers to motivate followers or subordinates. Gordon maintains that people have their own motives. The responsibility of the nurse executive is to provide a motivating environment in which people can carry on the work of the organization. A motivating environment is one that provides opportunities for personnel to *(1)* express and satisfy their own motives and *(2)* contribute to the achievement of organizational goals.

A nonmotivating environment produces disillusionment, job dissatisfaction, and role conflict. Role theory is structured on the observable fact that there are prescribed relationships and activities for specified roles; for example, a traffic police officer is expected to direct traffic, and a secretary is expected to type the boss's letters. There is little agreement in our society as to the expectations for the role of a nurse. An ambiguous role, coupled with an abundance of diverse job descriptions, compounds the problem and interferes with the maximum development of potential.

Today's mobile, intelligent, aggressive, and talented nurses need leaders who can help them identify personal and professional goals. They need administrators with enthusiasm, sensitivity, and creativity in patient care and nursing administration; administrators who understand the difficulties involved in simultaneously pleasing patients, physicians, and administrators. The nurse leader with such qualities seeks to create an environment in which professional nurses are motivated to practice at their highest level (Nyberg, 1982).

DEVELOPMENTAL PSYCHOLOGY AND HUMANS BECOMING

Developmental stages occur over the life span. The concept of developing, as opposed to that of aging, implies a human becoming rather than a human being. The essence of this distinction is captured in the words of Carl Rogers (1969): "I should like to point out one final characteristic of these individuals as they strive to discover and become themselves. It is that the individual seems to become more content to be a process rather than a product." Career development is a lifelong process, and career planning programs are based on the concept of humans becoming, not simply being.

Continued learning is the cornerstone of career development, and the recognition of staff members' learning abilities and educational interests is an important part of administration. The potential for learning remains intact over the life span (Arenberg & Robertson, 1974). Until the mid-1960s, however, it was almost universally assumed that adults past their twenties suffered an enormous loss of intelligence and learning ability (Thorndike, Bergman, Tilton, & Woodward, 1928). More recent studies have shown that the basic ability to learn changes little, if any, with advancing age. Changes in physical status, reaction time, hearing, vision, motivation, and speed of performance affect performance on timed tests (Zahn, 1967). Retention of the ability to learn favors active participation in a climate of positive motivation in which individuals can continue to pursue the enhancement of their skills and to seek to become something better than they are.

Developmental theories are useful in providing the administrator with a perspective on adult learning capabilities. Erickson's (1963) theory of development, although predominantly confined to the years of childhood, offers the potential for generativity and integrity, rather than for stagnation and despair, in the last two stages of life. Robert Peck (1968) has developed a remarkable picture of the second half of life in describing middle and old age as productive years. This now famous description has stood the test of time, as it has been used by other developmental psychologists, including Bernice Neugarten and Howard McClusky.

Biology may influence the determination of societal roles, but it should not repress the development of human potential. Work may be carried out in either a meaningless or meaningful way. A meaningful use of time is possible only within the context of a meaningful life. In our society, career reentry for women may still occur after the age of 40 and, for both men and women, career change may occur at 50. This has tremendous implications for the nurse executive who seeks to make full use of a nursing resource in a creative way.

Many options are available in nursing, and the creative nurse executive takes advantage of the various combinations of full-time, part-time, or intermittent employment patterns currently available for staff. A skills inventory completed at the time of employment can provide a composite picture of an employee's educational life and work experience. Periodic review of use of skills with the employee can create an environment for reward and creative planning for future assignment (Smith, 1982).

DEVELOPING LEADERS AND FOLLOWERS

An important part of leadership is the ability to identify potential leaders. The willingness to nurture a potential leader at the risk of developing competition for one's own role is the mark of outstanding leadership. The nurturance of followers of institutional goals is one of the major challenges in organizations, for it is easier to set up personal friendships and loyalties. Identifying potential leaders based on personal friendships is a pitfall that nurse executives should avoid. Because friendship tends to blind one to a friend's faults, it is difficult for the nurse executive to objectively evaluate the performance of a friend.

Nurses skilled in clinical practice or education are often moved into administrative positions without the benefit of administrative preparation. Programs designed to develop administrators require integration with institutional performance improvement. To improve organizational performance, it is necessary to develop the institution or the institutional unit. The development of individual administrators is an important part of the overall schema.

Nelson and Schaefer (1980) argue that the development of individual administrators and institutional development are highly interdependent tasks requiring an approach that integrates the needs of both the institution and the individual. Such an approach involves the setting of institutional goals by top management, followed by the development of participating administrators to move toward those goals. Translated to nursing, programs designed to improve the administrative capability of clinical directors and head nurses do not improve the performance of the nursing department unless they are planned to integrate with nursing department goals.

The nurse executive can encourage self-development efforts by establishing, with the employee, individual performance objectives and periodic performance evaluation. The administrator's attention to his or her own self-development further encourages such behavior in others. A positive climate for developing leadership can emerge from requiring administrators to assume the responsibility for the growth and development of their staff and assigning individuals to administrative responsibilities appropriate for their experience and interests. The active involvement of the supervisor is balanced with the encouragement of self-evaluation and personal goal setting.

The concept of supervision as a professional growth-producing process is not new, but, except in public health nursing, it is not widely practiced in the nursing field. The supervisory process requires that each staff member receive one-to-one guidance much more often than once a year for performance evaluation. The nurse executive sets the example for this process through conferencing on a regular basis with each employee who reports directly to him or her. The conferences, of course, provide the opportunity for exchange of information, but they also give the nurse executive time to review objectives, performance, strategies, and problems with each key person. This time is also used for coaching the employee so that he or she can gain new skills and develop new approaches to old problems.

It must be recognized that each individual's capacity to develop is a highly personalized process and that the best tool for self-development lies in the ability to accurately assess developmental needs in relation to life and career goals. Thorne, Fee, and Carter (1982) suggest that ideal career development should match job requirements with the individual's psychological makeup, educational background, experiential skills, and career interests. Figure 12.1 portrays the individual career planning process they propose.

Kleinknecht and Hefferin (1982) also propose a model for career development programs that can help nurse executives identify opportunities for restructuring nurses' work experiences to make them more interesting and challenging. Figure 12.2 portrays that model, which includes nurse executive, professional nurse, and career counselor responsibilities. The program focuses on assisting nurses to develop and

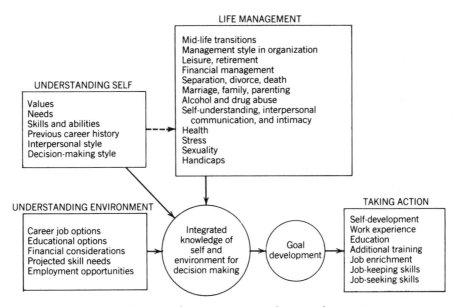

Figure 12.1 Individual career planning process. (From Thorn, I. M., F. X. Fee & J. O. Carter. (1982). Career development: A collaborative approach. Reprinted, by permission of the publisher, from *Management Review*, 71(9), p. 39 (September 1982 © 1982). American Management Association, New York. All rights reserved. Reprinted with permission.)

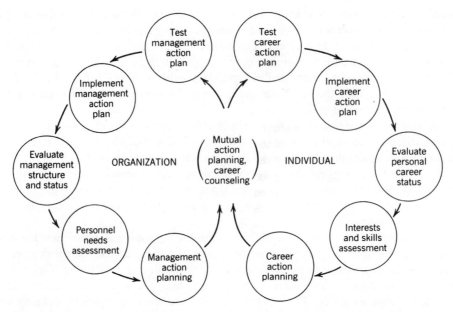

Figure 12.2 A dynamic career development program. (From Kleinknecht, M. K., & E. A. Hefferin. (1982). Assisting nurses toward professional growth: A career developmental model. *The Journal of Nursing Administration, 11* (July–August 1982), p. 32. Reprinted with permission.)

direct their own careers as well as on guiding them toward attaining self-knowledge of:

- Personal values, interests, and goals related to life and career planning.
- Endeavors and accomplishments related to life and work history.
- Life and work decision-making skills.
- Personal and professional growth needs and potentials.
- Career concerns and objectives. (p. 34)

Nursing career development programs serve a dual purpose: to help meet specific needs of the organization and the individual nurse and to provide the potential for expanding the reservoir of talent and motivation within the nursing division (Kleinknecht & Hefferin, 1982).

The followers of today will be the leaders of tomorrow. Setting the pace for the growth and development of the staff involves presenting an image of excitement and enthusiasm for excellence in the nursing department. Technology changes daily, but the need for nurses to develop and grow within a physically exhausting environment presents a major challenge to the nurse executive. The nurse executive has the responsibility to provide leadership in creating a climate in which nurses can practice at their highest level of expertise while continuing to develop as individual professional practitioners. The nurse executive alone cannot create this climate but has the knowledge and skills to lead the nursing division to this end.

MEETING NEEDS AND MAXIMIZING HUMAN POTENTIAL

Nothing mars the maximum development of human potential as much as burnout of either the nurse executive or staff members. Levinson (1981) describes the special kind of exhaustion that can follow the expenditure of intense energy with few visible results. People in such situations fell angry, helpless, trapped, and depleted. The experience is much more intense and devastating than ordinary stress. In seeking to create a professional practice climate, the successful nurse executive will seek to prevent burnout in self and staff by alleviating job stress and dissatisfaction in the early stages whenever possible.

In this regard, Stubbs and Parker (1979) have developed work setting examples and management practices to meet human needs as developed by Maslow. Their methodology translates to nursing as a caring philosophy on the part of administration. It includes caring about the career goals of staff and about how those goals mesh with the organization. It also includes caring about professional development opportunities, mentor relationships, and a creative environment that provides for review, guidance, reinforcement, and rewards for work as well as recognition and advancement. This philosophy can well serve as the guide for developing a motivating nursing environment.

Summary

By taking a human approach, the nurse executive can create an environment in which the development of human potential can be maximized. To do this, the administrator must take into account the difference between human beings and humans becoming. The work of Abraham Maslow and Howard McClusky provides a theoretical basis for the development of human potential in self, peers, and subordinates.

STUDY QUESTIONS

1. Define human potential and discuss its relationship to education.
2. Discuss the role of the nurse executive as teacher and learner.
3. Discuss how achieving one's maximum potential involves learning new behaviors.
4. List the hygienes (extrinsic factors) and motivators (intrinsic factors) and discuss how they are used in your operating environment.
5. Discuss the importance of performance-reward linkage and effort-performing linkage in expectancy theory. Be sure to include the importance of staff opinion in the performance of individual operations.

6. Discuss how to identify and develop a potential leader, with attention to a career development plan.

7. Differentiate between human beings and humans becoming.

References

Arenberg, D. L., & Robertson, E. A. (1974). The older individual as a learner. In S. M. Grabowski & W. D. Mason (Eds.), *Education for the Aging.* Syracuse, NY: ERIC Clearinghouse.

Deci, E. L. (1975). *Intrinsic motivation.* New York: Plenum.

Erickson, E. (1963). *Childhood and society.* New York: Norton.

Gordon, G. K. (1982). Motivating staff: A look at assumptions, *The Journal of Nursing Administration, 12*(11), 27–28.

Herzberg, F., Mausner, B., & Snyderman, B. (1959). *The motivation to work.* New York: Wiley.

Kleinknecht, M. K., & Hefferin, E. A. (1982). Assisting nurses toward professional growth: A career development model, *The Journal of Nursing Administration, 12*(7/8), 30–36.

Levinson, H. (1981). When executives burn out, *Harvard Business Review, 59*(3), 73–81.

Maslow, A. H. (1962). *Toward a psychology of being.* New York: Van Nostrand.

McClelland, D. (1961). *The achieving society.* New York: Van Nostrand.

McClusky, H. Y. (1974). Education for aging: The scope of the field and perspectives for the future. In S. M. Grabowski & W. D. Mason (Eds.), *Education for the Aging.* Syracuse, NY: ERIC Clearinghouse.

Nelson, G. M., & Schaefer, M. J. (1980). An integrated approach to developing administrators and organizations, *Journal of Nursing Administration, 10*(2), 37–42.

Nyberg, J. (1982). The role of the nursing administrator in practice, *Nursing Administration Quarterly, 6*(4), 67–73.

Peck, R. C. (1968). Psychological developments in the second half of life. In B. L. Newgarten (Ed.), *Middle Age and Aging.* Chicago: University of Chicago Press.

Pfoutz, S. K., Simms, L. M., & Price, S. A. (1987). Teaching and learning: Essential components of the nurse executive role, *IMAGE, 19*(3), 138–141.

Pritchard, R. E. (1975). A philosophy of teaching applied to administration, *The Journal of Nursing Administration, 5*(7), 38–40.

Robbins, S. P. (1980). *The administrative process* (2nd ed.). Englewood Cliffs, NJ: Prentice-Hall.

Rogers, C. (1969). *Freedom to learn.* Columbus, OH: Charles E. Merrill.

Skinner, B. F. (1953). *Science and human behavior.* New York: Macmillan.

Smith, M. M. (1982). Career development in nursing: An individual and professional responsibility, *Nursing Outlook, 30*(2), 128–131.

Stubbs, I. R., & Parker, E. R. (1979). Motivating for management effectiveness, *Legal Economics, 5*(5), 38–40.

Thorn, I. M., Fee, F. X., & Carter, J. A. (1982). Career development: A collaborative approach, *Management Review, 71*(9), 27–28, 28–41.

Thorndike, E. L., Bergman, E. O., Tilton, J. W., & Woodward, E. (1928). *Adult learning.* New York: Macmillan.

Vroom, V. H. (1964). *Work and motivation.* New York: Wiley.

Zahn, J. C. (1967). Differences between adults and youth affecting learning, *Adult Education, 17*, 67–77.

CHAPTER 13

Managing Fiscal Resources

Joanne L. Lound

Highlights

- **The operating cycle**
- **Financial and managerial accounting**
- **Assets, liabilities, revenues and expenses**
- **Revenue centers and cost centers**
- **The fiscal year**
- **Reimbursement methods**

To be a manager or administrator is to face the reality that resources are limited and choices must be made as to what will be produced and how it will be produced. Implicit in the task of managing fiscal resources is that managers and administrators are held accountable for the resources that are entrusted to them and they are expected to make the most appropriate use of resources. This suggests that they will strive to use resources in a way that is both efficient and effective. Recall that efficiency is the ratio of input to output, and the number that is produced by this computation is only meaningful relative to some standard of comparison with which it can be compared; someone must decide what that standard will be. Whereas efficiency refers to the relative productivity of a resource, the quest for effectiveness raises a different issue: What will be produced with the resources that are available? Again, human judgment is required to make the decision.

It should become clear that managing fiscal resources has both a technical and a policy component. This chapter is largely concerned with the technical component, which is presented in terms of accounting principles, reimbursement rules, budgeting, and management reporting. The policy component is concerned with values and judgments regarding the organization's goals as well as the strategies and structures that are chosen to implement them. How will the work of the organization be divided into operating units and how will the overall effort be coordinated? The technical component takes place within the policy environment, at times shaping that environment and at other times being limited by it.

A complete explication of the complexities of health care financial management is beyond the scope of this chapter. The intention here, instead, is to provide a framework for managing fiscal resources. The center of this framework is the operating cycle supplemented by specific areas that are likely to be most relevant to nurse executives. When you finish this chapter you should have a greater understanding of (1) the basic operating cycle of an organization, (2) selected accounting and fiscal management concepts that form the basis of many fiscal management routines and decisions, (3) reimbursement systems and how they shape and constrain internal management processes, and (4) budgeting and variance analysis processes.

THE OPERATING CYCLE

A basic accounting concept is that an organization is a "going concern"; that is, it intends to continue to operate for an indefinite period of time. As a going concern, we assume that an organization has an overall mission that defines the nature of its activities. The survival of an organization depends on the ability to create and sustain an operating cycle. By this we mean the ability to:

1. translate the organization's mission into fairly specific operating goals and objectives;
2. assess the demand for services it intends to provide;
3. transform or convert resources into a product or service and deliver that service to the patient;
4. realize an amount from the "sale" of those services that is adequate to replenish resources that were used up in the process, thus allowing the cycle to repeat itself.

The translation of an organization's mission into concrete goals is a function of the strategic planning process. Key considerations in the strategic plan are (1) how well it reflects the realities of the external environment and (2) how it seeks to respond to that environment.

A second feature of the cycle, demand for services, depends on the health status of the community and how health status is recognized and translated into demand, a topic that is beyond the scope of this chapter. The strategic planning process should help to define the type of demand that is to be met to determine what services will be provided. Once this has been agreed to, the budgeting process is used to forecast demand and to determine the appropriate mix of resources necessary to meet that demand. One thing we do know about demand is that in recent years, changes in reimbursement have made health care more competitive; that is, the demand for services is much more sensitive to the prices charged. The section on reimbursement elaborates on this topic.

Nurse executives are most directly involved and therefore should be most influential in the process steps of transforming resources and delivering services. Their decisions along with other departments will determine the ultimate cost of services and the pricing structure. In the absence of philanthropy or other sources of revenue, charges for services must reflect underlying costs if the organization is to recover enough resources to enable it to continue to do business.

The final step in the process, collecting payment for services, is generally not within the purview of nurse executives. However, the success of this activity has a significant influence on cash flow and overall availability of resources to the organization. We will not spend time on this area except to note that the inability to collect revenue on a timely basis may result in an increased cost burden of uncompensated care and interest expense. If the organization must borrow money to pay its bills until the patients pay their bills, it will have less flexibility in operating existing programs or initiating new ones. Some parts of the organization will be charged with reducing the "number of days revenue in accounts receivable" to assure an adequate cash flow. An organization may be successful in delivering services in a cost-efficient manner but it will not survive if it is not able to collect for services on a timely basis.

Understanding the basic concept of the operating cycle is fundamental to any manager who must function within it or who wishes to influence the process. This section concludes with a discussion of accounting terms and concepts. Those who are comfortable with these concepts already may wish to go on to the next section.

Financial Accounting and Managerial Accounting

The purpose of the **financial accounting** system, simply stated, is to keep track of resources and to make periodic reports summarizing financial transactions. This system has as its goal meeting the internal needs of top management in assessing the overall position of the organization or the reporting requirements of external agencies such as bondholders, other major creditors, or major purchasers.

Managerial accounting builds off the same information collected for financial accounting purposes, but its goal is to provide information that is aggregated at different level of the organization. A management accounting system should allow individual managers to focus on the activities that affect their areas of responsibility. Standards for financial accounting reports are often defined by external agencies and may be industry specific to assure comparability. On the other hand, managerial accounting formats are usually internally determined by the needs of the managers and administrators. The capability of the financial information system and the degree to which those who design the information systems understand the needs of line managers and administrators are important factors in the overall utility of the management accounting system.

Assets, Liabilities, Revenues, and Expenses

An **asset** is an item that has value to the organization because of its potential to satisfy a demand. Assets are categorized by their "liquidity," that is, how quickly they can be converted to cash in the event that cash or cash equivalent resources are needed to remain in business. Buildings and equipment, also referred to as "fixed assets," are the least liquid because they are usually specialized for a particular provider and are the most difficult to convert to cash without losing some of their book value.

Liabilities represent debts or amounts owed. They arise because most organizations do not operate on a cash basis; that is, they may delay payment to vendors beyond the usual payment period allowed or they may borrow money for short periods of time to meet current obligations, such as buying supplies or paying salaries. They may borrow for longer periods of time to acquire equipment or buildings. The concept of assets and liabilities allows an entity to record as assets the cost of resources to which they have legal title, even if they are not fully paid for; liabilities represent amounts owed on an asset such as the balance of a mortgage. The difference between total assets and total liabilities is referred to as "net worth." Net worth increases either because assets appreciate in value or because they were used to produce revenue that exceeds the value of the asset that was consumed in its production. Those concerned with the performance of an organization will be interested in evaluating assets, liabilities, and net worth at a particular point in time, as well as from period to period, to determine whether the changes in these items represent an improvement or deterioration in financial condition. A situation where liabilities exceed assets, that is, a negative net worth, may mean that creditors will be less willing to provide resources to the organization without some additional assurance that they will recover their investment. They may do so only if the organization is willing to pay a premium, such as a higher interest rate or cash in advance. Both approaches add to the cost of doing business and, based on price, make it more difficult to compete.

Revenue refers to the amounts recognized from the sale of a product or service. In health care, the term "sale" is not generally used to refer to the delivery of professional services. **Gross revenue** is the price that is charged for the item. Note that the recording of revenue in the accounting records is a separate process from the actual recording of the cash that is ultimately received. The difference between these two numbers provides useful information for management that would otherwise be lost if we measured revenue in terms of cash received. The difference between gross revenue and cash received may be due to discounts negotiated with purchasers or uncompensated care, which itself may have a variety of sources. The causes of the amounts "written off" should be evaluated to determine whether they are justified, since these items reduce available cash.

Expenses are recognized as the value of assets are used up or consumed to produce services or products. For example, as supplies are taken from inventory for use in patient care, they are recognized in the accounting records as expenses. Accounting for the expenses associated with wages and salaries is slightly different. Human resources are not generally recorded as assets on the books. Once an individual is hired and is performing the work of the organization, two accounting transactions occur simultaneously: a liability for wages is incurred during a pay period and the asset that is technically being purchased in increments of payroll hours is recognized as an expense without ever appearing on the books as an asset.

Recognizing the expense associated with the use of buildings and equipment, which have useful lives of several years, is accomplished by the concept of depreciation or amortization. **Depreciation** reflects the gradual deterioration of a fixed asset and allows the organization to recognize its costs gradually over the life of the asset. A simple example is one in which a $10,000,000 piece of equipment with a 10-year life represents a "straight line" depreciation expense of $1,000,000 per year that must be recognized as a cost and included in the prices charged for services. Depreciation may be accelerated in some cases, allowing the cost to be recovered faster. To reduce the need to borrow money and incur interest expense when equipment and buildings need to be replaced, some organizations will **"fund depreciation."** This means that the price charged for a service reflects depreciation expense, and cash realized from the revenue that is generated is set aside to be used to replace the item when it becomes fully depreciated.

Revenue Centers and Cost Centers

Patient billing is frequently based on a "fee-for-service" system; that is, a separate charge is made for each item of professional or ancillary service to the patient. A revenue center is any unit that makes a charge for service. For example, separate charges will usually be made for laboratory tests, pharmacy items, operating room use, and respiratory therapy services. These departments are distinguished from "cost centers," which do not issue a separate charge for their services. In the past, increases in costs or expansions in services in these departments were justified by the ability to increase prices. These include, for example, housekeeping, maintenance, dietary, and registration. The cost of these services must be allocated to the revenue-producing departments so that they can be reflected in and recovered through the pricing structure. Is nursing service a revenue center? Generally, not unless the service is billed as a separate item; instead, its cost is included under charges for "routine services," which includes a variety of costs.

The issue of revenue centers and cost centers may become less important if the fee-for-service method of reimbursement is replaced by a single charge for each admission to the hospital or each visit to an outpatient clinic, regardless of services performed. One major payer, Medicare, has already implemented this approach for inpatients. If this method were implemented for all payers, there would be little reason to allocate overhead costs to the traditional revenue-producing departments. All departments would then need to focus on improving internal efficiency. Institution-wide incentives would exist to decrease rather than expand procedures.

The Fiscal Year

Simply recording transactions, as is done by the financial accounting system, will have little meaning unless a time period is specified. A fiscal year is a 12-month period for which transactions are summarized. It does not necessarily need to coincide with a calendar year. Although a business may intend to be in operation indefinitely, establishing a fiscal year reporting period allows owners or trustees to make an assessment of its effectiveness and financial performance at regular intervals. As previously noted, in many cases, annual financial statements are more than a convenience and may be required by external parties. Although not legally required to do so, many organizations break the year down further into quarterly or monthly reporting periods so that results of operations can be assessed and corrective action can be taken on a more timely basis.

Accrual Accounting

Establishment of a fiscal reporting period requires that, for accounting purposes, we behave as if the business were "closed out" at the end of the period. Every attempt is made to reflect all revenue that has been generated as of the end of the period, even though, in fact, it may not actually be recorded until a later time. For example, if revenue from a patient bill is not recorded until the patient is discharged, revenue would not be recorded in the proper period. Accrual accounting requires that the records be adjusted to reflect revenue "as if" the patient had been discharged at the end of the reporting period. The same procedures apply to recording expenses. All significant expenses must be estimated for the period in which they occur, even though the paper work may not be available until sometime after the year end. This means that the organization "holds the books open" until all these expenses can be documented or reasonably estimated. A good example of an accrued expense, also referred to as a liability, is payroll expense. Quite often, the date of payment does not fall neatly at the end of a fiscal period. The portion of the payroll paid after the end of the period that applies to the prior period is accrued into the period where it was actually incurred. Accruing revenues and expenses into the proper fiscal period allows for "matching" of revenues and expenses in the period to which they apply. This adjustment is important if performance is to be compared from period to period.

REIMBURSEMENT METHODS

In the 1990s, health care administrators at all levels are feeling besieged to reduce costs after years of an expansion that far exceeded the rate of growth in the rest of the economy. Budgets have become more stringent. Practices long established for the organization and delivery of patient care are now being challenged by those who pay the bills. A brief review of the old reimbursement rules is important in understanding how to adapt to the new.

An important feature of health care reimbursement is that most patients are not usually directly responsible for paying the cost of health care. Major "third party" payers have assumed this responsibility. These include:

- Medicare, a federal program for patients 65 and over and for individuals who are disabled.
- Medicaid, a program financed jointly by the state and federal government for patients who meet tests of low-income levels; eligibility and types of services provided often vary by state.
- A number of commercial insurance companies provide coverage for various services to individuals either through their employment, as fringe benefits, or as individual policy holders.
- Blue Cross (for hospital service)/Blue Shield (for physician services) provides "group" coverage, generally through an employment relationship as a fringe benefit. Blue Cross is distinguished from commercial insurers because it contracts with individual hospitals that agree to treat patients at reimbursement rates and rules agreed to in advance.

By far, the most important payers are the state and federal governments and businesses that purchase Blue Cross or commercial insurance coverage as fringe benefits for their employees. The significance of the multiple, major payers is twofold: first, to the extent that they represent large groups of patients, they are able to negotiate prices for services and other rules as to what they will pay for; second, the terms and conditions vary from payer to payer, a situation that must be reconciled internally by the provider as they plan for services.

Services to patients covered by Blue Cross, Medicare, and Medicaid were initially reimbursed based on actual costs incurred with some adjustments for unallowable costs. This method of reimbursement created incentives for hospitals to expand services, regardless of how much demand there was for their services; the cost of excess capacity was factored into the cost paid by these major third parties. A highly simplified illustration is one in which Medicare patients represented 30 percent of the patients served. Under the previous cost-based reimbursement system, the Medicare program would reimburse the hospital for 30 percent of its costs regardless of how efficiently those resources were used. The system for reimbursement has changed, however; distortions created by the cost based reimbursement system still persist.

The new system of reimbursement implemented by Medicare in the early 1980s gradually replaced cost-based reimbursement and in its place, introduced a system that forces hospitals to be more cost efficient and to compete among themselves for patients. The first change introduced by Medicare was to develop a reimbursement formula that was based on an average cost-per-case, adjusted for a severity measure. If hospitals were able to deliver services for less than the price allowed by Medicare, they could keep the difference but if they exceeded the price, they were at risk for the excess cost. This system was quickly replaced by the Diagnosis Related Grouping (DRG) system, which provided a more refined system for recognizing differences in severity among patients. This system created incentives to reduce length of stay and procedures and to increase admissions. Every department became, in effect, a cost center for purposes of Medicare reimbursement. Although the DRG system applied only to Medicare patients, other payers began to follow suit in developing DRG-like systems. Large purchasers attempted to negotiate discounts for services for hospitals that were eager to increase their admissions to make up for the drop in occupancy. They also sought to make better use of facilities, which meant that fixed costs could be spread over more activity. The result for hospitals is that old ways of doing business no longer work in the new competitive environment.

Health Maintenance Organizations (HMOs) are another external force that has created pressure on the internal management of hospitals. An HMO actually combines the delivery of services with financing or insuring the cost of care. An HMO assumes the risk for the cost of health care for an enrolled population in exchange for a flat fee "per member per month." This clearly provides incentives to keep enrollees healthy and, if they do need health services, to use the least costly services available. In areas where HMOs have significantly "penetrated" the market, hospitals find that they must often take extreme measures: first, to compete against HMOs to retain their share of the fee for service business; and second, they must also compete for the inpatient hospital business that HMOs must provide their patients.

BUDGETING AND MONITORING RESULTS

The financial accounting process provides a historical record of transactions. This record allows owners of resources to assess the "results of operations." The budgeting process is, on the other hand, an opportunity to plan and shape those results. There are three types of budgets:

1. The **capital budget** is used for planning the replacement or addition of building and equipment. This budget generally covers a period of 3 to 5 years because of the cost involved and the time required for planning these acquisitions. The capital budget has significant implications for the future direction of the organization. Investment in capital assets represents "sunk costs," decisions that are not easily reversible if conditions in the environment change.

2. The **cash budget** forecasts the sources and uses of cash to determine borrowing needs and investment potential.

3. The **operating budget** brings together forecasts of demand, estimates of operating costs, and the pricing structure necessary to achieve financial goals. This budget usually covers a period of 1 to 3 years, with greatest attention to the first year where estimates are more reliable.

All three budgets are completed within the context of a longer range strategic plan for the organization. In addition to being related to a strategic plan, all three budgets are interrelated with each other:

> The capital budget will influence the type of service and activity level. Deciding to invest in more outpatient operating rooms instead of an MRI will have different implications for the operating budget.

> Funding the acquisition of building and equipment in the capital budget will depend on the cash budget; if borrowing is necessary, the operating budget must bear the burden of the interest expense that will be incurred. New capital assets will also result in additional depreciation, which must be covered in the prices charged for services.

> The operating budget will reflect planned efficiency in the use of resources and will determine the pricing structure and the ability of the organization to compete for market share.

It is important to keep in mind the interrelationship of these budgets; however, we will focus here on the operating budget because this is where nurse executives' knowledge of the patient care process should be most valuable.

Where does an organization begin with the budgeting process? At least three questions must be answered, possibly by different parts of the organization:

1. What services will be provided? For many areas the answer will be the same as in previous years, unless a decision has been made to add or discontinue a service or to change the service dramatically. These decisions are generally made at the strategic planning level of the organization based on information from the external environment as well as an assessment of internal strengths and weaknesses.

2. What level of activity and mix of patients are forecast? By mix, we mean some measure that differentiates patients based on care needs. Severity of illness is one measure. Operating budgets are based on forecasts for a "relevant range" of activity. The upper end is bounded by the capacity of fixed assets and the availability of a trained staff. Over the long run, the relevant range can be expanded by planning for increased staff or investing in fixed assets as part of the capital budget. Given that fixed assets are in place for the period of the current operating budget, the lower end of the range is fixed by some minimum level of baseline staffing. Staying within the relevant range depends on service availability, including facilities and staff, and the ability of the organization to market its services. Nurse executives may have very little involvement in marketing efforts but are expected to be able to plan services for the level and mix of patients who present themselves.

3. How will the services be provided to meet the level and mix of activity? If the forecasts of level and mix of activity are provided on an annual basis, perhaps with a breakdown by month with an overall intensity or measure of mix, it is the job of nursing administration to plan staffing to meet the level and mix of patients on a shift by shift basis. It is at this point that the line between budgeting and day-to-day management becomes blurred.

The less predictable the variation in activity from day to day, the more challenging it will be to meet patient care needs without having an excess of nursing resources on hand. Patient scheduling systems help to smooth out demand. However, scheduling systems that require patients to wait too long for an appointment may mean loss of patients to competitors who are able to serve the patient faster. Nursing resource pools, which provide temporary staff, or permanent staff who float between units as needed provide some flexibility. However, there may be implications for both cost and quality.

The cost of professional nursing time is the major resource that nursing administration is responsible for. Budgeting for nursing services requires three things: *(1)* the ability to classify patients at the time of their service according to their need for nursing services; *(2)* the ability to predict the mix of patients who will demand services; and *(3)* the creation of a standard for the amount of nursing time that will be required to provide the services that are predicted.

Although budgeting can be a daunting exercise, it is only the beginning of the process of managing resources. To be useful, budgets must be monitored to determine whether goals are being achieved or whether corrective action is needed to avoid financial disaster. The process of variance analysis is used to identify problems in performance and, also, problems in standards that may be unrealistically high or low, making them meaningless for purposes of managing resources.

An understanding of the assumptions and standards used to develop budgets is important in performing variance analysis. Because the budget is built on several assumptions, the actual results should be examined in light of these assumptions. At the time the budget assumptions are made, it is important to understand who is considered accountable for variations. For example, assume that a budget for 1 month is based on the expectation of two types of patients:

1. We expect to serve 1,000 type I severity patients who, we anticipate, will require 4 units of nursing care for a total of 4,000 units of nursing care for this group of patients. (A unit of nursing care is defined in terms of a fixed number of minutes, which need not be specified here.)

2. We expect to serve 2,000 type II severity patients who require 6 units of nursing care for a total of 12,000 units of nursing care for these patients.

Assume also that nursing administration has estimated that it can provide a standard unit of nursing care as called for by these patients at $10.00 per nursing care unit. This amount has been computed to include vacation and sick time as well as other paid time off. This portion of nursing costs is assumed to vary with activity so that as volume changes, we expect that costs will also vary. As a result the total variable costs are as follows:

$$1,000 \text{ type I} \times 4 \text{ units} = 4,000 \text{ units at } \$10.00 = \$ 40,000$$
$$2,000 \text{ type II} \times 6 \text{ units} = 12,000 \text{ units at } \$10.00 = \$120,000$$
$$\text{Total: } 3,000 \text{ patients} \qquad 16,000 \text{ units} \qquad \$160,000$$

Nursing services also has a separate component of fixed or overhead costs of $30,000 per month for this unit. These represent administrative costs that are not tied to the level of activity but are fixed for a relevant range of 2,000 to 5,000 patient visits. In this particular budget, the total of type I and type II patients is 3,000, which results in an allocation of fixed cost per unit of $10.00 ($30,000/3,000 = $10.00).

The total variable and fixed cost for 1 month for this unit is

$$\$160,000 + \$30,000 = \$190,000$$

If actual expenses for the period are $200,000, a variance of $10,000 exists. Further analysis indicates the following:

Type I services = 500 patients seen (500 less than budget)

Type II services = 2,500 patients seen (500 more than budget)

Total patients seen = 3,000 (no variance but mix varies)

Nursing salary costs = $168,000 ($8,000 over budget)

Nursing overhead costs = $32,000 ($2,000 over budget)

The first step in the analysis is to apply the budget assumptions to the actual level of activity by patient type. Given the mix of patients, we would expect they would require the following services:

$$500 \text{ type I } @4 \text{ units each} = 2,000 \text{ units} \times \$10.00 \qquad = \$20,000$$
$$2,500 \text{ type II } @6 \text{ units each} = 15,000 \text{ units} \times \$10.00 \qquad = \$150,000$$
$$\text{Total expected cost of nursing service variable costs} \qquad = \$170,000$$

Because the actual nursing salary costs were $168,000, this unit actually experienced a favorable variance of $2,000 after "adjusting for volume", ($170,000 − $168,000).

Further analyses should be made to determine whether the $2,000 variance is due to efficiency in the number of units used (i.e., does type I require less than 4 units or does type II require less than 6 units) or whether it is due to savings in nursing salaries (i.e., the cost was less than $10.00 per unit of service). It is also possible that the difference is made up of some combination of positive and negative variances in both items.

In addition to producing a numerical analysis, an assessment should be made as to whether the conditions that produced the variances are likely to persist. The $2,000 negative variance in administrative overhead needs to be examined to determine whether it is a permanent trend, so that if "annualized" over the full 12-month period it would accumulate a year-end negative variance of $24,000.

Variance analysis is a tool for analyzing the use of resources and identifying the need for corrective action. It is an integral part of the budgeting process and should be recognized as a tool for setting standards and monitoring expectations.

Summary

Managing fiscal resources implies not only authority over resources but accountability for the productive use of those resources. The task is an integral part of every manager's job. In health care, it is more challenging because of the dramatic changes that have resulted in more stringent reimbursement rules. With fewer slack resources and greater uncertainty in the new competitive environment, managers are called on to manage to "a finer tolerance." This is particularly challenging for nursing services because they provide much of the direct patient care that is the heart of the health care endeavor. To be accountable and responsive to patient needs, nurse executives must have an understanding of both the technical aspects and the larger policy environment where value judgements are made in developing assumptions and standards for the appropriate use of resources. This chapter has attempted to present the technical aspects of reimbursement, budgeting, and variance analysis in the context of the larger environment. Nurse executives are challenged to keep both the technical and policy aspects in mind as they assume greater roles in managing health care resources.

References

Anderson, O. W. (1990). *Health services as a growth enterprise in the United States since 1875* (2nd ed.). Ann Arbor, MI: Health Administration Press.

Beck, D. F. (1980). *Basic hospital financial management.* Rockville, MD: Aspen Systems Corporation.

Bolandis, J. L. (1982). *Hospital finance, a comprehensive case approach.* Rockville, MD: Aspen Systems Corporation.

Broyles, R. W. (1982). *Hospital accounting practice,* vol. I, *Financial accounting.* Rockville, MD: Aspen Systems Corporation.

Cleverly, W. O. (1978). *Essentials of hospital finance.* Germantown, MD: Aspen Systems
    Corporation.
Finkler, S. A. (1984). *Budgeting concepts for nurse managers.* New York: Grune & Stratton, Inc.
Horngren, C. T. (1978). *Introduction of management accounting* (4th ed.). Englewood Cliffs,
    NJ: Prentice-Hall, Inc.
Starr, P. (1982). *The social transformation of American medicine.* New York: Basic Books, Inc.
Williams, S. J., & Torrens, P. R. (1980). *Introduction to health services.* New York: John
    Wiley.

CHAPTER 14

Conflict Management in Personal and Professional Life

Highlights

- **Conflict management**
- **Characteristics of conflict**
- **Sources of conflict**
- **Functional and dysfunctional conflict**
- **Strategies for conflict resolution**

Conflict and conflict resolution within the framework of professional nursing administrative practice will be addressed in this chapter. Nurse executives must cope with the competing pressures and demands of hospital administrators for cost effectiveness, of medical staff for competent nursing assistance, and of nursing personnel for improved wages, benefits, and working conditions. Although continued conflict can and does produce stress in nurse executives, it can also provide an opportunity for the individual and organization to change and grow.

Conflict is an inherent part of an individual's personal and professional life. It is inevitable. Conflict may result from divergence of opinion, incompatibility, transmission of erroneous information, or competition for scarce resources. Although often envisioned as a negative manifestation of human interaction, conflict can have positive as well as negative aspects. How conflict is perceived and managed is the essence of whether the process is productive or unproductive to the individual or organizational system. The concepts, theories, and processes related to conflict and conflict resolution have been the subject of extensive and intensive study.

Conflict has a variety of definitions. Robbins (1974) depicts conflict as "all kinds of opposition or antagonistic interaction. It is based on scarcity of power, resources or social position, and different value structures" (p. 362). This definition is based on the premise of awareness. Individuals must first perceive a conflict situation before they can study it. Such awareness is especially pertinent for the practitioner, for whom conflict implies interpersonal, intergroup, and intragroup interactions.

Leininger (1974) views conflict as "opposing viewpoints, forces, issues, and problems which confront individuals, groups, and institutions, having been generated from a variety of internal and external personal and group forces" (p. 18). Whereas, Archer and Goehner (1982), in their definition, emphasize resource allocation because when a situation involves "two or more competing individuals or groups wanting more resources than their 'fair share' or than is available, or have different ideas about how something ought to be done, the stage is set for conflict" (p. 85).

PHILOSOPHICAL AND HISTORICAL BACKGROUND OF CONFLICT MANAGEMENT

Early classical writers on management, the traditionalists, considered conflict a destructive force and believed it was the role of the manager to eliminate conflict from the organization. This philosophy dominated the literature until the 1940s. Traditionalists felt that if a staff member created a conflict situation by disagreeing with the views of management or co-workers, then that person must be discharged from the organization. Because the reason for dismissal was rarely discussed, others were encouraged to abide by rules and regulations.

In contrast with the traditionalists, the behavioralists held the view that, although harmful, conflict was inevitable. In the behavioralist philosophy, conflict in complex organizations was accepted, and an attempt was made to rationalize its existence. This was done by devising measures to reduce, rather than to eliminate, conflict. Such measures focused entirely on the development of conflict resolution techniques. This reasoning eventually led to the view that conflict could be turned to beneficial use. Robbins (1974) espoused that a positive approach was needed if conflict was to be of value to an organization. The most current philosophy is that of the interactionist.

Interactionists recognize the need for conflict and encourage opposition as a creative force that must be stimulated as well as resolved. Indeed, they are concerned when conflict is inadequate or absent and in need of greater intensity. The interactionists believe that organizations that do not encourage conflict increase the probability of or lack of motivation, creative thinking, and effective decision making. They point out that companies have failed because few staff members questioned decisions made by management; in such cases, apathy allowed inadequate decisions to remain in effect because of a conflict-free management group.

Social scientists and humanists have studied conflict and conflict behavior, particularly since World War II. They have identified four major approaches to understanding conflict:

1. The study of interpersonal conflict is spearheaded by psychiatrists, psychiatric social workers, and psychiatric nurses. This type of conflict can and does occur within the individual. Ambivalence as well as disordered perception, feeling, and behavior are usually evident. These symptoms are associated with psychiatric problems.

2. The interactional sociological approach focuses on group behavior and interactional phenomena in decision making within a group.

3. The anthropological approach emphasizes the stresses of culture acclimatization, value and cultural conflicts, and conflicts related to personality and the social environment.

4. The economic-political approach emphasizes conflicts related to political concerns, power games, coalitions, and political and economic processes.

Leininger (1974) predicts the evolution of another approach to conflict theory in the health care professions, one concerned with transdisciplinary and intradisciplinary conflicts and problems. It is in this area that nurse executives must be knowledgeable in identifying, managing, and resolving conflict. They must not only deal with conflict effectively and use it constructively, but must also stimulate it if none is apparent. Lewis (1976) notes that "we should visualize a continuum, with too much conflict at one end and too little at the other. At some point between these extremes, the quantity of conflict is functional and valuable. This point is determined by management and will not necessarily be the same for any two organizations" (p. 18).

CHARACTERISTICS OF CONFLICT

Baldridge (1979) noted that the situations that provoke conflict can be described by four general characteristics. The first is known as the iceberg phenomenon, in which an apparent problem serves to draw attention to other critical issues under the surface. The superficial problem is raised as a pretense for bringing more fundamental issues to light. For example, an initial problem related to staffing, such as nurse assignment patterns, may actually be merely the externalization of a much more basic issue: the wish to gain participation in decision making at the staff nurse level.

The second characteristic situation is related to issues that cause large-scale conflict that tends to have a unifying effect on diverse interest groups. This has occurred in almost all campus resistance movements, in which individuals usually have no common interest other than being bound by the current conflict situation.

Third, conflict is often the result of rising expectations, rather than the presence of intolerable conditions. Nurse executives need to be cognizant that major concessions and improved conditions can induce a high level of expectation and thus actually provoke new conflict with the repetition of a similar pattern.

Fourth, the issue in conflict often has moral overtones that justify and legitimize radical action. Individuals use issues such as sex discrimination and nurse power as ultimate goals to justify almost any short-range excesses. At the other end of the organizational spectrum, however, the same tactic is used by nurse executives when they demand autonomy in their negotiations with the governing boards of health care agencies.

TYPES OF CONFLICT

Although, as we have seen, conflict situations have similar characteristics, the forms of conflict are highly diverse. They may be categorized as intrapersonal, interpersonal, intergroup, or interorganizational in nature. *Intrapersonal conflict,* which was mentioned earlier as a psychiatric phenomenon, is incongruous to an individual's role; there is lack of conformity between people's goals and what is expected within the framework of their roles. "Intrapersonal conflict exists in the cognitive and affective realms of an individual's mind. Thus, an individual may perceive that he or she is conflicting with the organization or other employees, but the conflict, in fact, exists only in that person's mind, not at a behavioral level" (Zey-Ferrell, 1979, p. 299).

However, intrapersonal conflict can be the underlying cause of *interpersonal conflict.* For example, emotionally distressed persons bring to their jobs feelings that relate to their private lives. Preoccupation with personal problems can produce less concentration on work-related responsibilities and decision making. The behavior due to mental processes, especially for the nurse executive, can be the source of interpersonal conflict among peers, subordinates, and co-workers of other disciplines.

Interpersonal conflict arises between two or more individuals or within a group. For example, withholding information may create a conflict between a nurse executive and her assistant. Conflicts among division heads, staff nurse and physician, and committee members may occur for the same reason.

Interpersonal conflict may be inherent in a person's role when there is disagreement between the values and beliefs of the occupant of the role and the expectations set forth by others. In many health care institutions in the 1990s, the nurse executive is accountable and responsible for the practice of nursing. However, disagreement can occur if one professional challenges the practice decisions of a member of another profession. Kalisch and Kalisch (1977) refer to a common source of conflict in the traditional behavior pattern between physicians and nurses as "physician's dominance and nurse's deference." This hierarchical attitude and expectation is found not only at the practice level but extends through executive-administrative levels.

In the capacity of executive-level administrator, Kelley (1977) maintains that the role of nurse executive is extremely difficult to enact because "that role is often stereotyped and contradictory, with multiple split opinions on its power and authority. A top-level nurse administrator . . . [is] surrounded by different sets of behavioral expectations to satisfy from groups higher up, lower down, and on the same level in the structure" (p. 157). Studies conducted by Arndt and Laeger (1970) and Halsey (1978) both concluded that conflict and role strain existed for the nurse executive resulting from pressure to respond to role prescription from a variety of sources.

It is vital that nurse executives examine their role conception. Executives should take an activist's position in regard to that role, making it the sort of role they perceive it to be, rather than merely fulfilling the role others expect or anticipate. An attempt to subscribe to the latter philosophy can be a source of intrapersonal conflict.

Intergroup, or *interorganizational, conflict* arises between two groups, such as in the form of interdepartmental issues. Disagreements and the transmission of erroneous information between departments, such as between medicine and nursing, are common sources of this type of conflict. Such conflicts are depicted as harmful by management, but Argyris (1976) points out that "instead of trying to stamp out intergroup conflict as bad and disloyal, the executives must learn how to manage it so that the constructive aspects are emphasized and the destructive aspects deemphasized" (p. 23).

SOURCES OF CONFLICT

Power, defined as the ability to influence others, may be a major source of conflict. Frost and Wilmot (1978) emphasize that, because it is always interpersonal, power exists only in a human context and is, in a sense, "given from one party to another in conflict" (p. 52). Within this context, power is not an actual show of force, but it is the perceived potential of one party to exert influence on another party, depending on the values and nature of the relationship of those involved. Individuals and groups have power when they have access to information and have control of resources and support services to carry out tasks.

French and Raven (1968) describe five situations in which one person has power over another. These five bases of social power are reward power, coercive power, legitimate power, referent power, and expert power. The basis of reward power is the ability to offer rewards. Thus, an individual is made to perceive that compliance with the wishes of another will lead to positive rewards. Coercive power, the opposite of reward power, is exercised in such a way that one individual perceives that another can mediate punishment for him or her. Legitimate power is based on agreement and values held in common, enabling one individual to exercise power over the other by consent. Referent power is based on identification with the ideals of an individual and the wish to emulate that person. Expert power is present when a person is perceived to have superior knowledge or skill in a particular field.

Because of position, knowledge, profession, and organizational context, the nurse executive may acquire and use all of the types of power described. The nurse executive should neither avoid nor overplay the use of power, nor fail to use it for ethical and legitimate purposes. Others are aware of potential resources of power, and the administrator who uses overkill in a power conflict risks loss of effectiveness. Thus, the administrative nurse must frequently come to terms with conflicts between personality, professional ideals, and the needs of the institution.

By position and title, the nurse executive's legitimate power and authority is generally recognized throughout the organization. However, the precise scope of this power and authority may be an area of conflict. An issue in many health care facilities is who controls the practice of nursing. The director of nursing has the authority, but the extent of power may be limited to resolving problems that occur within the department. Unless the director has other powers to augment his or her legitimate power, legitimate power may not be sufficient for the administrator to decide a nursing practice issue related to the overall organization or to other disciplines.

The nurse executive also has substantial reward and coercive power based on the right to hire, evaluate, promote, and discharge individuals. The nursing director needs to be sensitive to the fact that power is only a part of the continuing relationship between the supervisor and the supervised and that power is not an acceptable substitute for skillful leadership and motivation.

The nurse executive has expert power derived from two sources: professional nursing knowledge and administrative skills. In the past, these two types of power were not always compatible and were a source of intrapersonal conflict. With the acceptance of nursing administration as a legitimate area of nursing practice this should not be an important source of conflict. Simms, Price, and Pfoutz (1985) explored the role of the nurse executive in acute, home and long-term care, and educational settings. Results of this study yield the postulation that a new administrative role, the nurse executive, is emerging in acute, home care, and educational settings. The role requires advanced education and a high degree of leadership and management competence intricately linked with clinical nursing knowledge and research.

The role also demands teacher/learner skills with the nurse executive modeling behaviors that can be learned by others. Because conflict is almost always personalized by all participant parties it seems essential for personal behavioral change to occur if a state of dynamic conflict fluidity is to be achieved. In a healthy organization, conflict is stimulating and scientific debate of diverse ideas can lead to multiple creative ventures.

Referent power, based on personal characteristics, may or may not be strong enough to induce others to emulate the nurse executive. However, referent power can be diminished when the nurse executive develops hostile, defensive personality patterns.

Nurse executives who are knowledgeable about the various types of power and power bases and how they are used are better able to function in an enlightened position and provide a climate for more effective leadership. They need to make informed and high-risk decisions that may be potential sources of conflict. As members of the executive team in health care delivery settings, nurse executives must take risks and move into positions of power. Much of the power that executives gain is derived from their access to information. The nurse executive who is aware of the information network of the organization realizes there are formal channels that transport information to the decision makers. Legitimate access and the authority to command information are important tools for the nurse executive.

Marriner-Tomey (1988) describes some additional sources of conflict. One is a situation in which individuals involved in solving a problem do not have the same information. They define the problem differently, place different values on various aspects, or have divergent views of power and authority. For example, the presumption of power on the part of the physician to influence or control nursing practice is potentially a conflict-generating situation. The possibilities for conflict increase with the number of levels in the organizational hierarchy and the number of specialities. Conflicts of interest arise in competition for scarce resources and ambiguous jurisdictions, creating unclear authority or subordinate status. The latter may occur, for example, in matrix organizations when sources of conflict are generated.

ASSESSMENT OF FUNCTIONAL AND DYSFUNCTIONAL CONFLICT

Health care organizations are often classified as complex organizations. In complex and highly diversified organizations, conflict is inevitable and even desirable. Inappropriate responses to conflict can be unhealthy for individuals and groups within the organization. It is imperative that nurse executives reduce or increase conflict and tension to tolerable levels and channel the energy created by conflict situations toward constructive goals.

Conflict in and of itself can be a positive or negative force. It is the use or misuse of this force that determines its effect and relative value. Robbins (1974) implies that the demarcation between functional and dysfunctional conflict is neither clear nor precise. He indicates that no level of conflict can be adopted at face value as either acceptable or not acceptable. If the conflict supports the goals of the organization and improves the organization's performance, it is a functional or constructive form of conflict. Whereas, those interactions that hinder organizational performance are defined as dysfunctional (p. 362). A conflict may be dysfunctional at one time in a given setting, as perceived by individuals at a certain level within the organizational hierarchy, or may be considered functional at another time in a different setting by individuals at the top level in the organization. For example, a conflict may occur over an administrative decision to implement a nursing information system, especially if the staff nurses were not involved in the decision, and they perceive this change as an increased burden. However, management's rationale for the change was that data on the population served by the organization would be more readily available and accessible and would facilitate planning for needed services.

Characteristics do exist that assess actual conflict and functional from dysfunctional conflict. McFarland, Leonard, and Morris (1984) propose an assessment guide that can be used to determine interpersonal or intergroup conflict within the organization and whether a given conflict is functional or dysfunctional (see Figure 14.1). They emphasize that conflict assessment can help formulate a conflict diagnosis in the organization or subsystem or both. They also emphasize that at times the level of conflict may be either too low or too high within the work group. If the level of conflict is too low, it may be necessary for the nurse executive or manager to stimulate conflict. Whereas, if the conflict is too high, it becomes necessary for the executive to apply conflict resolution strategies. The authors propose an assessment guide that may indicate "too low or too high conflict levels." (See Figure 14.2). An affirmative response to the questions can be indicative of such conflict states. First, one should analyze the data collected from the assessment guide for actual conflict to formulate a conflict diagnosis. The data are then analyzed to determine the nature of conflict, whether it is too high or too low. The authors imply "that the conflict diagnosis can be stated to include the type of conflict and the related source, for example, dysfunctional interpersonal conflict related to differences in values, functional intergroup conflict related to differing subgoals, or too-high interpersonal conflict related to unequal access to resources" (p. 318). These conflict diagnosis statements along with an understanding of the nature of conflict can give direction to the selection of appropriate conflict management strategies.

Figure 14.1 Guide for assessment of conflict

Interpersonal or intergroup?

1. Who?
   • Who are the primary individuals or groups involved? Characteristics (values; feelings; needs; perceptions; goals; hostility; strengths, as past history of constructive conflict management; self-awareness)?
   • Who, if anyone, are the individuals or groups that have an indirect investment in the result of the conflict?
   • Who, if anyone, is assisting the parties to manage the conflict constructively?
   • What is the history of the individuals' or groups' involvement in the conflict?
   • What is the past and present interpersonal relationship between the parties involved in the conflict?
   • How is power distributed among the parties?
   • What are the major sources of power used?
   • Does the potential for coalition exist among the parties?
   • What is the nature of the current leadership affecting the conflicting parties?

2. What?
   • What is/are the issue/s in the conflict?
   • Are the issues based on facts? Based on values? Based on interests in resources?
   • Are the issues realistic?
   • What is the dominant issue in the conflict?
   • What are the goals of each conflicting party?
   • Is the current conflict functional? Dysfunctional?
   • What conflict management strategies, if any, have been used to manage the conflict to date?
   • What alternatives in managing the conflict exist?
   • What are you doing to keep the conflict going?
   • Is there a lack of stimulating work?

3. How?
   • What is the origin of the conflict? Sources? Precipitating events?
   • What are the major events in the evolution of the conflict?
   • How have the issues emerged/ Been transformed? Proliferated?
   • What polarizations and coalitions have occurred?
   • How have parties tried to damage each other? What stereotyping exists?

4. When/Where?
   • When did the conflict originate?
   • Where is the conflict taking place?
   • What are the characteristics of the setting within which the conflict is occurring?
   • What are the geographic boundaries? Political structures? Decision-making patterns? Communication networks? Subsystem boundaries?
   • What environmental factors exist that influence the development of functional versus dysfunctional conflict?
   • What resource persons are available to assist in constructive conflict management?

Functional or dysfunctional?

	YES	NO
Does the conflict support the goals of the organization?	[ ]	[ ]
Does the conflict contribute to the overall goals of the organization?	[ ]	[ ]
Does the conflict stimulate improved job performance?	[ ]	[ ]
Does the conflict increase productivity among work group members?	[ ]	[ ]
Does the conflict stimulate creativity and innovation?	[ ]	[ ]
Does the conflict bring about constructive change?	[ ]	[ ]
Does the conflict contribute to the survival of the organization?	[ ]	[ ]
Does the conflict improve initiative?	[ ]	[ ]
Does job satisfaction remain high?	[ ]	[ ]
Does the conflict improve the morale of the work group?	[ ]	[ ]

A yes response to the majority of the questions indicates that the conflict is probably functional. If the majority of responses are no, then the conflict is most likely a dysfunctional conflict.

Source: McFarland, G., H. Leonard & M. Morris. (1984). Nursing Leadership and Management (pp. 313–315. New York: John Wiley. Adapted by permission.

As nurse executives attempt to identify the issues and sources of conflict, the next logical step is to select the strategy or strategies for managing conflicts and to revisit their influence on and participation in the conflict.

STRATEGIES FOR CONFLICT RESOLUTION

A number of strategies can be used in an attempt to reduce conflict. It is important to select the conflict resolution strategy that is is most appropriate for the nature and type of conflict. Feldman and Arnold (1983) summarize four major strategies for intergroup conflict.

Avoidance

This type of strategy attempts to keep the conflict from surfacing at all. Examples would be to ignore the conflict or impose a solution. This conflict is temporary where concern for people and production is low. This may be appropriate if the conflict is trivial or if quick action is needed to prevent the conflict from occurring.

Defusion

Under this strategy, an attempt is made to deactivate the conflict and cool off the emotions and hostilities of the groups involved. Examples would include trying to

Figure 14.2 Guide for assessment of level of conflict

Is conflict too low?

	YES	NO
Is the work group consistently satisfied with the status quo?	[ ]	[ ]
Are no or few opposing views expressed by work-group members?	[ ]	[ ]
Is little concern expressed about doing things better?	[ ]	[ ]
Is little or no concern expressed about improving inadequacies?	[ ]	[ ]
Are the decisions made by the work group generally of low quality?	[ ]	[ ]
Are no or few innovative solutions or ideas expressed?	[ ]	[ ]
Are many work-group members "yes-men"?	[ ]	[ ]
Are work-group members reluctant to express ignorance or uncertainties?	[ ]	[ ]
Does the nurse manager seek to maintain peace and group cooperation regardless of whether this is the correct intervention?	[ ]	[ ]
Do the work-group members demonstrate an extremely high level of resistance to change?	[ ]	[ ]
Does the nurse manager base the distribution of rewards on "popularity" as opposed to competence and high job performance?	[ ]	[ ]
Is the nurse manager excessively concerned about not hurting the feelings of the nursing staff?	[ ]	[ ]
Is the nurse manager excessively concerned with obtaining a consensus of opinion and reaching a compromise when decisions must be made?	[ ]	[ ]

A yes response to the majority of these questions can be indicative of a too-low conflict level in a work group.

Is conflict too high?

	YES	NO
Is there an upward and onward spiraling escalation of the conflict?	[ ]	[ ]
Are the conflicting parties stimulating the escalation of conflict without considering the consequences?	[ ]	[ ]
Is there a shift away from conciliation, minimizing differences, and enhancing goodwill?	[ ]	[ ]
Are the issues involved in the conflict being increasingly elaborated and expanded?	[ ]	[ ]
Are false issues being generated?	[ ]	[ ]
Are the issues vague or unclear?	[ ]	[ ]

Figure 14.2 (*continued*)

Is job dissatisfaction increasing among work-group members?	[ ]	[ ]
Is the work-group productivity being adversely affected?	[ ]	[ ]
Is the energy being directed to activities that do not contribute to the achievement of organizational goals (e.g., destroying opposing party)?	[ ]	[ ]
Is the morale of the nursing staff being adversely affected?	[ ]	[ ]
Are extra parties getting dragged into the conflict?	[ ]	[ ]
Is a great deal of reliance on overt power manipulation noted (threats, coercion, deception)?	[ ]	[ ]
Is there a great deal of imbalance in power noted among the parties?	[ ]	[ ]
Are the individuals or groups involved in the conflict expressing dissatisfaction about the course of the conflict and feel that they are losing something?	[ ]	[ ]
Is absenteeism increasing among staff?	[ ]	[ ]
Is there a high rate of turnover among personnel?	[ ]	[ ]
Is communication dysfunctional, not open, mistrustful, and/or restrictive?	[ ]	[ ]
Is the focus being placed on nonconflict relevant sensitive areas of the other party?	[ ]	[ ]

A yes response to the majority of these questions can be indicative of a conflict level in a work group that is too high.

Source: McFarland, G., H. Leonard & M. Morris. (1984). Nursing Leadership and Management (pp. 316–317). New York: John Wiley. Adapted by permission.

"smooth things over" by playing down the importance and magnitude of the conflict or of established superordinate goals that need the cooperation of the conflicting groups to be accomplished. This strategy is appropriate where a stopgap measure is needed or when the groups have a mutually important goal.

Containment

Under this strategy, some conflict is allowed to surface, but it is carefully contained by spelling out which issues are to be discussed and how they are to be resolved. To implement this strategy, the problems and procedures may be structured, and representatives from the conflicting parties may be allowed to negotiate and bargain within the established structure. This is appropriate when open discussions have failed and the conflicting groups are of equal power.

Confrontation

Under this strategy, which is at the other end of the continuum from avoidance, all the issues are brought into the open, and the conflicting groups directly confront the issues with each other in an attempt to resolve the conflict. This is most appropriate when there is a minimum level of trust, when time is not critical, and when the groups need to cooperate to get the job done effectively (pp. 526–528).

Three basic strategies that individuals can use in interpersonal conflict, as well as intergroup and organization conflict resolution approaches are identified by Filley (1975) for dealing with conflict according to outcome. These are called *(1)* lose-lose, *(2)* win-lose, and *(3)* win-win approaches.

Lose-Lose

In a lose-lose approach to conflict resolution, neither party wins. One common approach is to compromise or take the middle ground in a dispute. Another is to pay off one of the parties in the conflict, which may take the form of a bribe. A third approach is to use a third party as an arbitrator. Another lose-lose strategy is when the parties in a conflict situation resort to bureaucratic rules or regulations to resolve the conflict. It is important to note that in all of these approaches, both parties lose. It is sometimes the only solution to the conflict situation, but it is generally a less desirable one.

Win-Lose

This strategy is commonly used for resolving conflict. In a competitive type culture, one party in a conflict situation attempts to assemble its forces to win, and the other party loses. Examples of win-lose strategies can be observed in supervisor and subordinate and line and staff relationships and labor-management disputes. In a win-lose strategy someone always loses, which may cause them to be bitter and revengeful.

Characteristics that are common to the win-lose and lose-lose situations include:

1. The conflict is a personal "we-they" conflict rather than a problem-centered focus. This is very likely to occur when two cohesive groups that do not share common values or goals are in conflict.
2. Parties direct their energy toward total victory for themselves and total defeat for the other. This can cause long-term problems for the organization.
3. Each sees the issue from her or his own point of view rather than as a problem in need of a solution.
4. The emphasis is on outcomes rather than definition of goals, values, or objectives.
5. Conflicts are personalized.
6. Conflict-resolving activities are not differentiated from other group processes.
7. There is a short-run view of the conflict, with settlement of the immediate problem as the goal rather than resolution of differences (Filley, 1975, p. 25).

Win-Win

A win-win strategy of conflict resolution is the most desirable especially from an organizational perspective. Innovation, creativity and energies are expended at solving the problems rather than demeaning the other party or parties involved. The needs and desires of both parties in the conflict situation are achieved, and both receive rewarding outcomes. These win-win strategies are usually associated with a favorable organization experience, improved decision making, and provide satisfaction to both parties in the conflict situation.

Techniques of Conflict Resolution

Negotiation   Negotiation is an indispensable tool for the nurse executive. However, the knowledge and skill to use this tool effectively has been limited to a degree in the health care field and in nursing in particular. Nevertheless, the responsibility of negotiating on behalf of the nursing division is a responsibility of the top level nursing executive. As Kelley (1983) stresses, "accomplishing organizational objectives according to an established timetable with a minimum of resources while influencing resolution of conflict is a major basis upon which nursing service administrators are evaluated and retained or released" (p. 427). Negotiation is given different meaning by various theorists. Strauss (1979) views negotiation as a cyclic interactional process that can be analyzed by three interacting elements. The first, process elements, includes such strategies as persuasion, trade-offs, appeals, demands, compromises toward middle positions, and mutual agreements. The second is the structural element, which incorporates the interacting parties in the negotiation process, the environmental setting, the timing of meetings, and the balance of power of the two parties. The last element is the negotiating situation itself. The interactive element comprehends the complexity and number of issues to be resolved, the experience of the negotiators, and the alternatives available to assure the continuance of negotiations.

Cohen (1980) presents another perspective on negotiation. He views it as a process of information, timing, power, and pressure to secure a commitment to change behavior. Power, the ability to use resources to achieve worthwhile goals, may include risk taking, competition, and persistence. Cohen stresses that successful negotiation is based on accurate and sufficient information gathered by critical listening, questioning, and reading cues. It is important to note that, to achieve agreement in negotiations, group tension must be reduced. Stress relief may be achieved by the following steps: *(1)* the maintenance of time limitations by both parties and *(2)* the application of pressure on the negotiator to take or avoid risks.

General guidelines to effective negotiations include belief in oneself as an able negotiator; willingness to seek assistance in problem solving, in the recognition that the objective is collaborative settlement as commitments made to individuals, not necessarily organizations; encouragement of an exchange of information; and the ability to assess and validate changing circumstances in the negotiating process.

Collaboration   I-win-you-win collaboration as a strategy or technique is closely related to negotiation, and the terms are sometimes used interchangeably when conflict resolution is discussed by different authors. However, collaborative theory supports the belief that people should bring their differences to the surface and delve into the issues to identify underlying causes and to find an alternative mutually satisfactory to both parties. The approach is based on the assumption that people will be motivated to invest time and energy in such problem-solving activity. The conflict is viewed as a creative, positive force that will lead to an improved state of affairs to which both sides are fully committed. When progress can no longer be made, a mediator (third-party consultant) may be used to assist the parties to arrive at a win-win position.

Collaborationists further argue that theirs is the preferable strategy for the good of an organization because *(1)* open and honest interaction promotes authentic interpersonal relations; *(2)* conflict is used as a creative force for innovation and improvement; *(3)* the process enhances feedback and information flow; and *(4)* the solution of disputes in itself serves to improve the climate of the organization by enhancing openness, trust, risk taking, and feelings of integrity (Likert, 1976).

Collaboration has been found to be most effective in situations in which there is *(1)* a high degree of required interdependence; *(2)* power parity, allowing the parties to interact openly, utilizing all of their resources to further their beliefs and concerns regardless of their superior-subordinate status; *(3)* potential for mutual benefits; and *(4)* the expectation of organizational support.

Nurse executives are frequently encouraged to develop leaderships skills that emphasize the resolution or suppression of conflict. At the same time, they often find that power is necessary to direct and coordinate day-to-day activities, compete for scarce resources, and attain goals. To perform these tasks effectively, however, nurse executives must understand and be able to plan strategies for dealing with conflict. They need to know how power is distributed within the organization and where they stand within the power structure to determine how to acquire the leverage needed to fulfill their role.

In the organizational hierarchy of a hospital, the two major power structures are the administration and the medical staff. These two groups are often inherently in conflict because of differences in their goals: the goal of the administrators is to realize an efficient, cost-effective organization, and that of the physicians to obtain optimum resources for their patients. In most hospitals, physicians do not have formal organizational authority over hospital employees, including nurses; yet, they do have power. Thus, an important task of the nurse executive is to increase the power of nursing without aggravating organizational conflict.

One route by which this objective can be attained is to emphasize the dependence of other organizational units of the hospital on nursing. For example, if the chief of pediatrics wants to open an intensive care unit for newborns, he or she must rely on the nursing director to staff it. The nursing director in turn must provide personnel not only in sufficient numbers but also with the necessary critical-care skills for quality patient care, ready and fully trained on the day the unit accepts its first patient. Rather than treating this accomplishment as a routine assignment to be expected of the position, the director should use the opportunity to make the hospital community aware of the importance of the nursing role to the realization of a goal. Further, the director should convey the idea that he or she has resources — that is, power — and is ready to use them to help or hinder the attainment of an objective of a member from another area in the hierarchy. Moreover, power may be augmented by gaining support from subgroups within a high-power group. Thus, by supporting the physicians, nurses can gain leverage in dealing with administrators who may be more interested in satisfying physicians than nurses.

Collective Bargaining as a Process Collective bargaining often produces conflict between nursing administration and the nursing staff. The principle questions related to the issue of collective bargaining are *(1)* whether it should serve primarily for economic gains and improved working conditions or whether negotiations should include patient care issues and *(2)* whether the professional organization, the American Nurses Association (ANA), should be the bargaining agent.

Staff nurses seem to be aware of the necessity of collective action to attain their economic goals and improve working conditions. The issues that remain in conflict are in the area of professional goals as to who shall control nursing, nursing practice, and quality outcomes. In the hospital setting the authority, responsibility, and accountability for hospital operations and patient care are vested in the hospital administration. Nurses are individually and legally accountable for their nursing practice, but because they are employees of a hospital, management in the person of the nurse executive is, in fact, responsible for the institutional quality of nursing care.

Many leaders of the nursing profession have published their views on the impact of collective bargaining on nursing. The thrust of arguments of those opposed to the principle is that the concept of collective bargaining is counterproductive to professionalism, whereas those in favor suggest that it is "an opportunity to develop a new model of labor relations which will benefit not only employees and management, but health care delivery as a whole." Cleland (1988) proposes a professional model for collective bargaining that is relevant for unionized and nonunionized organizations. This model places the State Nurses Association (SNA) collective bargaining activities in a separate organization, which might be called the Health Employees Union (HEU). Both the SNA and the HEU are controlled by a holding company that provides greater opening flexibility to pursue varying goals that enables nursing to improve its competitive stance relative to other unions and makes it possible for the SNA to broaden its base among nurses who are supportive of collective bargaining activities. Simms and Dalston (1984) eloquently state that the challenge before the nursing profession is "do not attempt to settle professional issues at the bargaining table or in the boardroom but settle these issues among professionals in collegial interchange over time" (p. 122).

An interesting alternative to collective bargaining is brokering. Johnson and Bergmann (1988) state that nurse executives have learned the value and necessity of being at the broker's table, which is a symbol representing full participation in organizational decisions. Brokering occurs at all levels in the organization and it involves negotiation, defines success situationally, and ensures that all are winners. The focus is less on who is right than the achievement of desired changes directed toward future goals. The authors encourage nurse executives to develop the brokering skills of their managers to be effective brokers. They stress that the development of effective brokering skills rests on the acquisition of power equity, political savvy, and knowledge of the organization's culture.

Still another approach to managing conflict is to create a participatory governance system in which workers and management share decision making that would cause major unrest if staff were not involved. A variety of shared governance models are being implemented to enhance participation in decision making (Deremo, 1989; Allen, Calkin, & Peterson, 1988; Porter-O'Grady, 1987).

Summary

Because conflict is an inherent part of an individual's personal and professional life, it is inevitable. Conflict, often viewed as a negative manifestation of human interaction, can have positive as well as negative aspects. How individuals perceive conflict may be influenced by the definition and theory they accept. There are three major philosophical views of conflict, first, the traditionalist, who views conflict as a destructive force that should be eliminated from organizations; second, the behavioralist, who views conflict as an inevitable occurrence that should be reduced or controlled; and last, the interactionist, who views conflict as a creative force that must be stimulated as well as resolved.

Four approaches to understanding the nature of conflict are *(1)* the interpersonal-psychological approach, *(2)* the interaction-sociological approach, *(3)* the anthropological approach, and *(4)* the economic-political approach. Each approach assumes different sources of conflict.

There are various situations that provoke conflict, such as the use of an apparent problem, which evokes a more critical issue to the surface; large-scale issues that tend to unify a diverse interest group; rising expectations; and moral overtones that justify radical action. The types of conflict that may be encountered are intrapersonal, or role conflict, interpersonal, and intergroup, or interorganizational. Power is viewed as one of the primary sources of conflict. This is particularly true when the disposition of power is seen as a "have" or "have-not" situation.

Many techniques or approaches may be used effectively for conflict resolution. Avoidance, defusion, containment, and confrontation are four major strategies that may be used for intergroup conflict. Three basic strategies that individuals can use in interpersonal, as well as in intergroup, for dealing with conflict include lose-lose, win-lose, and win-win approaches. Negotiation, collaboration, and collective bargaining are common techniques applied in conflict resolution. Each has its own advantages and disadvantages. Selection of the appropriate technique or conflict resolution strategy should be contingent on the characteristics of the situation.

The nurse executive must be cognizant of the particular circumstances underlying the presence of personal and/or organizational conflict. Rigorous analysis is essential before managerial intervention to facilitate conflict resolution.

THOUGHT PROVOKING QUESTIONS

1. Formulate a definition of conflict. Explain your rationale for this selection.

2. Compare and contrast the traditionalists', behavioralists', and interactionists' approach to conflict. Which approach do you favor. Why?

3. From your perspective, cite at least two examples and sources of conflict. What strategies or techniques for conflict resolution would you be likely to use? Explain.

4. Briefly describe a situation involving a nurse executive where there is conflict involving power and elements of the use of power. What is the actual or potential power base(s) of the participants? Describe the factors that influence the power base of the participants. Analyze ways in which an increase in power would either sustain or resolve the conflict situation.

5. Practice diversity by sincerely trying to listen to persons with whom you always seem to be in conflict. What do you learn from listening attentively?

References

Allen, D., Calkin, J., & Peterson, M. (1988). Making shared governance work: A conceptual model, *Journal of Nursing Administration, 11*(4), 37–43.

Archer, S., & Goehner, P. (1982). *Nurse: A political force.* Monterey, CA: Wadsworth.

Argyris, C. (1976). How tomorrow's executives will make decisions, *Think, 33*(6), 22–25.

Arndt, C., & Laeger, E. (1970). Role strain in a diversified role set: The director of nursing service, *Nursing Research 19*(3), 253–259.

Baldridge, J. (1979). *New approaches to management.* San Francisco: Jossey Bass.

Cleland, V. (1988). A new model for collective bargaining, *Nursing Outlook, 36*(5), 228–230.

Cohen, H. (1980). *You can negotiate anything.* Secaucus, NJ: Lyle Stuart Publishers.

Deremo, D. (1989). Integrating professional values, quality practice, productivity, and reimbursement for nursing, *Nursing Administration Quarterly, 14*(1), 9–23.

Feldman, D., & Arnold, H. (1983). *Managing individual and group behavior in organizations.* New York: McGraw-Hill.

Filley, A. (1975). *Interpersonal and conflict resolution.* Glenview, IL: Scott Foresman.

French, J., and Raven, B. (1968). The bases of social power. In D. Cartwright & A. Zander (Eds.), *Group Dynamics: Research and Theory.* New York: Harper & Row.

Frost, J., & Wilmot, W. (1978). *Interpersonal Conflict.* Dubuque, Iowa: William C. Brown Co.

Halsey, S. (1978). The queen bee syndrome: One solution to role conflict for nurse managers. In M. Hardy & M. Conway (Eds.), *Role Theory: Perspectives for Health Professionals.* New York: Appleton-Century-Crofts.

Johnson, J., & Bergman, C. (1988). Nurse managers at the broker's table. The nurse executive's role. *Journal of Nursing Administration, 18*(6), 18–21.

Kalisch, B., & Kalisch, P. (1977). An analysis of the sources of physician-nurse conflict, *Journal of Nursing Administration, 7*(1), 50–57.

Kelley, J. (1983). Negotiating skills for the nursing service administrator, *Nursing Clinics of North America, 18*(3), 427–438.

Kelley, J. (1977). The role of the top nurse administrator. *Proceedings, Nursing Administration: Issues for the 80s—Solutions for the 70s.* University of Minnesota. Battle Creek: W. K. Kellogg Foundation.

Leininger, M. (1974). Conflict and conflict resolution: Theories and processes relevant to the health professions, *The American Nurse, 6*(12), 17–22.

Likert, R., & Likert, J. (1976). *Ways of managing conflict.* New York: McGraw-Hill.

Lewis, J. (1976). Conflict management, *Journal of Nursing Administration, 6*(10), 18–22.

Marriner-Tomey, A. (1988). *Guide to nursing management* (3rd ed.). St. Louis: C. V. Mosby.

McFarland, G., Leonard, H., & Morris, M. (1984). *Nursing leadership and management.* New York: John Wiley.

Porter-O'Grady, T. (1987). Shared governance and new organizational models, *Nursing Economics, 5*(6), 281–286.

Robbins, S. (1974). *Managing Organizational Conflict: A Nontraditional Approach.* Englewood Cliffs, NJ: Prentice-Hall.

Simms, L., & Dalston, J. (1984). A professional imperative, *Hospital and Health Services Administration, 29*(6), 115–122.

Simms, L., Price, S., & Pfoutz, S. (1985). Nurse executives: Functions and Priorities, *Nursing Economics, 3*(4), 238–244.

Strauss, A. (1979). *Negotiations: Varieties, contexts, processes and social orders.* San Francisco: Jossey Bass.

Zey-Ferrell, M. (1979). *Dimensions of organizations.* Santa Monica, CA: Goodyear Publishing Company.

CHAPTER 15

Leadership in Care of Older People

Highlights
- **Standards of health care**
- **The frail older people**
- **The not-so-frail older people**
- **Mobility products**
- **Obstacles to a geriatric emphasis**

The rapid growth in the older population in this country is projected to be one of the most influential forces shaping the health care delivery system and society as a whole well into the next century. Americans over age 65 will increase from 25 million in 1980 to 66 million by 2040 according to projections by the U.S. Bureau of the Census in Projections of the Population of the United States: 1982 to 2050 (Figure 15.1). This represents a surge from 11 percent to 21 percent of the total population (Riffer, 1985). The question arises as to whether or not this group represents a vast group of untapped human resources or a burgeoning pocket of individuals in the upper age ranges who have the greatest need for social, income maintenance, housing, and health services. History will decide the outcome of this argument, but in the meantime, drastic changes in the thinking of health professionals (including nurse executives) must occur.

Traditionally, the health care field has been facility driven (Thomas and Bobrow, 1984). However, it is becoming increasingly evident that new programs must be

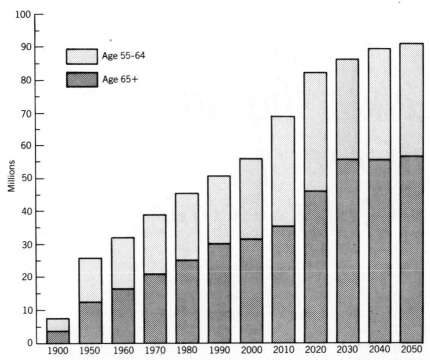

Figure 15.1 Number of persons aged 55 and over by age group, 1900 and 1950 to 2050 (data for 1980–2050 are projections). (From the National Center for Health Statistics.)

developed with creative solutions that go beyond bricks and mortar if the benefits of longevity are not to bankrupt America and other countries around the world. The majority of older people are active individuals who prefer to live at home in apartments, houses, and mobile homes. Although home health services have mushroomed, a major gap remains in the market for creative individualized services. A network of services is essential to the provision of a system that will support older people living at home. One of the most important linkages could be ambulatory centers that provide health maintenance information and activities as well as numerous social activities for clients and/or their families. Another is the nursing-home model that serves as a rehabilitation center. Walk-in ambulatory day centers and redesigned nursing homes may serve as the key to liberation of older people now and into the twenty-first century.

The application of assistive technology to the problems of older people will have two major effects (Haber, 1986). First, it will reduce the costs of care by providing additional help to older people so they can remain independent, and second, it will enhance the quality of life. Numerous devices, described later in this chapter, will minimize the problems of vision, hearing, musculoskeletal disabilities, proprioceptive loss, and the dementias. It is conceivable that many tasks now performed by nursing staff could be assisted by robotics. Nurse executives may wish to analyze critically current and emerging technologies that could not only enhance the quality of life of older people but could greatly affect the nature of nursing care.

The fastest-growing group is the old-old, those over 75 years. If the nursing profession is to respond adequately to the growing numbers of older adults, it must intensify its commitment to the special health and health-related problems of older people at every level of administration, education, practice, and research (Abdellah, 1981).

Since 1950, life expectancy in the older ages has increased at an accelerated pace (see Figure 15.2). Most of the increase in life expectancy before 1950 was due to decreasing mortality at the younger ages: growing numbers of people reached old age because of decreased mortality rates in the younger age groups. Since World War II, life expectancy at the older ages has increased at a faster rate than at birth.

It is anticipated that the number of older people will increase even more in the decades ahead. This is not an unreasonable or unwanted speculation when one considers the fact that for humans to travel to and live on other planets, a much longer life span will be required. As women disproportionately outnumber men in the older age group, one wonders what new social patterns will develop by the year 2000 (see Figure 15.3).

For health care professionals, including nurses, the impact of the increased aging population is one of major importance. The use of all health care services increases dramatically with age. Most older people have at least one chronic condition, and older people with multiple chronic diseases are common. The most common chronic conditions in old age requiring health care services are arthritis, hypertension, hearing impairment, heart conditions, orthopedic impairment, sinusitis, visual impairments, and diabetes (Figure 15.4). Therefore, chronic conditions have serious impact on care needs for those who require services ranging from daily personal care to hospitalization in acute or long-term care facilities.

The use of hospitals and nursing homes increases significantly with old age. The hospitalization rate for people 65 and older is two-and-a-half times greater than for younger people (Allan & Brotman, 1981). Although most people 65 and older are not hospitalized in any given year, older people will continue to account for an increasing share of total hospital usage.

The nursing home population has also increased remarkably. In 1963, there were 505,000 people living in nursing homes in the United States. The number has grown to 1.3 million, a 150-percent increase (Allan & Brotman, 1981). Less than 5 percent of all people over 65 are in nursing homes, but this figure increases significantly in the middle-old and old-old groups. Seven out of 100 people in the 75–84 age group and one out of five in the 85-plus group are in nursing homes. Women are likely to be present in larger numbers than men because there are more women in this age bracket.

The causes of death, and therefore the nature of health care, for old people are markedly different than for young people. Heart disease, stroke, and cancer account for three fourths of all deaths in the group aged 65 and older.

Thus, the demographic changes in our population project an increasing number of older people as well as an increased need for health care services. The significance of

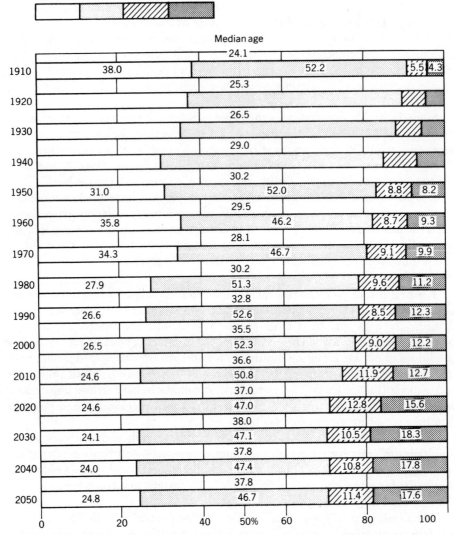

Figure 15.2 Distribution of the total population by age group, 1910 to 2050 (data for 1980–2050 are projections). (From the National Center for Health Statistics.)

long-term care — long considered less important than short-term care — will become fully recognized in the next decade. Long-term care encompasses a continuum of interrelated health and social services. It includes both institutional and noninstitutional services and requires coordination of public policies, funding, and case management to provide appropriate services for individuals with changing needs (Koff, 1982).

The concern for older people in today's health care world is not solely the result of the greatly increased number of them. Changes in federal legislation since the 1930s have contributed much to the economic status of the 65-and-over group. As a result of

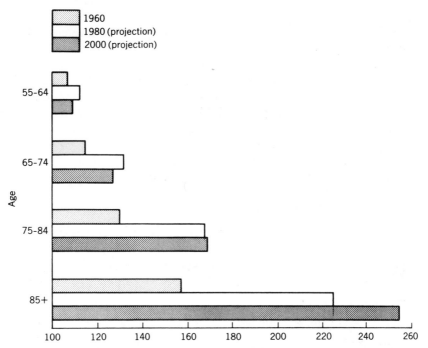

Figure 15.3 Sex ratios (women per 100 men) aged 55 and over by age group, 1960, 1980, and 2000. (From Bureau of the Census.)

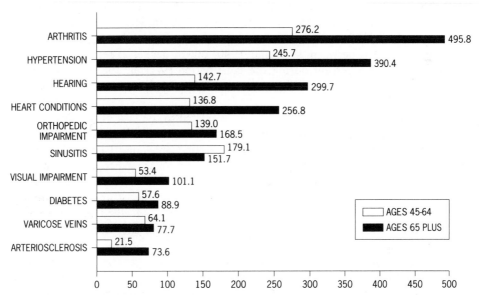

Figure 15.4 Top ten chronic conditions among the elderly, 1982 (rates per 1,000 persons). (From Belsky, J. K. (1988). *Here Tomorrow: Making the Most of Life After Fifty* (p. 7). Baltimore and London: Johns Hopkins University Press. Used with permission.)

the Great Depression, the Social Security Act was passed, establishing a retirement income system and a system of federal grants to states to provide financial assistance to the aged (Koff, 1982).

Nurses can expect to deliver care to increasing numbers of older people who can pay for health care either through private insurance or Medicare-Medicaid reimbursement. All facets of care are available, ranging from highly complex technological procedures to wellness-based, self-care, teaching-learning approaches. For most of the old-age group who are not incapacitated by disease, intellectual functioning and the capacity for learning neither cease nor diminish because of chronological age (Pierce, 1980). This fact allows nurses to develop creatively those options for nursing care that uniquely meet the nursing care needs of older people.

STANDARDS OF HEALTH CARE

There is a rapidly growing opinion on the part of all health professionals that older people should not be treated as separate systems, organs, and diseases. Rather, they should be treated by a single practitioner as complete people with individual medical, emotional, and social histories (Warfel, 1982). This single practitioner could provide:

- Accessibility to care.
- Competence of the practitioner.
- Caring focus.
- Affordable care.

Translated into reality, this mode of treatment would provide patient-centered care, with an emphasis on maintaining cost-effective, humane services. Older people today pay more out-of-pocket expenses for health care than when Medicare programs were first established. Even though federal expenditures for health programs increased by 35 to 40 percent between 1970 and 1980, out-of-pocket expenses paid by the elderly increased 295 percent during the same period (Warfel, 1982). Although 45 percent of the total health care bill is currently paid by Medicare, many items of need are excluded.

Much of the inefficiency in care delivery is related to the lack of optimal services geared toward the special needs of older people. Dr. Leslie S. Libow (1982), the medical director at the Jewish Institute for Geriatric Care, Long Island, New York, envisions the nursing homes as a respected place for treating people. He sees the nursing home as a major center of activity in the nation's health care scene and an extension of the university health sciences campus. Training of undergraduate and graduate students in medicine, nursing, social services, and allied health sciences would involve exposure to geriatric and nursing home patients.

In proposing a framework for improving the standards of care for aged people, Libow suggests that aging is the celebration of survival and geriatrics the fruition of the clinician. Increasingly, the nursing home — if not all long-term care facilities — is the place for that celebration and fruition to occur. Libow sees the nursing home image changing from a place in which to die to a respected place for treating people. Libow maintains that there is no respectable science and art of medicine without geriatric medicine and no true geriatric medicine without the nursing home.

High standards of care for older people are based on the belief that a continuum of care is affordable, available, and desired. Recent gerontological research has come to grips with the inconsistent findings of relocation research. Increased mortality is not a typical or usual finding in the geriatric relocation literature (Coffman, 1981). Increased mortality has occurred no more often than increased survival. Neither mortality effects nor postrelocation decline have been observed as often as has no significant change in postmove mortality rates.

Therefore, it is conceivable to imagine a full-service geriatric program that involves provision of services across settings from the patient's own home to a skilled nursing home to an acute hospital, and so on. Older people are no more limited to place of care than are younger people. Frequently, the acute care hospital is the point of entrance to the health care system, and it is at this point that nursing has the greatest opportunity to influence decisions about continuity of care and linkage with aftercare. Figure 15.5 presents a model of the type of geriatric health care system outlined by Libow (1982). A similar systems approach has been proposed by Denson (1992) as the result of tracing older people through the health care system. The nursing home as a rehabilitation site has been vastly underused (Adelman, Marron, Libow, & Neufeld, 1987). Unfortunately, standard hospital rehabilitation programs often reject the very patients who require rehabilitation prior to discharge. The frail older people are a very large part of this group. As hospitals seek to diversify, it becomes essential for nurse executives to design new nursing patterns that will promote continuity of care across various settings. To establish a rehabilitation unit in a nursing home is to depart from

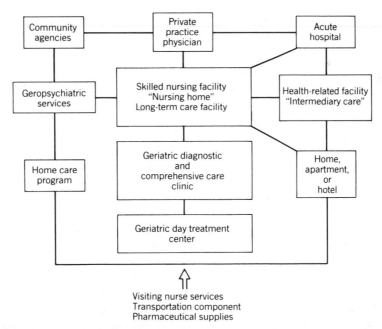

Figure 15.5 The geriatric health care system. (From Libow, L. S. (1982). Geriatric medicine and the nursing home. Reprinted by permission of *The Gerontologist, 22*(2), p. 139.)

the traditional role of the nursing home and offer a setting in which a full interdisciplinary team can excel. Rehabilitation in the United States has traditionally been applied primarily to persons in youth and midlife. The widespread association of aging with infirmity and the assumption that loss of function is normal in advanced age have contributed to denial of essential therapies. Rehabilitation could be imbedded in the total care program rather than an add-on, fee-for-service treatment. Health professionals must recognize that rehabilitation or its lack may be the determining factor in whether an individual will require care from others and what level and duration of continuing care will be required.

THE FRAIL OLDER PEOPLE AND SECONDARY AGING

In the medical world, where a disease-illness orientation is predominant, social-psychological theories of aging are less important than biological theories. The identification of the causes of the numerous physical and mental afflictions is the goal of research in the biology of aging. The average human life has increased mainly because infectious diseases have succumbed to antibiotics, immunization, and improved sanitation.

Various biological studies indicate that the cause of aging may not be outside us but within us. Simple descriptions of changes in the physical and mental characteristics of the aged are not sufficient to explain the aging process. A number of investigators are conducting experiments on cultured cells. Leonard Hayflick (Forbes & Fitzsimons, 1981), in California, has shown that cultured human fibroblasts double only a limited number of times before they deteriorate, lose their capacity to divide, and die. However, he does not think that people age because some of their cells lose the capacity to divide. Rather, he attributes aging to the loss of cell function that occurs before cells reach their limit for division. As cells malfunction, body organs and whole systems are affected and eventually die (Steinberg, 1983).

Other investigators attribute senescence to errors in cell operations regulated by DNA. The aging body's increasing susceptibility to disease may be directly related to declining levels of thymosin. The increase in disease in older people occurs during the same period that the thymosin-producing thymus gland shrinks with age. Other biological theorists espouse the wear-and-tear theory, the lipofuscin theory, the cross-linkage theory, and the immunological theory (Forbes & Fitzsimons, 1981).

One cannot help but think that theories of aging that focus on changes in individual cells are not comprehensive enough. Yet the nature of this kind of research and the interest in prolonging life at any cost necessarily affects physicians, nurses, and the decisions they make in caring for people. Many doctors and nurses still speak of finding a cure for old age, as if it is a disease rather than part of the life cycle. There always seems to be hope that some medication will be found to block the aging process.

In a sense, then, aging presents a negative picture to health professionals. In care settings, the loss of physical functions tends to blur the image of older people as lively, unique individuals. Students in nursing and medical schools must understand the function of all body systems; failure of these systems is viewed as an indication of the decline of the whole person.

Loss of function in primary aging occurs at varying levels in all organs and systems. Diseases, however, contribute a secondary aging effect and are the chief barrier to extended longevity. In primary aging, aging without disease, changes occur in audio-visual, neurological, cardiovascular, metabolic, renal, and respiratory function (Steinberg, 1983). When disease is present, more function is lost and at a faster pace.

Nurse executives are responsible for nursing practice, research, and education as they relate to professional nursing within the institution. Yet, little if any attention is directed toward the care of old people, who now account for 25 percent of all health care costs. According to Stryker-Gordon (1982), the health care system in the United States has two standards of care: one for the aged and one for younger patients. These problems of double standard are primarily due to failure of the nursing and medical professions to incorporate gerontological and geriatric knowledge into their educational curricula, research, and clinical practice.

In hospitals, nursing homes, and home care settings, there is a need for health care workers to prevent confusion, minimize dependence, and provide physical care for older patients. Skill in caring for the aged patient can be improved only if someone in a leadership position demands new standards of care. The nurse executive has wide influence throughout the institution and, aside from the physician, is the single person most likely to affect the care of large numbers of patients. Nurse executives can establish the goal of having better prepared nurses by sharing gerontological knowledge and providing resources with which staff nurses may enhance their skills.

Aging is not the same as disease. The aging process may slow some mental and physical functions, but it is the disease that causes death. Stryker-Gordon (1982) notes two major obstacles to the assumption of responsibility for improving the care of older patients: *(1)* a general misunderstanding by nurses of aging and *(2)* the fact that, because of the physicians' attitudes toward geriatric care, nurses cannot rely on physicians as the traditional source of expertise.

Nurses are in a unique position to influence care of older people. The frail, disabled, and dysfunctional older people are a particularly powerless and voiceless constituency (Moses, 1982). Burnside (1981) describes the frail older people as those who have reached a great age, over 75, and who have, during their long lives, accumulated multiple disabilities, chronic illnesses, or both. These changes, combined with an aging physiology, put such people at increased risk of physical and psychosocial impairments. The frail older person is under constant stress from within and without and has difficulty maintaining daily living activities. Maintenance of wellness is difficult and illness is frequent. Recognizing the real and potential physical changes in old age, nurse executives face a tremendous challenge in planning patient-centered care that requires recognition of environmental and learning needs.

THE NOT-SO-FRAIL OLDER PEOPLE[1]

When Palmore at Duke University compared trends in surveys conducted by the National Center for Health Statistics, he found less infirmity in 1980 than in 1970 and

---

[1]Note: This section has been adapted from a paper presented by L. Simms and S. Fink at the Exploration: Technological Innovations for an Aging Population Conference, Florida, Jan. 31–Feb. 1, 1989 (Simms & Fink, 1989).

less disability in 1970 than in 1960. As a group, older people are more fit and in better health today (Belsky, 1988). Many people are physically middle aged in their 60s and the "silver-haired marathon runner has overtaken the image of the passive older person staring into the sunset" (Belsky, 1988, p. 7).

Even older adults with functional impairments resulting from chronic disease and physiologic changes associated with the aging process can be and are more fit if they have been provided information about assistive technology. When impairments are the result of slow gradual changes rather than an acute episode, individuals are rarely aware of assistive devices that might enhance their functional ability. Enhancement of functional abilities both permits independent living and enables older people to participate in meaningful activities. Nurse executives are in a key position to assist the older population by sharing knowledge of available and developing technologies with the potential for enhancing independent function.

Assistive technologies for community-dwelling older adults range from everyday products that are readily available to the general consumer to specialized assistive devices and high-tech solutions such as robotics. Although the use of the word "technology" tends to focus attention on the more complex, it is important also to consider the potential uses of readily available consumer products. Advances in science and industry affect each of us in our daily lives. Technology has, in innumerable ways, enabled us to expend time and energies that would otherwise be spent in self-maintenance or home maintenance tasks on other pursuits. Opening our minds to the potential uses of everyday consumer products as well as products specifically designed for the disabled enlarges the options that can be offered.

Mobility Products

Older people who have difficulty with grasping and twisting motions can operate a lever more easily than a knob. Door knobs can be replaced with levers either by replacing whole mechanisms or by a lever that fits over the existing knob. Kitchen cabinets are easier to open when knobs are replaced with a c-shaped handle and pull catches replaced with a magnetic latch. Faucets in the kitchen and bathroom that require a grasping twisting motion can be replaced with a lever faucet. A universal turner is available that uses spring-loaded nylon cylinders to grip almost any knob or switch and enables their operation through a lever action. These are particularly useful for stoves, washers, dryers, and other appliances. The small knob-type switch on lamps is particularly troublesome, but a number of alternative adaptations are readily available. The timer can be set to ordinary times of use or a light-sensitive or motion-sensitive device can turn the light on automatically. Lamps also are now available that turn on when the base of the lamp is touched.

Loss of manipulative mobility in the hands may make it impossible for older people to write legibly or may make writing a painful task. The telephone provides one alternative to written communication. This may not be sufficient for people who depend on writing for continued professional activity or as a valued form of communication with distant friends. An electric typewriter with a light touch or a personal computer with word processing software may enable people to meet important goals. If older people cannot manage a standard keyboard, computer adaptations that allow the selection of letters or key words from a menu may be useful.

Specialized Devices

The number of specialized assistive devices available to older people is staggering. ABLEDATA, a computerized data base sponsored by the National Institute for Handicapped Research, lists over 6000 products (Szeto, Tingle, & Cronk, 1981). The difficulties lie in maintaining up-to-date information about these products, evaluating their potential usefulness for specific individuals, and funding when the cost exceeds the individual's resources. The American Association for Retired Persons (AARP) and the Western Gerontological Society have published a catalogue of items specifically selected to assist older people to live independently. It is difficult to determine from a catalogue description or picture whether an item is useful. Lending libraries of assistive devices and health fairs that allow for hands-on examination and trial would be useful approaches to educating potential consumers to the usefulness of various devices.

Computer technology has provided a number of options for home monitoring that can increase the security and convenience of older adults. Home-security devices that automatically signal a service or law enforcement agency if there is an intruder may enable people to feel safer. Thermostats are currently available that enable the programming of the desired temperatures for each day of the week with several temperature changes each day. Computerized monitoring-control devices can enable the person to control home heating, lights, other electrical appliances, and even door locks from a control panel that is centrally located or portable. The lifeline system, which is in operation in many communities today, enables the person to call for help by pressing a button on a lightweight transmitter that is designed to be worn. This transmitter is electronically linked to a health care institution 24 hours a day and sends an automatic signal if it is not reset by the person at predetermined intervals.

These devices are merely illustrative. Older people are often extremely creative in finding ways to adapt their own environments to make optimal use of their strengths and to meet personally meaningful goals. Nurse executives can be helpful to older people by keeping staff abreast of new developments in biotechnology and related fields. The creative nurse executive will support the development of new options and resources for maintaining independent function and enhancing the quality of life. Freedom from basic-coping needs can enable older people to reinvest their energies in continuing growth and development and meaningful activities rather than in disease-concentration behavior. (Becker & Kaufmann, 1988). The resourceful nurse executive will support the "skunk works" model present in innovative organizations by sponsoring ongoing innovation and invention task forces.

ASSUMING LEADERSHIP FOR CARE OF OLDER PEOPLE

The basic assumption underlying all rehabilitation, remotivation, and reality-orientation care models is that older adults have the ability to learn new behaviors. In the words of Howard McClusky (1971), who lived and functioned as a professor until the age of 82:

In general, then, we are justified in saying that even into the 70s and 80s, and for all we know as long as we live on the functioning side of senility, age per se is no barrier to learning. There is no one at any age, even the most gifted, who is without limitation in learning. Thus limitation per se—age related or otherwise—should not be our criterion for appraising the capacity of older people for education. We can teach an old dog new tricks, for it is never too late to learn. (pp. 12–13)

Stryker-Gordon (1982) has described essential steps for nurse executives in providing leadership in stimulating better care for older people. These include:

1. Read in the field and divest oneself of false beliefs.
2. Examine one's personal experience with older people.
3. Pursue continuing education.
4. Take on the challenge of making quality care for older people comparable with quality care for other individuals.
5. Develop a cadre of interested nursing staff who are able to make observations and obtain information from older people.

The authors would add:

6. Create geriatric clinician or clinical specialist roles that give institutional recognition to the importance of older adult care.

The lag between nursing knowledge and practice is greater for older people than for any other age group. Few nurses are prepared for geriatric care, and few nurses know that the aging process alone is not a cause of a patient's psychological condition; other causes might be drugs, nutrition, disease, or depression due to grief. The nurse executive has wide influence in an institution and is in a better position than any other person to affect the care of large numbers of patients. For every organization that becomes a center of geriatric expertise, higher expectations of care will be sought in other organizations.

The nurse executive role in nursing homes is at a significant crossroad. National efforts are under way to improve the expertise of nurse leaders through increased opportunities for education for leadership in long-term care (Lodge, 1983). Nonnursing leaders are losing power as their competencies and motives are challenged. Nurses are learning that they hold the expertise to meet regulatory agencies' demands and that it is the nursing profession that keeps the doors of the nursing home open (Eliopoulos, 1982).

The 1981 White House Conference on Aging (Benson & McDevitt, 1982) provided an additional stimulus for the nursing profession to offer leadership in the care of older people. Major emphasis was given to the importance of such nursing leadership in health care services. Nurses have already demonstrated leadership in establishing preventive health care services in nontraditional settings with a focus on wellness. Nurses have served as health care givers, counselors, and client advocates, and it is important now to direct such efforts to promoting health for older adults. Health was recognized at the conference as the chief determinant in improving quality of life for our senior citizens.

A variety of educational programs can be designed, irrespective of health care setting, that can improve the physical health, mental health, self-esteem, and independence of the aged person. Gershowitz (1982) suggests that the best mode for restoring psychological health and, indirectly, physical health is through remotivation techniques that encourage patients to use their own past experiences and skills in coping with the present. Prior life experiences, values, and interests can be used by a knowledgeable staff in assisting older adults to greater independence and improved quality of life.

Feier and Leight (1981) suggest that the intellectual and communication declines common in nursing home residents can be counteracted by engaging residents in meaningful activities. For old-timers in nursing homes, regularly provided experiences may no longer be of interest and cognitive performance may decline as a result. Studies carried out by Feier and Leight (1981) demonstrated that when learning experiences meaningful to residents were provided on a regular basis, functional capacity improved.

Sperbeck and Whitbourne (1981) support attention to functional competence and the need to teach staff how to work with older people and change behavior. Because institutional dependency has been found to be related to poor self-concept and low life satisfaction, it is important to investigate altering both behavior and setting to enhance resident autonomy. Nurses have a major role to play in identifying measures that will offset the effects of cognitive, elimination, audiovisual, and mobility problems. Regardless of disease processes, these functional disabilities commonly interfere with activities that could enhance self-esteem and encourage independence. The same principles of care apply in acute, long-term, and home care settings.

OBSTACLES TO A GERIATRIC EMPHASIS

A negative attitude toward older people is frequently cited as the major cause of disinterest in working with older people in any health care setting. Aging may be equated with disease or even death, both having negative connotations in our society. All societies deny death. This is manifested in various ways of ignoring the dying person or carrying on elaborate rituals to keep the dead with the living, as seen, for example, in the practices of keeping cremated ashes in the living room or preserving departed family members in cryogenic vaults. Belief in an afterlife is one of many societal supports, and the clear if unwritten goal in the institutions where most of us will die is to preserve life at any cost. In fact, modern medicine has added more to immortality than have all the theologians and church people in history combined. Physicians seem determined to do almost anything to keep a human system going.

Overcoming negative attitudes is difficult, for they are usually strongly held. In defining programs and goals with a geriatric emphasis, the nurse executive will have to facilitate learning behaviors that will produce positive attitudes. Despite the prevailing belief that old age is synonymous with a decline in creativity, Simonton (1990) proposes that a much more favorable outlook can be gained by reviewing the actual careers of artists and scientists in their later years. The author cites the work of Galileo, Goethe, Bach, Handel, Beethoven, Hawking, and Rosenweig as individuals who refused to let physical handicaps stop them from generating ideas. Creativity in the later years may be dependent on an individual's initial creative potential in earlier life and seems unrelated to age. The potential for late-life creativity has implications for planning health care services and in viewing human resources in care-giving roles. Perhaps every individual patient has untapped creativity and potential for living a meaningful life. It is up to the caregiver to spot this potential and to match nursing therapies with abilities. Depression is a major dysfunction in old age but is one that can be addressed with holistic patient-centered care that recognizes individual goals for creative activities.

Older adults are the biggest users of illness care in U.S. hospitals and nurse executives need to know and understand concerns of older adults. Knowledge of concerns could lead to establishing services that might be offered on an outpatient basis without hospital admission. Older adults comprise 20 percent of hospital admissions, 40 percent of inpatient days, and 30 percent of hospital discharges (Halbur & Freeberg, 1991). Recognizing that comprehensive geriatric programs are needed, Halbur and Freeberg conducted a survey of older adults' concerns in an urban community hospital. Handling changes in life and staying active and involved were high on the list of identified concerns of older people. The results further suggested involvement of older people in planning geriatric programs.

Contrary to popular belief, the economic situation of older people has improved dramatically over the past several years. Older people as a group have impressive financial assets in spite of areas of deep poverty. Aging of the population and the related requirements for home personal assistance have increased the demand for unskilled home care services, whereas the supply of acceptable quality, paid custodial home care is threatened by the increasingly precarious financial condition of providers (Kane, 1989). As hospitals seek new markets, the creative nurse executive must attend to the rapidly increasing need for housekeeping services at home in combination with skilled nursing services. A creative nurse executive could design a unique geriatric home care program that links housekeeping services with health care services in a product that has appeal for a large number of clients.

More than nine million older people live in rural areas of our country (Bender & Hart, 1987) and many of them suffer from some form of chronic disease. Nurse executives, seeking to develop marketable health promotion product lines, may well be interested in recognizing this group as they work to develop a positive geriatric emphasis. The present system of activities by agencies is based on a belief that old people are sick, disabled and poor, and unable to participate independently in society (Morris, 1989). Those who are actively concerned about the aged can play an active role in shaping the nature of change by devoting more attention to the positive side of aging to balance the past emphasis on dependency, helplessness, deprivation, and cure of disease.

OLDER WOMEN: A SPECIAL NEED

Nursing care programs often ignore the special health needs of older people, and, in particular, they may not even recognize the needs of older women. Lillard (1982) describes older women as economically disadvantaged, socially isolated, and negatively stereotyped. The medical profession takes a different view of men and women experiencing the same medical problems, and it is not uncommon for women to receive tranquilizers that are not appropriate. Ageism and sexism form a double-edged sword. Postmenopausal women have frequently outlived their culturally ascribed usefulness and frequently face additional negative attitudes toward feminine aging. The vast majority of elderly people are older women, and because the care of older people is primarily a nursing task, the opportunities for negative behavior are compounded if nurses do not have a geriatric interest.

Women are less apt to have supportive family groups (Simms & Lindberg, 1978). They become widowed before men, and they have fewer remarriage options. It is not socially acceptable for older women in our culture to marry men substantially younger than themselves. Health problems abound in older women, and few doctors seem interested in these problems. "Postmenopausal syndrome" and "senility" frequently cover up a medical diagnosis or lack of it.

Summary

Responsibility for care of older people as a significant part of the nurse executive's role has not been addressed in most organizations. Most staffing studies focus on high turnover rather than on the potential for nursing leadership in providing quality care for older people. Our society's concept of aging and the attitudes of health professionals and patients influence the development of optimal care programs. Nurse executives should encourage creative approaches to care, ranging from changing attitudes toward older people to designing programs that meet their special needs. They are also in a unique position to support the development of assistive technology.

STUDY QUESTIONS

1. How does the increasing older population relate to nursing administration and practice?

2. Why are population trends considered important aspects of society?

3. People are living longer in the United States today than at any other time in history. Explain how this affects the health care delivery system. Include the effects of Social Security and Medicare-Medicaid.

4. Describe holistic care. Give reasons why such care could be beneficial to the care of older people.

5. Explain Libow's position on nursing homes, and contrast it with your own concept of nursing homes.

6. Discuss the concepts of primary and secondary aging.

7. Explain the importance of distinguishing the aging process from a disease process and give the major reasons why aging is sometimes considered a disease.

8. Define frail older people.

9. List the steps essential for nurse executives to provide leadership in stimulating better care for older people.

10. Give reasons why it is vitally important that nursing personnel understand the concepts of geriatrics.

11. What is the most frequently cited reason for disinterest in working with older people? What are some of the others?

12. What is geriatric burnout?

13. List some of the special needs of older women.

References

Abdellah, F. G. (1981). Nursing care of the aged in the United States of America, *Journal of Gerontological Nursing, 7*(11), 657–663.

Adelman, R. D., Marron, K., Libow, L. S., & Neufeld, R. (1987). A community-oriented geriatric rehabilitation unit in a nursing home, *The Gerontologist 27*(2), 143–146.

Allan, C., & Brotman, H. (1981). *Chartbook on aging in America.* Washington, DC: U.S. Government Printing Office.

Becker, G., & Kaufman, S. (1988). Old age, rehabilitation and research: A review of the issues, *The Gerontologist, 28*(4), 459–468.

Bender, C., & Hart, J. P. (1987). A model for health promotion for the rural elderly, *The Gerontologist, 27*(2), 139–142.

Belsky, J. K. (1988). *Here tomorrow. Making the most of life after fifty.* Baltimore: Johns Hopkins University Press.

Benson, E. R., & McDevitt, J. Q. (1982). Health promotion by nursing in care of the elderly, *Nursing and Health Care, 3*(1), 39–43.

Burnside, I. M. (1981). *Nursing and the aged.* New York: McGraw-Hill.

Coffman, T. L. (1981). Relocation and survival of institutionalized aged: A reexamination of the evidence, *The Gerontologist, 21*(5), 483–500.

Denson, P. M. (1992). Tracing the elderly through the health care system: An update. *AHCPR Monograph. DHHS, PHS, Agency for Health Care Policy and Research (AHCPR).* Information and Publications Division, 18-12 Parklawn Building, Rockville, MD.

Eliopoulos, C. (1982). The director of nursing in the nursing home setting: An emerging dynamic role in gerontological nursing, *Journal of Gerontological Nursing, 8*(8), 448–450.

Feier, C. D., & Leight, G. L. (1981). A communication-cognition program for elderly nursing home residents, *The Gerontologist, 21*(4), 408–416.

Forbes, J. F., & Fitzsimons, V. M. (1981). *The older adult.* St. Louis: Mosby.

Gershowitz, S. Z. (1982). Adding life to years: Remotivating elderly people in institutions, *Nursing and Health Care, 3*(3), 141–145.

Haber, P. A. L. (1986). Technology in aging, *The Gerontologist, 26*(4), 350–357.

Halbur, B., & Freeberg, K. (1991). Older and wiser: A hospital-based comprehensive geriatric program, *The Gerontologist, 30*(6), 833–836.

Kane, N. M. (1989). The home care crisis of the nineties, *The Gerontologist, 29*(1), 24–31.

Koff, T. H. (1982). *Long-term care: An approach to serving the elderly.* Boston: Little, Brown.

Libow, L. S. (1982). Geriatric medicine and the nursing home: A mechanism for mutual excellence, *The Gerontologist, 22*(2), 134–141.

Lillard, J. (1982). A double-edged sword: Ageism and sexism, *Journal of Gerontological Nursing, 8*(11), 630–634.

Lodge, M. P. (1983). *Professional practice for nurse administrators in long-term care facilities.* Unpublished report of the American Nurses Foundation and the Foundation of the

American College of Nursing Home Administrators. Battle Creek, MI: W. K. Kellogg Foundation.

McClusky, H. Y. (1971). *Education*. Background paper for 1971 White House Conference on Aging. Washington, DC: U.S. Government Printing Office.

Morris, R. (1989). Challenges of aging in tomorrow's world: Will gerontology grow, stagnate, or change? *The Gerontologist, 29*(4), 494–500.

Moses, D. (1982). Nursing advocacy for the frail elderly, *Journal of Gerontological Nursing, 8*(3), 144–145.

Pierce, P. M. (1980). Intelligence and learning in the aged, *Journal of Gerontological Nursing, 6*(5), 268–270.

Riffer, J. (1985). Elderly 21 percent of population by 2040, *Hospitals, 59*(5), 41 & 44.

Simms, L. M., & Fink, S. V. (1989). Empowerment learning: Control of destiny in the later years. *Exploration: Technological Innovations for an Aging Population Conference Proceedings*. University of Wisconsin: Stout. Lake Buena Vista, Florida, Jan. 30–Feb. 1, 1989, 10–13.

Simms, L. M., & Lindberg, J. (1978). Women and the lengthening life span. In *The Nurse Person*. New York: Harper & Row.

Simonton, D. K. (1990). Creativity in the later years: Optimistic prospects for achievement, *The Gerontologist, 30*(5), 626–631.

Sperbeck, D. J., & Whitbourne, S. K. (1981). Dependency in the institutional setting: A behavioral training program for geriatric staff, *The Gerontologist, 21*(3), 268–275.

Steinberg, F. V. (Ed.) (1983). The aging of organs and the organ systems. In *Care of the Geriatric Patient* (6th ed.). St. Louis: Mosby.

Stryker-Gordon, R. (1982). Leadership in care of the elderly: Assessing needs and challenges, *Journal of Nursing Administration, 12*(10), 41–44.

Szeto, A., Tingle, L., & Cronk, S. (1981). Automated retrieval of information on assistive devices, *Bulletin of Prosthetics Research, 10*, 27–34.

Thomas, J., & Bobrow, M. L. (1984). Targeting the elderly in facility design, *Hospitals, 58*(4), 83–88.

Warfel, B. L. (October, 1982). *Information on aging*. Newsletter from the Institute of Gerontology, Wayne State University and the University of Michigan, no. 27.

Bibliography

U.S. Department of Commerce, Bureau of the Census. (1981). *Statistical abstract of the United States: 1981*. Washington, DC: U.S. Government Printing Office.

U.S. Department of Health and Human Services. (1981). *The need for long-term care: A chartbook of the federal council on aging*. Washington, DC: U.S. Government Printing Office.

PART IV

Facilitating Professional Nursing Practice

CHAPTER 16

Ethical Decision Making and Moral Judgments

Charlotte McDaniel

Highlights

- **Ethics defined**
- **Ethics and quality care**
- **Ethics and current practice**
- **Ethics and applied benefits**
- **Generic decision models**
- **Ethical decision models**

Ethics as a basis for clinical practice is important to nursing and to health care. The importance of ethics for the delivery of nursing care, however, is receiving increasing attention in nursing administration because of the contribution that ethics can make to a positive work environment and to the organizational culture of nursing practice.

Nursing administration as a professional practice for the delivery of health care is fundamentally a moral practice. Nursing administration is fundamentally moral because the delivery of nursing care is based on the interaction and interrelationships of patients as human beings and on decisions about them and their care (Beauchamp & Childress, 1989). Because morals and ethics are intertwined, nursing care is also an issue of ethics. Nurses make decisions in the daily implementation of their practice and in the management of patient care that affect and influence human beings and their lives. These important and often critical decisions are significant to nursing administration because nurse executives shape and sustain the practice environment of those nurses who are delivering patient care.

ETHICS DEFINED

Although ethics is variously defined, it is recognized as a branch of philosophy that addresses questions of right or wrong. Ethics is the rational and systematic examination of issues pertaining to right and wrong. "Ethics systematically explores what we ought to do by asking persons to consider . . . our ordinary actions, judgments, and justifications" (Beauchamp & Childress, 1989; xii). Similarly, ethics is "the search for and establishment of reasons for . . . conduct, including such things as actions, motives, attitudes, judgments, rules, ideals, and goals" (Ladd, 1978; 402).

A critical component to the study of ethics is a systematic approach that involves rational thinking; it implies an ability to think critically about moral and ethical issues. Essentially, this process is ethical decision making. Although distinctions can be made between morals and ethics, because the focus of this chapter is on decision making in applied ethics for the administration of nursing care, for the purposes of this chapter the two terms will be used synonymously. This is appropriate because nursing administration is based on decision making, and ethics pertains to rational decisions about ethical issues.

ETHICS AND QUALITY CARE

A sound sense of ethics, conveyed by ethical decisions, is essential to quality nursing care. It is important not only to professional nurses and to nursing, it is also important to the patient as the health care consumer. Patients understand and perceive an ethical system by the nature, the competency, and the quality of the care that they receive. Consumers formulate their understanding of the ethical nature of nursing by those individual and patient care dimensions of nursing practice.

Ethical practice is also important to nurse executives who are responsible for those nurses and, in turn, to other administrators to whom nursing reports. This is not to imply that current practices are unethical, but, simply that applied ethics is fundamental and important to quality nursing care and administration. Ironically, a well-grounded and ethically-based administration frames nursing practice, which, in turn, supports the professional practice of nursing administration. Thus, the interrelationship of these two — care and administration — are not only necessary to each other, they are essential to each other.

ETHICS AND CURRENT PRACTICE

Faced with an ethical dilemma, what do nurse executives do? How do administrators make decisions? Studies on ethics and administration in nursing report two general findings. One is that nurse executives experience ethical conflicts at work, usually emerging out of the conflicts between various components of the hospital (Sietsema &

Spradley, 1987). The second finding is that administrators rarely resolve ethical situations in systematic ways. For example, one method for making decisions is the use of "unstructured" (Christensen, 1988) approaches, meaning that nurse executives use a variety of approaches to resolve ethical dilemmas. Another study reports a "subjective" approach (Self, 1987) used by the administrator respondents; they relied on their own intuitions or experiences for resolving ethical clashes, in contrast to using ethical frameworks. These findings, nevertheless, suggest that models commensurate with the definition of ethics as a systematic and rational approach are needed by nurse executives to sustain them in their professional practice of nursing administration.

ETHICS AND APPLIED BENEFITS

Applied ethics may also benefit nursing personnel and the management as well as patients. Ethics is suggested as one way to bring consistency between the philosophy and practice of professional nursing (Christensen, 1988). Ethics can assist in examining the ever-present issues of power or authority of health care facilities (Erlen & Frost, 1991; Sullivan, 1986), or in rebalancing power in them (Jameton, 1984). It can assist in interdisciplinary communication by providing a common language. That language can offer a consistent background for exploring patient care solutions. Last, "ethical distress" is suggested as one factor in "reality shock," contributing to the turnover of nurses (Jameton, 1984). Administrative strategies that enhance ethics may counter turnover or burnout in nurses, thereby, improving nurse retention. For these reasons, strategies that enhance ethical practice and support nursing care in these settings are critical to the professional practice of nursing administration.

DECISION MAKING IN NURSING ADMINISTRATION

Generic Decision Models

Nurse executives must balance clinical and organizational imperatives in managing the professional practice environment. It is clear that the quality of the decision is critical to the well-being of an organization. Although the information required for patient care or administrative decision making may vary, the nature of the underlying decision process and its use in health care organizations is similar.

Alternative choices of action bridge the gap between a problem and a goal. The generation of alternative problem solutions assists in formulating a plan of action. Rarely, does a problem have only one solution. In fact, the challenge of administrative decision making in health care is to arrive at one best alternative among several competing ones. Basically, decision making is a cognitive process of choice that precedes the chosen behavior.

In thinking about decisions, it can be useful to differentiate the decision process from the decision itself. Although heuristic in nature, decision making can be divided into two parts, the process of the decision making and the content about which the decision will be made. This section examines general decision making as a foundation for ethical decision making. The focus is on the decision process.

The decision process is a series of interrelated steps for systematically and logically coming to a decision. It is analogous to other systematic processes that guide intellectual work, such as the scientific method or the research process. Decision making is the point in the process at which the choice, or selection of alternatives, is made and is often viewed as the culmination of the decision process.

Prescriptive Model   As shall be seen, that which differs is the components of the process. These vary depending on whether the underlying model for the process of decision making is prescriptive or descriptive. Prescriptive models, which derive from economic theory, rest on assumptions that a rational decision maker strives to reach *optimal* outcomes and the information is available to determine those outcomes. A prescriptive process includes the following steps to arrive at a quality decision:

1. Recognition and analysis of the problem or situation requiring a decision.
2. Identification of all feasible alternative solutions.
3. Determination of potential favorable and unfavorable consequences and their likelihood for each alternative considered.
4. Selection of the alternative that results in *optimal* outcomes.

Descriptive Model   In contrast, a descriptive model for decision making is based on how decisions are *actually* made. One of the most influential of these was formulated by Herbert Simon (1976). This type of model acknowledges that decision makers often have limited time or information on which to make a rational decision. This grounding in reality is particularly relevant to the busy nurse executive. Descriptive models lead to what Simon calls "satisficing" in which the decision maker searches for alternatives until one is found that provides an *acceptable* solution, rather than an optimal solution. Steps in a decision process based on the descriptive model of satisficing include:

1. Recognition and analysis of the problem or situation requiring a decision.
2. Development of criteria for an acceptable outcome.
3. Identification of alternatives.
4. Evaluation of whether the alternative will lead to acceptable outcomes.
5. Selection of a *satisfactory* alternative.

Other and less well formulated models are also used but are considered less likely to consistently produce good outcomes. For that reason this discussion will be limited to these two. However, two additional steps are often included as components of the decision process: implementation of the decision and the evaluation of the decision outcome. No decision process is considered complete without these final steps.

Ethical Decision Models

Applied ethics implies decision making. It involves the content of ethical theory applied to health care situations in a systematic, rational, and critical manner. In this case, the situations emerge out of the nursing administration of health care delivery. The aim is to analyze the situation to determine an ethically sound administrative solution. This process is fundamental to applied ethics in nursing administration.

Although applied ethics relies on the process of decision making, the content will differ and it may influence the process. To some extent, the content of ethics can influence the process of decision making. In most cases, however, a model of applied nursing ethics will be similar to the generic model discussed earlier.

Nursing Model for Process   A widely used model of ethical decision making for nursing has been formulated by Mila Aroskar (1980). It proposes three steps for ethical decisions: *(1)* obtain information or data, *(2)* consider questions from decision theorists, and *(3)* articulate the ethical theories.

Other models of decision making in nursing ethics are in the nursing literature. Although it is beyond the scope of this chapter to examine them all in detail, several models are briefly noted that the reader may explore further. Theoretical models using criteria are proposed (Silva, 1990); several (Curtin & Flaherty, 1982; Thompson & Thompson, 1985) address ethical decision making and moral judgments. However, there are common themes among these models. One of them is that a systematic and rational approach would be fruitful. Another implication is that there is no *one* way to resolve an ethical dilemma.

Ethical Content-Principles and Theories   The content of ethics can influence the process of the ethical decision making. The relationship between the process and the content of ethics is more sensitive than with generic decision models. The influence would depend on the choice of principles or theories as potential content. One may also combine and use both of them.

When philosophers have attempted to determine common features of a problem or case, they are often stated as principles (Beauchamp & Walters, 1989). Nursing has borrowed from biomedical ethics in its application of key principles as a "framework" or a set of parameters for examining ethical situations. Administrative decisions concerning, for example, allocation of resources, can be examined in the light of ethical principles it poses for the decision maker. Justice is a principle relevant to allocation.

There is no agreement on the exact number or set of principles; however, several emerge as major ones. They are beneficence, justice, and autonomy (Beauchamp & Walters, 1989). Briefly defined, beneficence is doing good, justice is also called fairness or equality, and autonomy refers to rights of self or others. Administrative situations can be examined in light of the principle that emerges as the central one in that situation. In many instances, a case may illustrate more than one principle. The principle becomes, then, a means of examining the situation and exploring its alternatives. Principles become a framework for examining ethical situations.

Theories of ethics can also provide content for ethical decision making. Although a variety of theories are used, there are several appearing frequently. These are the utilitarian, the deontological, and the egoist theories (Aroskar, 1980). Briefly, the utilitarian focuses on the consequences of a decision, the deontological addresses the act itself, and the egoist would be concerned with the best solution for oneself.

The theory selected for ethical examination can influence the process because the alternatives may need to be reexamined in light of the outcome. Also, the type of ethical situations confronted by nurse executives are often vastly troublesome with no clearly defined right or wrong answers. That is why a decision framework for ethics is so important to the professional practice of nursing administration.

ETHICS AND PROFESSIONAL PRACTICE
OF NURSING ADMINISTRATION

Confounding ethical situations that need nursing administration attention usually occur in the relationships among personnel. Ethical situations for nursing administration usually emerge out of the intra- or interdisciplinary relationships in health care settings.

Today's health care environment is changing rapidly, creating a turbulent and more ambiguous context for nursing practice. Major contributors to this constant change are the increasing amounts of technology that nurses are required to understand and to use in their work and the changes in reimbursement illustrated by diagnostic-related groups and prospective payment. Although increased technology is advancing health care and extending life, a side effect of these advances is the increasing number of ethical issues that the use of technology creates. The extension of life provides opportunity and challenge for ethical decision making about issues such as termination of life, withholding of treatment, or appropriate termination of treatment and discharge of psychiatric patients (McDaniel, 1992). Health care changes bring with them an increasing number of ethical situations that affect nurses, their work, and their professional relationships with those in health care. Those changes raise ethical issues for nursing work, affecting the relationships among nurses and among nurses and auxiliary personnel, physicians, and nurse executives.

Nursing Staff

Nurses face challenges in their daily practice that require decisions and judgments that are ethical in nature. Nurses also make ethical decisions about their work and patient care (Yarling & McElmurry, 1983), informed by professional, institutional, and group norms. These decisions require judgment about what is right and wrong and what is the best outcome in light of the ethical parameters.

Because one's ethical system is informed by the values of individuals, nurses may differ among themselves in the priority they place on a situation or they may differ in philosophy. There may be conflicts among nurses about the best way in which to resolve a conflict. These, in turn, create ethical conflicts of an intraprofessional nature. In these instances of ethical disagreement, the support and education provided by nurse executives is important to shape and sustain nurses, their practice, and their ethical decisions. It is here that a nurse executive can play an important role in facilitating resolution of ethical dilemmas.

Nurses and Auxiliary Personnel

There are also ethical situations emerging in the interactions between nurses and auxiliary personnel. Ethical conflicts may occur among the nursing service personnel, referring to nurses and their auxiliary co-workers, support services, or health-related personnel. Ketefian (1981) found that moral reasoning differed according to educational level. If there are differences in educational background among nursing service personnel, one can anticipate differences in moral reasoning. Understanding these perspectives and their influence on ethical dilemmas can assist nurse executives in developing supports and strategies for arriving at an ethical solution.

When nurses are responsible for the delegation and implementation of care provided by those under nursing service but who are not professional nurses, the responsibility itself may take on ethical parameters. Nurses may be reluctant to assume responsibility for auxiliary functions (Cohen, 1991). In the face of mounting nurse shortage and increased demand for care, auxiliary personnel may be pressed into delivery of care that is beyond the scope of their education and experience. Nurses, who rightfully perceive their responsibility for other personnel in differentiated practice environments, may be unsure about the level of accountability that they as nurses assume. These situations can pose ethical conflicts surrounding the work relationships among personnel in nursing service.

Nurses and Physicians

The range of ethical dilemmas may also extend to nurse-physician interactions. There are several reasons why these tensions occur. One reason is inherent in the structures of the typical hospital. Although there are trends for change, illustrated by the increasing number of group practices and health maintenance organizations (HMOs), physicians in the typical hospital are usually not employed by the facility and are remunerated by a fee-for-service structure. Nurses, in contrast, are frequently employed by the hospital for an hourly rate. A physician who sees more patients, likewise enjoys a parallel larger remuneration. Nurses receive no added remuneration from increased work loads. This fundamental difference in financial structure can be the basis for ethical conflicts. Facilities and physicians may desire to admit additional patients or it might be financially desirable to assign more patients to a unit and, thereby, to an individual nurse, than that nurse feels competent to attend. If additional nurses are not used, then the increase of patient load creates a larger profit margin but may compromise care. This is a relatively common situation that raises ethical issues (Flaherty, 1982).

Other conflicts occur. Physicians and nurses may place different importance on various aspects of the patient's treatment. Nurses and physicians may have different perspectives of patient care situations, emerging from different philosophical backgrounds and approaches (McDaniel, 1991). Nurses may assume an advocacy role for the patient, placing them in conflict with continuing treatments advocated by a physician. The imbalance of power experienced by nurses in the traditional hospital means that physician decisions carry more "weight." Thus, nurses may feel intimidated by those in positions of power, those with greater authority, or those who simply are more assertive (Erlen & Frost, 1991). Ethical frameworks, however, can assist in redressing these imbalances of power (Jameton, 1984) by reframing the examination of power and placing it in an ethical context. This reframing of power serves as a support to both nurses and nurse executives.

Nurses and Nurse Executives

Ethical conflicts can also occur between nursing staff and nurse executives. In many instances, these dilemmas occur because there are inherent differences in the perspectives that staff nurses and nurse executives hold. For example, staff nurses will usually assume what is termed a microlevel perspective, illustrated by concern for an individual patient or case. This perspective is commensurate with their level of responsibility for individual patient care. In contrast, an executive will assume, by virtue of position, a macroperspective, illustrated by concern for a whole unit or facility. Staff nurses, delivering care at the bedside, will view their patient care situation differently than their nurse executive(s). Although often overlooked as an inherent distinction, different levels of responsibility contribute to differing perspectives about the situation and its outcome. These perspectives need to be explored to arrive at an ethical and mutual understanding of the situation.

A common difference is illustrated in the assignment of nursing staff. Staff nurses may experience a shortage of qualified staff to deliver the quality of care desired. The shortage of nurses places those at the bedside in a compromising care delivery situation, an ethical issue (Flaherty, 1982). Shortage of nursing personnel is an ethical issue of resource allocation and pertains to justice as a principle.

Nurse executives, too, experience ethical conflicts when they must allocate fewer available nursing staff across more patients than actually provides adequate coverage. This situation is especially troublesome because it has implications for quality of care for patients as well as quality of care for nursing staff. The constrained economic environment within health care (Fry, 1986) contributes to the intensity of this relatively common situation. Nurse executives who experience this level of administrative and ethical conflict are often placed in a compromising situation with their own facility administrators as well. To support one's own administrator in the face of economic constraints and the need also to support one's staff and their patients is an ethical conundrum. The resulting hierarchical ethical conflict is one of the most difficult for nurse executives and, thereby, affects the professional practice of nursing administration.

Summary

Decision making is a cognitive process of interrelated steps for systematically and logically coming to a decision. It may be subdivided into the process and content of decision making. The process can be based on a prescriptive or a descriptive model. In applied ethics for administration, nursing models and ethics content are used. Situations requiring ethical administrative decisions may emerge from relationships among personnel in the professional practice of nursing administration.

References

Aroskar, M. A. (1980). Anatomy of an ethical dilemma: The theory, *American Journal of Nursing 80*(4), 658–663.

Beauchamp, T. L., & Childress, J. F. (1989). *Principles of biomedical ethics* (3rd ed.). New York: Oxford University Press.

Beauchamp, T. L., & Walters, L. (1989). *Contemporary issues in bioethics*. Belmont, CA: Wadsworth Publishing Co.

Christensen, P. J. (1988). An ethical framework for nursing service administration, *Advances in Nursing Science, 10*(3), 46–55.

Cohen, E. L. (1991). Nursing case management: Does it pay? *Journal of Nursing Administration, 21*(4), 20–25.

Curtin, L., & Flaherty, M. J. (1982). *Nursing ethics: Theories and pragmatics*. Bowie, MD: James Brady Co.

Erlen, J., & Frost, B. (1991). Nurses' perception of powerlessness in influencing ethical decisions, *Western Journal of Nursing Research, 13*(3), 397–407.

Flaherty, M. J. (1982). Insubordination-patient load. In L. Curtin & M. J. Flaherty (Eds.), *Nursing Ethics: Theories and Pragmatics*. Bowie, MD: James Brady Co.

Fry, S. T. (1986). Moral values and ethical decisions in a constrained economic environment, *Nursing Economic$, 4*(4), 160–163.

Jameton, A. (1984). *Nursing practice: The ethical issues*. Englewood Cliffs, NJ: Prentice-Hall.

Ketefian, S. (1981). Critical thinking, educational preparation, and development of moral judgment among selected groups of practicing nurses, *Nursing Research, 30*(3), 98–103.

Ladd, J. (1978). The task of ethics. In W. Reich (Ed.-in-Chief), *Encyclopedia of Bioethics, 1*. New York: Free Press.

McDaniel, C. (1992). Ethical issues in the restructuring of psychiatric services, *Issues in Mental Health Nursing, 13*(1), 31–37.

McDaniel, C. (1991). Ethics and the nurse administrator. In B. Henry (Ed.), *The Inquiry and Practice of Nursing Administration*. Kansas City, MO: American Academy of Nursing.

Self, D. J. (1987). A study of the foundations of ethical decision making of nurses, *Theoretical Medicine, 8*, 83–95.

Sietsema, R. N., & Spradley, B. W. (1987). Ethics and administrative decision making, *Journal of Nursing Administration, 17*(4), 28–32.

Silva, M. C. (1990). *Ethical decision making in nursing administration*. Norwalk, CT: Appleton & Lange.

Simon, H. (1976). *Administrative behavior*. New York: Free Press.

Sullivan, M-C. (1986). Professionalism and ethics in nursing, *Second Opinion, 1*, 103–123.

Thompson, J. E., & Thompson, H. O. (1985). *Bioethical decision making for nurses*. Norwalk, CT: Appleton-Century-Crofts.

Yarling, R. R., & McElmurry, B. J. (1986). Rethinking the nurses' role in "do not resuscitate" orders: A clinical policy proposal in nursing ethics, *Advances in Nursing Science, 5*(4), 1–12.

CHAPTER 17

Personal and Group Empowerment

Lillian M. Simms

Highlights

- **Visioning**
- **Group learning through action research**
- **Perceptions of work**
- **Work excitement**
- **Empowerment and effective practice**
- **Identifying work penetration points from unit data**

There are no more big daddies and big mamas to make everything right. The President of the United States cannot alone change the health care system. The Director of Nursing can no longer single-handedly make everything work efficiently and effectively. Tomorrow's leadership must see its prime duty as the empowerment of other people. The most vital requirements for a leader will be those of self-knowledge and inner balance, and a leader's major attribute will be to facilitate the empowerment of colleagues to be their own leaders. They will facilitate the person in the group who takes the initiative and becomes the point of entry of an idea. They will not squelch ideas, although they may differ in points of view.

The emergence of the phenomenon of transformation is providing a rare opportunity for leaders in nursing. Transformation provides a scenario for a new way of interacting, a new way of problem solving, and a means for developing a shared vision among health professionals in various settings. The seeds for transformation are in every organization awaiting a cultural climate that will encourage, support, and cultivate them. The essence of transformation is a "metanoic" shift and the realization of personal empowerment that comes from a group with a common vision (Adams, 1984). In metanoic organizations, people do not assume they are powerless and they believe deeply in the power of the individual to assume control of destiny. A growing number of organizations are developing prototypes for a metanoic model with five primary dimensions forming the basis of organizational philosophy:

a deep sense of vision
alignment around that vision
empowering people
structural integrity
the balance of reason and intuition.

How to go about doing this is not so easy. The purpose of this chapter is to discuss the meaning of personal and group empowerment, including an approach to building one's constellation of empowerment through individual assessment, visioning, and continuous learning. Those who wait for someone to hand them power will never know they have it. Power must be recognized from within.

EMPOWERMENT

The key to empowerment is self-development and appreciation of others. Kinsman (1986) speaks of self-development in the truest sense—intellectually, bodily, emotionally, and spiritually. Self-empowered leaders are "focalizers," those who focus the energies of the people in their areas. Focalizers, says Kinsman (1986), help to make decisions in a group but on the basis of input from everyone in the group. Lang (1988, p. 6) defines empowerment as "unleashing—to release from or as from a leash; to set free to pursue; to let loose; to give official power; to enable."

Personal and group empowerment are realized through personal mastery and continuous learning (Senge, 1990). The ability to focus on future dreams and goals is a cornerstone. One ought to have a purpose for living, and it ought to make a difference that one has lived. Work flows fluidly in enterprises when personal, group, and organizational visions are shared. Personal empowerment can be developed in many ways. One approach is to foster the idea of a continuously developing "dream plan." Figure 17.1 provides a mental model for personal empowerment. It is a picture of components of thoughts and ideas that can convey a positive view of the world. Your constellation may be somewhat different and your picture of each star in the constellation may be at a different level of development.

Kornbluh, Pipan, and Schurman (1987) defined empowerment learning as unlimited energy in an organization. Human learning is considered an organizational asset, and in transformed organizations, human learning and problem solving abilities are viewed as vitally important resources in empowering people—a continuous source of energy. Participation in transformation is seen as a process, not a goal. A zero-sum conception of power in command and control organizations assumes that power is a

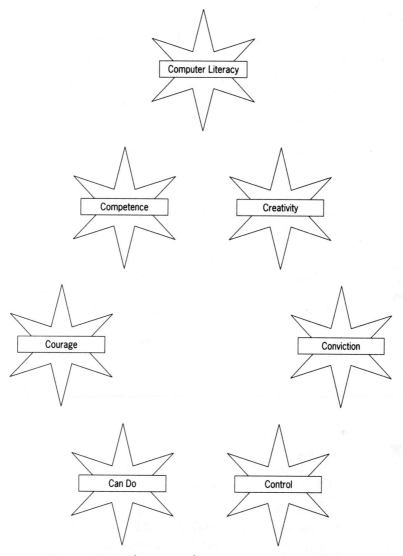

Figure 17.1 The personal empowerment constellation.

finite commodity in which some may gain only if others lose. A radically different approach is proposed—a "non-zero-sum model" of power in which the total amount of power is always expanding. Based on creation of a learning environment, workers are empowered to use their intellectual abilities to individual and organizational advantage. In this model, every worker counts and every worker exerts control over performance and quality of work and life variables. In transformed metanoic health care organizations, the goal is patient-centered care and it is everyone's responsibility to participate in building and advancing a shared vision.

VISIONING

Bennis and Nanus (1985) were among the first to discover that one of the outstanding characteristics of exemplary leaders is the ability to foster organizational learning. Individual visioning unfolds to become a common vision. The group's vision is not the vision of the most articulate or dominant individual but, rather, a distinct entity generated by the group and groups in an organization. Bennis and Nanus (1985) speak of the management of attention through vision. Kinsman (1986) speaks of vision as "powerful to the extent that it expresses one's underlying purpose." Vaill (1981) speaks of high performing systems whose members have pictures in their heads that are strikingly congruent.

Senge (1990) describes business and other human endeavors as systems, bound by invisible factors of interrelated actions that may take years to fully understand their effects on each other. Each organizational member is part of that lacework (or cobweb) and it is difficult to see the whole system as we tend to focus on isolated snapshots of the system. Personal mastery according to Senge (1990) is the discipline of continually clarifying and deepening one's personal vision, focusing energies, developing patience and seeing reality objectively. Personal mastery is the essential cornerstone of the learning organization. Because few organizations encourage the growth of their people, there is a pervasive sense of powerlessness in individuals and groups. Resource dependency theory should be advanced to resource discovery theories.

Personal learning and organizational learning are intertwined in building shared visions. Personal mastery begins with understanding the self and the ability to work with our internal mental models. The earlier chapter on making sense of organizations described the organizational window with a variety of images or window panes with differing perceptions of the organization. Building shared vision involves unearthing pictures of the future that form a mission and philosophy that is believed and shared by its members. Group learning is vital to shared vision because work groups or teams are the fundamental learning unit in modern organizations.

If you want to change the world, there is no time like the present. Lang (1988, p. 11) envisions a world in which we as nurses:

encourage an entrepreneurial revolution in nursing.

encourage true competition in the solution of health care problems.

experiment with nursing corporations and partnerships, and nurse-managed centers.

decrease physician resistance (to nursing practice).

increase malpractice and professional liability coverage options for nurses.

encourage incentives for resolution of dependency, maintenance of health status, and peaceful deaths.

As authors of this book, we envision a world in which professional nurses practice independently and collaboratively in the delivery of health care; a world in which nursing has its own recognized and credible technology of knowledge, skills, and equipment and is not totally dependent on other disciplines for energy and innovation.

EMPOWERING THYSELF

PART I. Curriculum Vitae

Name
Address
Phone and fax numbers
Current position
Academic history including school; degree; specialty; year of graduation
Professional experience
Research activities
Management activities
Publications
Professional papers presented
Honors and awards
Professional organizations
Community service
Other

PART II. Career Plan/Personal Vision

Important life milestones to date—e.g., early years; high school; college; work; etc.
Personal support system—e.g., people; pets; places; etc.
Personal learning style
Strengths/weaknesses
Dreams for the future
Ideas in process
Future life milestones/career points
Lifelong learning schedule to achieve career points (include projected time schedule) What do you need to learn to achieve career points?
Fit with current organizational vision (mission and philosophy)

Figure 17.2 Developing self-assessment and personal visioning skills.

Figure 17.2 provides a simple approach to nurturing personal empowerment. Imagine the untapped resources discovered in work environments where everyone learns self-assessment through the generation of a resumé or curriculum vitae. We have resource abundance in this country. We simply do not recognize it. Personal visioning can be learned through regularly appending one's curriculum vitae with a personal vision or career plan that simply sets out where you have been, where you want to go, and where you fit in your current organizational vision. It is an example of one's lifelong learning plan.

PERSONAL AND GROUP POWER

Power is difficult to define without bringing up images of coercion and domination. However, nurses must begin to understand power and empowerment to succeed in achieving their professional and organizational goals. Gorman and Clark (1986) defined nursing power as the nurse's ability to do, to achieve nursing objectives. This definition recognized that nursing power does not mean total control over patient care but rather collaboration with other health professionals. Kanter (1977) described organizational power as:

the ability to get things done, to mobilize resources, to get and use whatever it is that a person needs for the goals he or she is attempting to meet. In this way, a monopoly on power means that only a very few have the capacity, and they prevent the majority of others from being able to act effectively. Thus the total amount of power—the total system effectiveness—is restricted, even though some people seem to have a great deal of it. However, when more people are empowered—that is, allowed to have control over the conditions that make their actions possible—then more is accomplished, more gets done. (p. 166)

GROUP LEARNING THROUGH ACTION RESEARCH

Participatory research offers a strategy for group learning that is consistent with the assumptions of people-centered development (Brown, 1985). It encourages inquiry that focuses on local problems and pragmatic concerns that are reality based. Innovations developed by participants and researchers can catalyze developmental changes. Resultant cooperative relations can combine outside resources with local resources, bringing in commitment to learning new options and energy and skills for solving problems. Interaction with outside researchers links local participants with previously unexplored sources of information and outside alliances that can be sources of political and economic empowerment.

The action-research approach is dependent on participants learning and working together in unit assessment and planning for redesign. The key characteristics of participatory action research (Israel, Schurman, & House, 1989) are:

participation of employees in most aspects of the research and action; research process is not dependent on theoretical interpretation of the researchers.

cooperation of managers, employees, and researchers in a joint process.

a colearning process in which clinical managers, researchers, and employees develop an understanding of the situation under study.

system development in which participants develop the competencies to engage in the process of diagnosing and analyzing problems, planning, implementing, and evaluating changes, such as redesigning work or introducing technology.

an empowering process in which participant organization members gain increased influence and control over their work lives.

Participatory action research provides a legitimate model for creating the learning environment essential for this research design. Brown (1985) made a strong case for using people-centered development and participatory research as a means to maximize human resource development. Participatory action research asks adults to be interdependent participants and colearners rather than dependent and researcher controlled. The researchers learn skills for general problem solving, such as managing meetings, getting information, organizing work, or planning activities. The control of learning in participatory action research can seldom be predicted or planned in detail across projects and is participant-learner dependent rather than researcher-teacher controlled. Participatory research is a way to promote people-centered development in various systems that encourage local empowerment. This is especially relevant as we seek to transform nursing work environments and pave the way for patient-centered care delivery systems.

Examples of successful action research studies have been described in the labor and occupational studies literature. A substantial amount of data exist in Scandinavian documents, wherein the holistic conception of the work environment is considered paramount. Important American studies have been conducted by Deutsch (1988, 1989) in his investigations of workplace democracy and worker health resulting in the postulation of a learning/activation/learning process described in Figure 17.3. Kornbluh, Pipan, and Schurman (1987) reported positive findings on empowerment learning and control in workplaces in industry. Schurman and Israel (Schurman, 1989)

Desire for more learning (political learning) with larger scope of involvement and activation

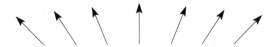

Active participation and work towards change in the workplace and beyond

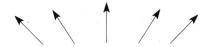

Attainment of broader knowledge and extension of learning

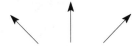

Activated interest in greater learning and more involvement

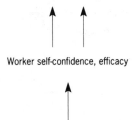

Worker self-confidence, efficacy

Skills building (e.g. hazard recognition and abatement) and competency

Figure 17.3 Learning/activation/learning process (movement upward and expanding the impact). (From Deutsch, S. (1989). Worker learning in the context of changing technology and work environment. In Lehmann, H., & S. Kornbluh (Eds.). *Socialization and Learning at Work* (p. 252). Brookfield, VT: Gower Publishing Co. Used with permission.)

have a highly credible record in involving workers as researchers and using action research methods in the study of occupational stress. Employee-based and union-initiated efforts to improve the work environment have worked well in various work organizations as well as hospitals.

DIFFERENT PERCEPTIONS OF WORK

Empowerment, personal or group, is related to feelings about work. Studies related to retention and turnover abound in the nursing literature and, in general, have had a negative impact on changing nursing work environments (Simms, Erbin-Roesemann, Darga, & Coeling, 1990). The lack of agreement on the meaning of work in the literature has resulted in a variety of definitions among theoreticians. Work is believed to be different than job with job satisfaction used to refer to affective attitudes or orientations on the part of individuals toward jobs (Blegen & Mueller, 1987). Work is something individuals and society take very seriously, although authors disagree on the meaning of work.

Schurman (1989) believes that the meaning of work is very complex, which is central to the notion that work has a different meaning for every individual, allowing for work to be identified as something other than satisfaction and excitement. Work is viewed as a central human activity in which mind and body unite in actions that not only provide sustenance for the life process, but also generate objects, material and ideational, which have meaning and value to both *self* and others. Attempts to link meaning of work to the organization of work, however, is weak in the literature. Instead, meaning of work is generally associated with job satisfaction, with the former regarded as a reflection of the latter. Sandelands (1988) makes the rare distinction between affect about the work (i.e., meaningfulness of work) and attitudes about the work (i.e., job satisfaction), which he argues are relevant to designing work organizations.

Authors of work-enrichment studies often fail to include in their assumptions the meaning of work to the individual. It is likely for individuals to view work as paid employment and not wish to have their jobs enriched. This may be because they have higher level needs met by other forms of work outside their jobs. Fein (1977) concluded that the need for fulfillment from one's job applies only to those workers who choose to find it in their employment. He contends that the vast majority of workers seek fulfillment outside their jobs. In addition, Hackman and Lawler (1971) found that employees with higher order needs satisfied, performed better and were more positive than those without the higher need satisfaction. Recently, Csikszentmihalyi (1990) described positive work experiences when people are in "flow," linking psychic energy with optimal goal achievement and the work experience.

The meaning of work has also been examined on intrinsic and extrinsic dimensions. Fein (1977) stated that the intrinsic nature of the work performed is not the main cause of the difference between satisfied and dissatisfied workers. Workers' dissatisfaction with their jobs is due less to the nature of work than to other factors such as pay, freedom, and nonwork-related problems. Hackman (1977) disagreed with this conclusion, in that society as a whole has achieved substantial increases in economic benefits, therefore, people today want jobs that provide intrinsic work satisfaction. Trist (1981) identified the intrinsic characteristics of the job as: variety and challenge, continuous learning, discretion or autonomy, recognition and support, and meaningful social contribution. The extrinsic characteristics were identified as: fair and adequate pay, job security, benefits, safety, and health. These are consistent with the hygiene factors described in earlier work by Herzberg, Mausner, and Snyderman (1959).

JOB SATISFACTION

Hackman (1977) described his basic job characteristics model of work motivation in terms of five core job dimensions. These dimensions create three critical psychological states that, in turn, lead to beneficial personal and work outcomes. Skill variety, task identity, task significance, autonomy, and feedback from the job were noted, with the first three contributing most to a job's meaningfulness. Psychological states include experienced meaningfulness of the work, experienced responsibility for outcomes of the work, and knowledge of the actual results of the work activities. Four outcomes are affected by the level of generated motivation, including high internal work motivation, high "growth" satisfaction, high general job satisfaction, and high work effectiveness.

Mueller and McCloskey (1990) have continued to seek to identify the rewards that keep nurses on the job through the development and validation of an instrument to measure job satisfaction. The McCloskey/Mueller/Satisfaction Scale (MMSS) has been found to have acceptable reliability and construct validity and may be used to measure satisfaction with extrinsic rewards, scheduling, family/work balance, co-workers, interaction, professional opportunities, praise/recognition, and control/responsibility. The work is clearly limited to job satisfaction and does not address the more global construct of work.

The organization of people's work may be a major determinant in shaping their health and well-being outside of work. Drawing on years of research on job redesign and work, Karasek and Theorell (1990) attempt to bridge the gap between medical science, psychology, sociology, industrial engineering, and economics to present an approach to the redesign of work organizations to make them more psychologically humane. The authors present a laudable perspective on integrating worker health analysis and job redesign. Citing weaknesses in Quality of Work Life research, the authors further propose job redesign strategies that will promote health-related job change. They further support studies of physiological changes among workers as part of any work intervention program. In a study designed to improve competence of patients and personnel, physiological monitoring and educational programs resulted in improvement in patient clinical outcomes and worker health and safety. Important factors in creating an excellent work environment include worker health and safety.

WORK EXCITEMENT

Recent work by the Simms Practice Excitement Project (PEP) team on work excitement has yielded a tool to measure work characteristics and work excitement. To test the model for work excitement, a self-administered fixed-alternatives questionnaire with previously generated key items was used to collect data on 268 nurses' perception of exciting aspects of work and level of excitement about work. Construct validity was obtained using cluster and factor analysis. Cronbach's alpha used to assess internal consistency of the three main questions concerning interest, excitement, and frustration with work yielded reliability coefficients ranging from .85 to .94. Based on these validation studies, work excitement was conceptualized as "personal enthusiasm and interest in work evidenced by creativity, receptivity to learning, and ability to see opportunity in everyday situations." Multiple regression analysis supported five factors as significant predictors of work excitement: growth and development (learning); work arrangements; variety of experiences; working conditions; and change.

The factor identified as growth and development or learning comprised the variables: taking on challenging problems and projects and solving or accomplishing them and seeing and participating in the growth and development of other nurses. This factor was positively related to work excitement, indicating that the more opportunities for growth and development and learning, the greater the level of work excitement. The second significant factor of work arrangements consists of the variables of inappropriate and understaffing; issues of time and getting work finished; and communication problems between nurses, physicians, and other nursing personnel. It is negatively related to work excitement, indicating that the higher the level of frustration with work arrangements, the lower the level of work excitement.

The third important factor, variety, consists of the variables of variety of experiences and availability of learning opportunities. The positive correlation suggests that the more variety and opportunity for learning in the work environment, the higher the level of work excitement. The fourth significant factor was that of working conditions; it comprised the variables of convenient hours, schedules, and money. This factor is negatively related to work excitement, thus indicating that the more frustrated one feels about working conditions, the less work excitement one has.

Finally, the factor of change was a significant predictor of work excitement. This factor contains the variables of fast pace, variety of activities, high acuity patients, and unpredictable, crisis situations. It is positively related to work excitement, indicating that the more change that takes place in the work environment, the higher the level of work excitement. In other unreported graduate student projects, level of knowledge, working with high technology in critical care settings, and computer use have been found to be significantly related to work excitement. Although self-esteem and internal locus of control were not supported in this phase of the preliminary work, the researchers believe they are important contributing variables and they will be under intense scrutiny in later work. A conceptual model and theory of work excitement are still in the developmental stage.

The conceptual framework (Figure 17.4) guiding the ongoing research is permeated with opportunities for learning for care givers and recipients. For example, self-care and the use of assistive technology can be learned and can make a tremendous difference in discharge readiness. Learning new behaviors on the part of caregivers can and should result in continuing clinical competence and other changes in behavior, such as acceptance of assistive technology and the ability to work in flexible groups.

Mastery of the major elements in any unit work or practice pattern redesign will include learning and using the structural concepts of patient characteristics, nursing

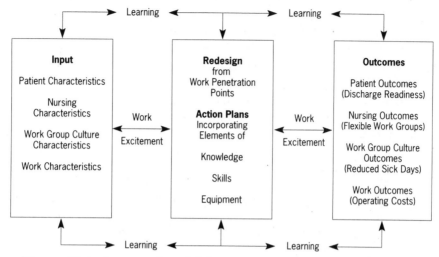

Figure 17.4 Conceptual model for participatory nursing work redesign.

resources, work group culture characteristics, and work characteristics (Beckman and Simms, 1992); the process components of an action plan; and clinical and workplace outcomes. The concept of work excitement, postulated in terms of person and work environment factors, is considered the catalyst for process and practice outcomes.

EMPOWERMENT AND EFFECTIVE PRACTICE

Inservice management training sessions can function as organizational rituals that maintain the status quo. Hirschhorn (1988) argues that managers and workers must enact sophisticated boundaries that help people to acknowledge the claims of outside stakeholders while protecting the coherence of the work group. By failing to do so, they may retreat from role, task, and organizational boundaries, thus creating a more irrational workplace than that found in an industrial milieu. The social defenses at work frequently create a distorted relationship between the group and its wider environment of customers, clients, and competitors. The "outside" is scapegoated or devalued in some way to preserve the "inside." A group dominated by its own social defenses retreats from the boundary it shares with its environment into its collective fantasies and delusions. Group development takes place when group members stop scapegoating others, when they cease using each other or outsiders to manage their shared anxieties. In so doing, they come close to confronting their primary task (Hirschhorn, 1988). In actual practice, this is difficult to do.

However, Gorman and Clark (1986) suggest that group empowerment is possible. During a 3-year period, the Nursing Knowledge Project conducted by Gorman and Clark (1986) examined how nurses applied their clinical knowledge and skills in the practice setting, identified barriers to nursing practice, and evaluated a series of training activities designed to increase nurses' power in practice settings. Four empowerment strategies emerged from their research (summarized as follows):

The practice of analytic nursing: nurses must routinely apply the same analytical skills that enable them to develop a patient's nursing care plan to the interpersonal and organizational problems they encounter daily in the hospital.

Engagement of nurses in change activities: nurses must plan and implement needed change in practice settings.

Strengthening collegiality: nurses must call on the support of their nursing colleagues and the extensive experience of other nurses for counsel and advice in the application of clinical knowledge and skills.

Extending administrative sponsorship: staff nurses must be provided the organizational know-how and support of administrative nurses in efforts to improve patient care. Through sponsorship, more senior nurses guide less experienced nurses to resolve difficult practice problems and link them to needed organizational resources.

Group learning was then encouraged through role-centered case analyses of reality-based unit case studies. The activities of the nurses became highly relevant and extraordinary and visible. In the training program, nurses working in heterogeneous groups, representing various parts of each collaborating hospital, acted as teams and selected common problems to address. The training program, therefore, included both educational and structural solutions for the problems of powerlessness experienced by nurses in the hospital setting. Educationally, the program was designed to empower the participating nurses by teaching them the analytic and interpersonal skills they needed to develop and implement plans for change. Structurally, it established new lines of communication between staff nurses and nurse executives, linking the nurses to needed resources and giving the nurses more control over working conditions.

The implementation of interdisciplinary groups centers on a nucleus of nurses, physicians, and health-care executives who appreciate the concept of collaborative work (Simms, Dalston, & Roberts, 1984). The core team should be bright, highly motivated, and closely linked with the recognized organizational leadership, both formal and informal. The core group educates, influences, provides role models, and demonstrates precepts through seminars, quality reviews, persuasion, contribution to the literature, and involvement in solving direct patient care problems. This core group is, above all, persistent, accomplishing what is achievable now, awaiting improved conditions, and then moving forward again.

AN EXAMPLE OF ACTION LEARNING THROUGH ACTION RESEARCH

Shared purpose/vision must be concerned with active movement from purpose to results. Support for action learning requires an organizational climate conducive to learning new knowledge and skills. One approach to action learning is through action research. In the ongoing Simms, Coeling, and Price redesign research, the researchers meet with unit staff and explain the overall process. Each unit serves as its own control group. The rationale for conducting periodic unit assessment to determine the effectiveness of current practice patterns and quality of patient care needs early discussion. The importance of data for decision making about changes in practice patterns becomes a nature follow-up of unit discussions. It is important to establish that unit staff will participate in data interpretation and decision making. Ground rules for maintaining respect for all group members and their opinions will be developed. Organizational mission, unit philosophy, conceptual elements of any practice pattern, flexible work groups, and quality care will be used as discussion themes at each site to lay the groundwork for introduction of assessment instruments.

The entire unit staff becomes part of the process, even though a task force of three to five people may be responsible for collection of data and completing the analysis. This task force includes staff nurses as well as the unit nurse executive. In fact, there can be several task forces conducting various parts of the unit assessment so that most or all staff members are involved in some way. Thus, unit-based participatory action research teams consisting of unit nurses and researchers will be established at each site and will be selected from volunteers who reflect the different unit skill mix. It will be noted that research teams will be flexible and will change over time so that all interested nurses can become intimately involved with the action research process. The following teams are the work groups, depending on the size of overall staff and different interests of the unit nurses and researchers:

Team A: Initial data collection team

Team B: Work penetration points identification team

Team C: Intervention planning team focused on discharge readiness

Team D: Action planning team

Team E: Follow-up data collection team

Team F: Data analyses and recommendations for future direction

Following introduction of the project and related activities to unit staff, patients will be verbally introduced to the project by a research team member on admission to the unit. The patient consent form will be used to guide the introduction so that all patients will receive consistent information. Patients will be asked to sign the consent form at the time of introduction to the study and will be given the discharge readiness questionnaire at discharge, to be returned in 1 week to the principal investigator.

Unit preparation, collection of baseline data on input and outcome variables, and identification of work penetration points related to discharge readiness will occur over a period of 6 months with data collection from unit staff nurses and nurse managers at all selected hospital sites. In all cases, it is anticipated that the team efforts will not encompass more than 2 months of work.

In sum, the procedure includes the following steps:

1. Unit discussion of mission, philosophy, conceptual elements of any practice pattern, flexible clinical work groups, and clinical outcomes. Technology will be discussed as will knowledge, skills, and equipment, the basic elements of any action plan.

2. Selection of unit task forces and introduction of study to patients.

3. Baseline unit data will be collected on:

   Current patient, nursing, unit work group culture, and work characteristics.

   Prevailing levels of discharge readiness among patients.

   Prevailing practice pattern (work group membership and arrangements).

Prevailing levels of work excitement among unit nurses.

Prevailing levels of work-related injuries and sick days among unit nurses.

Prevailing unit operating cost.

4. Group discussion of resultant data.
5. Development of a data-based action plan based on identified work penetration points.
6. Implementation of the action plan.
7. Follow-up evaluation of input and outcome variables.

IDENTIFYING WORK PENETRATION POINTS FROM UNIT DATA

The process continues with the identification of work penetration points identified from collected data. Resultant baseline data are combed for clinical and system variances that indicate unit-based work penetration points. Clinical variances are searched for and identified in the patient characteristics and discharge readiness data; systems variances are located in the work, unit culture, nursing resources, and unit nurse executive data. Unit data will be entered into a data base using spreadsheet software for easy and quick analysis. In this manner, unit nurses learn how to enter data, analyze data from group generated research questions, and to interpret spreadsheets.

Descriptive statistics are used to identify the key patient, nursing, work group culture, and work characteristics requiring immediate attention. The unit research teams generate a summary report describing their units and listing work penetration points that are of primary interest. Prioritizing work penetration points is essential, and the participatory action research teams can decide to address less urgent points at a later time. Some pretest units have identified learning needs related to inadequate knowledge for high-acuity patient care, lack of computer skills, and lack of freedom to leave the unit as immediate concerns. Other pretest units have identified other work penetration points.

For example, cultural analysis of one unit revealed a norm of frequently calling in sick, to the point of abusing the sick-time policy. A comparison of the preferred behaviors with current behaviors indicated the nurses wanted to be able to make patients more comfortable and to spend more time understanding patients' feelings. The work penetration point of altering attendance patterns was identified. The unit nurse executive (head nurse) worked with the staff to help them see that if there were fewer call-ins, they would have a more abundant and stable staff that, in turn, would provide more opportunities to spend time talking with patients and making them comfortable. As a result of this discussion, the staff made a conscious group effort to stop misusing sick time.

Cultural analysis of another unit revealed that it was not expected that nurses offer to help each other. Rather each worked alone to complete the work assigned to them. As budget cuts necessitated staff lay-offs and nurses had to work harder, the unit nurse executive noted a pattern of increased sick days related to back injuries attributed to nurses lifting and moving patients alone without help. A comparison of the preferred behaviors with current behaviors indicated the nurses wanted others to offer to help them more. The work penetration point of altering expectations related to helping each other was identified. Nurses were encouraged to make themselves more aware of their fellow nurses' work load and to take the initiative to offer to help them.

Cultural analysis of a third unit revealed a bimodal norm for attending in-services, attending college, discussing new ideas, and achieving clinical advancement. In other words, on this unit, some nurses valued these behaviors and other nurses rejected them. A new head nurse assigned to the unit noted how these divergent behaviors frequently lead to conflict on the unit. She identified the work penetration point of increasing commitment to continued learning. She made her norm of continuous improvement known to the unit. Within a matter of months, those nurses who did not value learning had resigned and the unit was becoming a stable, productive unit.

In sum, following the identification of work penetration points from unit assessment, unit staff determine an action plan for intervention and introduction of redesign of work, work groups, and/or practice patterns based on what they have learned through participation in the action research project. Work groups on the participating units then proceed to implement their individualized action plans with unit-designed interventions.

PARTICIPATORY ACTION PLANNING FROM ACTION LEARNING

Group-generated action plans are developed, considering collected baseline data, resultant work penetration points, and appropriate technologies (knowledge, skills, and equipment) to design interventions that can yield clinical and systems outcomes. Given knowledge of patient, nursing, culture, and work characteristics, the unit staffs consider the nature of the work to be done and the nursing and technological resources desirable and available to accomplish the work with the best advantage to patients. Consideration in developing the action plan is given to: What pieces of work can or should be done together or by one person? The work should not be characterized only in terms of tasks or time, but also as processes and activities. What work can be delegated to other people or technology? What work should be a patient/family responsibility? What work should be done differently? What work should not be done at all? *In other words, what knowledge, skills, and equipment are needed to redesign the unit work?*

Summary

Group empowerment emerges from personal empowerment, and personal empowerment is related to a sense of purpose and excitement about one's work. One's personal constellation of empowerment can be developed and fine tuned through systematically practicing visioning and self-development. One of the very best self-assessment tools is the simple resumé or curriculum vitae. The individual is the master of one's own life and the curriculum vitae is the history of one's professional life. To add the component of a lifespan career plan promotes the practice setting for envisioning who you may become and where

you plan to be over the next 50 years. Visioning skills are practiced frequently in childhood—they need to be continually honed in adulthood and in the later years. If you are envisioning collaborative initiatives, then learning activities must be planned to develop the skill and knowledge necessary for professional collaboration. Group empowerment emanates from group visioning and futuring and, ultimately, is measured in terms of performance and productivity.

References

Adams, J. D. (1984). *Transforming work.* Alexandria, VA: Miles River Press.

Beckman, J. S., & Simms, L. M. (1992). *Redesigning nursing practice patterns.* Ann Arbor: Health Administration Press.

Bennis, W., & Nanus, B. (1985). *Leaders: The strategies of taking charge.* New York: Harper & Row.

Blegen, M., & Mueller, C. (1987). Nurses' job satisfaction: A longitudinal analysis, *Research in Nursing and Health, 10,* 227–237.

Brown, L. D. (1985). People-centered development and participatory research, *Harvard Education Review, 55*(1), 69–75.

Csikszentmihalyi, M. (1990). *Flow—the psychology of optimal experience.* New York: Harper & Row.

Deutsch, S. (1988). Workplace democracy and worker health: Strategies for intervention, *International Journal of Health Services, 18,* 647–658. Also reprinted (1991). In J. Johnson & G. Johansson (Eds.), *The Psychosocial Work Environment: Work Organization, Democratization and Health.* Amityville, NY: Baywood Publishing Co.

Deutsch, S. (1989). Worker learning in the context of changing technology and work environment. In H. Leymann & H. Kornbluh (Eds.), *Socialization and Learning at Work* (pp. 237–255). Brookfield, VT: Gower Publishing Co.

Fein, M. (1977). Job enrichment: A reevaluation. In J. R. Hackman, E. E. Lawler, & L. W. Porter (Eds.), *Perspectives on Behavior in Organization* (pp. 269–281). New York: McGraw-Hill.

Gorman, S., & Clark N. (1986). Power and effective nursing practice, *Nursing Outlook. 34*(3), 129–134.

Hackman, J. R. (1977). The design of work in the 1980s. In J. R. Hackman, E. E. Lawler, & L. W. Porter (Eds.), *Perspectives on Behavior in Organizations* (pp. 458–473). New York: McGraw-Hill.

Hackman, J. R., & Lawler, E. E. (1971). Employer reactions to job characteristics, *Journal of Applied Psychology Monograph, 55,* 259–286.

Herzberg, R., Mausner, B., & Snyderman, B. (1959). *The motivation to work.* New York: Wiley.

Hirschhorn, L. (1988). Psychodynamics of the workplace. In L. Hirschhorn (Ed.), *The Workplace Within* (pp. 1–15). Cambridge, MA: MIT Press.

Israel, B. A., Schurman, S. J., & House, J. S. (1989). Action research on occupational stress: Involving workers as researchers, *International Journal of Health Services, 19,* 135–155.

Kanter, R. M. (1977). *Men and women of the corporation.* New York: Basic Books.

Karasek, R., & Theorell, T. (1990). *Healthy work.* New York: Basic Books.

Kinsman, F. (1986). Leadership from alongside. In J. Adams (Ed.), *Transforming Leadership.* Alexandria, VA: Miles River Press.

Kornbluh, H., Pipan, R., & Schurman, S. J. (1987). Empowerment learning and control in workplaces: A curricular view, *Zeitschrift Fur Sozialisationsforschung Und Erziehungssozio-logie (ZSE) J. Jahrgang/Heft 7*(4), 253–268.

Lang, N. (1988). Empower the nurse: A time for renewal. In *Nursing Practice in the 21st Century* (pp. 5–16). Kansas City, MO: American Nurses Foundation Inc.

Mueller, C. W., & McCloskey, J. C. (1990). Nurses' job satisfaction: A proposed measure, *Nursing Research, 39*(2), 113–117.

Sandelands, L. E. (1988). The concept of work feeling, *Journal for the Theory of Social Behaviour, 18*(4), 437–457.

Schurman, S. J. (1989). Reuniting labour and learning: A holistic theory of work. In H. Leymann & H. Kornbluh (Eds.), *Socialization and Learning at Work* (pp. 42–68). Brookfield, VT: Gower Publishing Co.

Senge, P. M. (1990). *The fifth discipline: The art and practice of the learning organization.* New York: Doubleday.

Simms, L. M., Dalston, J. W., & Roberts, P. W. (1984). Collaborative practice: Myth or reality, *Hospital and Health Services Administration, 29*(6), 36–48.

Simms, L. M., Erbin-Roesemann, M., Darga, A., & Coeling, H. (1990). Breaking the burnout barrier: Resurrecting work excitement in nursing, *Nursing Economic$, 8*(3), 177–186.

Trist, E. (1981). The sociotechnical perspective. In A. H. Van de Ven and W. F. Joyce (Eds.), *Perspectives on Organization Design and Behavior* (pp. 19–75). New York: Wiley-Interscience.

Vaill, P. B. (1981). *The purposing of high performing systems.* Paper presented at a conference on Administrative Leadership. University of Illinois, July, 1981.

CHAPTER 18
Strategic Planning

Eunice A. Bell

Highlights

- **The concept of strategic planning**
- **The process**
- **Internal assessment**
- **Defining the business-centered mission**
- **Role of nursing administration**

The purpose of this chapter is to examine the concept and the process of strategic planning as a critical function of nursing administration. Health care delivery in the 1990s is plagued by supply problems—oversupply and undersupply. The oversupply is represented by an excess number of hospital beds, a growing physician surplus, and an explosive increase in biomedical technology. The undersupply is reflected in the pattern of decreasing reimbursements based on limiting criteria, the continuing nursing shortage as a result of extraordinary need/demand, and the decreasing numbers of working Americans who support the social services systems. These supply factors directly and critically affect the financing and delivery of health care. Health care providers have responded to the financial crisis posed by the supply problems by investigating and adopting business strategies that are based on a proactive approach. Foremost among the current crisis strategies is the use of strategic planning.

THE CONCEPT

Drucker (1974) defines strategic planning within the context of business and industry as "a continuous systematic process of making risk-taking decisions today with the greatest possible knowledge of their effects on the future, organizing efforts necessary to carry out these decisions and evaluating the results of these decisions against expected outcomes through reliable feedback mechanisms" (p. 125).

Steiner (1979) defines strategic planning by declaring that "it is not an attempt to blue print the future in a static rigid manner. Strategic plans are subject to periodic review based on technology advances and other environmental changes" (p. 44). The strategic planning process in hospitals is described by Domanico (1981) as "the process whereby hospitals assess the total health care market and their true competitive position within the market to determine future directions while at the same time addressing community needs and satisfying regulatory requirements" (p. 25).

The terms "strategic planning" and "master planning" have been used interchangeably in the past. Flexner, Berkowitz, and Brown (1981) argue that the two are very different. Master planning has focused on facilities planning, either for new buildings or renovation of existing structures. Rising concerns in the 1960s about the proliferation of facilities led to governmental initiates such as the Health Planning Act (PL 93-641), which was intended to constrain unnecessary growth through the Certificate of Need legislation. These governmental restraints along with decreasing philanthropic funding and increasing construction costs resulted in a shift to program-focused planning—strategic planning. Theime, Wilson, and Long (1981) compared strategic and master planning and identified four features that differentiate the two. Flexner, Berkowitz, and Brown (1981) paraphrased the differences as:

1. a shift from a focus on production to one on people and population groups,
2. the definition of the organization's mission *following* a thorough external and internal assessment,
3. recognition of the importance of political as well as technical considerations, and
4. the need to integrate planning with ongoing management activities.

These important features form the framework of the strategic planning model (Figure 18.1). Strategic planning is the starting point for the strategy-driven management of hospitals. Smith (1987) contends that strategic management widens the domain of planning to strategy execution. Garner, Smith, and Piland (1990) differentiate planning from management in the following definitions "strategic planning is a commitment to defining formally the mission, objectives, and strategies for an organization by the top managers, the planning department and the Board of Directors. Strategic management incorporates a broader spectrum of members and is active, vibrant, changing, flexible" (p. 25).

THE PROCESS

Flexner, Berkowitz, and Brown (1981) identified the following steps in the strategic planning process:

1. assessment of external and internal environments and the organizational structure and process,

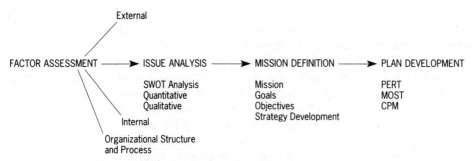

Figure 18.1 Strategic planning model.

2. examination of the issues critical to care delivery,

3. definition of a business centered mission, and

4. development of a plan designed around both facilities and program development.

The process is illustrated in the model (see Figure 18.1). The first step, assessment, is a complex and comprehensive activity. Assessing the external environment requires an examination of the following:

a. economic factors,

b. political issues,

c. market trends,

d. technology trends,

e. social/lifestyle trends,

f. regulatory factors,

g. competition/hospital image, and

h. manpower trends.

Economic Factors

Both a macro- and a microexamination of economic factors is essential. Macro analysis should include the national and international economic climate and the effect on health care consumers (both patient and physician), the manpower supply, and the payors (governmental, business, and private). Economic markers important to this analysis include the Gross National Product (GNP), the Consumer Price Index (CPI), and the rate of inflation/recession. At the microexamination level, assessment of state and local business climate, unemployment rates, and addition or loss of business/industry is needed. Assessment of change in payor mix based on changes in the business profile or the community would be helpful to the assessment process. Because economic factors are the key to the fiscal health of hospitals and their ability to deliver health care efficiently, assessment of the economic environment is a critical first step in the strategic planning process.

Political Issues

Political issues are a direct reflection of political party differences, thus national, state, and local elections may result in changes in priorities and directly affect health care delivery. Health care-related political issues that could impact strategic planning are abortion services, sex education for teenagers, daycare for working mothers, time off for childbirth and adoption, and time off for care of the acutely ill or terminally ill family member. Local political issues that impact care delivery include access to care for the indigent and homeless and care of increasing numbers of HIV-positive clients.

Market Trends

Market trends at the national, state, and local levels should be examined with care. Trends in alternate care delivery modes currently being trialed in other geographic areas could provide important data for strategic planners looking for a new service/program to address local needs. Investigation of new areas of marketing focus may be conducted using the following categories:

1. Consumer marketing—focused on attracting the patient directly to the hospital rather than indirectly through physician referral. This approach focuses on consumer preference for the physical plant, access to services, and type of services provided.
2. Packaged services marketing—packaging all services in one center, for example, oncology surgery, chemotherapy, radiation, marrow transplants, pain management, nutrition management, home care, and hospice care.
3. Program focused marketing—addressing broader concepts as Wellness-Centered Services and Women's Health Centers.

Close examination of the directions and strength of market trends as well as the diversity of market focus will provide the assessors with important data for strategic planning.

Technology Trends

Strategic planning requires an in-depth knowledge of advances in technology as they impact quality of care and the competitive position of the organization. This information may be obtained from local practitioners, researchers, professional groups, and commercial sources. In the assessment, it is important to determine the risks (medical and economic) attendant to adoption of a new technology.

Social/lifestyle Trends

Changes in society that impact health care delivery should be assessed. Increasing numbers of single parents and full-time working mothers, the returning-to-the-nest syndrome, the increasing housing options for older people, and the disabled are social changes that impact how, where, and when health care is to be delivered.

Regulatory Factors

Assessment of the impact of governmental regulation on the delivery of health care is crucial to the planning process. Changes in Occupational Safety and Health Administration (OSHA) rules may affect both the patient/consumer and hospital personnel. Environmental Protection Administration (EPA) regulations regarding hazardous waste, water, air, and soil pollution may profoundly affect the plans for new services. The Food and Drug Administration (FDA) control of diagnostic and treatment procedures and substances is an important regulatory function that must be addressed in planning new endeavors.

Further, regulation at the state and local levels may impact new programming. Health Service Agencies (HSAs), which review utilization and confirm the need for new equipment and facilities and state laws affecting reimbursement for services, have the greatest impact on strategic planning.

Competition/Hospital Image

An assessment of the competitive position of the institution in both the community and the region may be based on utilization data, such as the number of hospital days, percent occupancy, physician specialty mix, and case mix. Fiscal data to be compared might include current ratios, operating margins, and long-term debt to equity ratios. Changes in services, administrative teams, and facilities of competing hospitals provide further data for assessment of the competitive position.

The hospital image may be assessed via qualitative measures, such as patient satisfaction surveys, community focus groups, interviews with physicians and hospital personnel, and media coverage. Quantitative data may be obtained from retention rates for physicians, nurses, and allied health personnel.

Manpower

Information about local, state, and national manpower trends is needed for the external assessment. Nationally, the supply of physicians is maldistributed to larger cities and specialties. The national nurse shortage continues as a result of increasing demand for RNs in nonacute care settings and the higher nurse-patient ratios required in acute care facilities. Planning for new services, new care delivery systems, and new programs requires in-depth knowledge of the manpower available to staff the proposed changes. Such information is available locally from schools of nursing and medicine, local manpower studies, and professional practice groups. Nationally, information on manpower is available from governmental and professional agencies and publications.

The proposed external assessment data can be combined to provide a gestalt of the environment that will impact planning for the future. Smith (1987) reports that in the past 5 years, the environment has propelled hospitals into an externally oriented planning process.

INTERNAL ASSESSMENT

Flexner, Berkowitz, and Brown (1981) propose that an internal assessment by strategic planners would illustrate the hospital's strengths and limitations and the areas open to development. The assessment should include organizational culture, the communication process, and institutional demographics. The organizational culture can be examined via behaviors, norms, values, rules, and the philosophy. Luthans (1989) suggests that organizational behavior is based on a common language, terminology, and rituals. This is reflected in the interactions between and among groups. The perceived worth of groups to the organization is reflected in the relationships of such groups as physicians and nurses. Norms about work behaviors (how hard to work) may agree or disagree with the philosophy of the institution and organizational values of efficiency, quality of work, and dependability. Rules for getting along in the organization provide a framework for the climate, that is, a feeling that is derived from patient/worker interaction and that indicates the openness of employees to change. These data will be crucial to planners wishing to predict the success of proposed programs.

Effective organizational communication is crucial in developing new programs and, thus, assessment of the process is a primary need for strategic planning. Factors for examination are the patterns and channels of formal and informal communication, the efficiency and effectiveness of communication, and the nature of communications. An assessment of the organizational demographics will determine the human resources available as employees, volunteers, consultants, and collaborators. Further, data on age, gender, race, education, and experience will provide a detailed profile of the hospital resources.

ORGANIZATIONAL STRUCTURE AND PROCESS

Assessment of the structure will assist planners in determining how new services/programs may be best delivered. A decentralized organization may work well with one project. Another project may require central control or a matrix structure. The process by which outcomes are achieved should be evaluated. Leadership styles and the structure and function of groups are data that will assist the strategic planner.

EXAMINING THE CRITICAL ISSUES

On completion of the internal, external, and organizational assessment, the strategic planners prepare to examine the critical issues. The strategic analysis technique proposed by Stevenson (1976) uses data from the assessment for an in-depth analysis of institutional *strengths*, *weaknesses*, *opportunities*, and *threats*, known as SWOT. This analysis provides the basis for forecasting. Forecasters may use nonquantitative approaches such as intuition, judgement, hunches, experience, rule of thumb, listings, tables, or decision chains.

Quantitative approaches to forecasting include time series forecasts, econometric models, anticipatory surveys, correlation, and linear regression models. Whatever the forecasting technique, the decisions about future activities are based to some extent on value judgements and become political judgements in the strategic planning process. Again, strategic planning differs from master planning in the extent to which political decisions are primary. Woven through the critical issues development is the thread of negotiation. The power of major stakeholders must be assessed and the support for a particular issue or perspective obtained for a successful strategic planning process.

DEFINING THE BUSINESS-CENTERED MISSION

Once the critical issues are determined, the planners must articulate a business-defined mission that is goal oriented, action focused, and strategically advantageous to the organization. Flexner, Berkowitz, and Brown (1981) suggest that the business-defined mission represents the broad purpose of the institution, reflecting needs, wants, resources, and restrictions. Goals are set to exploit the opportunities and avoid the threats identified in the SWOT analysis. Optimizing goals, which are set at 3-, 5-, and 10-year intervals, motivate action and reflect organizational risk taking.

Strategy development is the next step. Kraegal (1983) suggests that planners select from alternate strategies, often developing clusters of strategies. She identifies three positions relating to strategy decisions — superior, equivalent, and inferior. The superior position addresses the organization's plan to use resources to develop new programs that will result in a superior position to the competition. The strategy position of equivalency seeks to maintain a competitive position. The inferior position allows the organization to cede primacy in a service to others.

The primary strategy of the 1990s for addressing the business-defined mission has been diversification. Ives and Kerfoot (1989) identify diversification as the strategy that attempts to spread financial risk by taking advantage of new market opportunities. Two major concepts of diversification are vertical and horizontal integration. Vertical integration can be forward directed (developing programs or services for health care beyond the hospital acute care focus): health screening and wellness centers are examples. Backward integration addresses raw materials or precursors needed in acute care delivery, for example, intravenous solutions and pharmaceuticals.

Horizontal integration strategies seek to enlarge the scope of practice by acquisition of like institutions in the area, linking several acute care agencies, or joining acute and nonacute facilities. The strategy seeks advantage from economies of scale, concentration of management, and increased access to capital.

DEVELOPING THE PLAN

The final step in strategic planning is the development of the plan. The planners have defined the problem, searched for alternate strategies, evaluated the alternates, and, finally, selected the strategies to be implemented.

The planning process is completed when a detailed comprehensive implementation model is presented. Planners may use tools such as Program Evaluation and Review Technique (PERT), Critical Path Method (CPM), and Management Operations Systems Technique (MOST) to graphically present planning, scheduling, and costing via a network.

Finally, evaluation is critical to the entire strategic planning process. Continuous evaluation of the effectiveness in achieving organizational goals and monitoring environmental conditions and trends is inherent to the concept of strategic planning. Strategies may require change in response to new opportunities and threats. Plans may be disrupted by changes in competition and regulation. Strategic planning promotes the flexibility necessary to promote and sustain the viability of hospitals in the turbulent environment of the 1990s.

THE ROLE OF NURSING ADMINISTRATION

Nurse executives are assuming increasingly stronger positions on the hospital administration team (Vestal, 1989). These chief nurse executives are regularly included in the institutional strategic planning function. In turn, nurse executives have used the strategic planning process at the divisional level with their team of nurse managers (Nash & Opperwall, 1988). Continuing the process, nurse managers have used strategic planning for their departments.

What do chief nurse executives contribute to the institutional planning process? Lukacs (1984) suggests that they contribute information about professional nursing services needed by customers. They identify client's needs for prevention and health promotion activities. For example, they focus on client needs for mobility, nutrition, counseling, and psychosocial support rather than disease-based needs.

The nurse executive shares data on the enlarged scope of nursing, that is, the increasing emphasis on health through screening, teaching, and counseling. The nurse executive identifies the nursing skill mix needed for a new program and identifies strengths within the department, that is, gerontology, pediatrics, Clinical Nurse Specialists. The nurse executive contributes information about the process of care delivery using the professional nurse and assistive personnel. The chief nurse executive assists the team to understand the role of nurses, the values nurses hold, and the nurses' perceptions of their value to the institution.

Overall, nurse executives reflect a care focus in the review of external, internal, and organizational structure. They contribute a nursing perspective to the business-defined mission, noting where nursing skills and abilities are required. They assist in the development of goals and objectives. They are the prime movers in operationalizing the strategies. When selecting among alternate strategies, they use political acumen to promote the best possible outcome. They use negotiation to win approval for programs that will be most successful. When final decision making occurs, they use highly developed skills of analysis for the selection of appropriate strategies. Finally, they direct the tactical planning mode as the second stage of planning and translate to the nursing division the mission, goals, objectives, and strategies. They then serve as leaders for divisional planning and transmit to unit nurse executives the skills to continue the process at lower levels. Finally in the implementation stage, they are the constant assessors, cheerleaders, and evaluators. Strategic planning demands long-term commitment of managers at all levels to match the organization to its environment. Nursing administration contributes to strategies planning at the organizational, divisional, and departmental level and contributes significantly to the successful operation of health care organizations in the turbulent environment of the 1990s.

Summary

Strategic planning has been discussed as the basis for strategic management of health care delivery. Major subconcepts include economic factors, political issues, market trends, technology trends, social/life

style trends, regulatory trends, and factors related to competition and manpower. The planning process encompasses definition of the problem, search for alternative strategies, evaluation of strategies, and selection of final approach. Nurse executives are intricately involved at unit and corporate levels in the strategic planning process.

References

Domanico, L. (1981). Strategic planning: Vital for hospital long-range development, *Hospital and Health Services Administration, 26*(4), 25–40.

Drucker, P. (1974). *Management tasks, responsibilities, politics.* New York: Harper & Row.

Flexner, W. A., Berkowitz, E. N., & Brown, M. (1981). *Strategic planning in health care management.* Rockville, MD: Aspen Systems Corporation.

Garner, J. F., Smith, H. L., & Piland, N. F. (1990). *Strategic nursing management.* Rockville, MD: Aspen Publishers, Inc.

Ives, J. E., & Kerfoot, K. (1989). Pitfalls and promises of diversification, *Nursing Economics, 7*(4), 200–203.

Kraegel, J. M. (1983). *Planning strategies for nurse managers.* Rockville, MD: Aspen Systems Corporation.

Lukacs, J. L. (1984). Strategic planning in hospitals: Applications for nurse executives, *Journal of Nursing Administration, 16,* 11–17.

Luthans, F. (1989). *Organizational behavior* (5th ed.). New York: McGraw-Hill.

Nash, M. G., & Opperwall, B. C. (1988). Strategic planning: The practical vision, *Journal of Nursing Administration, 18*(4), 12–16.

Smith, D. P. (1987). One more time: What do we mean by strategic management? *Hospitals and Health Services Administration, 32*(2), 219–233.

Steiner, G. A. (1979). *Strategic planning.* New York: Free Press.

Stevenson, H. H. (1976). Defining corporate strengths and weaknesses, *California Management Review, 19,* 51–66.

Thieme, C. W., Wilson, T. E., & Long, D. M. (1981). Strategic planning for hospitals under regulation, *Health Care Management Review, 6*(2), 35–43.

Vestal, K. W. (1989). Gainsharing: Rewarding nursing performance, *Journal of Nursing Administration, 19*(12), 10–11.

CHAPTER 19

Integrated Quality Management

Marylane Wade Koch

Highlights

- **Quality control: The industrial model**
- **Quality movement in health care**
- **Defining quality**
- **Components of integrated quality management**
- **Goals of quality management**
- **Trends in quality**

America has a new measurement for products and services: "quality." Consumers ask for "quality" in food, cars, and education. "Quality" is a nebulous term often defined by the perception of the consumer. Many have tried to define "quality." One thing is sure: health care cannot escape this measurement by consumers. The expectation of "quality" is foremost in the minds of health care consumers including patients, insurance companies, and the federal government—anyone paying the bill for health care services.

The health care provider must face the challenge of the question: "Can quality health care be delivered at cost-efficient prices?" The nursing professional must meet this challenge by implementing a process that addresses the multifaceted issues in providing "quality" health care. Although other businesses have implemented quality control programs, health care has been slow to respond in this area. Now, regulatory groups as well as the consumers demand it.

A new paradigm for the nursing professional includes integrated quality management: improving health care services through quality assessment and improvement, utilization management, infection control, and risk/safety management. The goal is "quality" care in the appropriate setting at reasonable costs with positive patient outcomes. The challenge to the nurse executive is empowerment of the professional nurse to demonstrate positive patient outcomes through integrated quality management. This promotes excellence, boosting the image of professional nursing to consumers and third party payors who decide what "value" health care service has in dollars. Professional nursing practice can make a difference in patient care outcomes, demonstrating "value" through integrated quality management.

QUALITY CONTROL: THE INDUSTRIAL MODEL

The history of modern quality control can be traced to Shewhart of Bell Laboratories. In the 1930s, Shewhart used the control chart to produce military supplies cheaply and in mass quantities. The applied statistics, called z-1 standards, were considered classified information (Ishikawa, 1985). Britain also adopted these standards.

When Japan was devastated by the War, the equipment and communications were poor. The United States government stationed there required implementation of quality control. In 1946, modern statistical quality control began to grow in Japan. Various leaders, such as W. Edward Deming and J. M. Juran, moved the country of Japan from a reputation of inferior products to one of superior products.

Both Deming and Juran later came to the United States and assisted American companies in organizing quality programs. Deming is well known for his 14 points that are key to any quality management program:

1. Create a constancy of purpose for service improvement
2. Adopt a new philosophy
3. Cease dependence on mass inspection
4. End practice of awarding business on price alone
5. Find problems. Constantly improve every process for planning, production, and service
6. Institute training on the job
7. Institute leadership for system improvement
8. Drive out fear for effective environment
9. Break down barriers between staff areas and departments
10. Eliminate slogans, posters, and numerical goals, asking for improved productivity without providing methods
11. Eliminate numerical quotas for workforce
12. Remove barriers to pride of workmanship
13. Institute a vigorous program of education and self-improvement for everyone
14. Create a structure in top management that will push every day for the above (Deming, 1982)

Juran has emphasized that quality must be implemented from the top down. He defined seven steps for management to follow for quality improvement:

1. *Awareness* of the competitive challenges and your own competitive position
2. *Understanding* of the new definition of quality and of the role of quality in the success of your company
3. *Vision* of how good your company can really be
4. *Plan* for action. Clearly define the steps you need to take to achieve your vision
5. *Train* your people to provide the knowledge, skills, and tools they need to make your plan happen
6. *Support* to ensure changes are made, problem causes are eliminated, and gains are held
7. *Reward and recognize* to make sure that successes spread throughout the company and become part of the business plan (Vasilash, 1988)

QUALITY MOVEMENT IN HEALTH CARE

Many nurse executives associate quality assessment and improvement with the Joint Commission for the Accreditation of Health Care Organizations (JCAHO), created in 1952. Actually, the quality health care movement actualized much earlier with Flexner and Codman in the early 1900s. In 1912, Codman designed and implemented the first medical "audits," an early form of outcome monitoring. When the American College of Surgeons formed their accreditation body in 1919, standards development, education, and practitioner competence were included. This group later became JCAHO. Quality assurance standards were made mandatory in 1981 with revisions in 1984.

JCAHO (1987) announced plans to revise the accreditation process. This revision has become known as the Agenda for Change. This Agenda is a major research and development process to improve JCAHO's ability to assist and evaluate health care organizations in provision of daily quality improvement. The Agenda includes educational and communications initiatives. Standards are more descriptive and less prescriptive. In short, the Agenda moves JCAHO in the position to evaluate not *can* the organization provide quality health care (structure and process) but rather *does* the organization provide quality health care (outcome) (JCAHO, 1987).

In March 1989, JCAHO approved 12 principles for organizational and management effectiveness in accredited organizations. These principles define the need for Continuous Quality Improvement (CQI) in strategic planning, performance appraisals, budgeting, and role expectations. The governing board, management, and clinical leaders are charged with developing values that encourage CQI. Evaluations for consumers, such as payors, patients, and employees, must be used in this process.

In January 1990, JCAHO approved 12 principles for CQI. CQI is described as "dynamic" in the preamble. The underlying principle is respect for the values, needs, and concerns of the consumers. These principles include such areas as philosophy and culture, mission, leadership, CQI systems, performance appraisals, education and training, and organizational relationships. The standards for these principles are being finalized.

DEFINING "QUALITY"

"Quality" has been defined in many ways. The Japanese Industrial Standards define quality control as "a system of production methods which economically produces quality goods or services meeting the requirements of consumers" (Ishikawa, 1985). Modern quality control combines this with the use of statistical methodology. Ishikawa (1985), a foremost authority, states, "To produce quality control is to develop, design, produce, and service a product which is economical, most useful, and always satisfactory to the customer." A definition that has received wide acceptance is "fitness for use" (Juran, 1989).

Donebedian (1980), a leader in medical quality assurance, initially defined quality as "that kind of care which is expected to maximize an inclusive measure of patient welfare, after one has taken account of the balance of expected gains and losses that attend the process of care in all its parts." JCAHO (1990) define quality as "the degree to which patient care services increase the probability of desired patient outcomes and reduce the probability of undesired outcomes, given the current state of knowledge." Others contend that quality is consumer perception: the degree to which the customer is satisfied with the product or service. Quality, then, is meeting or exceeding customer expectations.

QUALITY MANAGEMENT

Today, more health care organizations have a Total Quality Management (TQM) program for Continuous Quality Improvement (CQI), the term used by JCAHO. Quality management is different from a "fire-fighting" philosophy because it is organized, systematic, planned, and proactive. Quality management, or improvement, must be a **planned** change. Juran (1989) describes quality improvement as "the organized creation of beneficial change; the attainment of unprecedented levels of performance . . . a break-through."

TQM, or CQI, is the process of continuously improving the quality of products or service in any business. The anticipated results are increased customer satisfaction, more profit and market share, better productivity, and decreased costs through better resource utilization. Whatever the term used, the goal is the same: to expand traditional quality processes to include all clinical, administrative, and support functions to improve the quality of health care.

Most health care organizations have a quality assurance (QA) program. This program provides systematic monitoring and evaluation of patient care delivery. Organizations may also have infection control, risk and safety programs, and utilization management in place. What is often missing is the integration of all quality management components into nursing practice in the clinical and administrative settings.

COMPONENTS OF INTEGRATED QUALITY MANAGEMENT

Integrated quality management includes but is not limited to:

1. Quality assessment and improvement,
2. Infection control,
3. Utilization management,
4. Risk/safety management.

These areas, although unique and separate in some ways, have many commonalities. It is believed that each area is so dependent on the other that the whole is enhanced by integration. Webster (1984) best defines the interaction as "synergy," or "the combined action of 2 or more substances or agencies to achieve an effect greater than that of which each is individually capable." An integrated QM program can be the competitive strength of any health care organization.

Quality Assessment and Improvement

Quality assessment (QA) is the more recent updated process known previously as quality assurance. QA is the systematic, monitoring and evaluation program that identifies problems, designs solutions, and performs follow-up activities to make sure no new problems occur. JCAHO has standards that address this component of quality management. QA monitors both the quality and appropriateness of patient care. The carefully designed QA process can provide many opportunities for improvement of patient care or health care system processes.

QA evolved from the basic assumption that health care professionals have the responsibility for self-regulation. Health care professionals must assume the process of governing themselves to provide quality care. Some say Florence Nightingale was the first QA nurse, as she identified the health care problems, designed solutions, and performed follow-up activities in the Crimean War. QA is an integral part of integrated quality management.

The JCAHO QA standard defines a 10-step process for health care organizations to follow to assist in developing a useful QA program.

Step 1: Assign Responsibility　The governing board has ultimate responsibility for patient care. However, the daily operations are delegated down to each person in the organizational structure. Each person shares in the improvement of quality patient care and is responsible at that defined level.

Step 2: Delineate Scope of Care　The scope of care is determined by *who*, *what*, *when*, and *where* the care and services are provided. Each department must define the types of patients served; the conditions or diagnoses treated; types of practitioners providing the services; sites where services are provided; and the times of service delivery.

Step 3: Identify Important Aspects of Care　With limited resources, the important aspects of care must be reviewed and priority given to those with the greatest impact on patient care. JCAHO suggests prioritizing by:

HIGH VOLUME (HV): Occurs frequently or affects large numbers of patients.

HIGH RISK (HR): When patients are at risk for serious consequences or deprived of desired benefit if care is not provided in an appropriate, timely way.

PROBLEM-PRONE (PP): Tends to produce problems for patient, family/significant other, or staff.

Assign important aspects of care to one or more of these categories to decide the priority of monitoring and evaluation. All aspects must be identified but the nursing department may not actually implement QA for all each year.

Step 4: Identify Indicators   An indicator is a quantitative measure that can be used as a guide in the monitoring and evaluation process. This indicator does not measure quality in a direct way but rather screens for the need for further evaluation. Each important aspect of care needs at least one indicator.

Indicators can be structure, process, or outcome related. *Structure* indicators are those that measure the organization's ability to provide quality care, such as availability of resources or qualifications of professional nurses. *Process* indicators evaluate the way care is delivered, such as nursing process, patient teaching, or discharge planning. *Outcome* indicators monitor results, such as adverse reactions or customer satisfaction.

Step 5: Establish Threshold for Evaluation   Establishing a threshold for evaluation is a predetermined level of analysis that triggers further evaluation. Most simply, it is the level of acceptability. For some sentinel events, those that do not normally occur with frequency, the accepted threshold is 0 percent. These events, such as maternal death, must be investigated every time it occurs as this is an abnormal adverse outcome. Another indicator, such as performing admission assessments within 4 hours of admission, might be set at a threshold of 95 percent. Threshold levels are set based on seriousness of the event and its implication to quality care.

Step 6: Collect and Organize Data   Collecting and organizing data is the most labor-intensive step in this process. For each indicator, the QA plan must identify the data sources, collection methods, sampling techniques, frequency of collections, and responsibility for both collection and organization of the data. Identifying and using existing data sources, such as the medical record, log records, or incident reports, will decrease the time and resources needed.

Data can be collected concurrently, retrospectively, through interviews, by observation, or any combination of these. Retrospective review is least effective as there is no time for effective intervention once the patient care is done and the patient is discharged. Observation and interview are the most time consuming.

Step 7: Evaluate Care   To develop an effective action plan, accurate data must be obtained and interpretation analyzed to show trends or patterns in care that can be improved. Evaluation can be performed by a group, task force, or committee. The goal is to point out causative factors, not individual performance, such as knowledge deficit, behavior problems, or system deficiencies.

Step 8: Take Action to Improve Care   If an opportunity for improvement in patient care has been identified, an action plan is initiated. To effect positive change, this process must not be seen as punitive. The plan must identify *who* or *what* is expected to change, *who* is responsible for this change, and *when* this change is to occur. Often, the plan will be multidisciplinary as nursing interacts with so many departments in the organization.

Step 9: Assess Actions and Document Improvement   This step calls for assessment of the action plan and documentation of improvement. To do this, the original indicators and data collection tools must be used; otherwise, the results will be skewed. This step asks the question: "Did we make a difference in patient care?" If not, there must be reassessment of the opportunity for improvement and a change in action plan. This is an important step in documenting quality improvement.

Step 10: Communicate Information   In the QA plan, define all lines of communication for QA results. Communicating the documented outcomes of the action plan encourages integration of quality improvement information within nursing departments and within the organization. Communication of results is important if nurses are to see that planned change can improve patient care. This further encourages participation as the nurse sees value in the QA process.

Infection Control

Infection control is probably the oldest component of integrated quality management (QM), its beginnings dated B.C. Infection control has as a basic tenet, the understanding of communicable disease as causing illness through specific agents or toxic substances. Basic transmission modes and causes of communicable disease are important concepts for the practicing health care professional.

Trending and reporting infection control information is necessary to integrated QM. The type of surveillance and its scope can be determined by QM reports such as nosocomial rates or clean wound infection rates. Incidence and prevalence data can be determined through QM studies with appropriate follow-up and actions taking place. Although infection control is a unique component, it is nonetheless a necessary one to an integrated QM program.

Utilization Management

Utilization management (UM) is the planned, organized, directing of the health care resources in a cost-efficient manner, contributing to the quality of patient care and goals of the organization. In the past, UM was known as utilization review (UR) for, indeed, this process was just that—chart review for evaluating the use of medical services, procedures, and facilities against predetermined criteria. UM identifies and resolves problems that can cause inappropriate use of scarce health care resources.

Although required by the Social Security Amendments of 1965, UM gained a respected place in QM during the 1980s with the advent of DRGs. JCAHO developed an UM Standard in 1980. The Peer Review Organization (PRO) was established by the federal government to monitor the quality and appropriateness of patient care services. One example of UM is inappropriate scheduling of services that may cause a delay in patient treatment. Discharge planning is an important part of UM as is case management. UM complements the other components of QM by appropriate management of health care resources. UM has as its goal the appropriate level of care for each patient, thereby managing resources.

Risk/Safety Management

Risk management (RM) is the part of QM that demonstrates ongoing assessment of potential and actual organizational losses. Often, these risks can be equated into dollars lost or saved for the organization. The RM program is designed to avert losses and minimize exposure. Trending of incident reports is one important way RM contributes to QM process.

Safety and security problems fall under RM. There must be emphasis on preventive maintenance programs and disaster planning for the health care organization. RM works with other areas to secure QM data that enhances the process, such as patient advocacy programs, patient education, and patient satisfaction surveys. RM is an important part of QM as it works with other QM processes to maintain a safe environment with minimal risk to both patients and health care providers.

Each area of integrated QM is important and can stand alone for its unique purposes. As integration and consequent synergy occurs, however, each builds on the strength of the other. Quality assessment and improvement trends are available to RM to reduce the chance of losses through adverse outcomes. Utilization management uses the QA and RM reports to manage health care resources judiciously for better quality care. Infection control or safety concerns become indicators for QA and planned change can be evaluated. It is the interrelationship that gives such strength to the integrated QM concept.

GOALS OF QUALITY MANAGEMENT

The goal of most health care organizations is to provide "high quality health care," as defined in the mission statement. Quality management strives to create a culture where positive, honest communication can take place. Processes are put in place to monitor and evaluate problems, decrease the spread of infection, use resources appropriately, guard the organization from loss, and protect the consumer from adverse outcomes.

Quality management shows the consumer he or she is getting equitable value for the cost. A quality reputation can mean increased market share from customer satisfaction. Quality management can also help educate the consumer to what is reasonable for affordable costs. The goal is to provide the appropriate level of care needed for the specific consumer at a reasonable cost with a positive outcome.

STRATEGIES FOR INTEGRATING QUALITY MANAGEMENT

Most nurses prefer one area of integrated QM to the others. Perhaps the nurse has had experience with quality assessment and improvement or infection control. Another likes risk management and can readily point out patient and visitor needs. Still others seem "naturals" at finding ways to use resources more efficiently. To more integrated QM into the practice setting, however, each nurse must understand the basic principles of all areas and how they interrelate. This helps broaden the perspective of the individual nurse and improves the comprehensiveness of QM in nursing practice.

The accountability for QM rests at each level of nursing, from staff to nurse executive. To integrate QM into all practice settings, a new paradigm must be the vision of nursing administration. Early in the professional nurse's experience, the components of QM must be introduced and applied to basic nursing process. Educators and managers themselves must learn to value QM and become mentors for the nurse. Plans of care must address all components to produce positive patient care outcomes.

Nurse executives must recognize the impact of QM on advanced nursing practice. In JCAHO's Agenda for Change, the leadership standards hold the advanced practice nurse accountable for assessing and planning quality care. Nurse executives and advanced practice nurses can discuss the fears and positive outcomes that QM can bring with the staff and nurse managers. Staff and manager orientation can include the basics of QM, setting expectations for performance appraisals. Nurse executives must stay current with trends by reading and disseminating current literature related to QM. Research and publishing must be encouraged as nurses experience positive change with integrated QM.

Quality management can be interdepartmental and collaborative. Working with other professionals will bring more options for defined concerns with both patients and processes. Learning to value differences is an important part of integrated QM. Quality management offers many opportunities for collaborative practice both within and outside the practice of nursing.

TRENDS IN QUALITY MANAGEMENT

The trends in health care for QM are numerous. Today's consumers are more educated and have more expectations. Some of the trends that nursing professionals face in the present and future practice environment are directly related to QM.

Nursing Research

The nurse executive has the professional responsibility to promote and support nursing research. Nurses are both consumers and producers of research. The nurse executive must make research the cornerstone of professional decision making.

Quality management interfaces well with nursing research. Data collection and analyses are important parts of QM as well as research. All components of QM — quality assessment and improvement, utilization management, infection control, and risk/safety management — have some elements of research. The monitoring and evaluation of integrated QM clearly complements nursing research.

Quality management research can assist the nurse in documenting the clinical impact of professional practice to the external payors and regulation groups. Nursing research can assess the effectiveness of nursing interventions in outcome monitoring of the patient care part of QM. This type of study, combined with risk management and infection control, can demonstrate that professional nursing can make a difference in patient care outcomes.

Nursing research done in the area of health promotion is another natural fit for QM. As nurses confirm the impact of healthy lifestyles on disease prevention, third party payors and consumers may spend their health care dollars in health promotion provided by nurses. Nurses can make a difference in prevention of infection, such as

AIDS, by teaching universal precautions. Research on high-risk populations and necessary intervention may change the course of this devastating illness and produce positive outcomes. Again, QM has direct interface with nursing research.

Research dissemination and utilization is essential to quality health care in nursing practice. Research is concerned with the process and the outcome, as is QM. Nurse executives can foster the environment that encourages nursing research through integrated QM. Studies can include cost and effectiveness of nursing care and implications for patient safety. Agencies that use QM in nursing research will have a competitive edge in both staff retention and establishing preferred provider relationships.

Nursing Ethics

Bioethics is the term used to define the application of ethics to society and human life. This is a major area of concern in the current environment. Some health care concerns that relate directly to QM include:

- Treatment of dying patients
- Mercy killing, mercy deaths, and euthanasia
- Organ transplants
- Birth control, sterilization, and abortion
- Genetics, fertilization, and birth
- Human experimentation and informed consent
- Allocation of limited health care resources
- Confidentiality of the professional relationships (Thiroux, 1986)

The right-to-die issue continues to face health care professionals. The Cruzan case brought the concern to Congress for legislative action. On June 25, 1990, the Supreme Court issued the first right-to-die decision in favor of Nancy Cruzan. From this landmark case came legislation to regulate health care providers who accept federal payments. They must explain and offer an advanced directive to patients admitted for any service in any setting. This initiative, the Patient Self-Determination Act, mandates the patient has every opportunity to receive information and understand all options while still competent. This must be documented in the patient record. It is only one example of the challenge of ethics that can be addressed through a QM process. This poses some interesting risk and safety issues in health care. The Act indirectly addresses efficient use of limited health care resources.

Mandatory testing and disclosure of HIV is a major concern in health care today. The American Nurses Association (ANA) has issued a statement that supports strict adherence to universal precautions and infection control measures as the only way to stop AIDS transmission. Because of cost and unreliable AIDS testing, it is not practical to mandate testing and disclosure. There is no way to police the AIDS virus. Only teaching and effective safe practices by humans will curtail this debilitating disease.

In all of the examples mentioned previously, there are definite *risks* and *safety* issues to both patients and health care providers. These ethical dilemmas will impact the utilization of health care resources, **utilization management**. Many involve **infection control** principles, such as organ transplants and AIDS transmission. Finally, both positive and adverse outcomes will be demonstrated through monitoring and evaluation of **quality assessment** and **improvement**. Quality management plays a major role in nursing ethics.

Computerization

The nurse executive who wants to manage manpower effectively while integrating QM into practice will value computerization. Computers are useful in data management and analyzation. Risk management incident-report data can be trended more easily with computerization. Quality assessment and improvement data can be stored on the computer for regular analysis. Infection-control surveillance reports are conveniently available to the practitioner for easy reference on computer. Computerization can improve the efficiency of trend reporting, an important part of QM.

Marketing

As health care reimbursement decreases, providers must compete with other providers for limited dollars. Marketing is an important part of strategic planning for the nurse executive. Marketing plans identify the needs, preferences, and perceptions of consumers. Quality management can assist the nurse executive in designing the marketing plan.

Integrated QM includes measuring a beginning, benchmarking, of preferences and perceptions. The improvement outcome is measured, providing guidance to the nurse executive for effectiveness of marketing strategies. Some common measures of marketing effectiveness are use of services, employee and consumer satisfaction, turnover rates, and revenues and expenses. The nurse executive who has the professional goal of providing quality health care services has initiated a marketing goal as well. Demonstrated quality can attract and retain customers and payors.

Nursing Agenda for Health Care Reform

More than 40 nursing agencies have joined ANA in support of the Nursing Agenda for Health Care Reform (1991). Nurses have always supported access, quality, and affordable costs in health care delivery. This agenda defines methods of immediate reform to relieve the many ills of the current health care delivery system.

The agenda outlines restructure of the health care system to use the most cost-effective providers and therapeutic options in an appropriate setting (utilization management). A public plan would be offered to the poor and individuals-at-risk because of preexisting illnesses, such as AIDS (risk management and infection control). Steps would be taken to reduce costs through case management and prudent resource allocation based on policies developed from outcome research (quality assessment and improvement).

In short, integrated QM supports the agenda through:

- Provider availability
- Consumer involvement
- Outcome and effectiveness monitoring
- Review mechanisms
- Managed care
- Case management.

Summary

Professional nursing and QM have compatible goals. The nurse is the healthcare professional nearest the consumer for the most consistent periods of time. Integrated quality management empowers nurses to practice their professional philosophy. It gives nursing the image boost needed in today's environment, promoting research and professional autonomy.

A result of QM is increased organizational self-esteem, as professional nurses feel excited about the quality of care they provide. The increased morale makes retention and recruitment easier for nurse executives. Both the consumer and the provider benefit from QM.

The challenge to the nurse executive is to be a visionary in redefining the organizational culture that supports, encourages, and rewards professional excellence, demonstrated through QM in patient care delivery. The tools and principles of QM must be incorporated into daily nursing practice, whatever the setting. The time of opportunity for professional nursing has come; with integrated QM nurses can demonstrate their value and impact on positive patient care and organizational outcomes for health care into the present and future environment.

QUESTIONS FOR DISCUSSION

1. How does the JCAHO Agenda for Change impact nurse executives and professional nursing practice?

2. What are the chief components of integrated quality management? Give an example in one practice setting.

3. What are some strategies the nurse executive might use to integrate quality management into nursing practice?

4. Describe how integrated quality management relates to trends in nursing research, nursing ethics, computerization, and marketing.

5. What are the implications for Nursing's Agenda for Health Care Reform and quality management?

References

American Nurses Association. (1991). *Nursing's Agenda for Health Care Reform.* PR-3, 220M.

Deming, W. E. (1982). *Quality, productivity, and competitive position.* Cambridge: Massachusetts Institute of Technology Center for Advanced Engineering Study.

Donebedian, A. (1980). *Exploration in quality assessment and monitoring: A definition of quality approaches to its assessment.* Ann Arbor, MI: Health Administration Press.

Ishikawa, K. (1985). *What is total quality control? The Japanese way.* Englewood Cliffs, NJ: Prentice-Hall.

JCAHO (1990). *Accreditation manual for hospitals, 1991.* Chicago: author.

JCAHO (1987). *Overview of the joint commission's agenda for change.* Chicago: author.

Juran, J. M. (1989). *Juran on leadership for quality: An executive handbook.* New York: The Free Press.

Thiroux, J. P. (1986). *Ethics: Theory and practice* (3rd ed.). New York: Macmillan.

Vasilash, G. S. (1988). Buried treasure and other benefits of quality, *The Juran Report, 9,* 30.

Webster's II New Riverside Dictionary (1984). Boston: Houghton Mifflin.

CHAPTER 20

Advancing Nursing Research in a Professional Practice Climate

---

Highlights

- **Role of the nurse executive**
- **Researchable nursing problems**
- **Collaborative research**
- **Developing a nursing research emphasis**
- **Applications of research to practice**

The purpose of this chapter is to present nursing research as an essential component of a professional nursing practice climate. Nurse executives play a key role in promoting the application of nursing research to practice by stimulating staff involvement in research and promoting a climate in which research can occur. Executives are not necessarily researchers, but they must be knowledgeable about research methodology and must be willing to set the stage for research to occur. In other words, nurse executives must be willing to promote research-based nursing, for they are in key positions to influence the amount and nature of the research undertaken by nursing staff, faculty, and students (Simms, Price, & Pfoutz, 1987).

ROLE OF THE NURSE EXECUTIVE

Considerable confusion exists among nurses regarding the differences between the conduct of research and the utilization of knowledge from research (Haller, Reynolds, & Horsley, 1979). Although increasing numbers of nursing service departments are hiring nurse researchers, the role of the nurse-executive is to foster a climate in which nursing studies can be conducted and nursing research findings can be applied to practice.

The nursing service executive who plans to establish a nursing research program is faced with selling the concept to nursing staff. Egan, McElmurry, and Jameson (1981) suggest that the nurse executive must defend the notion of concluding a feasibility study while questioning the value of introducing a research program. There is still a common attitude in institutions that a research program is a nicety rather than an essential tool for data-based decision making. Furthermore, nursing staff may still view those conducting research as away from practice and not reality based.

Fine (1980) proposes that nurse executives can market the concept of nursing research to their staff by using the same methods that work on Madison Avenue: demand analysis and market segmentation. Says Fine, nurse executives must deal with negative demand, no demand, and latent demand for nursing research:

- Negative demand: research and related actions are disliked.
- No demand: most of the nurses are uninterested or indifferent to nursing research.
- Latent demand: a great number of nurses recognize the need for research, but none is being carried out.

According to Fine, the nursing service executive must identify the nursing group with the greatest latent demand for nursing research and systematically develop its interests. In doing so, the executive is following the guidelines for market segmentation, which is defined by Kotler (1976) as dividing a potential market into fairly homogeneous parts and selecting any part as a target.

Lindeman and Schantz (1982) stress the importance of stimulating staff to write good proposals based on good, researchable questions. These questions must be answerable by observable evidence or empirical data and should involve a relationship between two or more variables. The effect of primary nursing on quality patient care can be tested. The question "Should unit X change to primary nursing?" cannot be tested.

Increasing numbers of nursing service departments are hiring nurse researchers, establishing research departments, and fostering nursing research through application of findings to practice (Ventura & Waligora-Serafin, 1981). The models vary from agency-based programs to various types of collaboration with schools of nursing and other health-related schools. The particular model used should provide the best fit with the agency and the administrative style of the nursing service executive.

The role of the nurse executive in promoting research-based nursing, therefore, is one of leadership. It may not be necessary to develop an in-house research program if abundant resources are available from other disciplines. Whether the nursing division is a research utilizer or a combined research conductor and utilizer, the steps of the research process must govern the decision to study, not to study, or to apply data from another study. Too many administrators attempt to match solutions with problems without fully understanding the problem to be solved or studied.

In selling the concept of research throughout the agency, the nurse executive must encourage staff to understand and participate in research-related activities (Hefferin, Horsley, & Ventura, 1982). Such activities include and are not limited to emphasis on nursing process and quality assurance, attendance of research conferences, and participation in ongoing studies, either as subjects or data collectors. To introduce research findings into practice, the nurse executive must be able to evaluate research, using self-skills or obtaining the expertise of a nurse researcher capable of evaluating research.

The final role of the nurse executive is that of defender of practice changes. Many nurses see research as irrelevant to their practice, and the administrator often finds it necessary to justify decisions for changes in practice as well as to reallocate resources if necessary.

Thus, the nurse executive is conceived to be the leader, the pacesetter, the climate creator, the evaluator, and the defender of research-based practice. It is necessary for administrators to have research skills, and doctorally prepared nurses are increasingly moving into administrative roles. To utilize the skills and work of others in orchestrating professional nursing practice, it has become essential for all nurse executives to have, at a minimum, data management and research appreciation skills.

RESEARCHABLE NURSING PROBLEMS

Nursing problems surface in many possible ways, but basically they are related to patient care. Although most nursing staff will not have the qualifications to conduct research, they can be encouraged to participate in generating priority nursing problems. It is then up to the nurse executive to seek the most appropriate resources for studying problems.

Clinical, educational, and administrative problems can be brought into focus for study by using the research process. Elevating the area of concern from the mundane to the abstract is the first step in conceptualizing the area of study. This can be done by raising questions researchable within the areas of practice or questions that can be answered by other research. The research process, with all its detailed steps, is summarized in Table 20.1.

The importance of using the expertise of qualified nurse researchers cannot be overemphasized. At least one doctorally prepared nurse is essential to the conduct and utilization of quality nursing research. As professional nursing practice becomes increasingly based on empirical research findings, it is important that rigorous studies be conducted or used in changing practice or making clinical decisions.

Nursing problems requiring investigation may be clinical, administrative, or educational. Agency needs for research may vary, but the nature of the nursing problems should have commonality across institutions. Clinical nursing problems requiring special emphasis within the field are those related to mobility, eating, continence,

TABLE 20.1 The Research Process

Research Process	Scientific Steps	Technical Steps
Formulate the problem	Formulate the problem	
Review the literature	Review the literature	
Formulate the framework of theory	Formulate the framework of theory	
Formulate hypotheses	Formulate hypotheses	
Define the variables	Define the variables	
Determine how variables will be quantified		Define how variables will be quantified
Determine the research design		Determine the research design
Delineate the target population		Delineate the target population
Select and develop a method of collecting data		Select and develop a method of collecting data
Formulate a method of analyzing data		Formulate a method of analyzing data
Determine how results will be interpreted (generalized)	Determine how results will be interpreted (generalized)	
Determine a method of communicating results		Determine a method of communicating results

(From Abdellah, F. G., & E. Levin, (1979). *Better Patient Care through Nursing Research*, 2d ed. (pp. 97–99). New York: Macmillan. Used with permission).

cognition, and skin integrity. New clinical studies may be generated, or developed studies from other settings may be replicated.

Administrative studies of importance for nursing usually relate to the care given, as opposed to the nursing process or the activities investigated in clinical studies. Productivity and staffing pattern studies fall in this category, as do staff morale and satisfaction investigations. Another possibility for administrative study is the descriptive measure of technical and professional roles in nursing. Quality-of-care research overlaps both clinical and administrative questions.

A much neglected area for research within nursing divisions is that of evaluation of in-service educational programs. The questions arise as to whether continuing education makes a difference in behavior and whether it affects competency. Many types of issues are emerging today related to competency measures for relicensure and institutional licensure. The correlation of basic educational preparation to job performance needs much study.

COLLABORATIVE RESEARCH

To be effective in any given setting, nursing research must be a collaborative effort using intra- and interinstitutional resources. Collaboration between nurses in practice and academic settings and integration of nurses into the broad scientific community are essential to a sound research focus (Jacox, 1980).

Horsley (Hefferin, Horsley, & Ventura, 1982) and Hinshaw and colleagues (Hinshaw, Chance, & Atwood, 1981) have pioneered collaborative research programs. A collaborative research development model requires clinicians and researchers to be equally functioning team members in the development of clinical nursing research proposals. The importance of a collaborative research program is predicated on the following assumptions:

1. Too little practice-relevant clinical nursing research is conducted.
2. Practice-relevant research findings are too infrequently and slowly absorbed into practice.
3. Clinical nurses have too little influence on nursing research.
4. Collaborative research conducted by clinicians and researchers is more applicable to practice than to noncollaborative research. (Loomis & Krone, 1980)

Clinicians, administrators, educators, and researchers can collaborate and negotiate to produce sound, practice-based research that yields relevant, accurate information for practice decisions and contributes to nursing knowledge. Nurses in all of these roles are all responsible for making nursing professional. Hefferin, Horsley, and Ventura (1982) suggest that each collaborator has a unique role to play in the team effort:

- Clinician: identifies problems
- Administrator: facilitates nursing research
- Researcher: studies the problem and formats findings in clinical terms
- Educator: assists nurses through systematic review of research and translates criteria for evaluating research in terms clinicians can use

Intra- and interinstitutional collaboration goes beyond nursing to include the expertise of physicians, health-services-related engineers, biologists, psychologists, and sociologists as appropriate. Although nursing needs to develop its own knowledge base, it is apparent that, as an applied science, the profession can benefit from interdisciplinary and nursing-related research from other fields.

Positive and negative factors influence the development and maintenance of coi laborative research programs. Positive factors include institutional commitment to quality, patient-centered care, and widespread enthusiasm and interest with the nursing division for professional nursing practice. Negative factors of influence may include:

1. Unclear policies related to staff nurse participation in nursing research (Hodgeman, 1981).
2. Differing goals of scientific inquiry and clinical decision (Hinshaw, Chance, and Atwood, 1981).
3. Differing goals for research held by clinician, administrators, and researchers (Hinshaw, Chance, and Atwood, 1981).
4. Viewpoint held by nonnurse professional colleagues that nurses are not scientists or researchers (Brogan, 1982).

The support of hospital or agency administration and medical staff for a collaborative research program cannot be overestimated. The control of research subjects and resources clearly can influence the longevity and quality of any research program.

DEVELOPING A NURSING RESEARCH EMPHASIS

Before the development of a nursing research emphasis or program, the preferred model must be selected. Five distinct models exist; each has different merit for different agencies based on available resources:

1. University-based model: research is initiated and designed by scholars in schools of nursing, conducted in laboratories or health care agencies, and reported in research journals with opportunity for wide-spread application to practice (Loomis & Krone, 1980).
2. Agency-based model: an agency hires a researcher to assist in developing a study or hires a permanent, full-time researcher to stimulate in-house research (Loomis & Krone, 1980).
3. Collaborative university — agency-based model: the nurse researcher is director of both research programs and utilizes the skills of faculty researchers and agency staff.
4. External consultant model: a nurse researcher is hired for specific studies.
5. Nursing Development Unit model: a cluster of units on which clinical research can be tested (Ashurst, Clarke, Evitts, Lacey, & Snashall, 1990).

Readiness for a research emphasis must be assessed. Egan, McElmurry, and Jameson (1981) recommend specific criteria for testing readiness for a practice-based research department (see Table 20.2). One might add to those criteria the commitment to professional nursing practice, for without it, quality research cannot occur.

Chance and Hinshaw (1980) suggest three critical factors that can facilitate the initiation of a program:

1. The research-oriented attitude of the nurse executive
2. The existence of a research environment in the nursing department
3. The values and flexibility of both the hospital and the nursing department organizational structure.

The attitude of the nurse executive is critical and is the most important of the three factors. Once the commitment is made to establish a research emphasis and the model selected, a nursing research and review committee needs to be established (Fuhs & Moore, 1981). This group works closely with the director for nursing research in establishing a philosophy and goals consistent with ANA standards for nursing practice and with the orientation of the institution.

Obtaining funding for a proposed research emphasis depends on the creativity of the nurse executive. Depending on institutional receptivity to nursing research, the emphasis may be openly established. Other, back-door approaches include linkages with a quality assurance role, research consultation, or adjunct appointments for faculty researchers.

APPLICATIONS OF RESEARCH TO PRACTICE

A commitment to research is not enough to maintain an in-house research emphasis. Conducted or utilized nursing research must be seen as validating the effectiveness of

TABLE 20.2 Criteria for Assessing Readiness for a Practice-based Research Department

Condition	Criteria
Subject participation	Sufficient numbers of research topics to maintain a studies program over time.
	Acceptability of participation in research studies by patients.
Professional participation	Nucleus of personnel with some experience and interest in research.
	Presence of incentives for personnel to participate in research.
Market factors	Organizational expectations for systematic investigation into unsolved problems.
	Acceptability of systematic studies in nursing.
Organizational systems	Complementarity of a research program with established structures and functions.
Economic factors	Presence of various mechanisms for funding systematic studies.
	Identifiable benefits to be accrued from systematic studies.
Legal and statutory provisions	Presence of mechanisms to assure protection of human subjects.
	Presence of mechanisms and guidelines for approval of research projects.
Facilities and resources	Availability of essential facilities and resources necessary for the conduct of systematic studies.
Contributions to educational research endeavors	Presence of systems, procedures, and support for student research.
	Identifiable study topics appropriate for students.

(From Egan, E. C., B. J. McElmurry, & H. M. Jameson, (1981). Practice-based research: Assessing your department's readiness. *Journal of Nursing Administration, 11*(10), 29. Reprinted with permission).

nursing care and as an important means of improving nursing practice (Gulick, 1981). If research is relevant to practice, says Jacox (1980), it will be accepted and used by practicing nurses.

Application to practice can occur through data-based decision making or clinical practice activities. Decisions to alter staffing patterns can be research based. Selection of nursing care delivery models can and should be research based. The continuation or abandonment of decubitus care methodologies should be based on results of investigative studies. Quality of patient care must be evaluated in terms of outcomes as well as processes. Patient classification systems have little use unless linked with clinical and administrative decision making. Systematic evaluation of practice modes not only improves the quality of practice but also the quality of patient life.

Perhaps the best application of research to practice is the establishment of the testing, questioning, thinking environment in which professional nurses feel comfortable in asking, "Is this the best way, is there a better way?"

UTILIZATION OF NURSING RESEARCH

Fawcett (1980) suggests that only when professional nursing practice is based on knowledge validated by research will nursing gain independence as a profession. As long as nursing is viewed as an occupation, institutional policies and politics will keep nurses second-class citizens. The only way to generate nursing knowledge, so essential to professional status, is through scientific nursing research: the study of nursing phenomena. Nursing practice relies too heavily on other disciplines. It is time to develop our own research.

Research in isolation is meaningless, and theory in and of itself is irrelevant. If nursing research is to be palatable in practice, it must be presented in terms that are understandable and useful for implementation. Nursing theories developed and tested through research must become part of the language of nursing. As nursing practice becomes increasingly based on empirical research findings, it is important to conduct rigorous studies to assess current nursing practice or to evaluate changes in practice (Kirchoff & Kvig, 1981). A systematic review of existing nursing research and the establishment of innovation protocols for nursing practice have been described by Haller, Reynolds, and Horsley (1979). Although much has been done in this regard, research findings are not always useful for implementation nor are they always understandable. The participatory action research approach described in Chapter 17 offers much promise for stimulating participation in and utilization of research.

Summary

In the final analysis, it is left to the nurse executive to use nursing research and introduce research findings into practice. This is accomplished through the establishment of a professional practice environment that promotes involvement of staff in research activities and demands that clinical nursing policies and procedures are research based. Once the environment of research-based practice is established, it is no longer necessary to treat the concept as a separate goal, for, as in all professions, it becomes internalized in behavior.

LEARNING ACTIVITY

1. Identify three clinical or systems problems on your unit(s).
2. Develop an action research approach for studying these problems (see Chapter 17).

References

Abedellah, F. G., & Levin, E. (1979). *Better patient care through nursing research* (2nd ed.), (pp. 97–98). New York: Macmillan.

Ashurst, A., Clarke, D., Evitts, A., Lacey, J., & Snashall, T. (1990). Creating a climate for the development of nursing, *Nursing Practice, 4*(1), 18–20.

Brogan, D. R. (1982). Professional socialization to a research role: Interest in research among graduate students in nursing, *Research in Nursing and Health, 5*(3), 113–122.

Chance, H. C., & Hinshaw, A. S. (1980). Strategies for initiating a research program, *Journal of Nursing Administration, 10*(3), 32–39.

Egan, E. C., McElmurry, B. J., & Jameson, H. M. (1981). Practice-based research: Assessing your department's readiness, *Journal of Nursing Administration, 11*(10), 26–32.

Fawcett, J. (1980). A declaration of nursing independence: The relation of theory and research to nursing practice, *Journal of Nursing Administration, 10*(6), 36–39.

Fine, R. B. (1980). Marketing nursing research, *Journal of Nursing Administration, 10*(11), 21–23.

Fuhs, M. F., & Moore, K. (1981). Research program development in a tertiary-care setting, *Nursing Research, 30*(1), 24–27.

Gulick, E. E. (1981). Evaluating research requests: A model for the nursing director, *Journal of Nursing Administration, 11*(1), 26–30.

Haller, K. B., Reynolds, M. A., & Horsley, J. A. (1979). Developing research-based innovation protocols: Process, criteria, and issues, *Research in Nursing and Health, 2*(2), 45–51.

Hefferin, E. A., Horsley, J. A., & Ventura, M. R. (1982). Promoting research-based nursing: The nurse administrator's role, *Journal of Nursing Administration, 12*(5), 34–41.

Hinshaw, A. S., Chance, H. C., & Atwood, J. (1981). Research in practice: A process of collaboration and negotiation, *Journal of Nursing Administration, 11*(2), 33–38.

Hodgeman, E. C. (1981). Research policy for nursing services, Parts 1 and 2, *Journal of Nursing Administration, 11*(4,5), 30–36.

Jacox, A. (1980). Strategies to promote nursing research, *Nursing Research, 29*(4), 213–217.

Kirchoff, K. T., & Kvig, F. J. (1981). A strategy for surveying practice in institutional settings, *Research in Nursing and Health, 4*(3), 309–315.

Kotler, P. (1976). *Marketing for Nonprofit Organizations.* Englewood Cliffs, NJ: Prentice-Hall.

Lindeman, C. A., & Schantz, D. (1982). The research question, *Journal of Nursing Administration, 12*(1), 6–10.

Loomis, M. E., & Krone, K. P. (1980). Collaborative research development, *Journal of Nursing Administration, 10*(12), 32–35.

Simms, L. M., Price, S. A., & Pfoutz, S. K. (1987). Creating the research climate: A key responsibility for nurse administrators in acute, long-term and home care settings, *Nursing Economic$, 5*(4), 174–178.

Ventura, M. R., & Waligora-Serafin, B. (1981). Setting priorities for nursing research, *Journal of Nursing Administration, 11*(6), 30–34.

PART V
Managing Resources

CHAPTER 21
Mobilizing Existing Resources

Highlights

- **Recruitment, retention, and turnover**
- **The perceived nursing shortage**
- **Competency and relicensure**
- **Traditional practice patterns**
- **A new approach to redesigning nursing practice patterns**
- **The flexible work group**

The purpose of this chapter is to discuss an approach to mobilizing existing nursing resources according to levels of expertise, considering work and education experience. Practice patterns are discussed in terms of organizational variables, nursing resources, and patient care needs and a flexible work group model is proposed.

Trying to understand recruitment and retention problems in nursing today is like looking for a straw in the wind and trying to describe its path. The wind keeps shifting, and a tornadic gust threatens to blow the whole issue out of our sphere of influence, if not out of nursing's area of responsibility. Many hospitals and health care agencies have moved in the direction of nonnursing control of nursing recruitment and retention through the establishment of human resource departments that control hiring and firing of all health personnel.

Nursing is a focal point for the delivery of patient care in all health care delivery settings. Failure to change or implement differentiated practice patterns, may be the result of a lack of understanding of nursing resources and of the appropriate use of nurses according to experience and expertise.

Differentiated practice distributes nursing work according to care giver and care coordinator activities, and undifferentiated practice is a real barrier to full professional practice (Goertzen, 1991). This is frustrating to nurses who are often seen as focusing on menial tasks while their real, modern-day contribution is much more advanced. No recognition is given to the various educational levels for nurses and the expectations for performance are indistinguishable for AD and BSN nurses. The special skills of the master's and doctorally prepared nurses often go unrecognized and unused.

A serious barrier to professional practice in large, complex organizations is depersonalization (Simms, Dalston, & Roberts, 1984). Little consideration is given to joint practice or to developing models for patient centered care. Nurses are often treated as elements of production rather than intelligent, dedicated professionals. Differentiated practice promotes more efficient and effective distribution of talent according to educational preparation and experiential competency. As a model for intelligent distribution of nursing resources, it serves as a catalyst for patient-focused care.

NURSING RESOURCES

Nursing resources have been defined by Beckman and Simms (1992) in terms of selected variables, all of which have relevance for care assignment and quality care. Table 21.1 identifies and explains the various nursing resource components, ranging from staff mix and preparation to commitment, stability, availability, and special training. This conceptualization provides a broad perspective on the components of a nursing resource configuration. These components are covered in greater detail later in this chapter in the discussion of practice patterns.

RECRUITMENT, RETENTION, AND TURNOVER

Historically, nursing has experienced high turnover and cyclical shortages. In 1982, discussions of the nursing shortage were especially rampant. By 1984, the economy and the advent of prospective payment had changed the entire picture of recruitment and retention. Because of the large number of nurses in the work force, recruitment became an irrelevant issue, and retention of high-quality, satisfied nurses seemed to be a possibility for the first time in many years.

Recruitment refers to all those activities carried out by a nursing or personnel department to attract nurses to a particular work setting for purposes of interviewing and hiring. Retention activities designed to keep nurses in the work setting have received less than appropriate attention. Dramatic attempts have sometimes been undertaken to recruit regardless of qualifications. The problems that have led to nursing shortages and the difficulties of retaining nurses have not been addressed on a large scale by nursing and the health care industry.

According to Wolf (1981), administrative philosophy and policies contribute more than any other factors to a high turnover rate, which is the direct result of inadequate attention to retention and staff satisfaction. Wolf further describes salary and job conditions as the leading causes of high turnover. Salaries by and large are simply not at the same level as those of other workers with comparable education in our society. In addition, there is little difference in nursing pay scales according to level of

TABLE 21.1   Nursing Resources Variables

Variable	Range	Definition and Explanation
Mix by shift ratio Day Evening Night	Ratio	Five-week average count of RNs/LPNs/aides per shift transformed into a standardized ratio
RN/staff ratio Day Evening Night	Ratio	Five-week average count of RNs/other staff per shift transformed into a standardized ratio
RN/patient ratio	Ratio	Average number of patients per RN over a five-week period by shifts
Part-time/full-time ratio	Ratio	Five-week average of part-time to full-time nursing personnel, all shifts transformed into a standardized ratio
Staff stability: Turnover	0–100%	Proportion of staff replaced each year, separately for RN, LPN, aides
Absenteeism	0–12%	Proportion of staff absent each day, separately for RN, LPN, aides
Staffing instability	0–100%	The proportion of unit staff who change their unit or shift each day; shown for RN, LPN, and aides separately for the day shift
Staff availability	No range	An index of the labor market availability of different categories of nursing personnel
Preparation ratio	Ratio	The ratio of Master's + BSN, to DIP (diploma) + associate's degree (AD), to LPN + aide in the total nursing staff on the unit
Experience ratio	Ratio	The average number of years of experience on the unit for Master's + BSN, to DIP + AD, to LPN + aide
Special training	No range	An estimate of the extent of special training, separately by RN, LPN, and aides, in five skill areas relevant to practice pattern decisions
Staff development resources	No range	A descriptive statement based on responses to questions about staff development

(From Beckman, J. S., & L. M. Simms. (1992). *A guide to Redesigning Nursing Practice Patterns* (p. 9). Ann Arbor, MI: Health Administration Press. Foundation of the American College of Healthcare Executives. Used with permission).

preparation and experience. Aiken, Blendon, and Rogers (1981) also cite the limited growth in nurse's salaries as a prime factor in retention and turnover difficulties. They further suggest that as nurses' incomes rise in relation to those of other workers, more nurses become available for hospital employment, and vacancy rates decline.

What why do nurses quit their jobs? The following reasons have been observed by the authors over time and have been documented in the literature by many others:

- Scarcity of nursing leaders who are knowledgeable about governance
- Low salaries and little reward for experience
- Low prestige
- Much responsibility and little recognition

- Inflexible hours and schedules
- Excessive overtime
- Anger expressed by physicians toward nurses
- Gap between education and practice
- Lack of autonomy
- Too much work
- Quantity of assignments interferes with quality
- Frequent reassignment to unfamiliar units
- Assignment to units not compatible with skills
- Poor physician-nurse relationships
- Incompetent and unsupportive supervisors
- Lack of opportunity for advancement
- Lack of administrative support

There may be other contributing factors, but these issues appear over and over again in the literature. Equal pay for equal work is no doubt a major influencing variable, as the gap between nurses' and physicians' incomes has widened dramatically over the past several years (Aiken, Blendon, & Rogers, 1981).

High turnover and inactivity rates among nurses have long been a major concern to hospital administrators coping with staff nurse shortages and with increasing pressures for hospital cost containment (Weisman, Alexander, & Chase, 1981). Recently, the literature on turnover has become voluminous, and studies may be categorized as one of two types. First, there is the literature that explicitly identifies turnover as the dependent variable to be explained. Second, there are studies that treat turnover as one of several dependent variables to be explained. In general, the turnover models propose a sequence of events whereby employees become dissatisfied with their jobs, start to search for alternative positions, evaluate the alternatives, and decide to leave the organization (Taylor & Covaleski, 1985). The major weakness of these various explanatory models, however, is probably their lack of inclusiveness, which has led to low explanatory power and has made it impossible to assess accurately the relative importance of the various determinants of turnover (Price & Mueller, 1981).

The findings of Weisman, Alexander, & Chase (1981) and Price and Mueller (1981) revealed that nursing turnover may be viewed as the product of a predictable process. Weisman's team found that specific job and nursing unit attributes influence perceived autonomy, job satisfaction or intent to leave; only intent to leave and shorter job tenure had significant direct effects on turnover. In addition, the study showed autonomy was most strongly associated with perceptions of head nurse responsiveness, suggesting that autonomy may be related to individual relationships between staff nurses and head nurses.

THE PERCEIVED NURSING SHORTAGE

In recent years, much attention has been focused on the critical shortage of nurses, particularly in hospitals. For the following reasons, it is difficult to understand why a shortage is perceived to exist (if, indeed, one does any more):

1. There has been an overall decline in the growth of hospitals over the past three decades. Since 1950, the ratio of hospital beds to population has dropped by one third. (American Hospital Association, 1980).
2. Since 1950, the general hospital occupancy rate has declined significantly (American Hospital Association, 1980).
3. Since 1950, the nation's output of nurses has doubled (USDHHS, 1980).

Johnson and Vaughn (1982) found no statistical evidence of significant leakage from the profession. On the contrary, they observed that most evidence provided to support a shortage is based on anecdotal material. Over the past 10 to 15 years, there has been steady growth in the supply of nurses. There has also been an increase of newly licensed nurses. Seventy-five percent of all nurses are employed, an increase from 55 percent in the 1960s. Even though nurses may vacate positions temporarily during childbirth, they do return. The current supply of nurses should be visualized as a dynamic, constantly changing, constantly growing entity.

Various reasons are cited for the perceived shortage of nurses. Johnson and Vaughn (1982) called attention to the high probability that employee demand for nurses has been increasing and continues to increase at a rate faster than the supply of nurses is increasing. This may be due to the higher acuity rate in all settings and the technological revolution in the delivery of care.

Rose (1982) described the problem as one of intensity of annual institutional turnover, which ranges from 35 to 60 percent nationwide. The supply of nurses is also influenced by payment mechanisms. With the emphasis on cost containment, government ceilings on care costs simply do not allow for the number of nursing positions needed or desired. Moreover, the women's movement continues to influence the selection of nursing as a career, as women may increasingly choose professions in medicine, law, dentistry, the sciences, or the ministry and are no longer bound to those in teaching or nursing.

Aiken, Blendon, & Rogers (1981) equated the perceived shortage to the dramatic increase in nurses' participation in temporary service agencies to maximize their incomes and control their working hours. Agencies have proliferated in response to the increased need for temporary services and the decline in relative income for nurses. In addition, nurses wish to have more control over their working hours. One often forgotten reason for the perceived shortage is that the differential cost of a nurse over other personnel is so small that hospitals may be substituting nurses in jobs that could be done by nonnurses.

Beyers, Mullner, Byre, and Whitehead (1983) believed that not enough attention is paid to job promotion and career advancement, which provide functional turnover patterns, as opposed to the dysfunctional turnover when employees leave the agency. Temporary vacancies exist with functional turnover that should not be counted or depicted as a nursing shortage.

One final reason for the perceived shortage is the incomplete use of the vast nursing expertise in schools of nursing around the country. There are opportunities for faculty practice in acute, long-term, and home care settings that could be attractive to schools of nursing, but, to date, nurse executives and educators have not taken the initiative in exploring such options. A contract for services or a shared consultation model could be developed in most settings.

COMPETENCY AND RELICENSURE

If a clear identification of nursing services is really important under prospective payment, perhaps an analysis of nursing jobs will become as mandatory as continuing education is in many states. Some questions to be answered in such analysis include: What is the work of nursing? What should it be? Who should be doing which parts of the work? What will be the competencies of the workers? How will the nurse workers maintain competency according to their level of expertise?

Most states have health occupation legislation covering nursing practice and licensure provisions that specifically address professional nursing. In the state of Michigan, for example, the practice of nursing is defined as "the systematic application of substantial specialized knowledge and skill derived from the biological, physical, and behavioral sciences, to the care, treatment, counsel, and health teaching of individuals who are experiencing changes in the normal health processes or who require assistance in the maintenance of health and the prevention or management of illness, injury, or disability" (State of Michigan Public Health Code, 1978). The registered nurse engages in the practice of nursing; the practice of licensed practical nursing is considered a subfield of the practice of nursing performed only under the supervision of a registered nurse, physician, or dentist. Incompetence means a departure from or failure to conform to minimal standards of acceptable and prevailing practice for the health profession, whether or not actual injury to an individual occurs.

Although the laws in most states clearly describe the differences in levels of competency between registered and practical nurses, controversy continues to rage about substitution of LPNs for RNs. Inevitably, nursing must come to grips with the idea of a standard education for a professional activity. Although "BSN or equivalent" is frequently used to state a position requirement, no personnel department would ever argue for an MD or equivalent as the minimum requirement for a physician's appointment.

Over the years, nursing has evolved from the services of a trained nurse who learned skills at the bedside to those of a profession with standards of education and practice and recognized accountability to the public. Credentialing at graduation from accredited institutions suggests that minimal criteria with respect to faculty, facilities, and program have been met. Nurse executives set the standards for who will do what in nursing in their settings. They need to consider the basic educational and experiential competency of the participants, among other factors, before deciding on a particular organizational structure or practice pattern (Michigan Nurses Association Task Force, 1978; McClure, 1990).

Fragmented, irrelevant discussions prevail nationwide concerning competencies for registered nurses (Clayton, 1983). It is important that nurses be competent in their assigned roles. However, these assigned roles cannot be determined in educational settings away from the work environment. The technological revolution has created a situation in which education is far behind practice. Nurse executives are the professionals in the best position to see the needs of the patients and the organization.

Johnson (1983) described competency by the standards of the state of New Jersey as "being functionally able to perform duties of an assigned role. The functions are performed having drawn conclusion for this action from a sound knowledge of related sciences. The judgments made are based on a logical assessment of a given situation. Both deductive and inductive reasoning are imperative to competent practice."

The licensed practical nursing role is a dependent role. For minimal-level competency in today's dynamic health care system, the practical nurse should be prepared at the associate degree level. Registered nurses should be prepared at the baccalaureate level and should have studied supervision and management. As nurse executives conduct job and nursing staff analyses, they need to have competent nurses and nurse assistants to develop practice patterns designed for quality, cost-effective care delivery.

It is no longer acceptable to deny the legal accountability of the professional nurse by creating such titles as primary or team leader or modular nurse. Prospective payment legislation demands a quantification of nursing services. The first unknown to be defined in the equation is *nurse*. The nurse executive has the best key to solving the following:

$$n + \text{practice pattern} = \text{quality care}$$

The practice pattern is easy to identify once a clear decision has been made about n (nurse).

Nurse executives must create practice environments that address the best use of nurses, associate degree through doctorate. Nursing practice patterns based on the creation of new titles without attention to the competence of the participants lack credibility. Institutional licensure is greatly feared as the antithesis of independent professional licensure. If nurses do not assume responsibility for practice as defined in most state practice acts, it may be only a matter of time before institutional licensure takes over as a method of competency maintenance for relicensure.

TRADITIONAL PRACTICE PATTERNS

During the past three decades, an extensive literature has developed on the subject of nursing practice patterns, reflecting the importance of the use of nursing personnel in providing care in hospital settings. Nurses were "assigned" to work rather than considered as participants in a practice pattern. One type of assignment pattern focused on specialization and division of labor, or functional nursing. This type of assignment pattern evolved in response to political and economic factors that demanded a redistribution of registered nurses during World War II and included the creation of new nursing personnel categories such as licensed practical nurse and the nurses' aide. Functional nursing focused on getting the greatest amount of task work done at the least cost in time and training. This pattern was accomplished by assigning specific tasks—categorized or ordered according to degree of difficulty and importance to patient well-being—to nursing personnel with corresponding skill levels. The use of multiple personnel to provide elements of a patients' care requires a level of coordination and decision making best handled within a formal unit structure with a well-defined hierarchy.

Following the focus on specific technical excellence as the basis of assignment patterns, was an emphasis on integrating nursing personnel of varying skill levels into a democratic, close-knit team. Team nursing represents another way of adjusting care to the influx of auxiliary workers and was created to improve patient care by using the diverse skills of team members under the close guidance of registered nurses. This pattern shifted much of the authority for making nursing decisions to a lower level in the nursing hierarchy: the registered nurse team leader who assumes responsibility for care given by other team members.

One recent pattern to develop places the responsibility for nursing care management within the direct care giver. Primary nursing requires that the registered nurse's activities change from care manager-personnel organizer to care manager-care implementer. Nurse aide activities are refocused away from direct contact with the patient and toward equipment and supplies. The services of the licensed practical nurse are not used in this pattern or fall somewhere on a continuum from direct patient care to direct assistance to the registered nurse. Decisions in the care process are usually made by a single care giver and are facilitated through horizontal consultation with peers, rather than with line authority. Primary nursing has been the basic nursing practice pattern used in community health nursing.

Each practice pattern has had its day of popularity, and no one best way has emerged for all settings. Indeed, within the same pattern, there is no clear description of nursing responsibility. Within the primary nursing pattern, the time duration in which a primary nurse plans and gives care to a patient might span hospital admission to discharge or be limited to a patients' length of stay on a particular nursing unit. Within a given day, primary nurse responsibility for care management may vary from 8 to 24 hours. In team nursing, the team leader might carefully match patient needs to team member skills so that each patient must cope with only a limited number of personnel, or the team leader could functionally assign tasks within the team itself, with less concern for the number of personnel rendering direct care to an individual patient. In functional nursing, the picture of variation is less clear, for few nursing departments now identify with this structure. Yet one can recognize this structure in hospitals, where there are separate positions for activities such as discharge planning, patient education, parenteral infusion, and so on.

A NEW APPROACH TO REDESIGNING NURSING PRACTICE PATTERNS

The purpose of the nursing practice (formerly assignment) patterns study at the University of Michigan was to develop useful tools for nurses in management and clinical practice who are faced with nursing practice pattern decisions. The project included *(1)* development of instruments to measure nursing practice patterns, patient characteristics, nursing resources, and organizational support; and *(2)* the publication of a nursing practice user's manual (Munson, Beckman, Clinton, Kever, & Simms, 1980; Beckman & Simms, 1992).

This demonstration project collected data in four hospitals. Preliminary work was essential to the quality of the project and included:

1. Development of a conceptual framework within which the definition of the elements of a nursing pattern could be developed.
2. Literature review of about 270 items selected for their potential contribution to an understanding of the linkage between patient characteristics, nursing resources, and organizational support and appropriate nursing practice patterns.
3. Development of connective propositions from the literature review that could translate the data into appropriate recommendations for a unit's nursing practice pattern.
4. Development of the instruments.

In developing the essential instruments, the study group found it useful to go beyond the traditional nursing practice patterns (functional, team, or primary) and to think of three major dimensions in any nurse utilization pattern: patient characteristics, nursing resources, and organizational support. More recent work by Simms and Erbin-Roesemann (1992) has yielded a fourth major dimension, that of work characteristics and work excitement.

Conceptual Framework

Practice patterns on any patient unit may be seen as a link between problems, as presented by different patient populations, and purpose, as expressed by professional standards and purposes of the organization. Figure 21.1 shows the framework within

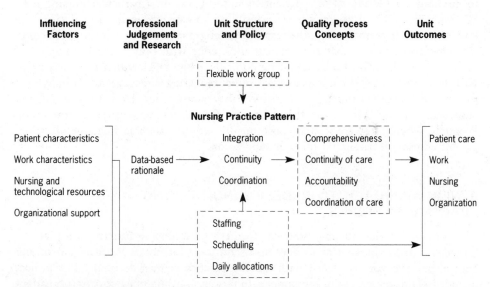

Figure 21.1 Nursing practice pattern conceptual framework. (From Beckman, J. S., & L. M. Simms. (1992). *A Guide to Redesigning Nursing Practice Patterns* (p. 4). Ann Arbor, MI: Health Administration Press. Foundation of the American College of Healthcare Executives. Adapted by permission.)

which the definition of the elements of a nursing practice pattern were developed. Four quality attributes identified by Horn and Parker (1975) were used as the basis for the conceptual framework: comprehensiveness, accountability, continuity, and coordination. Instruments were developed to measure the influencing factors of patient characteristics, nursing resources, and organizational support.

Within the nursing process, two basic activities are recognized: care giving and care planning, or management. Care management includes assessment of patient requirements for nursing care, formulation of nursing diagnosis, stating outcomes of care and nursing interventions, and evaluation. Care giving refers only to the implementation of nursing interventions. Table 21.2 highlights the four central elements of a nursing practice pattern.

These elements vary across practice patterns. Care management integration (CMI) would be relatively high in a functional practice pattern and in a primary nursing pattern where one person plans. In a team practice pattern in which the team changes sides of the hall every week, care management continuity (CMC) would be lower. Nursing care integration (NCI) would be high in most primary nursing patterns, lower in team, and lowest in functional, with the greatest number of care givers.

Additional integration, continuity, and coordination variables were conceptualized to complete the profile. Note in Table 21.3 the elements of integration, care management, continuity across settings, and the coordination elements of care-cure, patient services, and intershift coordination.

TABLE 21.2 Nursing Practice Patterns Concepts and Variables: Definitions and Relationships

Concept	Structure Variable
Comprehensive care	*Integration*
Nursing care is complete and inclusive; all aspects are well integrated on each shift for each patient	The degree to which nursing care of a patient is unified or divided on each shift, measured by the number of personnel managing care, giving care, or both
Continuity of care/Accountability	*Continuity*
Nursing care over time is consistent over shifts, unit stay, and agency stay	The degree to which the patient's care and care management is continuous or shifted among nursing personnel during unit and agency stay
The obligation for meeting total nursing care needs resides with an identifiable nurse	
Coordination of care	*Coordination*
The management of all patient care activities meets patient needs	The person, method, and/or medium used to plan and organize a patient's care within a shift, across shifts, and between nurses and medical staff, patient services

Note: Both concepts and variables are defined and measured from the perspective of the individual patient. These concepts and variables are adapted from Munson, Beckman, Clinton, Kever, and Simms (1980). The concepts were from original work by Dr. Barbara Horn and describe the nursing ideals or goals being sought. The structure variables describe the elements of the nursing unit practice pattern structure that relate to achievement of the concepts. These operationally defined variables are measurable and may vary over time and across units. It is important to note that achievement of the concepts is possible with various levels of the related variables, depending on influencing factors and related adjustments of other practice pattern variables.

(From Beckman, J. S., and L. M. Simms. (1992). *A Guide to Redesigning Nursing Practice Patterns* (p. 4). Ann Arbor, MI: Health Administration Press. Foundation of the American College of Healthcare Executives. Adapted by permission.)

TABLE 21.3 Elements of Nursing Practice Patterns

Variable	Abbreviation	Basis for Variable Definition
Nursing care integration	NCI	The proportion of total care given by the person providing the most care
Care management integration	CMI	The number of persons managing the care process at a given time
Plan-do integration	PDI	The proportion of caregivers also involved in the planning of care
Nursing care continuity	NCC	The average number of caregivers for a patient over a 7-day period
Care management continuity	CMC	The average number of care planners for a patient over a 7-day period
Care management continuity across settings (transfer)	CMCt	Whether a care planner is responsible for a patient before or after patient's stay on the unit
Nursing coordination	NC	An index that records the most common pattern of on-unit coordination of nursing care activities for a patient; method, level, and model of care delivery are indicated
Intershift coordination	ISC	An index that records the medium of communication by which intershift coordination is achieved; level and method are also indicated
Medical services coordination Patient services coordination	MSC PSC	Two indices that record the most common pattern of the nurse's direct involvement, and the proactiveness* of that involvement, in coordinating other inputs to the patient's care requirements from physicians (MSC) and from other professionals (PSC); the level and medium for coordination are included

Proactive: taking the initiative in coordination activities; for example, contacting other personnel, making referrals, problem solving. *Reactive:* not initiating; a passive or simply cooperative response to coordination initiatives from others.
(From Beckman, J. S., and L. M. Simms. (1992). *A Guide to Redesigning Nursing Practice Patterns* (p. 5). Ann Arbor, MI: Health Administration Press. Foundation of the American College of Healthcare Executives. Adapted by permission.)

By collecting specific data on patient, work, nursing, and organizational characteristics, a nursing unit can determine the type of practice pattern actually in use. It is also possible to look at patient characteristics and consider which elements of the nursing practice pattern are most closely related to the needs of the patients. For example, a patient with high psychosocial support needs may benefit tremendously from a high level of nursing care integration, that is, care provided by a single person. In contrast, the patient with multiple and complex care requirements may benefit from the care of several specialists.

Based on nursing resources, it is also possible for a unit to consider whether it is appropriate to move toward greater care management integration, a different level of care management continuity, or a different type of intershift coordination. In summary, the elements of a nursing practice pattern can be prioritized in order of importance according to the availability and competence of the nursing resources.

A great advantage in using this approach is the opportunity to look for the weak and strong points in organizational support. For example, it is difficult to have high levels of care management continuity when nurse staffing or scheduling systems provide a constant rotation of the nursing staff within a hospital. Scheduling and staffing policy are intricately related to nursing practice pattern decisions.

The findings in the Michigan studies suggest a better way to look at practice patterns. The identification of the key elements of the nursing practice pattern lead to the development of data collection instruments specific to four variables: patient characteristics, work characteristics, nursing resources, and organizational support. The new study further demonstrates that this type of information can be quantified and displayed in a format that can be used to defend an existing pattern or a change to a new pattern.

Implications   This research has had several implications. By providing an effective way to acquire a data base, the nurse executive can better evaluate high cost practice patterns, can select a particular component for concentrated study, or can more logically make comparisons across units. This study further suggests the need to view staff satisfaction and RN/LPN ratios as important aspects of nursing resources.

Implication for Turnover Problems   Primary nursing may be a better system for organizing care, but its effectiveness is not uniform for all types of nurses, even on nursing units in the same hospital. Shukla (1982) found that on matched units, where nurses had similar educational backgrounds and experience, differences in quality of care between primary and team nursing disappeared. This raised the question as to what makes the real difference in quality and satisfaction: the competency of the nurse or the nursing practice pattern.

Betz (1981) also found that nurses were not always more satisfied with primary nursing. Betz compared three team nursing units with three primary nursing units over a year and discovered that primary nurses were less satisfied than team nurses, depending on educational level. Primary nurses had difficulty delegating responsibility, utilizing personnel, and setting priorities. BSNs showed the greatest drop in satisfaction when moved to team nursing.

In the long-term care setting, Eliopoulos (1983) explores the use of the registered nurse in a professional manner. She believes it is an unrealistic goal in long-term care to increase the ratio of registered nurses, in light of the number of tasks that can be delegated to nurse assistants. Her preferred approach is the team practice pattern.

In a large research hospital survey, Carlsen and Malley (1981) determined that neither team nor primary nursing afforded sufficient opportunities for self-fulfillment, decision making, or independent judgment. Neither system provides sufficient opportunities to meet self-actualization needs. The need for primary nurses to be supervised was an unexpected finding.

In dealing with higher turnover, the nurse executive must not assume that primary nursing is the answer. Jumping on the primary nurse bandwagon may be possible only if qualified, baccalaureate-prepared nurses are available for the primary nurse role. Shukla (1982a) suggested that when nurse competency is controlled, the primary nursing structure does not provide more direct care than does the team or the modular structure. On the contrary, the primary nursing structure provides the least amount of direct care, suggesting that the competency of the nursing staff may have a greater impact than the structure. An additional finding in Shukla's work was that the modular structure is most productive. Registered nurses did not perform as many nonprofessional or indirect care tasks. Modular nursing has been defined as a mini-team, as it provides the features of both team and primary nursing practice patterns. The RN works in a subunit, or module, with an LPN or aide but does not follow the same patients if they are transferred to another subunit.

Other important issues in dealing with turnover problems are purported to be:

1. The propensity to leave the organization (Friss, 1982).
2. Inadequate information about leavers and stayers (Duxbury & Armstrong, 1982).
3. Interest in flexible hours with more leisure time and social opportunities (Vik & Mackay, 1982).
4. Need for role transition guidance (Dear, Celentano, Weisman, & Keen, 1982).

Perhaps most important is the element of support services. Nurses are more satisfied and more likely to stay in organizations where support services are adequate and they do not have to carry out extensive nonnursing tasks.

THE FLEXIBLE WORK GROUP

The flexible work group model, is based on the idea of assembling a patient care team according to the needs of patients. In this model, the housekeeper is a member of the work group. The patient and family members may also be members of the work group. The model combines the best of functional, team, and primary or case management ideas and allows the creation of work groups that can expand or decrease in size, depending on patients' needs. The flexible work group is defined as a patient-centered care team that is capable of responding or reforming when the nature of the work changes. Leadership is fluid and responsive to changing patient needs.

Reforming is a process of continuing engagement and disengagement in flexible work group patterns that facilitate the most favorable pattern of care for the patient. As the patient is regarded as an integral member of the work group as well as the focus or purpose of the work group's existence, in a flexible model, direction and decision making about required work may be a naturally occurring right of the patient or, for that matter, of any other member. Leadership is fluid or free in movement for action. It accrues from the best mix of a flexible team member's skills with the dominant needs of the patient with movement toward recovery or maintenance or promotion of health.

Where ill health is in irreversible progression, then a flexible work group team marries the location, the source, and the provision of care to the optimal comfort (physical, emotional, social, and spiritual) of the patient. The team's existence is validated only by the purpose for which it is formed. Central to that purpose is the planning of care in the realities of that purpose, the individual in need within the family, and all the constellation of variables in a particular lifespace (M. Idour, personal communication, 1990).

The flexible work group may also reflect cultural diversity. Cultural diversity is an untapped resource in meeting client needs. To facilitate care planning, client culture can be matched with at least one work group member who is from the same culture (Henkle & Kennerly, 1990).

Summary

The nurse executive should support the competency of nurses by building on the educational preparation appropriate for their roles and by using practice patterns selected through data-based decisions. Such an approach to using nursing resources differs from that found in traditional nursing texts. The availability of nursing personnel, coupled with organizational and patient characteristics, should dictate nursing practice patterns. Selection of any model without considering these variables is usually a contributing factor in dissatisfaction and high nurse turnover.

References

Aiken, L. H., Blendon, R. J., & Rogers, D. E. (1981). The shortage of hospital nurses: A new perspective, *American Journal of Nursing, 81*(9), 1612–1618.

American Hospital Association (1980). *Hospital Statistics: Data from the American Hospital Association 1979 Annual Survey.* Chicago: American Hospital Association.

Beckman, J. S., & Simms, L. M. (1992). *A guide to redesigning nursing practice patterns.* Ann Arbor: Health Administration Press.

Betz, M. (1981). Some hidden costs of primary nursing, *Nursing and Health Care, 11*(3), 150–154.

Beyers, M., Mullner, R., Byre, C. S., & Whitehead, S. F. (1983). Results of the nursing personnel survey, part 2: RN vacancies and turnover, *Journal of Nursing Administration, 13*(5), 26–31.

Carlson, R. H., & Malley, J. D. (1981). Job satisfaction of staff registered nurses in primary and team nursing delivery systems, *Research in Nursing and Health, 4*(2), 251–260.

Clayton, G. M. (1983). Identification of professional competencies. In N. L. Chaska (Ed.). *The Nursing Profession.* New York: McGraw-Hill.

Dear, M. R., Celentano, D. D., Weisman, C. S., & Keen, M. F. (1982). Evaluating a hospital nursing internship, *The Journal of Nursing Administration, 12*(11), 16–20.

Duxbury, M., & Armstrong, G. D. (1982). Calculating nurse turnover indices, *The Journal of Nursing Administration, 12*(3), 18–24.

Eliopoulos, C. (1983). Nurse staffing in long-term care facilities: The case against a high ratio of RNs, *The Journal of Nursing Administration, 13*(10), 29–31.

Friss, L. (1982). Why RNs quit: The need for management reappraisal of the "propensity to leave," *Hospital and Health Services Administration, 27*(6), 28–44.

Goertzen, I. E. (1991). *Differentiating nursing practice into the twenty-first century.* Kansas City, MO: The American Academy of Nursing.

Henkle, J. O., & Kennerly, S. M. (1990). Cultural diversity: A resource in planning and implementing nursing care, *Public Health Nursing, 7*(3), 145–149.

Horn, B. J., & Parker, J. C. (1975). Reorganization of nursing resources in hospitals. Unpublished manuscript. Ann Arbor, MI: University of Michigan School of Public Health.

Idour, M. (1990). Personal communication from visiting scholar from Massey University, New Zealand.

Johnson, H. (1983). Maintaining competency: A call for collaboration, *Issues, National Council of State Boards of Nursing, 4*(2), 3.

Johnson, W. L., & Vaughn, J. C. (1982). Supply and demand relations and the shortage of nurses, *Nursing and Health Care, 3*(9), 497–507.

McClure, M. L. (1990). Introduction. In I. E. Goertzen (Ed.). *Differentiating nursing practice into the twenty-first century* (pp. 1–11). Kansas City, MO: American Academy of Nursing.

Michigan Nurses Association Task Force (1978). *Position paper on competency for relicensure of Michigan nurses.* East Lansing, MI: Michigan Nurses Association.

Munson, F. C., Beckman, J. S., Clinton, J., Kever, C., & Simms, L. M. (1980). *Nursing assignment patterns.* Ann Arbor, MI: Health Administration Press.

Price, J., & Mueller, C. W. (1981). A causal model of turnover for nurses, *Academy of Management Journal, 24*(3), 543–565.

Rose, M. A. (1982). Factors affecting nurse supply and demand: An exploration, *The Journal of Nursing Administration, 12*(2), 31–34.

Shukla, R. K. (1982). Primary nursing: Two conditions determine the choice, *The Journal of Nursing Administration, 12*(11), 12–15.

Shukla, R. K. (1982a). Nursing care structures and productivity, *Hospital and Health Services Administration, 27*(6), 45–58.

Simms, L. M., Dalston, J. W., & Roberts, P. W. (1984). Collaborative practice: Myth or reality, *Hospital and Health Services Administration, 29*(6), 36–48.

Simms, L. M., & Erbin-Roesemann, M. A. (1992). Chapter IV. Work characteristics questionnaire. In J. S. Beckman & L. M. Simms, *A Guide to Redesigning Nursing Practice Patterns* (pp. 61–77). Ann Arbor, MI: Health Administration Press.

State of Michigan Public Health Code (1978). Article 15, Occupations Part 172, Nursing.

Taylor, M. S., & Covaleski, M. A. (1985). Predicting nurses' turnover and internal transfer behavior, *Nursing Research, 34*(4), 237–241.

U.S. Department of Health and Human Services, Division of Health Professions Analysis. *Supply of Manpower in Selected Health Occupations, 1950–1990.* DHHS publication no. (HRA) 80-35. Washington, DC: U.S. Government Printing Office.

Vik, A. G., & Mackay, R. C. (1982). How does the 12-hour shift affect patient care? *The Journal of Nursing Administration, 12*(1), 11–14.

Weisman C. S., Alexander, C. S., & Chase, G. A. (1981). Determinants of hospital staff nurse turnover, *Medical Care, 19*(4), 431–443.

Wolf, G. A. (1981). Nursing turnover: Some causes and solutions, *Nursing Outlook, 29*(4), 233–236.

Bibliography

Hofmann, P. B. (1981). Accurate measurement of nursing turnover: The first step in its reduction, *The Journal of Nursing Administration, 11*(11–12), 37–39.

Munson, F., & Clinton, J. (1979). Defining nursing assignment patterns, *Nursing Research, 27*(4), 243–249.

Weisman, C. S. (1982). Recruit from within: Hospital nurse retention in the 1980s, *The Journal of Nursing Administration, 12*(5), 24–31.

CHAPTER 22

Facilities Planning

Judith A. Bernhardt

Highlights

- **Role of nursing in facility planning**
- **Facility planning and design process**
- **Physical and functional evaluation**
- **Construction documents, the bid-award process, and construction**
- **Postoccupancy evaluation**

The purpose of this chapter is to provide basic knowledge of the process and content of planning the physical environment for health care facilities. Conceptualization of the physical environment has resulted in the recognition that staff functioning and patient recovery are affected by the human organization within health care facilities. Because the delivery of nursing care extends into and is dependent on all other areas in a health care facility, the importance of effective nursing administration in facility planning cannot be underestimated.

For any administrator, planning is an essential component of the administrative process and includes the major activities of setting objectives, determining policies and resources, making decisions, and assuring that the desired outcomes are achieved. Planning is the first conceptual skill required in an administrative role and is the dominant process in the design and construction of health care facilities. A useful way of thinking about planning is to consider both strategic and tactical planning.

Strategic planning encompasses long-range goals and objectives for an organization, whereas tactical planning focuses on goals and objectives in more detail and for a shorter time span. In the health care environment, strategic planning includes such tasks as describing an institution's mission and role, determining the scope of services and the level of care to be provided, and choosing the site location and design for a new health care facility. Tactical planning includes budgeting, identifying staffing ratios, and determining patient admission and scheduling procedures (Arndt & Huckabay, 1975). The function of facilities planning is to strategically conceptualize and plan how an individual health care environment will function in the future. To plan facilities strategically is to commit to the risk of conceptualizing about the future, because buildings are substantial investments that will stand for long periods of time.

THE ROLE OF NURSING IN FACILITY PLANNING

Nurse executives have a significant role in the facility planning process because of their clinical experience related to the technical and sophisticated nursing and medical services provided today. Nursing accounts for more than 50 percent of a hospital's payroll, and total payroll constitutes more than 50 percent of all hospital operating costs. Nursing merits active involvement throughout the planning process to produce management and operating efficiencies. The very nature of nursing's role as nursing service's representative and patient advocate makes it a source of invaluable experience and insight about nursing practice, the flow of materials and people, functional requirements of space, and environmental issues important to nursing staff, patients, families, and other health care providers. All of these elements can be enhanced or hindered by the design of the environment (Ryan, 1975).

The planning and design of building programs require a decision-making process that involves several levels within an organization. For major building programs, there is usually a director of planning who functions as the representative of hospital administration, a planning committee, special committees with broad and diverse user representation, and the governing board, which retains ultimate authority and responsibility for the entire building program. Smaller building programs and renovation projects may compress these decision-making levels. Nursing has an opportunity to provide input into the organization at the levels where strategic program management and operational planning occur throughout the planning and design process.

The task of strategically planning health facilities is generally accomplished by a planning committee typically composed of representatives from various departments or disciplines. Nursing administration must be represented at this level, where needs and future programs of the organization will be determined. At the same time, nursing can develop its own internal organizational structure to designate the appropriate staff who need to be involved on any special committees to influence the management of the program design and provide educated direction on nursing practice and function. Such organization is important whether the facility planning project is large or small, for the design portion of the process itself demands significant time commitments to the development, review, and approval of final design schemes.

For a large replacement project spanning a number of years, consideration should be given to establishing and assigning a full-time nursing representative to serve as a consultant and a link between the nursing staff and the architect, providing knowledge about the impacts of the physical environment on nursing practice.

Additionally, the facility planning arena introduces nursing to the world of planners, architects, engineers, and health consultants and brings with it techniques and terminology that are relatively new and unfamiliar. The nurse consultant must learn such techniques and terminology through daily interaction with these planning professionals to be able to communicate in planning jargon, anticipate information needed by the architect in each design phase, and evaluate design schemes. Well-prepared and relevant functional spatial requirements for nursing have a good chance of successfully becoming incorporated into the final design.

The following responsibilities are essential to the role of nurse consultant:

1. Coordinate the involvement of nursing in the planning and design decision-making processes.
2. Gather data and prepare documentation to facilitate decision making.
3. Examine and evaluate innovative design concepts, care delivery organization, and new technology, and make recommendations related to planning objectives.
4. Review program plans and assist in the definition of nursing practice requirements.
5. Act as liaison to interpret terminology and professional concerns between the staff, consultants, and external planning and regulatory approval agencies.
6. Monitor the design and construction for consistency with the original planning concepts. (Grubbs & Short, 1979)

Because the profession of nursing serves as a patient advocate, there are a number of patient and family needs that can be coordinated by nursing in facility planning. Nursing care is approached from a holistic view that recognizes the physical, spiritual, psychosocial, and developmental needs of patients, with the patient, family, and community central to nursing's concern and program implementation. The design or plan of the health care environment, therefore, should support patient and family needs for a therapeutic milieu. However, more often than not, health care facilities are designed primarily to meet health professionals' needs for efficiency of practice and often fail to provide an environment that supports recovery (Kraegel, Mousseau, Goldsmith, & Arora, 1974).

Although there is currently a dearth of information in the literature directly pertaining to hospital design and human behavior, nursing can, through experience, sensitize planners and architects to environmental design and behavior as it affects not only staff, but patients and their families as well. The needs of patients and their families basically relate to the degree of control they have over an otherwise stressful environment. Six such needs have been identified:

1. The ability to find one's way between destinations.
2. The ability to control what is likely to be seen and heard as a result of space relationships.
3. The ability to regulate the amount of interaction with others, visually and acoustically.

4. The security and safety of the environment.

5. The convenience with which various amenities and destinations can be reached.

6. Special needs because of age or physical or mental limitations.

Incorporating these needs into design enhances the delivery of quality patient care (Reizenstein, Grant, & Simmons, 1986).

THE FACILITY PLANNING AND DESIGN PROCESS

Whether in building a new health care facility or accomplishing major additions or alterations to an existing facility, optimal long-term outcomes are achieved when those involved have a basic understanding of the planning process and a concept of design objectives (Hardy & Lammers, 1977; Munn & Saulsbery, 1992). This section describes the process phases and discusses ways in which nursing can positively influence the phases (see Figure 22.1).

Mission and Role Study

The first phase of the planning process defines the facilities mission and role for at least 10 years in terms of programs, physical facilities, and general space requirements for departments of all types. Recently, health facilities have employed independent, professional consultants to develop long-range role and program plans. The mission and role study has the dimensions of a community-wide survey and includes such elements as patient origin studies, population projections, utilization trends, length of stay, patient days, average daily census, and bed requirements. The study includes the examination of plans of other health care providers in the area, community characteristics, the effects of legislation, and its primary, secondary, and tertiary care roles on a defined area-wide basis.

At the same time, required health care resources, the role of the health care facility in education and research, and long-range personnel requirements are evaluated. On completion and acceptance by the facility of this survey of health care needs and the services to be provided, capital costs and the ability to finance the project must be determined by a financial feasibility study. Effective nursing involvement later in the design process as it relates to types of patients and services to be provided requires that nursing be part of the prior development of long-range goals for the facility and be aware of the impetus for the building project (Hardy & Lammers, 1977).

The mission and role study is also necessitated by the high degree of regulation of the health care environment. Nursing may be involved in collecting and analyzing data to convince review agencies of the need for and economics of the project.

Physical and Functional Evaluation

The basic purpose of the physical evaluation is to determine the degree of physical obsolescence of the existing facility, identify major code violations, and project the facility's usability in the future. The functional evaluation assesses the facility's ability to serve as an efficient work place for personnel and to provide a supportive environment for patients and their families. The methodology used to functionally evaluate a

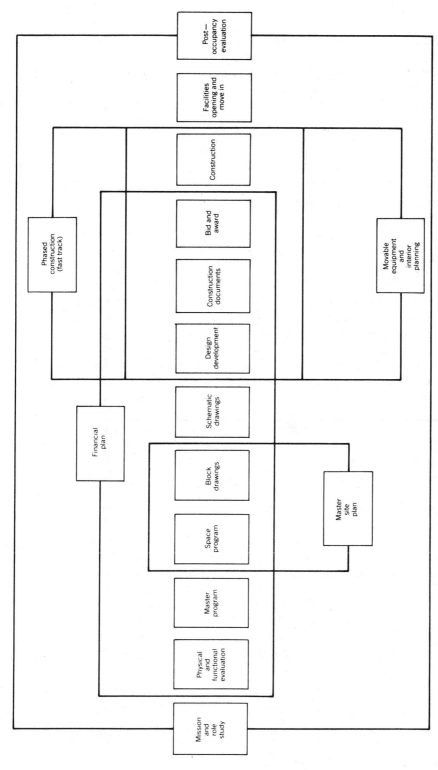

Figure 22.1 The planning and design process continuum. (From the Office of Planning, Research and Development. The University of Michigan Hospitals, Ann Arbor, MI.)

facility compares functional attributes with adopted criteria. *Minimum Requirements of Construction and Equipment for Hospitals and Medical Facilities*, HEW Publication (HRA) 79-14500 and pertinent state rules and regulations serve as the basis for criteria.

In addition to the codes and regulations, a number of functional concepts provide standards for evaluating functional features. The more common concepts include:

1. Viewing the whole facility as a single, efficient system.
2. Physical relationships required between departments.
3. Room size and shape needed to accommodate function.
4. The ability of the facility to expand.
5. Space and equipment flexibility.
6. The degree of automation.
7. Separation of cleaned and soiled zones.
8. Privacy accommodations for patients.
9. Building circulation patterns. (Hardy & Lammers, 1977)

The functional concept of flexibility deserves much emphasis. For a health care facility, flexibility is critical in allowing for changing techniques of professional practice, alteration of department layouts to meet those changes, and addition of new departments in the future.

If a major design effort is to be undertaken as a result of the physical and functional evaluation, then usually at this phase of the planning process, a project team is formed, roles of the members are defined, and the decision-making process is clarified. This is when a well thought-out process of designating staff or nursing committees for ongoing involvement in the remainder of the process can also be developed. It is not unreasonable to request that a nurse consultant or several nurses be assigned to the project team on a major renovation or replacement project. For minor projects, a consistent point of contact in nursing can be designated to coordinate and provide input at each major phase in the project.

The importance of this involvement cannot be overemphasized. The quality of a facility planning and design effort in the remaining phases depends on those assigned to plan the building in detail and on the architect who will design it. Health care facilities are composed of complex relationships, flows of people and supplies, technological requirements, and operational procedures. These relationships necessitate a series of planning and design decisions and compromises to create a project that balances user needs, is aesthetically pleasing, and is of reasonable cost and optimal utility. To achieve these goals, it behooves nursing to be an integral part of the decision-making process and assist in determining which program planning and design compromises minimally affect the functions required to care for patients.

Master Program

The master program phase of planning health care facilities precedes actual design efforts. The master program describes the concepts on which a facility will operate and specifies functions in terms of procedures, required equipment, and numbers and categories of space users. The projected number of procedures or tests is based on the number of admissions, patient days, and clinic visits projected in the mission and role study.

Master programming is one of the most important planning activities. The master program is reviewed by external regulatory agencies and becomes the major approved policy document. It serves as a guide for the architect, the manager responsible for constructing the facility, administration, and the people who will use the space. This programming effort, once the province of the design architect, is now frequently conducted by planners familiar with health care functions. Titled functional planners usually have a background in hospital management, and many are trained by consulting firms that specialize in both health care programs and facility planning.

A number of nursing-related operational concepts require decisions at this stage (Hardy & Lammers, 1977):

1. Types and mix of patient rooms (single, double, four-bed)
2. Centralized versus decentralized supply processing and material distribution systems
3. Size of nursing units
4. Presence or absence of a nursing station
5. Type of care delivery
6. Degree of automation for processing data
7. Degree of centralization for laboratories and pharmacies.

It is in this part of the planning process that the nurse executive can make a significant contribution by using designated nursing planning resources to describe and document for the planners the planning objectives and design concepts that are not only required but desired to implement nursing practice in a new setting.

The planning objectives and design concepts can begin with a description of the patient population and the philosophy of delivering nursing care within the overall mission and role of the health care facility. Such objectives include but are not limited to the operational concepts previously described.

Once the philosophy of care and the patient population are identified, it is useful to identify the program goals and assumptions for nursing, including definition of terms. An example of a program goal is to maintain a system of decentralized nursing administration. Once all the goals have been listed, with objectives stated for each, the operational and physical space requirements to implement each goal can be identified. Examples of operational and physical space requirements for the goal of decentralized nursing administration are to locate units with similar patient populations in close geographical proximity and to require office space for each head nurse on the unit for which he or she is responsible (Peterson, 1977).

As part of the master program, it is valuable if the documentation of planning objectives and design concepts for nursing itself are stated in a format that all parties can understand. To assist in the description of these objectives and concepts, the nurse consultant, designated nursing personnel, or both should review layouts of nursing areas and systems in other health care facilities. Such a review can be accomplished through carefully documented visits to other health care facilities; reviews of hospital, medical, and design journals; and operational analyses to prepare adequate documentation to support the proposed space requirements. An example of an operational analysis that may need to be performed is to describe and document the rationale for desiring a certain size nursing unit.

Space Program
A space program is a listing of every room or area to which a function is assigned in a proposed construction project. As a direct derivative of the master program, a space program is used to communicate facility needs to the architect and is frequently prepared by a functional planner. The traditional space program lists the type of room required within a unit or department and the quantity, size, and functional requirements of each. The space program should provide the architect with a clear understanding of not only what function is to be performed in the space, but the quantity and type of personnel required for the function, in addition to the equipment and environmental needs. The listing of rooms follows the order of the master program, and rooms are grouped by department, functional entity, or both (see Table 22.1).

Several factors influence the space program phase. Different conclusions about the dimensions and space identified by the functional planner for a room can be arrived at during the actual design by different architects. For example, an intensive care patient care room programmed for a certain size might need a generous width to allow adequate clearance at the foot of the bed during a cardiac arrest. However, the architect might believe that the length dimension is more important for the medical gas outlets and equipment required at the bedside. Thus, one important requirement might be needlessly compromised at the expense of another, equally important functional requirement.

Another factor influencing the space program includes minimum square footage assignments or the amount of space stipulated by most state and federal regulatory agencies for certain functions. Although these minimum requirements must be met for licensure, certain spaces need to be larger to accommodate specific functions; for example, a teaching hospital would require spaces to accommodate students. Finally, construction budgets influence space assignment size. When budgets are restricted, space sizes for rooms are usually at their functional minimum; when budgets are unrestricted, optimal space sizing can be achieved. Nursing can provide assistance in monitoring those essential spaces that may be in danger of becoming dysfunctional under budget constraints (Hardy & Lammers, 1977).

A carefully prepared master program and a well-defined space program can assist in achieving functional rooms and spaces for a health care facility, which enables administration to make many important design-related decisions without repeating the trial-and-error process often encountered in design.

Block Plan Drawings
Block plan drawings represent the beginning of design, the point at which the architect translates the program and space descriptions into simple drawings of blocks of space. Block plans graphically depict a facilities evaluation of necessary functional

TABLE 22.1 Example of a Partial Space Program for a Nursing Unit

Room Type	Functional Requirements	Quantity	Square Feet per Space	Total Square Feet
Family waiting room	Provide seating for 12 people at 15 square feet per person. Should have exterior windows and window to corridor. Close to drinking fountains and phone. Locate two toilets adjacent to but not inside room. Conversational environment. Provide for hanging coats, boots, and so on.	1	180	180
Single-patient room	Bed, access to bed, visitor seating space, patient chair space, exterior window, wardrobe for clothing, adequate circulation at foot of bed for equipment, accommodate flowers, tack board, patient clock.	16	130	2,080
Double-patient room	Same as single. Note: adequate clearance between beds.	8	200	1,600
Patient bathroom	One for each patient room, toilet with bed pan flusher, shower, lavatory, bed pan storage, staff shelf for specimens, patient shelving for toilet articles, wheelchair accessible, night light.	24	40	960
Nursing station	Space for charting, forms, and communication for six to eight people. Counter for computer terminal capability and chart rack. Space for telephone, nurse call, patient locator, tack board, clock, pneumatic tube station. Visual surveillance of corridor. Adjacent to medication station, physician dictation, and conference room. Provide good acoustical attenuation.	1	300	300

adjacencies between departments; for example, the emergency room should be located near the intensive care units to minimize travel distance for critically ill patients. The block of space for each department and the departments it relates to are shown by building level, along with major corridors and elevators. Alternative ways in which these blocks of space that make up the building can be designed are then evaluated as to how well they fit on the site designated for the facility.

At this phase, three-dimensional models are useful in demonstrating alternative building forms to assist in the selection of optimum relationships and configurations. Because the nursing unit is the major determinant of the building's shape, the architect first focuses on its location within the building. Nursing can assist the architect by providing criteria on departmental adjacencies important to nursing and on functional requirements that will influence the shape of a nursing area. Criteria of importance include nursing travel distances between spaces and the location of supplies for those spaces.

As block plan drawings are developed, a master site plan is formulated. This process encompasses selection of a site, analysis of the site, and development of drawings to visually portray the buildings and uses of all parts of the site. A site plan is the rational selection of a location to accommodate all construction envisioned during a 15-to-20-year future period for a health care facility. The plan reflects vehicle and pedestrian traffic flows, parking, building configuration, placement, organization, and landscape details. With the advancement of technology in health care, provisions for flexibility of site use and expandability of structures is an important part of the facility planning process (Hardy & Lammers, 1977).

The block plan phase is also the stage in the design process at which the building and evaluation of full-size mock-ups of various fully equipped rooms are of extreme importance. In planning and designing health care facilities, no other adequate substitute exists for seeing spaces in three dimensions. Users of the space can be involved at this point in evaluating function and predicting the operational quality of certain spaces, building materials, equipment, and furnishings. Mock-ups can also be of significant value to administration in introducing the new facility to the community. In fact, mock-ups should be installed permanently in the new facility as an in-service education tool for everyone from health care personnel to maintenance and housekeeping.

As part of the initial design phase, a mock-up program can be undertaken in several steps:

1. The project team and architect can evaluate two-dimensional drawings (sketches or floor plans).
2. Visits can be made to mock-up displays prepared by manufacturers of specific health care equipment.
3. The team can study three-dimensional scale models of specific spaces and participate in evaluating full-scale mock-ups with actual or simulated equipment and furnishings. Full-scale mock-ups can be built in the existing facility or in a nearby building and can be constructed for a small percentage of the overall project budget, particularly if planned from the onset.

A space can be considered a prime candidate for mocking up if:

1. The space recurs frequently in the design.
2. The space is complex and needs to be visualized to understand its functional relationships with people, equipment, and other spaces.
3. A mock-up is the best way to acquire, evaluate, and transmit meaningful user input about the space.

4. The capital and operating costs of the space are great.

5. The space is expensive to renovate after occupancy.

Spaces that might be mocked up include a general and an intensive care patient bedroom, a nursing station, an examination room, and an operating room. If full-scale room mock-ups are not financially feasible for a project, three-dimensional models should be used as a fallback predesign evaluation tool (Rogoff, Couture, & Bernhardt, 1979).

The first step in evaluating full-scale mock-up rooms is to develop performance criteria for how the space is expected to function; for example, there should be adequate space in a two-patient room at the foot of the bed to allow the second bed to be removed during a cardiac arrest without unduly disrupting the arrest procedure. The next step is to determine what tools will be used to evaluate the spaces, for example, questionnaires, interviews, and checklists. Activities that will routinely occur in the space can be role-played or simulated and can be photographed or videotaped to document which aspects of the design function well and which do not. With clear documentation, designers and the project team can address the findings and modify the design accordingly. Performance criteria and evaluation methodologies can also be used to test equipment, material, and furnishings.

Schematic Drawings

In schematic drawings, a detailed version of block plans, the shape of every room in each department is outlined. In addition to showing the corridors shown in the block plans, schematic drawings also reflect mechanical spaces, such as ventilation and pipe shafts and the location of building-support columns, stairs, and doors. All the assumptions about the equipment and furnishings that will be provided in each space must be known during the schematic phase (see Figure 22.2).

With the nursing units' location already established in the design of a new building, the relationship of spaces and flow of staff, patients, and materials within a department is determined during this phase. Nursing can prepare performance criteria for the unit in terms of number of people using the spaces, degree of privacy or openness, visual and acoustical needs, and control and monitoring requirements. If mock-ups are being used, this design information should be incorporated in the mock-ups, along with the criteria for the other spaces, and communicated to the architect.

The nurse consultant, the nurses on the units, or both can work with the architect to develop multiple schemes and options for laying out the spaces. Previous research and visits to other facilities can assist them in choosing from a range of options. The clearer the nursing design guidelines, the easier it is to develop alternative schemes and to evaluate the design that best meets original planning objectives.

Although the best time to decide which planning, design, and construction approach to take is before the facility planning and design activities are undertaken, the approach nevertheless must be selected no later than at the completion of schematic drawings. The two types of design and construction approaches are conventional and "fast track." In the conventional approach, construction is not begun until all the design and contractor documents are completed for the entire building.

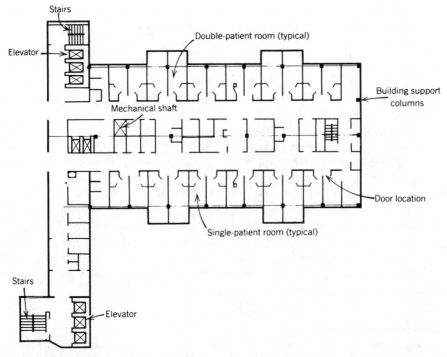

Figure 22.2 Example of schematic drawing of a patient unit. (From the Office of Planning, Research and Development. The University of Michigan Hospitals, Ann Arbor, MI.)

In a fast-track approach, construction begins on certain elements of the project while planning and design continues on other elements; for example, the lower portion of the building may be constructed while the nursing units are still being designed in detail. The theoretical advantage of fast tracking is an earlier construction completion date, which saves time and money. For health care facilities, fast tracking can force actions to keep the project on schedule in an industry where decision making is not always timely (Hardy & Lammers, 1977).

If a fast-track approach is used, the development of goals and objectives by nursing early in the master programming phase is especially crucial to avoid fragmented, reactive design decisions. Schematic drawings may allow some adjustments to the scope of the project, but at their completion, the scope and functional relationships of departments and rooms are usually fixed.

Design Development

Once decisions are made regarding functional space locations and basic departmental configurations as reflected in single-line schematic drawings, the architect begins to determine the details of design for each room. The drawing dimensions are more precise for all spaces than in a schematic design.

To determine the detailed design of each room, the project team collects detailed data about the physical requirements of each space. Examples of physical requirements include equipment, characteristics of the materials to be used, lighting types and levels, medical gases, mechanical and electrical systems, nurse call systems, telephone, intercom, and dictation and pneumatic tube systems.

It is not uncommon for rooms, doors, and even corridors to be relocated at this phase as mechanical and structural systems are better understood and evaluated by the engineers. Continued nursing input during this phase is important because design relocations can significantly change how some rooms function. The mock-ups can assist in evaluating these changes as well as to further test detailed room requirements. For example, for the layout of the head wall in patient rooms, the exact height, location, and quantity of gases, outlets, and equipment can be evaluated to determine the impact on efficient patient care delivery and bed placement within a patient room.

During the design development phase, definitive planning occurs for major movable medical equipment, such as dialysis machines and operating room tables. Finalizing the placement of such equipment is necessary to determine the precise room dimensions and the location of plumbing fixtures and electrical outlets. Interior design planning also begins during design development and entails decisions about color, wall and flooring materials, signs, furnishings, artwork, and plants. Input from nursing and from mock-ups or other research can contribute to the creation of a functional and aesthetically pleasing environment (Hardy & Lammers, 1977).

CONSTRUCTION DOCUMENTS, THE BID-AWARD PROCESS, AND CONSTRUCTION

Construction documents consist of the design specifications, working drawings, and conditions for construction that are incorporated into a contract. They represent the facility's decisions throughout the process and specify the dimensions and layout of what will be built. During this phase, the final details are worked out between the architect and the engineers. As problems are identified, design decisions are reevaluated and modified. If significant architectural or functional changes are required in patient care and related spaces, a review by nursing can verify that the changes are acceptable, based on functional goals and objectives.

During the bid-award phase, competitive bids are taken, and contracts are negotiated and awarded before construction commences. Again, changes can occur with respect to materials and equipment. Alternative materials and equipment are listed to increase competition for better prices. Such alternatives must be acceptable to nursing, because the contract will be awarded to the lowest bidder. Many times, substitutions beyond the acceptable alternatives are proposed by contractors and administrators as a way to reduce costs. This fact emphasizes the need for well-documented specifications on how staff expects all items to function. Nursing can provide input to assist in evaluating whether a substitution is appropriate, based on the construction cost, operating cost, depreciation, appearance, and functional requirements.

The most critical task for the project team during the construction phase is to make sure that the construction work proceeds according to the intent of the drawings and specifications and that it is on schedule and stays within budget (Hardy & Lammers,

1977). Contractors who are not aware of the original goals and concepts of the project might attempt to make changes that may directly affect the appearance and functioning of patient care areas, such as changes in the location and type of fixtures. Meetings with the project team and construction site tours can assure continued nursing participation during this phase.

Facilities Opening

During construction and before opening, the health care facility as a whole must turn its attention to both how people will function in the new design and plan the move. A smooth transition from old to new can require a minimum of 1 year or more of advanced planning, depending on the size of the project.

Therefore, there is a need to develop a move-in schedule, write policies and procedures, and orient employees to any new functional concepts and equipment that are part of the new facility. If this is not done, existing and new employees, because of an incomplete understanding of the facility's design, may attempt to carry over the current methods of functioning from the old facility to the new facility. In all probability, the new facility will have been designed to accommodate very different ways of operating (Hardy & Lammers, 1977). Moving into a new wing or a new patient tower is no simpler than moving into a new facility across town, as both situations involve the same process (Ryan, 1975).

POSTOCCUPANCY EVALUATION

Postoccupancy evaluations of building and spaces have two major purposes. The first is to provide feedback to functional planners and designers on how well the spaces function based on the original design goals. The second purpose is to gather data that can be applied to future design. The evaluation should be done within the first year after occupancy and consist of an objective assessment using a variety of research methods.

The research methods include gathering quantitative data on the number of users and uses of space and collecting qualitative data, such as data on the attitudes of people using the space and photographs depicting the behavior of the users. If there is consistency with the original design concepts and these concepts are still appropriate, then the design can be considered a success. Learning about what is inconsistent allows for immediate improvements and for information that can contribute to future design (Zimring & Reizenstein, 1981). Nursing has much to gain by being involved in postoccupancy evaluation from the standpoint of enhancing future practice and achieving a therapeutic environment.

Summary

Facility planning and design is a process that moves from macroscopic conceptual planning to the more microscopic details of design for renovations or new construction of health care facilities. This process is a complex one with many constraints. Yet nurse executives should not

be overwhelmed by the task. The most important people in the process are the administrator and the staff who have the final responsibility for developing and implementing the program and then for using the building or spaces. Therefore, it is critical that the nursing staff be knowledgeable about and actively involved in the planning and design process from beginning to end. Nursing knowledge and involvement can assist in anticipating and solving problems, which will lead to better design of health care facilities for staff and patients in the future.

References

Arndt, C., & Huckabay, L. (1975). *Nursing administration: Theory for practice with a systems approach.* St. Louis: Mosby.

Grubbs, J., & Short, S. (1979). Nursing input to nursing unit design, *Journal of Nursing Administration, 9*(5), 25–30.

Hardy, O., & Lammers, L. (1977). *Hospitals: The planning and design process.* Rockville: Aspen Systems Corporation.

Kraegel, J., Mousseau, V., Goldsmith, C., & Arora, R. (1974). *Patient care systems.* Philadelphia: Lippincott.

Munn, E., & Saulsbery, P. (1992). Facility planning — A blueprint for nurse executives, *Journal of Nursing Administration, 22*(1), 13–17.

Peterson, M. (1977). *Nursing ad hoc planning committee final report.* Ann Arbor, MI: the University of Michigan Hospitals.

Reizenstein, J., Grant, M., and Simmons, D. (1986). *Design that cares: Planning health facilities for patients and visitors.* Chicago: American Hospital Publishing, Inc.

Rogoff, D., Couture, P., & Bernhardt, J. (1979). *Staff analysis on mock-ups.* Ann Arbor, MI: Office of Planning, Research and Development, the University of Michigan Hospitals.

Ryan, J. (1975). The nursing administrator's growing role in facilities planning, *Journal of Nursing Administration, 5*(9), 22–27.

Zimring, C., & Reizenstein, J. (1981). A primer on postoccupancy evaluation, *American Institute of Architects Journal, 70*(13), 52.

CHAPTER 23

Nurse Staffing and Scheduling

Yvonne Marie Abdoo

Highlights

- **The evolution of nurse staffing systems**
- **Patient classification as a component of staffing systems**
- **Current staffing systems**
- **Work measurement in nursing**
- **Scheduling and workweek patterns**
- **Next generation nurse staffing systems**

One of the most critical issues confronting nursing service administrators today is nurse staffing. Staffing policies and needs affect the nursing department budget, staff productivity, quality of care provided to clients, nursing staff morale, and even nurse retention. At the same time, nurse staffing requirements are affected by overall hospital policies and by nearly every other department in the organization, including admitting, lab, x-ray, dietary, and the like. Thus, it is essential that nursing service administrators thoroughly understand the components and issues in nurse staffing.

Nurse staffing is a term often used but subject to a variety of interpretations. For purposes of this discussion, nurse staffing is a broad area composed of three main components: planning, scheduling, and allocation. Planning encompasses determination of the number of nursing personnel needed over a long-term period. The scheduling component entails assigning nursing staff for specific time periods by shift, based on patient care needs. Allocation of nursing staff involves staffing assignments or readjustments on a daily or shift basis.

A great wealth of information has been written in the realm of nurse staffing, but the articles tend to recount personal experiences and to describe trial-and-error, rather than scientific, approaches. Aydelotte (1973) asserts that:

Nurse staffing methodology should be an orderly systematic process, based upon sound rationale, applied to determine the number and kind of nursing personnel required to provide nursing care of a predetermined standard to a group of patients in a particular setting. The end result is prediction of the kind and number of staff required to give care to patients. This prediction of the number and kinds of personnel to give patients nursing care 24 hours a day, 7 days a week . . . is no small task. The aim is to provide, at reasonable cost to the general public the agency serves, a standard of nursing care acceptable to its clientele and the nursing staff serving it. (p. 3)

The planning or staffing methodology phase should be based on quantifiable, measurable data. This systematic nurse staffing determination must include the following variables: *(1)* an assessment of patient care needs (patient classification), *(2)* an assessment of required nursing time to meet patient needs (nursing work load determination), and *(3)* an algorithm that uses the first two variables. Average occupancy and seasonal fluctuations in the occupancy rate are also helpful supplemental variables.

Deviation from the intuitive approach to a systematic research approach can be achieved only after those involved in nurse staffing decisions thoroughly understand the history of nurse staffing, its trends, its complexity, and its needs.

THE EVOLUTION OF NURSE STAFFING SYSTEMS

Nurse staffing systems have evolved since early 1960 when Connor (1961) published a research report, based on his earlier doctoral dissertation, on the utilization of nursing staff. A major result of Connor's work was the development of a three-category patient classification tool in which a hospital's medical and surgical inpatients are identified by the unit's head nurse as category I, self-care; category II, partial or intermediate care; or category III, intensive or total care. Guidelines describing the typical characteristics of a patient in a particular category were developed for the head nurse to use in categorizing patients.

An average nursing time for each patient category was determined through work-measurement studies, and each of the average times was found to be significantly different from each other when tested statistically. A staffing algorithm using a patient care index (I) was developed

$$I = .5\,N_1 + 1.0\,N_2 + 2.5\,N_3$$

where I is the patient care index, N is the number of patients in each category, the constants represent the amount of direct care in hours, and the subscripts represent the specific clarification level (Connor, 1961).

Connor noted even in 1960 the effect of the variation of patient needs on the nursing work load. The nursing work load varied only slightly if the number and distribution of patients by classification were constant. "On the other hand," noted Connor, "if the number of each class of patients is also variable, we may expect wide variation in total daily demand on staff. It is, therefore, important to determine how the classes of patients vary within the census, for this, in conjunction with the average times required, would permit the estimation of variation in nursing staff requirements for a single ward or in the hospital" (Connor, Flagle, Hsieh, Preston, & Singer, 1961, p. 33).

The Commission for Administrative Services in Hospitals [CASH] (Des Ormeaux, 1977) adapted the work of Connor and his colleagues (1961) from the Johns Hopkins University, using additional systems analyses and other industrial engineering techniques to prepare a staffing manual to assist hospitals in determining their own nurse staffing requirements. The components of the staffing system include: (1) a three-level patient classification tool (self-care, partial care, and total care), (2) standard time allowance for the performance of each nursing procedure or task, (3) census data (the number of admissions, discharges, transfers, and occupied beds), and (4) the number and types of personnel employed on a nursing unit. The following reports, as summarized by Aydelotte (1973), can then be generated:

- Actual staffing plan (as it is in operation)
- Recommended staffing plan
- Report of accumulated hours, giving the amount of time for each worker and each task
- Work distribution sampling
- Recommendations for redistribution of the procedure (the work).

Other staffing systems (Georgette, 1970; McCormick, Roche, & Steinwacks, 1973; Cochran & Derr, 1975; Minetti & Hutchinson, 1975; Center for Hospital Management Engineering, 1978), developed during the 1960s and early 1970s for specific hospitals, adapted the work of Connor (1961) to fit a particular institution's specific needs. Although a modification of the classification tool might occur—for example, expanding the tool from three patient category types to four or five types with descriptive criteria, the basic methodology remained the same. The average amount of nursing care time needed was calculated from the patient classification input and converted to the average number of nursing staff needed to provide nursing care. The variances of the average nursing care time and nursing staff were not determined.

PATIENT CLASSIFICATION AS A COMPONENT OF NURSE STAFFING SYSTEMS

The component of traditional nurse staffing systems essential to all facets of the total system is patient classification. Classification may be defined as the ordering or arrangement of objects or properties conceptually, physically, or in both ways. This process has long been used in many fields and is evidenced by various taxonomies that have been developed in most sciences.

According to Sokal (1974), taxonomy is the theoretical study of classification, including its bases, principles, procedures, and rules. Taxonomy actually includes two phases: classification and identification. Identification encompasses assigning previously unidentified objects or concepts to the proper or correct class according to an established classification system. Thus, taxonomy is the science of how to classify and identify.

The major purpose of classification is to describe the structure or relationship of the constituent objects to each other and to similar objects and to simplify these relationships in such a way that general statements can be made about classes of objects (Sokal, 1974), which should facilitate the understanding of users. Another goal of a classification system is ease of manipulation or retrieval of information, because complex relationships are often simplified by a classification schema. Classification systems also facilitate economy of memory by summarizing information about relationships and attaching a specified label.

PATIENT CLASSIFICATION TOOLS

Since 1960, patient classification tools have been developed to categorize or group patients according to their prospective nursing care requirements for a specified period of time. Because the health needs — and, as a result, the nursing needs — vary from patient to patient, tools have been developed to predict the nursing time required based on the identified patient needs at a given time. According to Giovannetti (1978), the "concept of patient classification entails the categorization or grouping of patients according to some assessment of their nursing care requirements over a specified period of time" (p. 3). The main purpose of these early patient classification tools or instruments was to predict nurse staffing needs on a shift to shift basis.

Determining and agreeing on assessment criteria are not simple feats, however, because there are several ways of viewing patients' requirements for nursing care. A major issue that must first be resolved is whether the assessment categories should focus on health maintenance, illness problems, or degree of independence in meeting one's own health or illness needs. Abdellah and Levine (1965) discussed the concept of patient classification as an area of interest for nurse researchers in 1965. Patient classification was defined as a scaling scheme in which the underlying continuum can be conceptualized as expressing a quantitative statement of a patient's requirements for nursing services. These may range from no requirements at all — representing a condition of maximum self-help ability — to the other extreme, total requirements for nursing services — representing a condition of minimum self-help ability. One may also visualize the continuum as levels of wellness. The degree or amount of nursing care required by the patient is not necessarily positively correlated with the level of wellness; one cannot say that the less well the patient, the more nursing care he or she will require. For example, a terminally ill patient may require fewer nursing services than a person with a fractured leg (moderate level of illness).

The early patient classification systems documented in the literature (e.g., Connor et al., 1961; Chagnon, Audette, Lebrun, & Tilquin, 1978; Norby & Freund, 1977; Norby, Freund, & Wagner, 1977; Meyer, 1978a, 1978b) are based on defining the patient's physical needs during hospitalization and tend to exclude psychosocial and long-range health maintenance and sustenance needs. Various nursing models have evolved since 1970—for example, those of Kinlein, Orem, Rogers, and Roy—that do not view the patient according to an illness or disease state, as in the traditional medical model, but, rather, look at the whole person, including the person's health maintenance and promotion needs and his or her relationship to the total environment. Since the advent of these conceptual frameworks, patient classification criteria based solely on physical needs have been criticized by nurses.

Thus, establishing the viewpoint for a patient classification system is not simple. The issue has been compounded by the expanding and changing role of nursing, lack of nursing research on the topic, and reexamination of the patient's health illness status since 1970. A perusal of the published patient classification schemes indicates that the majority have been developed for adult populations in acute care settings and focus on determining the degree of patient dependency on nursing personnel to meet the patient's basic needs.

Once the viewpoint for the development of the patient classification system has been decided, problems with generics and semantics can arise. Common categorization schema of many patient classification systems currently in existence use three or four general groupings, for example, self-care, partial care, and total care; or minimal care, standard care, intensive care, and critical care. The terms by themselves, however, are not self-explanatory or mutually exclusive. What is the distinction between the intensive and critical care categories used in a particular patient tool? Thus, it is imperative that clear, detailed explanations describe the various classification groupings so that any existing ambiguity might be minimized.

It is important to realize that patients in a particular classification are not necessarily identical but, rather, possess many similarities related to the defined classification characteristics. Neither are the given classes mutually exclusive, although some authorities believe this is desirable. According to Giovannetti (1978), "each class should be mutually exclusive—classes should not overlap. However, it has already been shown that some overlapping is usually *unavoidable* because of variations in viewpoint which must be accommodated" (p. 9).

Sokal (1974), on the other hand, points out that classifications need not be hierarchic, and the clusters may overlap (intersect). "From studies in a variety of fields, the representation of taxonomic structure as overlapping clusters or as ordinations appears far preferable to mutual exclusivity. By ordination, we mean projection of the operational taxonomic units (OTUs) in a space of fewer dimensions than the original number of descriptors. When tested by any of several measures of distortion, ordinations in as few as two or three dimensions frequently represent the original similarity matrices considerably more faithfully than do dendrograms" (Sokal, 1974, p. 1121).

There are a wide variety of patient classification instruments currently in use in hospitals throughout the United States. It is sometimes facetiously remarked that there are as many different tools as there are hospitals. The tools vary in format and length. Patient classification schemes have several common characteristics:

1. Categories are used that describe patient characteristics or critical indicators of a patient's nursing care requirements that might encompass any or all of the following, as mentioned by Aydelotte (1973):

(a) Capabilities of the patient to care for himself or herself

(b) Special characteristics of the patient related to sensory deprivation

(c) Acuity of illness

(d) Requirements for specific nursing activities

(e) Skill level of personnel required in the care

(f) Patient's geographic placement or status in the hospital system

2. Most schemes include class designations ranging in number from three to nine, with descriptive statements regarding patient characteristics for each level. Examples of labels assigned to classes are self-care, partial care, and complete care; or I (minimum care), II (average care), III (more than average care), and IV (maximum care). The patient is then categorized as either a I, II, III, or IV based on the most characteristics the patient exhibits.

3. Physiological dimensions of nursing care are definitely designated, whereas psychosocial, religious, and cultural behavioral needs or requirements are generally not considered.

4. Most systems define nursing care times that can be assigned to activities in the appropriate class or category designation.

5. Many patient classification schemes have not been tested for validity and reliability.

When examining a patient classification instrument, one should critically analyze whether it recognizes professional nursing activities other than technical tasks. Connor's work in 1960 (Connor, 1961), the first published work in this area, emphasizes technical, or task, components of nursing care. But Connor's classification must be considered in the context of what nurses did at that particular time in nursing history. An increasing number of tools are now designating emotional support needs and teaching needs. If emotional support and teaching needs are checked off for every patient, however, without any way to differentiate the amount of teaching and emotional support needed to determine the nursing time required, then teaching and emotional support could actually be considered mathematical constants and could be built into the time allowances for the particular classification levels.

One should also realize that a very complex patient classification tool may not be any more accurate or reliable in determining the number of nursing staff needed than a very simple system. The necessity of reading lengthy directions may lead to utter frustration and increase the number of mistakes made when trying to follow the directions. The amount of time required to complete the classification tool must also be considered. Important goals for a patient classification instrument are *(1)* internal consistency, or a high interrater reliability; *(2)* simplicity of use; and *(3)* minimal time and cost for the users.

Abdoo (1987) demonstrated that it is difficult to quantitatively support the 90 percent agreement level for a patient classification instrument, as is usually recommended in the literature (Giovannetti, 1985). The desirable level indicative of achieving interrater reliability is dependent on the type of patient classification instrument used, and should be based on the number of disagreements that can be tolerated before a difference in patient care demand (and the resulting nurse staffing requirements) occurs. On certain days when the percentage agreement dropped below 90 percent in certain classification categories, a significant difference in nursing staff occurred, whereas at other times, a significant difference did not occur ($p = .10$). It appears that orientation may be the more important item to attain agreement. The patient care demand requirements increase for each orientation level (with the specific classification instrument used in this study), because there is an inference that if a patient is not oriented to time, place, and person, then he or she will require more nursing assistance. The major factors that contributed to the lack of agreement between raters were incomplete or incorrect information and differences in professional judgments (Abdoo, 1987).

It is important to note that most patient classification tools have been developed for acute medical-surgical patient populations prior to changes in reimbursement practices for inpatient care and expanding outpatient services. Changes have occurred in the mix of patient acuity and length of stay has decreased. It is also important to note that most of these patient classification systems are not necessarily generalizable to critical care, psychiatric (Eklof & Qu, 1986), maternity (Killeen, 1986), community health, pediatric patients, ambulatory care, or outpatient services (Hoffman & Wakefield, 1986; Johnson, 1989), home care, or long-term care settings. Although modifications of acute care patient classification tools have been made for long-term care settings, the frequency (daily versus weekly versus biweekly, etc.) of classifying patients needs to be carefully evaluated as well as the associated nursing care demand times for each classification level.

OVERVIEW OF CURRENT STAFFING SYSTEMS

During the 1970s, several commercial staffing systems were introduced that have gained popularity. The Medicus system (Norby & Freund, 1977; Norby, Freund, & Wagner, 1977; Freund & Mauksch, 1975) uses a computer-read classification tool with weights assigned to each of approximately 25 classification indicators. An algorithm using the sum of the weights for the inpatient census and coefficients obtained from regression analysis from previous work determines the number of nursing personnel needed to provide the care. Although the classification tool was computer-read using Scan-tron sheets, the original system did not operate in real time. Some hospitals now have the nursing staff classify the patients on-line (directly on the computer screen), whereas other institutions batch the classification sheets and obtain monthly reports for budgeting purposes.

From the work of Poland, English, Thornton, and Owens — the PETO group — evolved the GRASP (Grace-Reynolds Application Study of PETO) nurse staffing system (Meyer, 1978a, 1978b; Clark & Diggs, 1971). The patient care units (PCUs) used are obtained from the patient classification tool for inpatients, and PCUs for incoming admissions are also estimated. New admissions are assigned a bed on a nursing unit with the lowest PCU count to achieve an even distribution or work load among the nursing units. The system, although initially not designed to run on computers, now has a computerized version available.

Chagnon et al. (1978) developed a patient classification tool listing 129 possible nursing interventions, each having an estimated weighting for a 24-hour period. The number of staff needed (P) is determined using the following equation

$$P = \left(\frac{S + TUP}{360} \right)$$

where P is the number of staff needed for a particular shift, S is the patient care time, TUP are the tasks performed unrelated to individual patient care time, and 360 is the amount of productive time available by a staff member, with time for breaks, meetings, and so on subtracted from the total paid work time (Chagnon et al., 1978). The census form, which includes the number of patients on the unit and their classification is completed before each shift and submitted to the nursing office to facilitate decisions to balance supply and demand of nursing staff.

It is interesting to note that the published staffing systems derive the number of nursing personnel needed to provide care but do not quantitatively deal with the variance in the number of nursing hours needed. In most cases, the unit is staffed at the mean, and the variance in nursing time demand around the mean is not calculated. Although Connor (1961) discussed how variation in patient needs affects the nursing work load and the GRASP system attempts to reduce the variation in nursing work load by admitting the patient to a bed where there is available nursing time, no attempt has been made to estimate the variance.

Hancock, Segal, Rostafinski, Abdoo, DeRosa, and Conway (1981) have developed a computer-aided nurse staffing system that operates in real time and considers the variation within nurse staffing requirements. The system uses a patient classification schema adapted from Trivedi (1975, 1976) using the ambulation, bathing, feeding, and orientation categories with three possible levels — 1,2,3 — as the initial indicators of nursing care requirements. This schema results in 3^4, or 81, possible basic classification configurations, each with its own mean nursing time and variance in nursing time to reflect the nursing work load of medical patients, and another 81 means and variances for surgical patients. Intravenous therapy, catheter care, dressing care, and isolation are included in a special procedures section, because these activities have been found to reflect a high amount of nursing time.

The development of nurse staffing systems arose from the concern of most nursing departments of whether there are enough personnel to provide the necessary nursing care. But does the fact that actual staff equals or exceeds recommended staff mean that patients receive the necessary nursing care? Unfortunately, this cannot be concluded for several reasons. It is important to realize that inexperienced personnel, lack of productivity, inadequate support services, and unpredicted patient crises affect the accuracy of the predicted number of nursing staff. Overstaffing does not assure that the patients receive more attention. Ongoing and retrospective audits are necessary to evaluate the nursing care services provided.

WORK MEASUREMENT IN NURSING

The determination of the amount of nursing time required by each patient for every shift is an essential but by no means simple component of a staffing methodology. Nursing has relied primarily on industrial engineers and engineering work measurement techniques to quantify nursing actions, but there are often problems with the values obtained. For example, many of the allocated time values for patient care deal only with technical tasks. Abdoo (1987) delineates factors that contribute to difficulties in conducting work measurement studies to quantify nursing time:

1. The industrial engineer or nonnurse observer does not recognize the assessment, evaluation, and psychosocial aspects of the nurse-patient contact, and the nurse often does not convey these components of professional nursing practice to the industrial engineer, due to the nurses' unfamiliarity with work measurement techniques.

2. It is often difficult to differentiate between the start and completion of a nursing activity. For example, while giving a patient a bath, the nurse interacts with the patient. How much of the time spent with the patient should be allocated to the technical task of bath giving and how much to assessment and interaction?

3. Although often referred to as time-study or efficiency experts, industrial engineers cannot easily measure the time spent in assessment and interaction. Measurement of repetitious, technical tasks can readily be done, but determination of times involving professional judgment and skills is much more difficult.

4. There is a lack of uniformity in the methods used by nursing personnel in performing technical procedures.

5. The procedure often is not completed from start to finish without some type of interruption occurring (e.g., physician, another patient, nursing staff, or visitor asking for information).

Hudson's dissertation, summarized in Aydelotte (1973), presents:

Criteria that support the classification of nursing work as nonrepetitive. He also examines questions relating to variations in task prediction time, to procedure development, and to the incentive problem. Hudson found it difficult to encourage individuals to complete task assignments within the time predicted for their accomplishment. He concluded that a task's time variation was due not only to the individuality of the patient and his condition but also to the individuality of the nurse, her concept of nursing practice, and the preconceived notion of how to perform it. Adherence to a present plan or procedure was not seen by nursing personnel as either essential or desirable. The work sequence and pace were set by other kinds of priorities. (p. 27)

Improvement and refinements in determination of nursing activity times can only occur if the nurse has a basic understanding of work measurement principles so that effective collaboration with industrial engineers will occur. Four basic work-measurement techniques have been used in nursing studies to determine the time involved in nursing activities (Williams, 1977):

1. Time study and task frequency
2. Work sampling of nurse activity
3. Continuous observation of nurses performing activities
4. Self-reporting of nurse activity.

Lindner (1989) discusses Methods-Time Measurement (MTM), which was developed in the 1940s for industrial applications, and how a newer method, Methods

Time Measurement-Universal Analyzing System (MTM-UAS), can be used to break down nursing activities into small elements. "In order to develop a time standard for any task, it is necessary only to combine the small elements in the order necessary to complete the task. The order, or sequencing, in which these elements are combined is referred to as the "method" for the activity. . . . By adding the time required for each small activity, total time for the process can be determined . . . " (p. 46).

Difficulties encountered by nursing in using industrial-based work-measurement methods to measure nursing practice are as follows:

1. Many of the allotted time values deal with technical tasks, because the industrial engineer or observer does not recognize the assessment, evaluation, and psychosocial aspects of the nurse-patient contact. Thus, a patient who requires technical tasks could very likely be rated in a higher category than one who requires psychosocial or teaching activities.

2. In developing a patient classification system, some nursing departments borrow the nursing times from the classification systems of others. It is important to realize that the times for one agency may not be accurate for another, because the nursing policies and procedures, unit architecture, experience of the nurse, and methods of implementing the work can vary from agency to agency.

3. Many systems use the mean time for a task without any consideration of the variance. Abdoo, Hancock, Luttman, & Rostafinski (1979) have found that nursing tasks often vary widely with who performs the activity and the method used. For example, report time on *one* studied unit ranged from 15 to 90 minutes, with a mean of 30 minutes.

4. The educational and experience background of the observee is often not considered, nor is a differentiation made among the levels of RN, LPN, and nurse assistant or aide.

5. Times obtained by nurses self-recording the nursing actions they performed may not be accurate because it is difficult to perform accurately and time the work as one is actually doing it. If observers had been used, however, observer bias could also occur. The observers would need to be trained in time studying nursing activities and tested for interrater reliability.

6. Most studies do not consider:
   (a) The appropriateness of the nursing intervention occurring at the time of intervention.
   (b) The staffing situation at the time of the study (over-, under-, or satisfactorily staffed).
   (c) Whether primary, functional, or team nursing was in effect.

At present, there is a lack of research dealing with these issues to support what differentiations should be made.

In summary, determination of accurate nursing activity times is very complex but extremely important, because it, along with a reliable and valid patient classification system, should serve as the foundation for the determination of the number of nursing staff required.

SCHEDULING AND WORKWEEK PATTERNS
FOR NURSING PERSONNEL

Once the long-range determination of the average or minimum number of nursing personnel necessary for daily patient needs has been made, the personnel scheduling can begin. At first glance, scheduling seems to be an easy task of marking days on and off on scheduling sheets. In reality, however, effective scheduling is a science as well as an art. The most overwhelming problem is the interrelatedness between the staffing determination and the scheduling function, because the weekend and holiday-off policies have a direct impact on the necessary number of budgeted nursing positions to provide daily coverage. For example, if the policy is every other weekend off and a minimum of four nurses are needed daily on the day shift, then additional nursing positions are needed to provide the necessary personnel on weekends and required days off. Weekend staffing policies also have direct impact on the nursing budget, because the number of extra personnel needed will vary with the number of weekends off in a given scheduling period. Other institutional policies, such as handling of overtime, shift rotation, and number of different shifts that can be worked in a week, also affect scheduling.

Various scheduling systems have been published and deserve consideration: cyclic, supplemental, block, and computerized. There does not appear to be much difference between cyclic and block scheduling, except that the assignment pattern of the former repeats itself in cycles. One advantage of the cyclic method is that the staff can determine their schedule far in advance if the system is strictly adhered to. Requests for certain days off can also be eliminated, because the nursing personnel would be responsible for switching their days off with someone else. Both cyclical and block scheduling lend themselves easily to computerized scheduling.

The practice of float, or supplemental, scheduling has been used intermittently. At one time, float nursing pools were common in hospitals, but they were eliminated as nursing departments were forced to cut their budgets. The pendulum seems to have swung in the opposite direction with "dial-a-nurse," or agency nursing, coming into the picture. Many of these nursing agencies are businesses owned and managed by nurses to provide contract staffing. Although many nursing service departments initially used these contractual services, some nursing departments decided it would be more cost effective to create and/or reinstitute their own float pool to supplement daily nursing needs. A number of factors must be considered for a successful float pool: selection of float personnel, job satisfaction, inservice education, method of unit assignment, support system, and other factors. The use of float nurses is a viable, cost-effective option when used properly. Trivedi (1976) discusses how float nurses can be used during the allocation (daily scheduling), or "fine-tuning," phase.

Computerized nurse scheduling was originally conceived as the cure-all for the monotony of nurse scheduling as well as a cost-effective solution to scheduling problems. A nurse or staffing clerk would no longer be needed to do the technical task of scheduling personnel. Cyclic scheduling lends itself naturally to computerization because, after defining the constraints, the algorithm repeats itself. But manual staffing systems that honor employee requests for days off, require shift rotation, have a nursing shortage, or have high personnel turnover are not as amenable to computer programming. Warner (1976) describes his methodology for more flexible staffing options with a main-frame computer; it is based on building in a large number of assumptions and definitions in the computer program algorithm. Warner's system initially appeared successful but still required human handwork afterward to fine-tune the schedule. For example, on Tuesday, there may be only four nurses assigned (the defined minimum number needed), whereas on Wednesday, seven nurses might be assigned to the same unit. This computerized scheduling system, originally developed by Warner to work on a computer main-frame system, was later converted by Warner to work on personal computer based. The computer algorithm was refined to better allocate the nursing staff, and this microcomputer operated system is being marketed as ANSOS.

With the decreasing cost and, at the same time, improving capability of microcomputers, computerized scheduling systems such as ANSOS, NURSPREF (Applied Interactive Management Corporation, 1987), etc. have evolved and are being used in acute care settings. Cost savings are difficult to determine with computerized scheduling systems as one must consider the hardware, software, and, also, associated personnel costs to set up and maintain the system. Some have tried to cost justify the purchase, installation, and maintenance of a scheduling system because the number of Fulltime Equivalent (FTE) personnel needed later to maintain the system will decrease. One must still plan on having the equivalent of one FTE to work with the individual head nurses or unit personnel to maintain the system for about a 400-bed institution. When staff vacancies are minimal, a good staffing clerk can produce a good schedule as efficiently as can a computer. When staff vacancies are high, a computer cannot replace the human judgment necessary to adjust the nursing resources to provide adequate staffing coverage.

Innovative practices from industry regarding the length of the workday have also affected nursing. Debate continues over 8-hour, 10-hour, and 12-hour workdays as well as one-week-on, one-week-off patterns. The 10-hour workday has been found to work best in areas where continuous 24-hour coverage is not essential. If 24-hour coverage is required, then a mechanism must exist to provide an additional 4 hours of coverage. Two advantages of the 10-hour workday are extra days off in the workweek and decreased transportation-related expenses. Potential child-care difficulties, fatigue, and handling of call-ins are some of the disadvantages. In addition, workers may not be used in the best manner when overlapping shifts occur, which can result in extra staffing for a 2-hour period.

Twelve-hour shifts easily provide the necessary 24-hour coverage. Advantages are similar to those of the 10-hour day, whereas the disadvantages could be more severe; for example, the employees may notice more fatigue and staff may not be able to work overtime to cover a call-in.

Although compressed workweeks have been gaining popularity in nursing settings, more research is needed regarding employee fatigue, employee productivity, cost effectiveness, and fatigue-produced errors. Each method must be examined regarding:

1. Adaptability to institutional personnel and payroll policies and procedures.
2. Impact on nonnursing departments.

3. Willingness of the nursing staff to work nontraditional hours.
4. Cost savings, if any, not only to the employer, but also to the employee (e.g., 4-day workweeks eliminate 1 day's work of driving).
5. Present overtime worked by nursing staff on 8-hour workdays.

Because these five considerations can vary from institution to institution, one ideal workday length for every agency may not exist. There may not even be unanimous consensus for all units within one institution.

Shift rotation is another important component of nurse scheduling. The preferred trend at present is to hire staff for each of the shifts, but because there is often difficulty finding enough personnel to work afternoons and midnights, the day-shift personnel must often rotate. Felton (1975) has written an interesting report concerning her findings related to the effects of shift rotation on physiological body rhythms: "The temperature and potassium levels did not return to the before-night rotation levels even 10 days post night duty . . . In addition to averaging one and a quarter hours less sleep during the day when subjects worked at night, five factors were related to a higher disruption of the quality of their sleep and restfulness: (1) trouble staying asleep, (2) trouble sleeping because of noise or environmental temperature, (3) fatigue, (4) difficulty switching from night to day shift, and (5) requiring a week to adjust bowel habits after night duty. One factor was related to lower disruption: satisfaction with the regular work schedule" (Felton, 1975, pp. 18–19). More studies regarding shift rotation of nurses and circadian rhythms as well as comparisons of the physiological effects among day-to-night, day-to-afternoon, and afternoon-to-night rotating shifts are needed. One implication thus far is that it is better for a regular day-shift employee to work several consecutive night shifts rather than to work a day-night-off, day-night-off type of rotation.

The issue of centralization adds another dimension to the scheduling and staffing issue. Proponents of decentralization feel that this approach conveys an interest in the individual needs of the employee, whereas the employee may feel he or she is only a number when dealing with a centralized scheduling office. A centralized scheduling office can usually provide a better balanced schedule in terms of personnel for each shift, whereas a decentralized system may have difficulty providing adequate coverage on certain shifts, especially if the unit is totally responsible to provide its own personnel. The question arises as to which type of scheduling is more cost effective and which is better able to use the needed nursing staff, based on the patient classification data.

NEXT GENERATION NURSE STAFFING SYSTEMS

The development of patient classification, nurse staffing, and nurse scheduling systems was summarized in the previous sections. Questions arise as to whether current systems meet the needs of nursing service departments and where these systems should be going to meet future needs. Advanced computer technology; diagnosis-related groups (DRGs); fee-for-services arrangements; increasing emphasis on productivity, cost-effective nursing care delivery, and total quality management, are factors that have had and will continue to have the greatest impact on the development and current use of nursing staffing systems.

Computerized patient classification, staffing, and scheduling systems have become more common as the personal computers have become increasingly powerful, and there is less need to have these systems run on hospital main-frame computers. Giovannetti and Johnson (1990) discusses a "second-generation patient classification system, ARIC (Allocation, Resource Identification and Costing), incorporating innovative design features made possible with recent software advances." This system provides unit-specific classification information and ongoing reliability and validity monitoring capabilities.

If one looks critically at the current systems in place, one sees that they tend to be fragmented systems developed for a very specific purpose, rather than separate pieces that can easily interface with other specialized systems to result in a completely integrated (closed feedback loop) system. The patient classification tool was originally developed to classify patients, which then, in turn, can be used to predict demand for nursing care time. That information, however, does not typically interrelate with the purchased computerized scheduling package, unless the daily patient classification summary data for a nursing unit is manually reentered into the scheduling system. The question also arises as to whether a patient classification tool is actually needed if computerized nursing care plans can be developed with associated nursing care times as part of the computerized clinical nursing information system, which then allows the amount of nursing care time required by each patient to be calculated. It is the opinion of this author that this is the direction that patient classification and nurse staffing systems should be taking, rather than trying to develop a patient classification instrument that will satisfy both the nursing staff and nurse managers. If automated or computerized nurse charting is also available, then the nursing care that the patient needs can be compared with the documented nursing care that the patient receives. Budd and Propotnik (1989) describe a patient classification system driven by computerized nursing notes, developed at LDS Hospital, that determines appropriate staffing and also bills patients directly for nursing services.

Daily patient acuity information, the resulting nursing staff predicted necessary to deliver patient care, and the actual staffing with the computed variance in predicted number of staff needed versus actual, can be used by nurse managers for decision making, budget forecasting, and in quality assurance programs. The predicted number of staff should be compared with actual staffing on a daily, weekly, and monthly basis. The information should also be aggregated by day of the week, which could help allocation of staffing during scheduling. For example, if a surgical unit consistently shows less staff needed than usually provided on Tuesday, the scheduler may be able to adjust future schedules accordingly.

The relationship between patient classification (acuity) and DRGs as well as the feasibility of fees for services, based on nursing care provided, are being studied in a number of institutions (Giovannetti, 1985). The major problem has been that the patient classification data, if computerized, has been typically stored as aggregate data (summed over the total number of patients) for a specific patient care unit either by day or by each shift, rather than storing each patient's individual classification configuration for every classification occurrence for that patient.

Summary

Nurse staffing consists of several components: planning, scheduling, and allocation. The planning or staffing methodology phase should be based on quantifiable, measurable data. This systematic nurse staffing determination must include the following variables: *(1)* an assessment of required nursing time to meet patient care needs (patient classification, *(2)* an assessment of required nursing time to meet patient needs (nursing work load determination), and *(3)* an algorithm that uses the first two variables.

The predicted number of nursing staff can be used for personnel scheduling, budgeting, and productivity tracking. A variety of scheduling options are currently used by nursing departments: computerized, compress workweek (with 10-hour and 12-hour workdays); cyclical, block, and float, or supplemental; and centralized or decentralized. It is important to realize that what works well in one institution or even one unit may not work well in a different institution or unit. Although many nurse staffing systems have evolved over the past 30 years, computer technology, DRGs, fee-for-services arrangements, changes in financial reimbursement practices for delivered client care, and the evolution of computerized nursing management and clinical information systems will have further impact on the development and use of future staffing systems.

References

Abdellah, F. G., & Levine, E. (1965). *Better patient care through nursing research.* New York: Macmillan.

Abdoo, Y. M. (1987). A model for nurse staffing and the impact of inter-rater reliability of patient classification on nurse staffing requirements. (Doctoral dissertation, University of Michigan, 1987) *Dissertation Abstracts International, 48*(2).

Abdoo, Y. M., Hancock, W. M., Luttman, R., & Rostafinski, M. (1979). *Determination of nurse staffing requirements: A case study.* Unpublished doctoral dissertation, report, University of Michigan, Ann Arbor.

Applied Interactive Management Corporation (1987). *NURSPREF.* Seattle, WA: Author.

Aydelotte, M. K. (1973). *Nurse staffing methodology: A review and critique of selected literature.* (*DHEW Publication No. (NIH) 73-433*) Washington, DC: U.S. Government Printing Office.

Budd, M. C., & Propotnik, T. (1989). A computerized system for staffing, billing and productivity measurement, *Journal of Nursing Administration, 19*(7), 17–23.

Center for Hospital Management Engineering (1978). *Nurse scheduling: An examination of case studies, proceedings of a forum.* Chicago: American Hospital Association.

Chagnon, M., Audette, L. M., Lebrun, L., & Tilquin, C. A. (1978). A patient classification system by level of nursing care requirements, *Nursing Research, 27*(2), 107–113.

Clark, E. L., & Diggs, W. W. (1971). Quantifying patient care needs, *Hospitals, 45*(18), 96, 98, 100.

Cochran, J., & Derr, D. (1975). Patient acuity system for nurse staffing, *Hospital Progress, 56*(11), 51–54.

Connor, R. J. (1961). A work sampling study of variations in nursing work load, *Hospitals, 35*(9), 40–41.

Connor, R. J., Flagle, C. D., Hsieh, R. K., Preston, R. A., & Singer, S. (1961). Effective use of nursing resources: A research report, *Hospitals, 35*(9), 30–39.

Des Ormeaux, S. P. (1977). Implementation of the CASH patient classification system for staffing determination, *Supervisor Nurse, 8*(4), 29–35.

Eklof, M., & Qu, W. H. (1986). Validating a psychiatric patient classification system, *Journal of Nursing Administration, 16*(5), 10–17.

Felton, G. (1975). Body rhythm effects on rotating work shifts, *Journal of Nursing Administration, 5*(3), 16–19.

Freund, L. E., & Mauksch, I. (1975). *Optimal nursing assignments based on difficulty. (Final Project Report USPHS 1-R18-Hs001391)* Washington, DC: U.S. Government Printing Office.

Georgette, J. K. (1970). Staffing by patient classification, *Nursing Clinics of North America, 5*(2), 329–339.

Giovannetti, P. (1985). DRGs and nursing workload measures, *Computers in Nursing, 3*(2), 88–91.

Giovannetti, P., & Johnson, J. M. (1990). A new generation patient classification system, *Journal of Nursing Administration, 20*(5), 33–40.

Giovannetti, P. (1978). *Patient classification systems in nursing. (DHEW Publication No. (HRA) 78-22)* Hyattsville, MD.

Hancock, W. M., Segal, D., Rostafinski, M., Abdoo, Y. M., DeRosa, S., & Conway, C. A. (1981). A computer-aided patient classification system where variation within a patient classification is considered. In C. Tilquin (Ed.), *Systems Science in Health Care.* Toronto: Pergamon Press.

Hoffman, F., & Wakefield, D. S. (1986). Ambulatory care patient classification, *Journal of Nursing Administration, 16*(4), 23–30.

Johnson, J. M. (1989). Quantifying an ambulatory care patient classification instrument, *Journal of Nursing Administration, 19*(11), 36–42.

Killeen, M. B. (1986). A patient classification tool for maternity services, *NLN Publication,* (20-2155), 293–306.

Lindner, C. (1989). Work measurement and nursing time standards, *Nursing Management, 20*(10), 44–48.

McCormick, P., Roche, J. M., & Steinwacks, D. M. (1973). Predicting nurse staffing, *Hospitals, 47*(9), 68,73–77.

Meyer, D. (1978a). *GRASP: A patient information and work load management system.* Morganton, NC: MCS.

Meyer, D. (1978b). Work load management system ensures stable nurse-patient ratio, *Hospitals, 52*(5), 81–85.

Minetti, R., & Hutchinson, J. (1975). System achieves optimal staffing, *Hospitals, 49*(9), 61–64.

Norby, R. B., & Freund, L. E. (1977). A model for nurse staffing and organizational analysis, *Nursing Administration Quarterly, 1*(4), 1–13.

Norby, R. B., Freund, L. E., & Wagner, B. A. (1977). A nurse staffing system based upon assignment difficulty, *Journal of Nursing Administration, 7*(9), 2–24.

Sokal, R. R. (1974). Classification: Purposes, principles, progress, prospects, *Science, 185*(4157), 1115–1123.

Trivedi, V. M. (1976). Daily allocation of nursing resources. In J. R. Griffith, W. M. Hancock, & F. C. Munson (Eds.), *Cost Control in Hospitals.* Ann Arbor, MI: Health Administration Press.

Trivedi, V. M., & Hancock, W. M. (1975). Measurement of nursing work load using head nurses' perceptions, *Nursing Research, 24*(5), 371–376.

Warner, D. M. (1976). Computer-aided system for nurse scheduling. In J. R. Griffith, W. M. Hancock, & F. C. Munson (Eds.), *Cost Control in Hospitals*. Ann Arbor, MI: Health Administration Press.

Williams, M. A. (1977). Quantification of direct nursing care activities, *Journal of Nursing Administration, 7*(8), 15–18.

CHAPTER 24

Building Effective Work Groups

Sandra R. Byers
Lillian M. Simms

Highlights

- **Work context**
- **Hospital context**
- **The effective unit workplace**
- **Unit nursing work**
- **Unit ethos**

Building effective nursing work groups in various settings requires knowledge and skill with planning, coordinating, delegating, and dealing with conflict. The need for effective teamwork is self-evident, and the problems of coordination and cooperation require a sophisticated understanding of teams and groups. Interdisciplinary health care team management requires knowledge of the dynamics of different practice patterns and effective strategies for managing teams, task forces, and task-directed groups. This chapter presents an approach to the study of work groups and workplace environments to plan and build effective work groups.

Planning is a conceptual activity and may be defined as predetermining a carefully detailed course of action that will enable the organization, unit, or individual to achieve specific objectives or goals. Planning requires the ability to think, to analyze data, to envision alternatives, and to make decisions. Planning is essentially a decision-making process and the steps are similar to those of the nursing process. They include assessment of the system or subsystem, including goals and objectives; assessment of present strengths and weaknesses; establishment of assumptions and *prediction of* what will influence activities; determination of alternative courses of action; identification of priorities; and selection of a course of action.

Coordination may be described as organizing the work of nursing care within each shift, between shifts, and between nurses and other health professionals. Delegation is a complementary function of direction. Effective delegation implies that a nurse shares a segment of responsibility, delegates a specific segment of corresponding authority, and demands accountability. Conflict is an inherent part of all organizations, units, and work groups. Within a health care organization, conflict may result from divergence of opinion, incompatibility, transmission of erroneous information, or competition for scarce resources. Although frequently viewed as a negative manifestation of human interaction, conflict in work groups can have positive as well as negative aspects. The redesign of work groups can be used as a tool for developing shared values and building effective and flexible work groups (Beckman & Simms, 1992).

WORK CONTEXT

Nurses are employed in diverse settings: hospitals, community agencies, long-term care, private practice, and ambulatory clinics, which have an impact on the design of work groups. This diversity has resulted in a variety of employee-employer-consumer contracts that frame the different degrees of independence, accountability, authority, and types of services provided by the nurse and the corresponding work group. In addition, these contracts, formal or informal, assume the underlying understanding every professional has with clients to provide competent and appropriate service and to be compensated for these services. For example, the nurse in the community-based environment frequently delegates physical care and many basic treatments to family members that in the hospital environment are carried out by the nursing staff. Medications are given by family members in the home and some records are kept by family members.

In the hospital setting, it is assumed that the majority of all care must be performed by employees. In contrast, the work group in the home environment has quite different levels of responsibilities, independence, and accountability. In long-term care settings, both the work group's care plans and actual care place more emphasis on the chronic nature of the patient's disease and the physical, social, and emotional needs of the patient over time. Therefore, the work group members may be more consistent as the patient's progress and needs change less dramatically. In the hospital, although "total patient" is the framework for developing the patient's plan of care, the acute needs of the patient will take precedence.

THE HOSPITAL CONTEXT

One critical way to understand nursing work groups is to examine the hospital and unit context, even though the majority of clients receive care outside of hospitals. The majority of nurses work in a hospital and are assigned to work on a specific clinical unit.

Hospitals are large, complex organizations with unique characteristics. One of the ways hospitals are unique is they employ a large number of professional nurses. Professionals tend to have loyalties to their professional association outside the hospital. They have a mission that is based on their commitment to society, not to the organization. Complex organizations are usually bureaucracies characterized by rules, a division of labor, a hierarchy of authority, specialists, line and staff positions, a separately designated administrative staff, records, and "closed-systems thinking" (Fuszard, 1983; Daft & Steers, 1986).

In the current hospital environment, the cost of services has been increasingly emphasized. Singleton and Nail (1984) explain hospital structure, organization, and relationships from a financial perspective. In "big business," usually the consumer is clearly the purchaser and payer of service. In the hospital, the consumer is the patient who must be admitted for the purchase and receipt of services ordered by the physician. The physician is not a formal partner in the business enterprise but is responsible for ordering the product of care for the patient. Nurses and others employed by the hospital are responsible for implementing the care prescribed and the care within their practice domain. The payers, usually government agencies or private insurers, have a great deal to say about the amount of payment for the health care and the conditions under which the care is provided (Singleton & Nail, 1984). Therefore, the quantity and the quality of the services provided to patients are influenced and monitored by another body, essentially outside the hospital environment. This kind of control creates a complex environment for hospitals that must adjust numbers of personnel and programs to fit with revenue resources.

Strauss, Fagerhaugh, Suczek, and Wiener (1985) describe hospital organization in practical terms and identify complexities in the system. They describe contemporary hospitals as:

variegated workshops-places where different kinds of work are going on, where very different resources (space, skills, ratios of labor force, equipment, drugs, supplies and the like) are required to carry out that work, and where the divisions of labor are amazingly different, though all of this is in the direct or indirect service of managing patients' illnesses. (Strauss et al., 1985, p. 6)

The workplace and nurses' work were examined by Melosh (1982) in relationship to the physician's role and women's history, labor history, and sociology. She viewed nurses as subordinate to physicians by custom and law, yet second in command on the hospital unit and closely associated with physicians' prestige and power. She described nurses' occupational culture as "a tradition of pride in manual skills, of direct involvement with the sick, of respect for experience and often a concomitant mistrust for theory" (Melosh, 1982, p. 7). She perceived a conflict and a strength between nurses' "culture of apprenticeship" and the traditions of professional ideology in controlling and defining their work (Melosh, 1982, p. 207). The apprenticeship approach is the way for nurses to affirm their skills and define their work and maintain the profession's ideals of the patient as the center of nurses' work and the basis for nursing's legitimate authority. From this perspective, Melosh posits that nursing autonomy is doomed unless it is linked to broader issues of hospital work.

The work of nurses is imbedded in the structural and role relationships within the hospital environment. Aiken (1983) suggests six fundamental tensions between hospitals, physicians, and nurses. These tensions are *(1)* The nurses' sphere of authority has not changed since World War II, even though nurses are now in command of much of the available clinical expertise to care for the seriously ill and make judgments about appropriate use; *(2)* Physicians work fewer hours and are available less for consultation (in the hospital). The authority of the nurse to act in the absence of the physician has not been redefined; *(3)* Nurses have not been recognized for their new level of clinical decision making with the increase in older and more seriously ill patients; *(4)* An increase in medical subspecialties has resulted in numerous physicians involved in a patient's care, fragmentation of care, and the potential of costly and dangerous duplication or omission of services. The role of the nurse to synthesize and monitor multiple diagnostic and treatment regimens has not been recognized; *(5)* Nurses are the coordinators of all the support services involved with the care and safety of a patient, yet they have no authority to deploy or redirect these services to carry out the responsibilities; and *(6)* Nurses, largely females and now looking at many professional career options, do not find working conditions in hospitals professionally satisfying. These six tensions, which Aiken terms incompatibilities, suggest that nurses lack recognition and status within the hospital. They may also indicate the need for the nursing profession to communicate to others about what nurses can and do accomplish.

THE UNIT WORK CONTEXT

Whereas the clinical unit in community care is the home, the clinical unit in most hospitals is defined by a designated physical space and labeled according to a type of medical specialty. Patients admitted for care are placed in private or semiprivate rooms. Hospital employees and nonhospital employees come and go on the unit, depending on their assigned responsibilities. Each clinical unit is quite isolated and has unique characteristics. Physical structure, organizational structure, management, culture, and work-related variables have constituted the study of the clinical unit in the past.

The workplace of the nurse has received national attention from The American Academy of Nursing in its Task Force on Nursing Practice in Hospitals report, *Magnet Hospitals, Attraction and Retention of Professional Nurses* (American Academy of Nursing, 1983) and the *Secretary's Commission on Nursing Final Report* (USDHHS, 1988). Hospitals that were judged to have outstanding records of nurse recruitment and retention were then labeled "magnet hospitals." This report has been used extensively by nurse executives in trying to correct their own nurse recruitment and retention problems.

The *Magnet Hospital* report identified positive work environment characteristics and encouraged hospitals to design programs incorporating them. They are *(1)* a visible, accessible, and participatory administration; *(2)* knowledgeable and strong leaders who support their work and care about their working conditions; *(3)* a collaborative organizational structure with mutual goal setting; *(4)* staffing patterns that recognize the need for adequate quantity, quality, and mix of expertise of staff; *(5)* personnel programs and policies with flexible work schedules, competitive salaries, and benefits; *(6)* active recruitment and retention programs; and *(7)* professional practice support and a drive for quality with models of delivery that support nurse autonomy, constructive feedback on the quality of care, and knowledgeable nursing care consultants available. Nurses in these hospitals, identified for their outstanding recruitment and retention programs, are recognized for their contributions to the total care of the patient and family and are consulted by physicians. Professional development is supported and includes strong orientation programs, inservice, and continuing education, formal education, and career development.

THE EFFECTIVE UNIT WORKPLACE

The Secretary's Commission on Nursing Report (USDHHS, 1988) contained 8 out of 16 recommendations addressing reorganization of the workplace. Briefly, the eight recommendations are *(1)* health care delivery should preserve nurses' time for direct patient care by providing adequate staffing levels for clinical and nonclinical support services; *(2)* innovative staffing patterns should use nurses' different levels of education, competence, and experience; *(3)* automated information systems and other new labor-saving technologies should be developed; *(4)* methods for costing, budgeting, and tracking nursing resource use should be developed; *(5)* involvement of nurses at all policy- and decision-making levels must occur; *(6)* the decision-making level of the nurse in cooperation with medicine should be recognized; *(7)* positive and accurate images of nurses' work should be promoted; and *(8)* the effects of nurse compensation, staffing patterns, decision-making authority, and career development on nurse supply and demand and health care cost and quality should be researched.

Fine (1982) proposes three applications for creating a work place for professional nurses aimed directly at organizational structure. They are *(1)* changes in staff nurse participation to include representation at board and administrative levels and at controlling and coordinating levels of nursing service; *(2)* changes in the structure of nursing to two levels, a coordination and control level and a technological level; and *(3)* changes in work autonomy to mean the client-professional relationship incorporates innovation, individual responsibility and communication, and socialization and resocialization efforts as necessary to maintain nurses' professional roles.

Lancaster (1985) suggests creating a climate for achievement by helping employees feel like somebody, establishing explicit goals, making expectations clear, providing feedback and reinforcement, eliminating threats, encouraging individual responsibility, and open communication.

Nurse retention is used as an indicator of the hospital's and unit's status. J. Alexander (1988) studied voluntary turnover rate of 1,726 registered nurses and licensed vocational nurses on 146 units within 17 hospitals. The dependent variable, voluntary turnover rate, was correlated with four unit organizational variables: "staff integration," defined as the ratio of RNs assigned to the unit to total patient care staff assigned to unit, extent of RN rotation among shifts, and ratio of full-time staff to all unit staff; "centralization," defined as RN influence in unit-related decisions and decision-making authority of the head nurse; "communication/coordination," defined as the frequency of contact and communication among nurses during the shift, frequency of patient care conferences, and explicitness of unit policies and procedures;

and "evaluation," defined as perceived accuracy of head nurse performance evaluation and the number of patient care hours performed by head nurse per week.

Results indicated four organizational categories significantly related to turnover: salience of evaluation, frequency of patient care conferences, shift rotation, and RN ratio. There was a positive correlation with shift rotations and a negative correlation with the RN ratio suggesting, "A collegial group of professional workers and some degree of organizational stability may be necessary to achieve organizational integration and consequently to reduce turnover" (J. Alexander, 1988, p. 69). He also contended that where there is formal communication, instrumental communication or informal communication occurs and positively influences turnover. For example, planned meetings and conferences, as patient care conferences, increase the opportunities for staff socialization and positively influences retention. Fair and accurate evaluations legitimize the RN role and, thus, reduce the conflict and alienation that may result in turnover.

Butler and Parsons (1989), Pooyan, Eberhardt, and Szigeti (1990), and Weisman, Alexander, and Chase (1981) studied nurse retention. Butler and Parsons focused on 212 nurses' perceptions of environmental factors, finding inadequate salary, lack of control over scheduling and patient care load, lack of recognition for clinical excellence, and lack of managerial support influencing satisfaction and retention. Pooyan and colleagues (1990) surveyed 1,250 nurses at three private hospitals, examining the relative contributions of work-related and demographic variables to turnover intention. Demographic variables of age, occupational tenure, education, and marital status did not contribute to nursing job changes in ways not accounted for by work-related variables. The results of Pooyan et al. were consistent with those of Weisman et al. (1981) in suggesting turnover-related variables that can be potentially controlled by management. These variables are satisfaction with promotion, pay, and supervisor, together with three work environment variables: role ambiguity, participation opportunity (e.g., how much "say" the nurses perceived they had in making job-related decisions regarding how to do one's job, the sequence/speed of work, and division of work responsibility as well as the amount of work), and performance constraints (shortage of nursing staff, unavailability of medical equipment/supplies, lab delays, too much paper work, and not having sufficient instructions). Satisfaction with promotion and perceived performance constraints were the first and second most significant predictors of turnover.

Alexander, Weisman, and Chase (1982) interviewed 789 nurses at a university-affiliated hospital and identified characteristics significantly influencing nurses' evaluations of their jobs. Nurse autonomy and nurses' opinions about physician task delegation were correlated with four personal characteristics: baccalaureate education, first position, length of employment, and internal control (degree to which an individual perceives his behavior is controlled by fate or by his own initiative or skill); and seven job-related characteristics: primary nursing, rotating shifts, position level, workload, head nurse scale (staff nurses' attitudes about the head nurse's leadership style and responsiveness), physician task delegation, and adequacy of professional time with perceived autonomy. Five variables significantly predicted perceived autonomy: baccalaureate education, internal control, primary nursing, head nurse scale, and adequacy of professional time. The head nurse scale measuring nurses' attitudes toward their head nurse's leadership style and responsiveness was the strongest predictor of perceived autonomy.

Williams (1988) reviewed the literature on hospital and unit design, spatial environment, sound, color, thermal conditions, and weather. These variables have had limited attention from researchers and appear to influence work and environment.

UNIT NURSING WORK

Nursing work has been studied extensively and described in a variety of ways by categorized activities, by physical skills required, by identified "hidden work," by "quality" nursing care characteristics, and by the philosophical and cultural foundations of nursing care.

Yocum (1987) studied practice patterns of over 4500 newly licensed nurses who responded to questions about nursing activities and client needs. The activity statements were worded in terms of what the nurse does rather than how, how well, or why the nurse performs the activity. The practice domain of the nurse was based on clinical practice area and education program attended. Nurses in medical/surgical clinical units scored high in performing routine nursing measures, monitoring clients at risk, preparing clients for procedures, and controlling pain. They scored low in meeting acute emotional/behavioral needs; staff development, management, and collaboration; and quality assurance and safety. Nurses were very low in categories specific to a setting such as parenting skills associated with teaching new mothers and fathers how to care for a new infant or the administration and teaching of immunizations with pediatric patients' parents. The middle group of categories for the medical/surgical nurses was protecting clients, planning/managing client care, helping clients to cope with stress, assisting clients with needs related to mobility, assisting clients with self-care, meeting acute physical needs, supporting client's family, and ensuring safety during intrusive procedures. The study found work setting (e.g., obstetrical, pediatrics, or rehabilitation inpatient units) and type of clients (whether young or old) influenced the frequency of the activities.

A time/task survey was conducted by The Hay Group in over 850 hospitals about nurses working on medical-surgical units ("Misuse of RNs," 1989). They found 26 percent of RN's time on average is spent in "professional nursing": physical assessments, care and treatments, monitoring patients' conditions, planning and documenting care. In a typical shift, 22 percent of the time was spent with support functions: patient education, family contacts, nursing communications, and coordination. The largest amount of time, 52 percent was spent in housekeeping details, answering phones, and ordering supplies ("Misuse of RNs," 1989). The investigators reported the reason these nurses stayed or left an institution was based on reasons directly and indirectly related to environment, job, and perceived opportunity for personal and professional growth.

Nursing work has been described using words such as "knowing," "caring," "intuitive," the "essence of nursing," or "hidden work" in contrast to the activities/task approach previously presented. Styles (1990) described good nursing care from the patient's perspective and suggested clients should know who is in charge of their personal care and what the plan of care will be. The knowledgeable and technically competent nurse distinguishes between what is nice and what is necessary for client's care and not only cares about the assigned clients but also cares for them. The nurse should be organized and attend to priorities, serve as patient advocate, and allow the patient as much control as possible. The nurse works with others to ensure the treatment progresses as planned and to minimize complications in preparation for discharge and recovery.

Wolf (1989) points out much of nursing work is hidden, thus decreasing societal status and perceived value. She studied a medical unit in a large urban hospital (1988), investigating four "nursing rituals": postmortem care, medication administration, medical aseptic practices, and change of shift report. Wolf observed that nurses pass on their nursing and patient care knowledge chiefly by word of mouth and by demonstration. Nursing in her opinion has both sacred and profane components and described it in terms of unseen work and dirty work. The unseen tasks are: common sense and caring work, system maintenance and safety work, interpersonal work, comforting work, privacy work (e.g., collection of private information and personal hygienic needs), sacred work (i.e., moral and ethical problems), and cognitive work. The dirty work is body work and death work. She believes nursing work should be made visible and not taken-for-granted. Strauss et al. (1985) describes the social organization of medicine in similar terms: machine work, safety work, comfort work, sentimental work, articulation work, and the work of patients.

The candid and challenging work of Reverby (1987) in *Ordered to Care* depicts nursing as a form of labor shaped by the obligation to care in a society that does not value or know how to evaluate caring. This obligation has resulted in it being described as "women's work," a "duty" encumbered with societal and ideological constraints and difficulties. She views nurses, historically, as individuals from different classes, with heterogeneous experiences and beliefs. This creates a unity and a language problem as efforts are made to mobilize the group toward professional goals. Caring is not only a subjective construct but it is work. Reverby (1987) challenges nursing via political endeavors, educational and practice clarification, and technological advancement to create the conditions under which caring is valued.

The work of Noddings (1984), Gilligan (1982), and Belenky, Clinchy, Goldberger, and Tarule (1986) can contribute to nurses' awareness and understanding of the complexity of work relationships by considering how the female orientation may affect those relationships. This literature sheds a positive perspective on the capabilities and strengths of women, which would be helpful for nurses to understand as they struggle for identity and a stronger image. Noddings (1984) explored caring from an ethical, aesthetical, and psychological perspective. She suggests one meaning of caring as the charge "to protect, maintain or be concerned about the welfare of something or someone" (p. 9). Gilligan (1982) suggests that women are raised and socialized with an ethic of care, of thinking in terms of the concrete other. Belenky et al. (1986) describe five ways women view reality and define truth, knowledge and authority. Women "know" by using intuition, personal meanings, and self-understanding. They connect with ideas and they seek understanding rather than control over ideas or proof that something is so.

UNIT ETHOS

Byers (1990) explored a hospital's unit ethos, defined as the norms and expectations characteristic of individuals within their work context, by studying 15 staff nurses. They completed questionnaires adapted from Quinn (1988) based on his Competing Values Model, described later. This model appeared meaningful in understanding the complex and competing dynamics on a hospital unit. Underlying beliefs and values are critical to the change process and this model helps to reflect those. In addition, nurses who are in the environment, performing the work, are the experts in judging the effectiveness of that work and in redesigning their work to meet patient care needs. A deeper awareness about how nurses understand their world of work and the norms and expectations in that world might contribute to new organizational models for nursing care delivery and impact retention. An assessment of unit ethos as perceived by the nurse and the work group, may reveal tensions with aspects of organizational life such as relationships with hospital administration, physicians, and nurse peers, disillusionment with the work, and inadequate information and communication systems.

Quinn (1988) was concerned about how experts think about effective organizations and tried to understand underlying assumptions causing the behavior. In Quinn's research about organizations, describing effective organizations led to longer and different lists of criteria, based on each organization. The outcome was the competing values framework, which acknowledges organizations as dynamic and confronted with change, ambiguity and contradictions (Figure 24.1). The model, briefly described, has intersecting horizontal and vertical axes, which create four quadrants. The vertical axis ranges from flexibility to control and the horizontal axis ranges from an internal to an external focus. Each quadrant represents one of the four major schools of organization theory: human relations, open systems, rational goal, and the internal process model. Each model has specific characteristics and is in polar contrast to the opposite corner, hence, the notion of competing values.

The model allows the organization to be explored from the perspective that these polar tensions exist in organizations and are not mutually exclusive. The human relations model stresses internal focus, with criteria as cohesion and morale, and values human resources training, whereas it is in contrast to the external oriented rational goal model that values output, productivity, and efficiency with planning and goal setting. Organizations want and need both ways of functioning, and they are not mutually exclusive. In the same way, the open systems model provides an external orientation, values expansion and adaptation, readiness, growth, competition, and resource acquisition. Its polar opposite, an internal orientation, is the internal process model that values continuity and consolidation with stability and control, information management, and communication. "The model can be used to diagnose and intervene in actual organizations" (Quinn, 1988, p. 50). The information can provide a realistic base for progressive change or adaptation in nurses' work.

The Organizational Effectiveness Questionnaire (Quinn, 1988) places the characteristics in eight groups, which in Byers' study (1990), was used to gain insights into the unit expectations that influence nurses' beliefs about their practice. For example, the average nurse score for participation and openness is 1.25 (in parentheses, Figure 24.1). This particular work group appeared effective and scored highest in commitment to work, positive morale, a clear idea of goals and direction, and participation

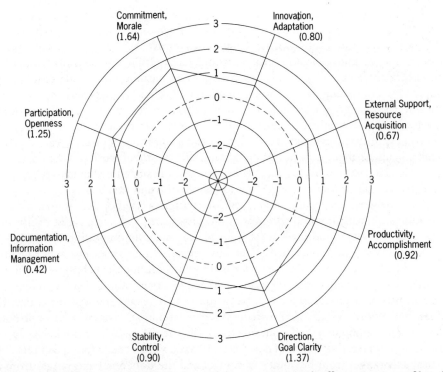

Figure 24.1 The competing values model: organizational effectiveness profile of a nursing unit. The average scores (in parentheses) of the 15 nurses are plotted for the eight organizational components. (Model from Quinn, R. E. (1988). *Beyond Rational Management* (p. 141). San Francisco: Jossey-Bass. Reprinted by permission.)

and openness. The low score was in documentation and information management. The nurses did not value these activities, which might impact a transition to computerization. Nurses who have these same values would probably remain on this unit and find this unit best for them. This type of information can be applied when designing nurses' work, in types of unit work group assignments, in recruitment and retention, and in any planned change.

Summary

The work place of most nurses is a physical unit that is frequently a closed sub-system of a larger hospital and houses a variety of workers and clients. The units are staffed by nurses who want adequate working conditions, rewards, and benefits, typical of most other workers in our society. The interactions between the mix of workers are complex relationships influenced by the expectations of each other and the way in which the work groups are organized. Nurses are torn between professional allegiance and allegiance to the organization as they continually change and reposition themselves in the organization. The degree to which most hospitals have become individual specialty units, triggered by the increase in complex technology and the specialized nursing care that is required, has influenced the structure of the organization in terms of the need for increased communication and integration.

Nursing studies that explore the affect of unit structure and the kind of integration and communication required at all levels in the organization continue to be essential. The Competing Values Model (Quinn, 1988) offers a way to study the work group and workplace environment. The information currently available on nurses' work and employment conditions suggested by the Byers' study described in this chapter can assist nurses in improving nursing services to patients in all settings. Using Quinn's effective work groups approach can stimulate new care delivery models and promote the delivery of effective and efficient patient-centered nursing care.

References

Aiken, L. H. (1983). Nurses. In D. Mechanic (Ed.), *Handbook of Health, Health Care and the Health Professions* (pp. 407–431). New York: Free Press.

Alexander, C., Weisman, C., & Chase, G. (1982). Determinants of staff nurses' different clinical contexts, *Nursing Research, 31*(1), 48–52.

Alexander, J. A. (1988). The effects of patient care unit organization on nursing turnover, *Health Care Management Review, 13*(2), 61–72.

American Academy of Nursing Task Force on Nursing Practice in Hospitals. (1983). *Magnet hospitals. Attraction and retention of professional nurses.* Kansas City, MO: American Nurses Association.

Beckman, J. S., & Simms, L. M. (1992). *A guide to redesigning nursing practice patterns.* Ann Arbor, MI: Health Administration Press.

Belenky, M. F., Clinchy, B. M., Goldberger, N. R., & Tarule, J. M. (1986). *Women's ways of knowing.* New York: Basic Books.

Butler, J., & Parsons, R. J. (1989). Hospital perceptions of job satisfaction, *Nursing Management, 20*(8), 45–48.

Byers, S. R. (1990). *Relationships among staff nurses' beliefs, nursing practice and unit ethos.* Unpublished dissertation, The Ohio State University, Columbus.

Daft, R. L., & Steers, R. M. (1986). *Organizations a micro/macro approach.* Glenview, IL: Scott, Foresman and Company.

Fine, R. B. (1982). Creating a work place for the professional nurse. In A. Marriner (Ed.), *Contemporary Nursing Management Issues and Practice* (pp. 96–109). St. Louis: C. V. Mosby Company.

Fuszard, B. (1983). Adhocracy in health care institutions? *The Journal of Nursing Administration, 13*(1), 14–19.

Gilligan, C. (1982). *In a different voice.* Cambridge, MA: Harvard University Press.

Lancaster, J. (1985). Creating a climate of excellence, *The Journal of Nursing Administration, 15*(1), 16–19.

Melosh, B. (1982). *The physician's hand work culture and conflict in American nursing.* Philadelphia: Temple University Press.

Misuse of RNs spurs shortage, says new study: "Only 26% of time is spent in professional care." (1989), *American Journal of Nursing, 89,* 1223, 1231.

Noddings, N. (1984). *Caring. A feminine approach to ethics and moral education.* Berkeley: University of California Press.

Pooyan, A., Eberhardt, B. J., & Szigeti, E. (1990). Work related variables and turnover intention among registered nurses, *Nursing and Health Care, 11*(5), 255–258.

Quinn, R. E. (1988). *Beyond rational management.* San Francisco, CA: Jossey-Bass Publishers.

Reverby, S. M. (1987). *Ordered to care. The dilemma of American nursing, 1850–1945.* Cambridge: Cambridge University Press.

Singleton, E. K., & Nail, F. C. (1984). Autonomy in nursing, *Nurse Forum, 21*(3), 123–130.

Strauss, S., Fagerhaugh, S., Suczek, B., & Wiener, C. (1985). *Social organization of medical work.* Chicago: University of Chicago Press.

Styles, M. M. (1990). Ten ways to know . . . , *Nursing and Health Care, 11*(6), 283.

U.S. Department of Health and Human Services (USDHHS). Office of the Secretary. (1988). *Secretary's Commission on Nursing, Final Report, Volume 1.* Washington, DC.

Weisman, C., Alexander, C., & Chase, G. (1981). Determinants of hospital staff nurse turnover, *Medical Care, 19*(4), 431–443.

Williams, M. A. (1988). The physical environment and patient care, *Annual Review of Nursing Research, 6,* 61–83.

Wolf, Z. R. (1989). Uncovering the hidden work of nursing, *Nursing and Health Care, 10*(8), 463–467.

Yocom, C. J. (1987). Practice patterns of newly licensed registered nurses: Results of a job analysis study, *Journal of Professional Nursing, 3*(4), 199–206.

CHAPTER 25

Human Productivity

Highlights

- **Definition of productivity**
- **Characteristics of high performing systems**
- **Methods of measuring productivity**
- **Low productivity**
- **Energizing responsibilities of the nurse executive**

The purpose of this chapter is to present the concept of productivity as an important human component of managing resources. Although productivity has not often been a concern of nursing, current cost constraints have made it an important issue. The idea of applying productivity concepts to nursing has not received wide acceptance. Standards, time studies, production rates, and other productivity concepts from industry have been resisted by nurse executives who believe that nursing is a profession and cannot as such be quantified. However, resistance must be followed by action. Nursing must be active in developing and testing methodologies that attend to relevant issues in productivity.

Is the concept of productivity relevant and applicable in nursing? Is the individual nurse free to contribute as much or as little as he or she desires? Or is there a basic required level of "output" for a specifically defined type of nurse? Does the nurse work as fast or as slowly as required by the ratio of staff to patients that happens to exist on a specific unit during a shift? If the nursing staff on a unit can accomplish all the necessary work when one nurse is off, why should the additional nurse be needed at all?

Unlike doctors, nurses are generally not paid more by seeing more patients or accomplishing more tasks. In some home care agencies, salary incentives based on the number of patients seen beyond a minimum are being used. Regardless of how much they "produce," nurses cannot usually make more income or receive further compensation. Nurses are often rewarded for quality by promotion or salary increases, but quantity of services is usually viewed only negatively. That is, if a nurse employee does not contribute an equal share to the unit work load, disciplinary action is threatened or taken by the nurse executive.

How much can an "average" nurse "produce" on a medical unit as opposed to a surgical unit? Is passing medications to 25 patients equivalent to changing dressings on 10 patients? Does a new graduate have lower productivity standards than a graduate of 10 years ago? What is the incentive for a nurse to strive for a productivity standard of five home visits a day or the completion of care plans on two newly admitted patients? What is a reasonable assignment in a long-term care facility?

The concept of productivity goes far beyond the idea of gaining greater output and being efficient. Today's nurses have different values and expectations from those of predecessors of a few years ago. The people issues can no longer be ignored. According to Bennett (1983), a great change has occurred in the work world. Workers are not less motivated. Their expectations of the work environment have risen. The quality of the human experience is of paramount importance and is linked to several factors: the work itself, the work environment, and personal factors.

Although hours and pay are still important, it is the human element that demands recognition. Like workers in factories, nurses in health care delivery settings raise the hue and cry, "I want to matter. *Know* that I am here." As Rosten (1978) states so eloquently: "I cannot believe that the purpose of life is to be 'happy.' I think the purpose of life is to be useful, to be responsible, to be honorable, to be compassionate. It is, above all, to matter, to count, to stand for something, to have it make some difference that you lived at all" (p. 4).

Skinner (1982) proposes four reasons why employees are not as productive, loyal, and dedicated to their companies as they could be:

1. Achieving wholehearted cooperation, energy, and commitment from large numbers of people is difficult, and managers are unrealistic in their hopes to do so.
2. Concepts concerning management of large numbers of people convey contradictory messages to managers.
3. Critical problems in corporate management of personnel are largely unresolved.
4. Some management assumptions undermine the efforts of managers.

Wholehearted cooperation, energy, and commitment demand the best of individuals, which, in the final analysis, depends on individual pride and creativity in spirit and work. Large groups cannot reach maximum productivity unless individuals are willing and eager to move beyond minimum expectations. Eagerness is a part of productivity but not the total concept.

DEFINITION OF PRODUCTIVITY

To improve productivity means to produce more with the same amount of human effort. Labor productivity is the efficiency with which output is produced by the resources used. The measurement can be person-hours worked or total hours paid for measurable output (Glaser, 1976).

This definition causes problems for measuring productivity in nursing because output is difficult to measure. In community health nursing, an output measure of home visits per day has been acceptable, but this cannot be the only one if productivity is an index of quality as well as quantity. Some objective means of determining what are acceptable productivity standards for nursing in various settings must be established.

CHARACTERISTICS OF HIGH PERFORMING SYSTEMS

Peter Vaill (1981, pp. 7–9) proposed the following characteristics of high performing systems:

Clear on their broad purposes and on nearer term objectives for fulfilling these purposes. They know why they exist and what they are trying to do and members have pictures in their heads that are strikingly similar.

Commitment to these purposes is never perfunctory, although it is often expressed laconically. Motivation is always high and energy focus is more important than energy level.

Teamwork is focused on the task, and members have discovered the aspects of systems operations that require integrated actions and have developed related behaviors and attitudes. There are firm beliefs in a "right organizational form," and a noticeable amount of effort is devoted to attaining and maintaining this form. Once members have found a form that works, they cling to it.

Leadership is strong and clear and it is not ambivalent. There is no question of the need for initiative or of its appropriate source, although it may not always be the same person. Leaders are experienced as reliable and predictable.

Fertile sources of inventions and new methods are within the scope of the task they have defined and within the form they have chosen.

They are clearly bounded from their environments, and a considerable amount of energy, particularly on the part of leaders, is devoted to maintaining these boundaries.

Avoid external control, scrounging resources from the environment nonapologetically. They produce what they want by their standards, not what someone else wants.

Above all are systems that have gelled, even though the phenomenon is difficult to describe. Demonstrate an intense human interdependency and fit of the various elements and practices of the system.

Vaill has based his propositions on the intensive study of individual cases. His propositions have relevance for nurse executives as they attempt to improve productivity in various environments.

UNITS OF PRODUCTION

To know what current productivity is, a nurse executive must have an objective measurement. Without such a measurement, the executive has little basis on which to plan changes in productivity level. What level of staffing is the optimum for what is needed to be completed each year, each month, each week, each day, and each shift? There are very few objective data to assist nurse executives in answering these questions.

In quantitative terms, productivity equals the relationship between resources and units of production:

$$\text{Productivity} = \frac{\text{resources}}{\text{units of production}}$$

The question arises in health service settings as to what constitutes nursing's unit of production. Dollars per patient day and hours per patient day continue to be the prevalent expressions in the health care field. Unfortunately, states Hanson (1982), neither dollars nor hours are human resources or adequate expressions of human resources. Dollars are units of exchange with which to purchase human resources and a constraint on the acquisition of human resources. Patient days are therefore not meaningful units of production.

A more realistic unit of production is patient contact hours, a true measure of nursing services. Patient classification systems can be a vehicle for measuring productivity by providing a quantitative measure of need for nursing services. With the advent of the Tax Equity and Fiscal Responsibility Act (TEFRA) legislation and related diagnosis related groups (DRG) mandate, productivity and cost containment have become top priorities for nurse executives.

Efforts to link patient classification with productivity have resulted in the development of creative tools for measuring nursing effort. For example, a midwestern hospital nursing service developed a patient classification tool that measures productivity in staffing of units on a daily and monthly basis and makes budgetary projections within cost containment restrictions. Linkage with quality patient care is also under study (Grant, Bellinger, & Sweda, 1982).

Besides units of production, the other frequently unknown variable in the productivity equation is human resources. According to Hanson (1982), four elements need to be considered:

1. Knowledge and skill
2. Energy (physical, mental, and emotional)
3. Motivation
4. Self-direction

A deficiency in one or all of the four elements has great impact on productivity. For example, failure to use nursing resources according to education and skill creates confusion and dissatisfaction among nurses. The blame for ineffective use of nursing resources cannot be placed on the educators. There must be a combined assumption of responsibility, with nurse executives seriously examining existing nurse-utilization patterns that are outdated and do not create a fit between professional nurse and job description.

METHODS OF MEASURING PRODUCTIVITY

A valid method of measuring productivity is necessary before any changes can be undertaken to change productivity. For community health nursing, one method that is useful and uncomplicated is the caseload/work load analysis tool developed by Easley and Storfjell (1979). This tool provides a measure of the nurse's productivity in relation to what is required in her caseload. The result is an objective comparison of what the nurse does do and what can be accomplished in the time he or she has available. The use of this kind of tool in an inpatient setting would be more complex but could be utilized.

Another method of indirectly measuring productivity was developed for an outpatient setting by Henninger and Dailey (1983). The method was developed to predict nurse staffing needs by means of assigning a standard value time to all direct and indirect nursing procedures. After forecasting the amount of work the nursing staff would be required to complete for the fiscal year, calculations were made to determine if the current staff level was sufficient for the projected work load.

In the inpatient setting, patient days have been used to apportion nursing costs among the diagnosis-related groups and calculate the amount paid for nursing care. The per diem method has not been satisfactory, and the New Jersey Department of Health initiated several studies under the direction of Grimaldi and Micheletti (1982) to develop another way to measure productivity and allocate nursing costs. The most viable are the relative intensity measures (RIMs) studies. The RIM researchers tried to develop an allocation method that would specifically relate the patient's use of nursing resources to his or her medical condition. Nursing resources are defined in terms of minutes of nursing care received; the larger the number of minutes, the greater the amount of resources consumed. These studies may be used to identify payment rates related to the specific diagnosis-related groups.

Leah Curtin (1983) describes another potential measure of productivity in her discussion of nursing care strategies (NCSs). In essence, these are detailed nursing care plans that include direct and indirect care needed and allow for variances in both the interdependent and the independent functions of nurses related to patients' severity of illness within each DRG. To determine the average amount of time needed to deliver nursing care for each DRG or NCS, patients should be classified daily according to the number and complexity of their nursing care needs.

LOW PRODUCTIVITY

Many subjective symptoms of low productivity may exist:

- Complaints of not enough staff
- High absenteeism
- Failure to complete patient care items on each shift

- Low number of home visits per day per public health nurse
- Complaints by medical staff
- Complaints by patients.

Some of these symptoms, however, may be the result of burnout or another phenomenon. The other complicating factor is that too little or too much staff can also result in low productivity.

One of the most frequently described barriers to productivity is burnout. Lavendero (1981) and Seuntjens (1982) describe burnout as a physically and psychologically debilitating condition brought about by work-related frustrations that results in lowered productivity. Low morale then produces negative feelings about self and the organization.

Seuntjens (1982) further describes burnout in terms of the following symptoms, all of which are detrimental to any organization:

Subjective	Moodiness
	Fatigue
	Anxiety
	Guilt
Behavioral	Increased accidents
	Impaired speech
Cognitive	Poor decision making
	Forgetfulness
Organizational	Absenteeism
	Turnover
	Low productivity
	Less commitment
	Job dissatisfaction
	Poor quality of care

For the burned-out nurse, the perceived nonimportance of self and the perceived lack of opportunity make any work or pay schedule unreasonable. The sense of accomplishment that comes from satisfaction from a job well done becomes nonexistent. Burned-out nurses lose respect for their superiors, and their personal lives become uncertain and disrupted. The nurse executive needs to assess the source of job-related stress and determine organizational strategies for stress management long before burnout and decreased productivity can occur.

Nowhere in the annals of administrative literature is there a more fitting description of the motivational crisis in organizations today than the Levinson (1973) description of "the great jackass fallacy." Levinson described the jackass fallacy as an unconscious managerial assumption about people and how they should be motivated. It results in the powerful treating the powerless as objects and the perpetuation of anachronistic organizational structures that destroy the individual's sense of worth and accomplishment.

Many nurse executives are fearful of losing control of their division and fall into the trap of insensitivity to human feelings and treating employees as objects. The first image that comes to mind in thinking of the carrot-and-stick philosophy is that of a jackass—characterized by stubbornness, stupidity, willfulness, and unwillingness to go where someone is driving it. People respond to the carrot-and-stick by trying to get more of the carrot while protecting themselves against the stick. This had led to the formation of unions, suspicion of management's motivational techniques, and outright sabotage of management's motivational efforts as well as organizational changes (Levinson, 1973).

When employees perceive that they are viewed as jackasses, they automatically see management as manipulative and resist. As long as those in leadership roles have a reward-punishment attitude toward motivation, they implicitly assume that employees are in a jackass position in relation to them. Levinson believes that this paternalistic attitude inevitably leads to decreased efficiency and productivity and increased absenteeism, theft, and outright sabotage.

ENERGIZING RESPONSIBILITIES OF THE NURSE EXECUTIVE

Some cost containment studies have shown that as much as 47 percent of a nurse's time is consumed in nonnursing tasks (Levinson, 1983). If nursing productivity is low, several avenues of study may be needed to determine the reasons, so that corrective actions may be taken. If study shows that much of nurses' time is spent in nonnursing areas, administration must also determine if it would be cost effective to hire other categories of personnel to assume the nonnursing duties, thus decreasing the number of nurses, or to maintain a percentage of nonnursing tasks in each nurse's assignment. If all nonnursing tasks were taken away from nurses (that is, if all of them could be identified), the need for nurses could conceivably be decreased by a sizable amount.

The nurse executive must weigh the need for professional judgment in nonnursing tasks and in relating them to patient care. Many categories of nonnurses can be trained to perform tasks, but only the professional nurse has the knowledge and experience to put the nonnursing tasks into the context of total patient care. Instead of being concerned with giving away tasks, the nurse executive may explore ways of eliminating tasks, spreading them more equitably across the nursing staff, or assigning them to personnel under the control of nursing.

The central objective of nursing administration is to maximize the use of human resources toward the achievement of maximum production. There is no automatic way to enhance worker motivation, the key factor influencing productivity and quality of performance. If nurse executives are to energize and create motivating environments, they must understand motivation theories. Amply discussed in Chapter 12, on human potential, motivation theories are presented in this chapter in their application to productivity. Theories of motivation provide frameworks and tools for assessing specific situations and generating creative ideas on how to develop productive environments (Gordon, 1982).

There is no such thing as an unmotivated person. All people are motivated. It is a challenge for nurse executives to speculate about why people behave as they do. Goals are accomplished through people and by people. Roles and positions do not interact; people interact, and they do so within their perceptual fields. A chasm of misunderstanding between the nurse executive and staff can result from difference in the economic, sociological, geographical, and environmental factors under which each person's perceptual field was formed (Kepler, 1980).

The work of nursing service is accomplished through the human element. As nurses move up the administrative ladder, there is less need to function at the technical level, but the administrator must never lose sight of the technical demands that must be met. Current nursing practice is highly technical, in keeping with modern times. Although the human body has not changed, the nature of treatments has changed as society has become increasingly computerized and mechanized.

Joiner, Johnson, Chapman, and Corkrean (1982) suggest that job enrichment can increase the potential for work satisfaction and help administrators attract and keep a high-quality nursing staff. Although job enrichment can be viewed as part of the energizing function, it must be remembered that not all nurses want enriched jobs: jobs that are high in skill variety, task identity, task significance, autonomy, and feedback. At different times and in different years, individual nurses vary in growth needs and in their interest in their jobs.

Hackman and Oldham (1975) have identified five core job dimensions that could contribute to job satisfaction in nursing. These are useful for the nurse executive in identifying jobs that have low motivating potential:

1. Skill variety: the degree to which job challenges the individual
2. Task identity: the degree to which the task provides for the completion of a job
3. Task significance: the degree to which the job has an impact on the lives of others
4. Autonomy: the degree to which the job gives the nurse freedom to act independently and use personal discretion
5. Feedback: the degree to which the job provides the nurse with information on job performance.

Sorrentino, Nalli, and Schriesheim (1992) examined the effect of head nurse (unit nurse executive) behaviors on job satisfaction and performance among staff nurses. Using a sample of 103 registered nurses, the results show significant correlations between unit head nurse behavior and job satisfaction and performance. The findings also suggest the importance of unit nurse executive responsibility in moderating the effects of job anxiety, unit size, and support. Head nurse direction without support was found to impact negatively on performance.

To energize one's staff is to know what those employees do, not to be expert in their jobs, but to know and understand their work. The executive should walk around the health care setting and stop and observe what individual nurses and patients are doing. This practice conveys to the employee not only that he or she has worth as an individual but also that the particular job or position has worth. This practice also serves as a tracking method for identifying points at which work can be changed. Recognition of the human element is of utmost importance in energizing the division of nursing staff.

Technical and Professional Roles

Does it matter whether technical and professional roles are clarified? Yes, it does matter, not because one role is better than the other, but because they are both important to the quality of patient care and nurses' work lives. Failure to use professional nurses according to their education and expertise is the first great evil in the health care world. Expecting too much of technically prepared nurses is the second greatest malady. There is no nursing shortage today, just a shortage in our thinking about utilization of nursing resources.

Johnston (1982) states that there is a great need to clarify the differentiation between technical and professional nursing roles. Graduates of 2-, 3-, 4-, and 5-year nursing programs are all eligible for the same license. Nurse executives hire them to do the same work at the same starting salary. Using the Rines model, Johnston tested the hypothesis that nurses differ in their use of the nursing process according to their educational preparation. The degree and nondegree nurses differed in several categories. The major implications of the study were that:

1. Unnecessary duplication of effort exists between the two groups of nurses.
2. The team nursing assignment pattern lends itself to the use of baccalaureate nurses as team leaders.
3. Primary nursing patterns could use the baccalaureate nurse as the primary nurse and ADs and diploma nurses as associates.

Nursing's Contribution

Budgets of health care agencies are based on projected revenues from, for example, the number of patient days, the number of procedures, and the number of home visits. Nursing contributes to these projected revenues because it contributes to the accomplishment of these objectives.

If there are not enough nursing staff for a hospital or unit, patients cannot be admitted. If, on the other hand, the projected number of patients is not admitted, not as many nurses are needed. Determining and implementing ways of balancing these factors are part of the productivity effort.

Other factors also contribute to a productive health care environment. For example, nurses need to contribute to such patient care decisions as those to transfer patients into and out of intensive care units, to assign special duty nurses, and to admit and discharge patients. Although most decisions are not controlled by nurses, nurses must be involved in those decisions that affect the use of nursing resources. Without this involvement, objective productivity measures may not be valid. Often, health care administrators make decisions based solely on fiscal data and are not aware of their impact on nursing productivity.

Performance Planning

Organizational humanism concerns human interest, values, and the dignity of human beings. The humanist believes that humans are complex, have shifting needs, and strive for perfection. According to Clark (1982), power should be exercised through collaboration and reason rather than imposed by coercion and fear. Performance appraisal processes can be constructive means for humanistic staff development. Quality performance evaluation of staff is done for, not to, staff.

Discontent and restlessness will soon develop in a person unless the individual is doing what he or she individually is fitted for. This Maslovian guide for management is the basis of performance planning appraisal. Performance planning, with follow-up appraisal, is a cooperative venture between the nurse executive and the employee, based on a genuine concern for each other's success (Council & Plachy, 1980). Properly used, the system encourages employee participation and goal achievement.

Performance planning is a way of enhancing communication between the nurse executive and the employee. Praise and helpful criticism can become a regularly scheduled part of evaluation meetings. Such meetings can also serve as valuable opportunities for the nurse executive to learn more about employees, to assess how they have changed, improved, or corrected their performance. It is also an opportunity to cooperatively plan future direction and encourage individual growth. Individual employees differ in growth needs; astute nurse executives recognize early on those individuals who have a desire to move forward. It is easier to fan a glowing flame of interest than to try to find a cinder in the ashes of discontent.

Any type of performance improvement system is meaningless unless the nurse executive has a sincere commitment to the constructive use of such a system. Management by objectives can be a meaningless paper exercise if it generates nonachievable objectives that are demoralizing and inhumane. On the other hand, realistic objectives can be the focus of the well-motivated, creative energies of nursing staff and middle managers. Quality performance appraisal can contribute to a productive environment.

Summary

Although productivity has not often been a concern of nursing, the current environment of cost constraints has given it high priority for nurse executives. Because nurse executives have not necessarily had control of nursing resources, both they and individual nurses have had little incentive to control costs and increase productivity.

Productivity is defined quantitatively and qualitatively. Patient classification tools can provide a framework for measuring productivity. Job satisfaction and a motivating environment are factors that contribute to productivity. Performance planning is an important energizing approach in dealing with low productivity.

STUDY QUESTIONS

1. Define productivity and discuss the factors that influence it in nursing.
2. Describe the symptoms of low productivity.
3. Explain resistance to productivity measures and the rationale for them.
4. What can be done about nonnursing tasks?

5. What recent developments have provided the major impetus to measure and increase nursing productivity?

6. Describe the factors that influence motivation and describe how motivation theories can be used to increase motivation.

7. Discuss the implications of differentiating the roles and performance of professional and technical nurses. Is this important?

8. Name some productivity measurement tools useful for nurses in implementing DRGs and discuss their application.

References

Bennett, A. C. (1983). *Productivity and the quality of work life in hospitals.* Chicago: American Hospital Association.

Clark, M. D. (1982). Performance appraisal, *Nursing Management, 13*(10), 27–29.

Council, J. D., & Plachy, R. J. (1980). Performance appraisal is not enough, *Journal of Nursing Administration, 10*(10), 20–26.

Curtin, L. (1983). Determining costs of nursing services per DRG, *Nursing Management, 14*(4), 16–20.

Easley, C., & Storfjell, J. (1979). *Easley-Storfjell instruments for workload analysis.* Ann Arbor, MI: University of Michigan.

Glaser, E. M. (1976). *Productivity gains through worklife improvements.* New York: Harcourt Brace Jovanovich.

Gordon, G. K. (1982). Motivating staff: A look at assumptions, *Journal of Nursing Administration, 12*(11), 27–28.

Grant, S. E., Bellinger, A. D., & Sweda, B. L. (1982). Measuring productivity through patient classification, *Nursing Administration Quarterly, 6*(3), 77–83.

Grimaldi, P. L., & Micheletti, J. A. (1982). RIMs and the cost of nursing care, *Nursing Management, 13*(12), 12–22.

Hackman, J. R., & Oldham, G. R. (1975). Development of the job diagnostic survey, *Journal of Applied Psychology, 60*(2), 159–170.

Hanson, R. L. (1982). Managing human resources, *Journal of Nursing Administration, 12*(12), 17–23.

Henninger, D., & Dailey, C. (1983). Measuring nursing workload in an outpatient department, *Journal of Nursing Administration, 13*(9), 20–23.

Johnston, S. (1982). The use of the Rines model in differentiating professional and technical practice, *Nursing and Health Care, 3*(7), 374–379.

Joiner, C., Johnson, V., Chapman, J. B., & Corkrean, M. (1982). The motivating potential in nursing specialties, *Journal of Nursing Administration, 12*(2), 26–30.

Kepler, T. L. (1980). Mastering the people skills, *Journal of Nursing Administration, 10*(11), 15–20.

Lavendero, R. (1981). Nurse burnout: What can we learn? *Journal of Nursing Administration, 11*(11, 12), 17–23.

Levinson, H. (1973). Asinine attitudes toward motivation, *Harvard Business Review, 51*(10), 70–76.

Levinson, H. (1983). What nursing administrators say about RIMs and DRGs, *American Journal of Nursing, 83*(10), 1466–1467, 1484.

Rosten, L. (1978). *Passions and prejudices.* New York: McGraw-Hill.

Seuntjens, A. D. (1982). Burnout in nursing: What it is and how to prevent it, *Nursing Administration Quarterly, 7*(1), 12–19.

Skinner, W. (1982). Big hat, no cattle: Managing human resources, Part 1, *Journal of Nursing Administration, 12*(7, 8), 27–29.

Sorrentino, E. A., Nalli, B., & Schriesheim, C. (1992). The effect of head nurse behaviors on nurse job satisfaction and performance, *Hospital and Health Services Administration, 37*(1), 103–113.

Vaill, P. B. (1981, July). *The purposing of high performing systems.* Paper presented at the Conference on Administrative Leadership, University of Illinois.

Bibliography

Rines, A. R. (1977). Development of objectives: Program level/course and unit. In *Preparation of Associate Degree Graduates.* New York: National League for Nursing.

PART VI

Communication

CHAPTER 26

Effective Communication

Highlights

- **Communication with self**
- **Anger**
- **Revitalization of self**
- **One-to-one communication**
- **Group communication**
- **Persuasion**
- **Public speaking**

The purpose of this chapter is to present communication as a concept and a basic management skill with emphasis on the personal aspects of communication.

What messages do I convey about myself to others? Everyday we convey our thoughts and ideas to others through our work and behavior. Gold (1978) describes communication as both a cause of consternation and an enigma. Bordon and Stone (1976) describe it as a contact sport, our only way of contacting others. Communication is the hub of existence and a basic self-tool for survival.

Everything written about communication would consume volumes. A meaningful distillate emerges in the words of Gold: "Whatever else communication is, its definition, scope and purpose, it is a process, and not simply one of language and all its component parts" (Gold, 1978). It is a process with a purpose that an individual consciously or unconsciously uses to affect others.

Each of us has a personality and an appearance like that of no one else in the world. This uniqueness is our most valuable attribute, and it represents a balance between our personal role identities and our professional role identities. All communications between nurses and others involve the two role identities, and they may come into conflict when personal goals conflict with organizational expectations (Bradley & Edinberg, 1982). In the fully functioning administrator, the two personalities merge.

Communication is the central part of everything done in administration. Communication, or lack of it, is one of the most frequently mentioned problems in a division of nursing. Nurse executives write for others to read and read what others have written. Everyday communication flows to and from the nurse executive by virtue of telephone, written materials, computer printouts, and meetings. The basic purpose of communication is to effect change in our environment, in others, and in ourselves.

COMMUNICATING WITH SELF

McGregor and Robinson (1981) present communications with self as the element of first importance in the communication matrix, followed by communication one-to-one and in small groups (see Figure 26.1). The most valuable tools for handling criticism and blame are the confidence and perspective one gains by knowing and communicating with oneself. To communicate with oneself necessitates taking time to think and dream. It involves introspection and self-awareness. It mandates coming to grips with oneself regarding who one is, how one presents oneself, what one thinks is important in life, and, in doing this, determining one's own philosophy of life. It means knowing one's own energy cycle and knowing what place at home or work provides the solitude needed for creative thinking. To be comfortable with oneself in solitude can be energizing.

Time for communication with oneself can be misused if spent in self-blame. Self-criticism is important and an important part of self-renewal if used appropriately. Set aside time on your calendar to think and dream. Take a walk, putter in the kitchen or garden, or sit in a rocking chair and stare engrossed in your own thoughts. Develop a curiosity about your own thoughts, ask yourself questions about an idea. Try to extract a logical decision from intuition. Recognize your brewing times — times when no ideas come forth and you know you are unconsciously mulling over an idea.

Read literature other than that required for your work. Read novels that will help you fantasize. Read science fiction. Above all, take time to appreciate your surroundings and environment. Come to know yourself and understand how you perceive your environment. The ability to think clearly in abstract terms emanates from the ability to communicate with yourself.

Anger

One area in which communication with oneself is very important is anger. Duldt (1981a) states that health professionals frequently encounter anger in their daily practice, yet it is rarely studied. Anger interferes with communication with others and above all with the self. Anger turned inward is a self-destructive process that can lead to depression and burnout (Figure 26.2 presents Duldt's description of the process of anger) (1981b). One needs to recognize the source of anger and explore the underlying reasons for it. Although many authors assume that anger must be worked out with the other person(s), this author believes the first step in resolution of angers is to talk to oneself.

Tasks and *tools* for communicating with:

	Self	One or a few others	Medium to large groups
Top managers	To set standards for self and others To define sense of direction for organization *Self-awareness, self-criticism* *Assess personal and organizational vulnerabilities* *Health habits, diet, exercise*	To use power prudently To stimulate excellence in interpersonal communication To raise levels of social skills To balance organizational and personal communication *Movement, accessibility, listening with eyes and ears* *Personal example, give recognition, praise, reward* *Ceremonial communication, informal exchanges*	To represent organization to general public and own industry or profession To communicate about survival, profitability To pursue quality *Membership, offices* *Staff: researchers, writers, coaches, liaison officers* *Briefings, practice, homework*
Middle managers	To make decisions on use of people and resources To accept and adapt to change To accept and use criticism To sort out and use facts, inferences and value judgements *Six-step decision process* *Fact, inference, opinion* *Reexamine personal goals and values*	To establish favorable interpersonal climate To build relationships with superiors, subordinates, and peers To keep bad-news channels open *Personal example, climate checklist* *Manager-subordinate interview guide* *Unblocking channels for good and bad news*	To maintain open climate To keep higher management informed To communicate within and outside the organization *Circulate, keep news fresh* *Schedule, rotate staff meetings* *Use "hip-pocket" talk*
Front-line managers	To know yourself To think systematically To keep an open mind *Make time to think* *Determine your objective and your audience* *Search for differences* *Eliminate absolutes ("all" and "none"); add "etcetera"*	To understand the basic communication tools To direct, motivate, appraise, counsel To tap the grapevine To use the telephone effectively *Speak, listen, write, read, act, observe* *Interview plan: listen, look to the future*	To communicate with staff, small and large groups To fulfill special assignments *Use meeting planning checklist, meeting do's and don'ts* *Follow outlines for assignments: introductions, awards, retirements*
Staff professionals	To relate priorities to results To start and finish on time To follow professional ethics *Balance effectiveness and efficiency with timing, costs, benefits* *Use energy cycle* *KALM: keep a little margin*	To be understood by nonprofessionals To stimulate interaction inside and outside To help by coaching and ghost writing when needed *Audience analysis: interests, language* *Use a "foot soldier"* *For the grapevine: sensitive ear, discreet tongue*	To present self and organization to outside To prepare for media quiz To make others look good *Monitor trends inside, outside; keep up* *Share current expertise* *Have "hip-pocket" talk ready* *Use professional, trade associations*

← L E V E L S ↓

←———— Numbers ————→

It is important to recognize that anger is an emotion, a state of arousal. Look at yourself in a mirror. Ask yourself what factors contributed to your state of anger. What did you do to bring about the condition? What did others do? What is the pattern of your anger? At whom is it most frequently directed? In what other ways could you react to the same situations? Most organizations recognize excess stress and burnout as interferences with good administration. Few realize the importance of understanding and using anger.

Venting your anger with yourself can occur in various ways. Talk to yourself. Write to yourself. Explain why you are angry. View yourself as objectively as you can. Pretend your best friend is in the same situation. What would you advise him or her to do? Map out a strategy for resolving the anger in the most constructive and least constructive ways. Set a time and date for resolving the problem. Allocate a set time each day for communicating with yourself about the problem, but do not allow yourself to spend more than the allotted time. Continual reworking of the problem can also be destructive.

Revitalization of Self

Another period of communicating with oneself is that special time between jobs when one has time to introspect and revitalize oneself. This may be an enforced period because opportunities did not develop as planned or because a position was phased out because of funding changes or reorganization. Increasingly, nurse executives are subject to severance because of conflicting philosophies with medical staff or hospital administration. This period of time can be very productive or very depressing, depending on one's approach.

Do not make excuses for what went wrong. Analyze the situation in terms of what you learned. Attempt to reopen your mind to all the facts that contributed to the situation. Use this time to sort out your thinking and make decisions about new goals. This can be a fruitful period in terms of self-analysis and self-assessment in terms of personal history. Organize your thoughts and plan to speak to others regarding your experiences. This will not only force you to redirect yourself in a positive manner but will also allow you to share your expertise with others.

One-to-one Communication

Nurse executives play a complex, intertwined combination of interpersonal, informational, and decisional roles. Mintzberg (1975) describes the administrator as the nerve center of the organizational unit. Administrators require "soft" information as well as "hard" data. Soft information can be gossip, hearsay, or speculation. It may be acquired on the telephone, in the office, in the coffee shop, in the restroom, or by the water cooler. First-rate soft information greatly enhances the quantity and quality of information stored in the brain of the nurse executive. Mintzberg (1975) stated that

Figure 26.1 The communication matrix. (From MacGregor, G. F., & Robinson, J. A. (1981). Reprinted, by permission of the publisher, from *The Communications Matrix*, © 1981 by G. F. MacGregor and J. A. Robinson. Published by AMACOM, a division of American Management Associations. All rights reserved.)

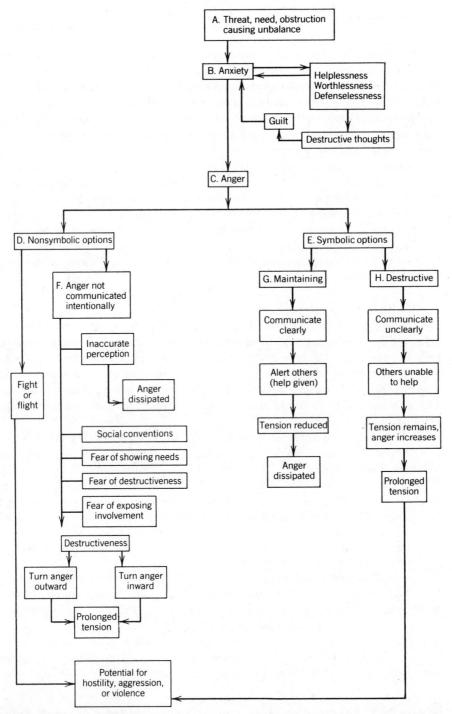

Figure 26.2 The process of anger. (From Duldt, B. (1981). Anger: An occupational hazard for nurses. Copyright © 1981, American Journal of Nursing Company. Reproduced from *Nursing Outlook, 29*(9), p. 514 (September 1981). Reprinted with permission from Mosby-Year Book, Inc.)

the executive may not know everything, but he or she typically knows more than any member of the staff.

One-to-one communication may be thought of in terms of giving and receiving information. The inexperienced executive may not fully realize the value of listening and may perceive one-to-one communication only as an opportunity for disseminating information and delegation. The effective executive spends more time listening than talking. Regularly scheduled one-to-one conferences with subordinates create a positive, healthy climate for interaction—a time for the executive to get to know the staff and a time for staff to understand the executive as a person with goals and ideals for change.

These conferences would be scheduled on a regular basis with all subordinates who report directly to the nurse executive. In addition to getting to know each other, the one-to-one conference serves several other purposes:

1. Updating each other on projects, problem areas, and other pertinent topics
2. Educating each other about clinical or administrative areas
3. Joint problem solving
4. Working on written material
5. Guiding and coaching the subordinate.

This last purpose is perhaps the most important function of the nurse executive who is interested in improving the functioning of the administrative staff. The nurse executive will need to assess each subordinate's strengths and areas for improvement and to encourage self-assessment. Part of each conference time is then spent on providing guidance in the areas for improvement. Various approaches will be needed in providing guidance, for example, discussion about options for problems, role-playing assertiveness, and suggesting literature to read. Of course, the employer will demonstrate growth in the role so that the guidance content of the one-to-one conferences is reduced over time.

THE INTERVIEW

Interviews are golden opportunities to assess the quality of another's attributes and determine the potential for perfect fit with the organization. It is also a time for the interviewer to present himself or herself as an administrator with a sense of direction and enthusiasm for a creative, stimulating work environment. The interview is a special form of one-to-one communication, allowing for both concentrated presentation of self and listening. As with any one-to-one conversation, the participants are particularly vulnerable to overdisclosure of information. The interaction mandates participation, for no others are present. The skilled interviewer prepares in advance, giving attention to topics to be covered or omitted.

GROUP COMMUNICATION

Nurse executives spend most of their time in communication, and committee meetings are increasingly becoming the most frequent group activity. The executive is also involved in large-group, formal presentations within or outside the organization. Public speaking as a special form of group communication is addressed later in this chapter. Small and medium-sized groups are usually task forces or committees established to advance management objectives and facilitate the work of the organization.

Stevens (1975) identifies a critical problem in wasted time through unproductive committee work. She states that chronically unproductive committees should not exist simply because participants enjoy themselves. Perhaps the committee does not need to exist or it consists of the wrong people. The nurse executive needs to decide which groups should exist and whether they should be standing or ad hoc groups. Stevens (1975) describes five different purposes for group meetings:

1. Tell: information transmitted to group
2. Sell: persuasion for acceptance of an idea
3. Seek information: information solicited from group
4. Brainstorm: collection of wide variety of ideas without judgment
5. Seek advice: opinions and judgments transmitted.

All contribute to the data base of the nurse executive and are assistive in decision making or implementing decisions. Although other skills are important in group meetings, those of listening, persuasion, and debate are especially important for the practicing nurse executive.

Generally, in administrative practice, the intermediate-sized group (five to seven members) should be used for problem and conflict resolution. The large group (over seven members) is useful for information giving and voting. The executive should avoid using two-to-three-member groups for conflict resolution and large groups for problem solving (Delbecq, 1979).

Organizing for a committee meeting is a skill that all nurse executives must possess and must teach by example. An organized agenda should include the topic, person responsible, action to be taken, and allotted time. If problem solving is the action to be taken, sufficient time must be allocated for discussion and debate. The executive will be aware if the group is not moving to resolution and can adjust the agenda. Another key factor in having productive meetings is to have members come to the meeting prepared. If materials are to be discussed, they should be distributed well enough in advance.

Persuasion

McGregor and Robinson (1981) define persuasion as any effort to influence or change the beliefs, attitudes, or feelings of another person. The principle purpose of persuasion is to influence change in a planned direction. An individual or group will be persuaded more quickly if the speaker has the group's attention and has personal and professional credibility. The nurse executive will attempt to persuade individuals as well as groups. In both cases, familiarity with concepts and evidence is crucial. Repetition of key words and phrases needs to occur with group members both inside and outside of scheduled meetings.

Nurse executives can learn through practice and appropriate workshops to be highly skilled persuaders. Attention to interpersonal skills, dressing to match the meeting environment, and the ability to argue without abrasiveness contribute to the effectiveness of the persuader. Dress for both comfort and personal style. The image one conveys is another message of persuasion.

Negotiation is the highest level of persuasion. Laser (1981) states that successful negotiation provides satisfaction to both parties and is termed partnering. Both participants emerge as winners in the "I win, you win" relationship. Other levels of persuasion described by Laser (1981) include:

Persuasion: I win, you lose.
Accommodation: I lose, you win.
Compromise: I lose, you lose.

Successful negotiation is the result of:

1. Confidence in presenting a proposal.
2. Timing (date and time of day).
3. Preparation of supporting materials.
4. Attention to verbal and nonverbal communication.
5. Advance orientation to topic (seeding an idea and nurturing its growth and development before final negotiation).

Skilled administrators develop the style of negotiating that is best for them. Testing and evaluating different approaches facilitate this development.

Debate

Effective nurse executives are comfortable in leadership roles, have the ability to deal with conflict, and can engage in effective dialogue while presenting data in support of their position (Gesse & Dempsey, 1981). It is increasingly important to be able to support and defend a position, even if it is unpopular. The ability to defend no cutbacks of the staff is a good example of an administrative decision requiring intelligent and creative persuasion.

Debate involves persuasion and argument at their best. Until recent times, debate was thought to be relegated to politicians. Budget meetings, curriculum meetings, in fact, all meetings resulting in controversial decisions benefit from hearty debate of the issues. Gesse and Dempsey (1981) recommend that debate be used as an important teaching and learning strategy in leadership role seminars. Effective debating requires that the speakers learn to select, conceptualize, and analyze a topic. They must further be able to gather supportive materials and prepare to deliver a talk that will convince others that an idea is sound (Archbold & Hoeffer, 1981).

VERBAL COMMUNICATION

Verbal communication may be thought of as the transmission of human ideas through either the spoken or the written word. Verbal communication can therefore be first- or second-hand, direct or indirect. First-hand, or direct, verbal communication comes out of the oral cavity without opportunity for editorial changes. Second-hand communication — in the form of reports, bulletins, schedules, rumors, assorted papers, and other media — has the potential for tampering with and editing the original data.

Administrators constantly have the problem of putting their words on paper. As Swift (1973) states, the administrator's words in memos and letters are almost always designed to change the behavior of others in the organization. Intelligent written communications are the result of thinking well, composing ideas, writing down the message, editing, and rewriting. Many nurse executives dictate the first draft and then edit and rewrite as needed.

Effective written communication is hard work. Swift (1973) suggests that, to write effectively, administrators must isolate and define the critical variables in the proposed message and then scrutinize the message for clarity, simplicity, and time. He describes writing as feedback and a way for the administrator to discover the self. It is the evidence of one's thinking. In other words, if administrators write well, they think well. If they learn to think well, it will be more likely that they will write well. There is no better way to foster creative thinking habits than to develop message-writing skill.

Fielden (1982) suggests that, to get messages across, one must vary writing style to suit each situation. Expert writers select a style that fits a particular reader and the particular writing situation. Situations are described as positive or negative, conveying good or bad news. Or they may convey a directive or information. Whatever the case, the writer chooses the appropriate words and format to produce the desired result.

The nurse executive must determine the desired effect and select a writing style that will achieve that purpose. Fielden (1982) suggests the following styles as examples:

1. Forceful: direct and active
2. Passive: low power and ambiguous
3. Personal: friendly and positive
4. Impersonal: nonuse of personal names
5. Colorful: flowery, many adjectives and verbs.

In addition, nurse executives should develop a vocabulary that personalizes all their messages.

NONVERBAL COMMUNICATION

Nurse executives are known by the clothes they wear and the company they keep. Nonverbal communication emanates from each person in personality style, choice of food, housing, office arrangement, priorities for appointments, and social habits. In other words, one's behavior travels as an advance guard every time one speaks in public or attends public activities. Everything an executive does is open for criticism, either positive or negative. Assessment of personal characteristics may be based on whether one is a cat or a dog person. Does one always go along with the crowd, or does one favor individualized activities? How much does the executive value personal privacy? Overemphasis on personal privacy may be viewed as detrimental to the organization. The effective executive uses nonverbal communication deliberately.

FORMAL AND INFORMAL GROUPS

To create a climate in which the nurse executive can maintain a flow of communication to and from staff, among staff, and to and from the rest of the organization is a major challenge. Useful information is everywhere, and the excellent nurse executive must access it either directly or indirectly. Get out and be seen, move around, listen to the grapevine, talk some but do not give away too much, listen a lot. Schedule and hold regular staff meetings. Attend required meetings most of the time.

Direct information generally is obtained through meetings of formal groups such as standing committees, boards, and other institutional groups requiring the presence of the nurse executive. The formal group situations also allow the nurse executive time for informal exchange with members of other disciplines.

Informal groups are characterized by irregularly occurring meetings between two or more persons without agendas. These tend to deal with immediate concerns, but often the topic is content for a larger range of problem resolutions. The nurse executive may find the informal group occupying a good deal of time if formal groups do not meet regularly with agendas to which everyone has a chance to contribute. Informal groups can bring out valuable information that does not always fit in the format of a formal meeting with a tight agenda. Informal, casual encounters may be arranged to break communication barriers with members of established formal groups.

COMPUTER TECHNOLOGY

The computer is a wondrous thing
A million benefits it can bring
It can store our files
Eliminate our paper piles
Save hours of calculation
And enable data manipulation

But if we don't manage this thing
A million headaches, it can bring.
We'll need a well planned approach
And ensure that our managers we coach
We'll need a user's point of view
And, boss, the whole thing depends on you.*

The key to using computers in nursing administration is understanding them. According to Worthley (1982), the basis of the problems encountered in using computers is the unenlightened use of technology. Although the technology is well developed, the management and use of computer technology is underdeveloped.

No administrator would think of running an office without a typewriter or a copying machine. Yet many nurse executives are not comfortable with computers and fail to see them as an exciting tool that can enhance their management skills. Worthley (1982) suggests that computers are resisted for many reasons:

1. Fear of losing jobs to computers
2. Professionals' fear of the loss of prestige and status as the result of computer usage

---

*Reprinted with permission from Worthley, J. A. (1982). *Managing computers in health care: A guide for professionals.* Ann Arbor, MI: AUPHA Press.

3. Resistance to control of information by machines
4. Belief that it is socially acceptable to resist computers
5. Fear of losing professional human-to-human contact
6. Previous negative experiences.

Historically, most new inventions have caused consternation and fear. People tried to stop the use of the first Model T Fords. The telephone was much feared, as were the first electric lights. Understanding nuclear technology is almost as difficult as understanding computer technology for many individuals. Both technologies have the capacity for easing human work, but both are constantly under challenge.

Harnessing computer technology in nursing has the potential for freeing professional nurses to practice nursing in its most humane form. Time-consuming record-keeping activities and the ordering of supplies can be extensively simplified using computers. Patient classification and care audits and staffing and scheduling activities are just a few of the communication activities that can be facilitated with computers. The most sophisticated systems establish patient files in computer memory and have provisions for adding information to those files on an on-line, real-time basis (Farlee, 1978). The able nurse executive should rate a computerized nursing information system as a high priority and take full advantage of institutional computer experts in planning implementation.

PUBLIC SPEAKING

Public speaking is an important and expected part of the nurse executive's role. Fully functioning administrators need to be able to speak in public forums, panel discussions, social gatherings, open board meetings, and various other formal gatherings. Impromptu talks and requests for one's opinion are part of the job. The ability to deliver formal scholarly papers is often a qualification for the job and also one of its duties.

Clear, effective public speaking can be mastered. It emanates from the ability to think clearly and set objectives. It emanates from a curiosity about the world of work and the world at large. It emanates from a strong internal sense of eagerness to share knowledge about a topic. One cannot present a topic that one is not interested in; one cannot present a talk of merit if one lacks self-confidence.

To prepare to be a speaker of worth, it is important to read, absorb, and create files for "bits" of information about a topic of interest. Several weeks before a scheduled presentation, communicate with yourself as to what you want to present. Write an outline for your talk, and edit and revise it until you are sure it meets the needs of your audience. Be comfortable with making changes as additional information causes you to believe changes are necessary. Until one becomes a practiced, accomplished, self-confident speaker, one should tape a practice session and review for clarity and tone.

Pay attention to clothing, for one's attire will convey a message, as will the speech given. Public speaking is a human-to-human process. The speaker must develop a sense of responding to cues in the audience. Are they listening? Can they understand you? Are you delivering a message? All effective communication implies messages sent and messages received.

Most nurse executives are expected to be able to give a variety of public presentations, ranging from orienting new staff, to progress reports, to scholarly papers based on research or literature review. All types of communication convey a message from the administrator and the institution and need to be thoughtfully prepared.

Summary

This chapter has presented communication as a concept and a basic management skill. The importance of communication with self and others in formal and informal groups is especially emphasized. Although computer technology is well developed elsewhere, the use of computerized information systems is not widespread in nursing administration. Harnessing this technology has the potential for freeing nurses to practice nursing in its most humane form.

STUDY QUESTIONS

1. To what extent do you communicate with yourself about work-related problems or issues?

2. How do you personally prepare for small group interactions?

3. Select a recent situation in which you interacted with several people in a formal group structure. How did you communicate verbally and nonverbally?

4. Considering your immediate peers, whom do you consider an effective communicator? Why?

5. How do you plan to nurture your computer utilization skills over the next five years?

6. Describe your public speaking style.

7. How computer literate are you? Do you use a computer in your everyday life?

References

Archbold, P. C., & Hoeffer, B. (1981). Reframing the issue: A debate on third-party reimbursement, *Nursing Outlook, 29*(7), 423–427.

Bordon, G. A., & Stone, J. D. (1976). *Human communication.* Menlo Park, CA: Cummings Publishing Co.

Bradley, J. C., & Edinberg, M. A. (1982). *Communication in the nursing context.* New York: Appleton-Century-Crofts.

Delbecq, A. L. (1979). *The art and politics of decision making.* Paper presented at the Michigan Nurses Association, May 11, 1979.

Duldt, B. W. (1981a). Anger: An alienating communication hazard for nurses, *Nursing Outlook, 29*(11), 640–644.

Duldt, B. W. (1981b). Anger: An occupational hazard for nurses, *Nursing Outlook, 29*(9), 510–518.

Farlee, C. (1978). The computer as a focus of organizational change in the hospital, *Journal of Nursing Administration, 8*(2), 20–26.

Fielden, J. S. (1982). What do you mean you don't like my style? *Harvard Business Review, 60*(3), 128–138.

Gesse, T., & Dempsey, P. (1981). Debate as a teaching-learning strategy, *Nursing Outlook, 29*(7), 421–423.

Gold, H. (1978). Communicating with others: One to one. In L. M. Simms & J. Lindberg (Eds.), *The Nurse Person.* New York: Harper & Row.

Laser, R. J. (1981). I win—you win negotiating, *Journal of Nursing Administration, 11*(11,12), 24–29.

McGregor, G. F., & Robinson, J. A. (1981). *The communication matrix.* New York: AMACOM.

Mintzberg, H. (1975). The manager's job: Folklore and fact, *Harvard Business Review, 53*(4), 49–61.

Stevens, B. J. (1975). Use of groups for management, *Journal of Nursing Administration, 5*(1), 14–22.

Swift, M. H. (1973). Clear writing means clear thinking means . . . , *Harvard Business Review, 51*(1), 59–62.

Worthley, J. A. (1982). *Managing computers in health care.* Ann Arbor, MI: Health Administration Press.

CHAPTER 27

Mentorship and Networking

Catherine Buchanan

Highlights

- **The role of mentors and sponsors**
- **What is a mentor?**
- **Mentors and mentor relationships**
- **Women and mentors**
- **Benefits of mentoring for the mentor and the protégé**
- **Becoming a mentor**

Nurse executives often do not consider networking or mentors in the development of a successful career. This is particularly true of nurses who occupy middle management positions in health care organizations. A powerful and influential person within an organization acting as a mentor or sponsor can make a crucial difference in providing visibility, credibility, and acceptance. The purpose of this chapter is to present the nature, characteristics, and consequences of mentor and networking and their application to nursing administrative practice.

Without question, women entering fields and professions that are traditionally male dominated are encouraged to enter under the aegis of a mentor. Wynter and Soloman (1989) coined the barrier that prevents women from moving up the career ladder to top level executive positions as the "glass ceiling." This subtle barrier often stalls women in middle management positions. They are able to view the next level but are unable to break the glass ceiling to advance their careers.

In their study of nurse executives Price, Simms, and Pfoutz (1987) substantiated the presence of influential persons in the professional and personal lives of their respondents. The value of role modeling, teaching, and encouragement surfaced as descriptions of career advancement assistance.

THE ROLE OF MENTORS AND SPONSORS

Mentorship has received increased attention as an important element in career development. It has been especially popularized in business literature as the means to a successful climb up the corporate ladder (Cook, 1980; Hennig & Jardim, 1977a; Kanter, 1977; Levinson et al., 1978; Lundig, Clements, & Perkins, 1978; Martin & Strauss, 1968; Roche, 1979; Shapiro, Haseltine, & Row, 1978; Warihay, 1980). Men, women are told, hold the key to success in their chosen occupations and professions because they are competitive, politically wise, and help each other via the "old boy's network." Further, if women are to succeed, they must be socialized into this network. This "tuning-in" process for both men and women is accomplished with the assistance of mentors, or sponsors.

Researchers interested in organizational behavior have identified the mentor phenomenon. The distinguishing function of the mentor is to access power and influence for the protégé. "A major influence determining who moves and how far is the action of the sponsor. When the sponsor rises, the protégé moves with him. Which career lines are chosen or available often depends on the action of a sponsor" (Martin & Strauss, 1968, p. 203).

Kanter (1977) describes an informal pattern of selection observed in her study of a complex business organization. Individuals in the fast lane were affiliated with sponsors who served as influential and powerful conduits for their protégés. Men and women who moved up without sponsorship were often stalled at some point in their career and denied admission to the inner circles of upwardly mobile elites. Sponsors not only prepare their protégés for upward mobility but also influence how they are received by those in higher echelons.

WHAT IS A MENTOR?

The term "sponsor" reached popularity in the 1960s and early 1970s. Today, the commonly accepted term is "mentor." "Sponsor," "mentor," and "role model" are often used interchangeably, but most would agree that mentoring is reserved for a relationship that is more special, intense, and enduring than that implied by modeling (Levinson et al., 1978).

It has been suggested that role modeling is not effective in helping women acquire reputations of influence and power. The strategies used by those who have achieved success may not be relevant to succeeding generations of women. Searching for the role model who encompasses all the attributes associated with success is discouraged. Instead, a combination of models may be more appropriate. This provides the novice an opportunity to choose the traits he or she wishes to emulate while rejecting others.

A patron system that embraces a continuum of support is proposed by Shapiro, Haseltine, & Rowe (1978). Mentor and peer pals are the two end points, with sponsor and guide as internal positions on the continuum. Mentor is the most intense and paternalistic relationship on the continuum. Social selection, ascription, and trust are characteristics of this relationship. Next is the sponsor relationship, defined as supportive but not powerful in terms of career advancement. This relationship tends to be encouraging, corroborating, and confidence building in nature. Guides, the next position on the continuum, function to steer individuals. They often provide helpful information about the system, pitfalls to avoid, and standard norms of behavior. Guides are usually administrative assistants or executive secretaries. They also function as gatekeepers who control access to the elite in an organization. Last on the continuum is the relationship between peers: peer pals. Peers share information of mutual interest, serve as a sounding board for one another, support one another, and generally develop relationships that help one another grow, progress, and succeed in career endeavors.

Dalton, Thompson, and Price (1977) advance a model of career organization consisting of four stages: apprentice, colleague, mentor, and sponsor. The apprentice stage is a dependent relationship that involves learning experiences. The collegial stage supports independence. The mentor is involved in helping the apprentice. The sponsor is an individual involved in the direction of an organization through policy formulation and the promotion of key people.

Yoder's (1990) concept analysis of mentoring reveals a more traditional version that she based on Bowen's (1985) definition:

Mentoring occurs when a senior person (the mentor) in terms of age and experience undertakes to provide information, advice and emotional support for a junior person (the protege) in a relationship lasting over an extended period of time and marked by substantial emotional commitment by both parties. If the opportunity presents itself, the mentor also uses both formal and informal forms of influence to further the career of the protege. (Yoder, 1990, p. 31)

According to Yoder (1990), role modeling, sponsorship, precepting, peer strategizing, as well as being one's own mentor should not be used interchangeably with the mentoring process. The emphasis in this analysis focused on the intensity of the relationship, psychosocial and personal commitment to the relationship by both parties, and the protracted period of time both persons are loyal to the process as being the hallmark of the concept of mentorship.

CHARACTERISTICS OF MENTORS AND MENTOR RELATIONSHIPS

Typically, mentors are highly placed in an organization. They are usually associated with the most powerful and influential people. Frequently they are men, simply because women are not in the higher management echelons in most organizations. Sometimes a mentor has more than one protégé within the organization.

Levinson et al. (1978) describes the relationship between mentor and protégé as a love relationship, intense, not sexual. It often occurs naturally and spontaneously. The experience is described as similar to falling in love in that it cannot be arranged or mandated. Many protégés describe their mentors as father figures, wise, loyal, trustworthy, and protective.

A comparison can be made between mentoring and Erickson's (1963) generativity stage of development. Human beings reach a stage in their development that requires them to give others the benefit of their life's experiences. It is the process of passing from one generation to another the values, standards, and norms of the former generation.

Ideally, a similar process occurs between mentor and protégé. Mentor passes to protégé values and standards that maintain continuity and stability of leadership within the organization. The mentor prepares the next generation of leaders.

Blackburn, Chapman, and Cameron (1981) describe this grooming process as cloning. The mentor fashions the protégé in his or her own image and likeness. This style of grooming occurs in the preparation of scientists. The novice scientist mimics the master in ways that benefit the continuity of scientific excellence. It is often through the eminence of the mentor that the work of the protégé is recognized.

Zuckerman's (1977) study of the Nobel laureates provides evidence of the valuable link between bright young scientists and their eminent sponsors. The socialization of the next generation of prize winners is the unofficial domain of the laureates in science. It is understood that the work of science is passed from one generation to the next. It is accepted that a laureate will guide and promote the successful achievements of the next generation of Nobel prize winners.

WOMEN AND MENTORS

Women need mentors at two crucial points in their lives: during the early stages of career development and during the final thrust to the top (Holcomb, 1980). The majority of nurses who remain at the practice level and work in hospitals need different sponsorship activities. These nurses need ongoing access to career guidance and informal informational counseling about the hospital system (Campbell-Heider, 1986).

Studies of women in top level management positions indicate that they had help from a mentor, usually a male boss (Hennig & Jardim, 1977b). In contrast, women who failed to establish upwardly mobile career patterns were without sponsors and other support relationships (Kanter, 1977). There are, however, some important considerations for women who engage in mentor-protégé relationships with men.

Cross-gender mentoring — as exists between a male mentor and a female protégé — is discouraged by some authorities (Levinson et al., 1978). Stereotyping is cited as one barrier that influences the relationship negatively. It is believed that commonly held attitudes about women may interfere with the effectiveness of the mentor: "she is bright but not committed," "she is too pretty to be committed to a career," "she will get married, get pregnant, and leave."

Another barrier involves the perception of peers and colleagues. Men and women fear being linked to illicit relationships in the workplace. Mentor-protégé affiliations can fall victim to the faulty perceptions of others, resulting in severe damage to reputations and careers. Organizations can remedy this potential threat by a willingness to recognize the mentor-protégé relationship as a positive and sound force in the preparation of leadership skills. This in turn is beneficial to the organization. Generation continuity and homogeneity of leadership is the prized objective of most organizations (Lundig, Clements, & Perkins, 1970; Darling, 1985a).

The final barrier in cross-gender mentoring is the fear of the mentor-marital triad (Epstein, 1970). The intensity of the relationship can be disruptive when marital partners are not clear about the intent and purpose of the protégé's relationship to the mentor. Working late, an occasional trip out of town, and the importance of the mentor in the professional life of the protégé are all potential problems in the triad.

It is by virtue of its intensity and focus that the mentor-protégé affiliation is the best method for grooming future leaders; by its very nature, mentoring can be both valued and feared. Unless mentoring, especially cross-gender mentoring, is a legitimate structure within an organization, both men and women are reluctant to risk its hazards. In spite of the risks, however, cross-gender mentoring has been successful. Women have reported enormous benefit from their work with male mentors (Cameron & Blackburn, 1981; Hennig & Jardim, 1977b; Sheehy, 1974).

A less intense, less personal relationship has benefits as well. Mentors and protégés can adjust their expectations of each other by maintaining only a professional interest in the relationship. Such a modified version of the more intense prototype can be effective in sponsoring efforts (Cameron & Blackburn, 1981).

MENTORING NURSES

The barriers and attitudes concerning the role of women in the workplace are concentrated in nursing. In addition to overcoming the barriers created by cross-gender mentoring already mentioned, nurses must overcome the stereotype attributed to their profession. The attitude that nurses should be content with traditional nursing roles and leave the task of comprehensive health and fiscal planning and management to those best suited — namely, hospital administrators and physicians — is a major barrier. This perception, commonly held by men in health care management, is often shared by nurses (Puetz, 1983).

Another common attitude is that nurses are educated to provide service. They are not expected to provide meaningful management direction for an institution. The nursing profession itself is ambivalent about nurse executive roles in health care organizations. This ambivalence is manifested by confusion about the best arrangement of clinical and management components in graduate programs preparing nurse executives. Nursing staff in health care settings are not supportive of nurse executives who cannot demonstrate clinical practice skills, but they also expect the executive to possess the necessary skills to access power and credibility in the higher echelons of management within the institution.

These attitudes constitute a barrier that thwarts the desire and progress of the nurse executive who is capable of assuming greater responsibility and career diversity. Although same-gender mentoring is advocated for both men and women and would seem to alleviate the problems and attitudes inherent in cross-gender mentor-protégé relationships, the dilemma posed by the employment of too few women in the upper echelons of management is a reality. Women, and especially nurses, are often stalled in middle-management positions because they lack visibility and opportunities for the men who are in power to see them behave effectively (Felton, 1978).

WOMEN MENTORING WOMEN

Women often are not supportive of each other's efforts in the workplace. Halsey (1978) uses the phrase "queen bee" to describe senior managers who lack interest in the careers of their juniors and give them little assistance in securing promotion and advancement.

The queen bee is unwilling to see her role as a sponsor of other women. She is motivated by self-interest and fear of losing a position that she believes she earned through her own hard work and initiative. Spitzer (1981) summarizes the queen bee syndrome in nursing as:

1. Identification with those in higher hierarchical positions.
2. Alignment with the establishment and resistance to change.
3. Projection of antifeminist beliefs about other women.
4. A need to run the show at the expense of other competent women. (p. 22)

Darling (1985b) refers to any negative mentor relationship as toxic. She categorizes these toxic mentor behaviors as avoiders, dumpers, and destroyer/criticizers. Antidotes to a toxic situation include identifying the nature and source of the relationship as well as any past unrelated experiences that are being attributed to the situation, understanding the mentor's current situation and needs so that exceptions can be applied, and finally balancing the relationship with other support networks if getting out of the relationship is not an option.

Most mentor-mentee rifts occur when the mentor has a position of authority over the mentee (Darling, 1985c). Conversely, this similar configuration in the relationship is necessary to promote the credibility and visibility of the one being mentored.

Research has shown that there is another side to the issue of women supporting each other. Warihay (1980) has found that the support giver and the support receiver have different perceptions of the amount of support given. Those in the upper echelons always report giving more than their junior colleagues report receiving. Such perceptions are troublesome, especially in situations in which there are few women at the top levels of management and many in the lower echelons. These perceptions inhibit women in top management from facilitating the career development of other women.

How men in nursing are affected by cross-gender and same-gender mentor-protégé affiliations is not precisely known. There is a paucity of data addressing the issue of male nursing careers and their mentorship experiences. Until the number of men in nursing increases substantially, nursing will continue to be identified as a profession of women. It is important to assume, however, that men in nursing administration are confronted with similar obstacles with respect to cross-gender mentor-protégé relationships. Same-gender mentor-protégé affiliations may be more favorable for the career promotion of men in nursing management, given the tendency of men in senior management ranks to support their junior counterparts.

BENEFITS OF MENTORING FOR THE MENTOR AND THE PROTÉGÉ

Benefits for the protégé include recognition, encouragement, and an opportunity to establish a confidential sounding board. Increased morale and productivity are often related benefits (Atwood, 1979). Honest criticism, informal feedback, nonjudgmental guidance, and an insistence by the mentor that the only performance is the best performance are vital to leadership growth. Knowing that one is being groomed for leadership by a recognized mentor is an experience that has no equal. The nurse executive who demonstrates a power stance beyond his or her expected role needs the support and direction of a recognized mentor who can smooth the way and access power and influence. The nurse executive's credibility and reputation require facilitation by another who is accepted and respected within the organization.

Benefits for the mentor include an opportunity to pass on one's values and standards, increasing the satisfaction that comes from helping another develop the attributes of leadership. The potential to discover oneself by helping others is not a new or different idea. The relationship can help the mentor fulfill professional responsibilities as a supervisor who is interested in those in the lower ranks. It also provides the mentor-manager a support system for policies and activities affecting people in the lower ranks of the organization with whom the protégé may have daily contact. Within the context of nursing administration, there exists for the mentor a nurse executive protégé who can execute a smoother, more cooperative management triad among nursing and support staff, nursing management, and agency administration. The perceived dichotomy between administration and service, which tends to polarize administrators and practitioners, can be ameliorated through the joint efforts of the mentor and the protégé. Such depolarization, in turn, benefits the organization.

CHOOSING MENTORSHIP

It is advisable for upwardly mobile men and women to seek a mentor. Several may be needed at various junctures in a career to serve as information conduits, provide support, and assist in developing leadership behaviors. The following questions and statements are intended to assist the nurse executive in assessing his or her need and desire for sponsorship in career development (Hall & Sandler, 1983). The questions can be altered to adapt to a particular institution or management level. They are not intended to be comprehensive; rather, their purpose is to stimulate a career-planning mode of thought:

1. What circumstances and situations within your organization are best suited for increasing your visibility?
2. What attitudes and behaviors are rewarded by your supervisors in your organization?
3. What are the organization's formal and informal criteria for promotion and salary adjustment beyond the nursing director level of management?
4. Who are the decision makers involved in your advancement in the organization?
5. Who speaks for you at board meetings and policy planning sessions when you are not invited or are unable to attend?
6. Who can nominate you for promotions, prizes, awards, or important committee assignments or simply indicate you are the best person to get a certain job done?

7. Who defends you when ideas and people come together in conflicting patterns? Who makes certain you are heard even when you voice unpopular or controversial ideas (someone to steady the boat you have just rocked)?

8. How is "inside information" disseminated, policy created, approval for successful change projects achieved, and important decisions regarding staffing, budget, salary, and so on made?

9. Who are the powerful and important people in your organization and who has their ear?

10. Does your organization's structure support role changes and extensions with respect to nurses and other professionals?

Being able to answer these questions in some detail provides the framework for a decision with respect to one's need for a mentor.

BECOMING A MENTOR

In deciding whether to become a mentor, one must consider what one can offer a protégé. Equally important is a consideration of the benefits one can derive from a mentoring relationship. What one can offer a protégé has a great deal to do with the allocation of one's time and energy.

The mentor may begin by providing the protégé visibility at meetings, business luncheons, and preparation and feedback sessions in conjunction with presentations and projects initiated by the protégé. Many men and women appreciate a mentor's assistance with appropriate dress, hairstyle, and body language. The management of career, marriage, and childbearing is a crucial area of conflict for women, and learning to juggle these competing responsibilities necessitates a support system, preferably from those with similar experiences. A mentor could provide knowledgable assistance with such problems. Thus, mentoring is lending one's personal help to a talented person. Ultimately, the mentor must be willing to put his or her reputation on the line for the protégé's sake (Moore, 1982). J. D. Watson, famed Nobel laureate, remarked, from the perspective of a young scientist, "It is extra-ordinarily important that you have a . . . patron because there'll be times when you are bound to strike it bad and you'll need somebody to convince people that you are not irresponsible" (Zuckerman, 1977, pp. 134–135).

The critical shortage of qualified, competent professional nurse managers in the higher echelons of health care administration suggests the need for the early identification of leadership talent and the sponsorship of that talent by other talented and respected nurses. In this era of rapidly changing health care demands, nurses must be trained to assume leadership roles. The time required to prepare competent leadership must be shortened and addressed as a professional responsibility. The talents of our current leaders must not be lost.

MENTORING ATTITUDES AND BEHAVIOR

Mentors must reconcile the differing perceptions inherent in the roles of mentor and protégé by making explicit the extent to which they can and will offer guidance concerning personal and professional issues. Some authorities suggest that the signing of a contract by both parties in agreement to the terms of the mentorship relationship assures clarity of purpose and direction (Hart, 1980). Whether the relationship is formal or informal, it is important to know its parameters and constraints ahead of time.

The mentor must provide feedback to the protégé as a function of the mentorship relationship. Such feedback should be framed in an objective context that presents praise and criticism as specifically as possible. The mentor should be prepared to stand by the protégé. The professional stature of the fledgling leader must be protected. At times, the mentor may give the protégé an added degree of credibility and growth advantage by letting others know the protégé speaks for the mentor. For example, the protégé can replace the mentor's contributions at meetings, presentations, and conferences.

Fagan and Fagan (1983) in their research discovered a strong link between job satisfaction and mentoring. They recommend that nurse executives encourage both informal mentoring and formal mentor programs to improve professional development within their organization.

As much as possible, the nurse executive–mentor should include other nurses in both professional and informal activities. Inviting a novice manager to a luncheon session with senior management people is an effective way to advertise the mentor's investment in the protégé. Mentoring need only consist of informing a junior colleague of available resources and being willing to support his or her professional endeavors. This support may consist of advice about job advancement, strategies, or an opportunity to rehearse the presentation of a project to a group of influential leaders in the organization.

The mentor must socialize the protégé into a competitive environment. Female nurses, like many women, are not prepared for this dimension of the workplace. In a sense, nurses are similar to the Nobel laureate who described his need for a sponsor to compete in the institution of science: "I knew the technique . . . I had a lot of knowledge. I had the words, the libretto, but not the music. What was missing was an opportunity to work with men of high quality" (Zuckerman, 1977, p. 123).

Nurses are firmly grounded in their knowledge of nursing care, but they are not equally schooled in the effective discharge of this function in a competitive environment. To establish successful career patterns, nurse executives need to increase their sphere of influence, project credibility, be accepted as important contributors, to the policy formulation of their institutions, and be treated as equals with other influential people in the system. Career advances in an organization require the socializing influence of a sponsor. The central purpose of mentoring is to provide the protégé with a competitive advantage so that ability can be transformed into effective leadership skills. For some, mentoring may not be possible, advantageous, or desirable. Whatever the nature of the support, however, we all need someone with whom we can share our hopes and career aspirations, a person who will promote our ideas and our best work and place us in a competitive sphere in which we can prove our abilities and worth. Mentors are in a real sense a necessary ingredient of self-actualization in the workplace. Maestro and pianist, master and artist, and rabbi and student have been paired throughout history so that the very best could give to the best in an effort to preserve the continuity of excellence. Although mentors are not a substitute for competence, commitment, ability, and hard work, these things alone, unfortunately, do not bring the success and reputation that women and men of ability deserve in the workplace.

THEORY OF NETWORKING

In addition to researching mentor affiliations as a strategy of promoting career advancement and opportunities, social scientists have investigated the phenomenon of networking. Data indicate that inclusion in a profession is associated with career success. A measurement of the degree of inclusion in one's profession is, in turn, associated with networking activities (Buchanan, 1984). Networking provides the visibility and means to disseminate one's ability, talents, and professional support to others.

Aldrich (1976) defines a network as the totality of all the units connected by a certain type of relationship and is constructed by finding the ties between all the members within a bounded system. Further, networks develop basically from two types of relationships: *(1)* family and close friends and *(2)* professional and other infrequent contacts.

The common networking bond between family and close friends is a similarity of beliefs, values, attitudes, and social origins. Support and information exchange characterize the bond between professionals and other social contacts. Granovetter (1973) categorized family and close friends as strong ties that exert a substantial influence on the behavior of those in the network. Communication patterns tend to be predictable, uniform, and repetitive. Members of such networks are usually few and, thus, have limited access to a wide variety of information sources.

Professional and social contacts are considered weak ties. Relationships within such a network structure exercise less influence on the behavior of members than do strong ties. Because communication patterns are less predictable, more varied, and not repetitive, weak ties provide greater opportunity for the communication of original and expert information. This pattern of communication and its potential for unlimited sources of information is the rationale for the strength of weak ties in facilitating career progress. Thus, the weak-tie theory supports the notion that mobilizing a large weak-tie network enables one to gain access to individuals, groups, and systems for the purpose of achieving occupational, professional, personal, and social goals.

MEN AND WOMEN AND NETWORKING BEHAVIOR

Kleiman (1980) considers networks "a step beyond role models and mentors, a necessary next step for women if they want to achieve their professional and career goals" (p. 6). Increasingly, women are turning to other women in an effort to gain professional visibility, exchange information, identify job opportunities, reduce isolationism for women in token positions, support one another in professional growth endeavors, and provide emotional reinforcement. However, networking is a relatively new experience for women. What men achieve quite naturally in their contacts and support of each other is not as commonplace for women.

Patricia Wyskocil, vice president and director of marketing for the First Los Angeles Bank, observes that "men bond naturally and network instinctively" (Kleiman, 1980, p. 8). Josefowitz (1980) suggests that "just as men relax in a very special way when alone with their own sex group, women too have a special bonding that occurs when they are together without men" (p. 101). It is equally important for men and women to network together in a mixed-gender support group, according to Josefowitz.

The discomfort a woman may feel entering a male-dominated group is identical to that of a man entering an all-female group. However, an effort must be made by both men and women to gain admission to networks within their organizational workplace and professional systems. Not only is work-oriented gossip shared at network meetings — which occur over lunch, after work, or on weekends — but so is important inside information. Through networking, alliances are developed, connections made, and concerns aired. Although it may not be easy to gain entry to certain networks or to subdue feelings of discomfort as a new member in some groups, the nurse executive must seek access to the most influential networks in the health care organization.

Nurses, in particular, encounter difficulty moving out of their sphere of comfort. This is in part due to the traditional separation of the nurse and the physician socially and professionally within health care settings and the lack of assertiveness that continues to be part of the subservient role of traditional nursing service.

Particularly relevant to nurse executives is the contention of Warihay (1980) that in some organizations where few women enjoy the career benefits of upper management, developing a new women's network may be premature. The women in need of support may far outnumber those available to give it. In addition, limiting sources of support to women would tend to narrow career mobility. Thus, any man or woman in one's organization who will be an ally and is supportive of women and men and their achievement perspective warrants inclusion in a network.

PROFESSIONAL NETWORKING

The importance of networking in achieving professional goals has been demonstrated in academe (Cameron & Blackburn, 1981; Buchanan, 1984). Data indicate that a linkage exists among career success, inclusion in one's profession, and networking activities. Successful nurse academicians report that involvement in professional networks is critical in establishing successful career patterns.

Nursing colleagues occupying prestigious positions as journal referees, publishers, grant reviewers, and officers of professional nursing organizations and groups are invaluable sources of professional support for the nurse academician. Networking among academicians is a time-honored institution. Crane (1972) calls such unstructured arrangements "invisible colleges." The dissemination of knowledge is the underlying purpose of such networks. Academicians network about their interests, projects, successes, and each other. These contacts form a valuable link among colleagues within the community of scholars.

Nurse executives must provide similar access to each other as well as senior and junior managers within the health care system. Puetz (1983) and O'Connor (1982) provide a comprehensive overview of the art of networking. They discuss attitudes, skills, and behaviors pertinent to the development of a network culture in nursing. These authors emphasize the necessity of supportive activity between professionals. Using the experience and understanding of others can reduce feelings of isolation and promote self-esteem when career progress is stalled or discouraged by others in an organization.

Networking requires a commitment based on professional competence, reliability, and credibility. O'Connor (1982) aptly points out that "networks provide suggestions, direction, guidance, and support, not solutions" (p. 40). Clarity and honesty based on what one can offer another or what one needs from others is vital to successful networking. In addition, incorporating cross-gender and varied professional representation in one's networking systems will greatly enhance and expand the likelihood of achieving professional goals.

Nurse executives have opportunities to network within their local, state, and national spheres of influence in nursing. This can be accomplished through professional organizations and groups or simply by making contact with others in the professional nurse and health care management community. One reason nurses are rarely invited to debate or report important health issues — as are physicians and other health care specialists — is that they lack professional networking skills. Nurses can also establish important weak ties across professions. For example, they can network with journalists concerning women's health issues, the problems of aging, or clarifying the media-imposed image of professional nursing.

When one needs the assistance and support of others, others often feel the same way. When individuals come together with mutual interests and concerns, a network is created. It is unnecessary to endure self-imposed isolation from peers and colleagues.

Summary

There are varying degrees of assistance identified as positive forces in the development of a satisfying career. Mentorship is one aspect of the patron system of support that nurses are encouraged to adopt. Nurse executives are vulnerable to the barriers women in the workplace encounter as they attempt to move into the higher echelons of power and influence within health care organizations. There is evidence to support the view that the assistance of a respected, influential person can be a critical factor in promoting successful career endeavors.

Until greater numbers of nurses achieve positions of authority in health care organizations, they must support each other and recognize the need for cross-gender mentor-protégé affiliations. In addition to sponsorship, nurses in leadership positions contact their peers and colleagues through networks. There are data to support the link between networking, inclusion in a profession, and career satisfaction and success. The individual must determine the most effective support system for promoting his or her professional stature and achieving successful career development.

THOUGHT PROVOKING QUESTIONS

1. Critically analyze the advantages and disadvantages of mentor-protégé relationships in a health care setting.

2. Develop a role description of the nurse executive as a mentor and as a protégé.

3. Identify various people within a health care setting most appropriate to mentor a nurse executive.

4. Evaluate the mentoring strengths and weaknesses of each potential mentor identified in question 3.

5. What is the nurse executive's role in creating and legitimatizing a positive environment for mentoring and networking?

6. Draw up a contract between mentor and protégé explicating the terms of the relationship and the responsibilities of each.

7. Critically evaluate the place of role modeling on the support continuum as it relates to the nurse executive.

8. Cite the paradoxical nature inherent in cross-gender mentor-protégé relationships.

9. Formulate a definition of mentoring applicable to the nurse executive's career advancement.

10. Explain the theory supporting the career advantage of participating in networks.

References

Aldrich, H. (1976). *Organizational sets, action sets and networks: Making the most of simplicity.* New York: Cornell University.

Atwood, A. H. (1979). The mentor in clinical practice, *Nursing Outlook, 27*(11), 714–717.

Blackburn, R. T., Chapman, D. W., & Cameron, S. M. (1981). Cloning in academe, *Research in Higher Education, 15*(4), 315–327.

Bowen, D. (1985). Were men meant to mentor women? *Training and Development Journal, 39*(1), 30–34.

Buchanan, C. (1984). *An investigation and analysis of the prevalence and effect of sponsorship in the academic career development of nurses.* Unpublished doctoral dissertation, University of Michigan, Ann Arbor.

Cameron, S. M., & Blackburn, R. T. (1981). Sponsorship and academic career success, *Journal of Higher Education, 52*(4), 369–377.

Campbell-Heider, N. (1986). Do nurses need mentors? *Image, 18*(3), 110–113.

Cook, M. (1980). Is the mentor relationship primarily a male experience? *Personnel Administrator, 24*(11), 82–84, 86.

Crane, D. (1972). *Invisible colleges.* Chicago: University of Chicago Press.

Dalton, G. W., Thompson, P., & Price, R. L. (1977). The four stages of professional careers: A new look at performance by professionals, *Organizational Dynamics, 6*(1), 19–42.

Darling, L. W. (1985a). Becoming a mentoring manager, *Journal of Nursing Administration, 15*(6), 43–44.

Darling, L. W. (1985b). What to do about toxic mentors, *Journal of Nursing Administration, 15*(5), 43–44.

Darling, L. W. (1985c). Endings in mentor relationships, *Journal of Nursing Administration, 15*(11), 38–39.

Epstein, C. F. (1970). *Woman's place.* Berkeley, CA: University of California Press.

Erickson, E. H. (1963). *Childhood and society* (2nd ed.). New York: Norton & Company.

Fagan, M. M., & Fagan, P. D. (1983). Mentoring among nurses, *Nursing Outlook, 4*(2), 80–82.

Felton, G. (1978). On women, networks, patronage, and sponsorship, *Image, 10*(3), 58–59.

Granovetter, M. S. (1973). The strength of weak ties, *American Journal of Sociology, 78*(6), 1360–1379.

Holcomb, R. (1980). Mentors and the successful woman, *Across the Board, 17*(2), 13–18.

Hall, R. M., & Sandler, B. R. (1983). *Academic mentoring for women students and faculty: A new look at an old way to get ahead.* Washington, DC: Association of American Colleges.

Halsey, S. (1978). *Role theory: Perspectives for health care professionals.* New York: Appleton-Century-Crofts.

Hart, L. B. (1980). *Moving up and leadership.* New York: AMACOM.

Hennig, M., & Jardim, A. (1977a). Women executives in the old-boy network, *Psychology Today, 10*(8), 76–81.

Hennig, M., & Jardim, A. (1977b). *The managerial woman.* Garden City, NJ: Doubleday.

Josefowitz, N. (1980). *Paths to power.* Reading, MA: Addison-Wesley.

Kanter, R. M. (1977). *Men and women of the corporation.* New York: Basic Books.

Kleiman, C. (1980). *Women's networks.* New York: Ballantine.

Levinson, D. J., Darrow, C. N., Klein, E. B., Levinson, M. H., & McKee, B. (1978). *The seasons of a man's life.* New York: Knopf.

Lundig, F. J., Clements, G. R., & Perkins, D. S. (1978). Everyone who makes it has a mentor, *Harvard Business Review, 56*(4), 89–101.

Martin, N. H., & Strauss, A. L. (1968). Patterns of mobility within industrial organizations. In B. G. Glaser (Ed.). *Organizational Careers: A Sourcebook for Theory.* Chicago: Aldine.

Moore, K. M. (1982). The role of mentors in developing leaders for academe, *Educational Record, 63*(1), 22–28.

O'Connor, A. B. (1982). Ingredients for successful networking, *Journal of Nursing Administration, 12*(12), 36–40.

Price, S. A., Simms, L. M., & Pfoutz, S. K. (1987). Career advancement of nurse executives: Planned or accidental? *Nursing Outlook, 34*(8), 236–238.

Puetz, B. E. (1983). *Networking for nurses.* Rockville, MD: Aspen Systems Inc.

Roche, G. (1979). Much ado about mentors. *Harvard Business Review, 57*(1), 14–16, 20, 24–28.

Shapiro, E. C., Haseltine, F. P., & Rowe, M. P. (1978). Moving up: Role models, mentors, and the "patron system," *Sloan Management Review, 20*(2), 51–58.

Sheehy, G. (1974). *Passages.* New York: Dutton.

Spitzer, R. (1981). The nurse in the corporate world, *Supervisor Nurse, 12*(4), 21–24.

Warihay, P. (1980). The climb to the top: Is the network the route for women? *Personnel Administrator, 54*(4), 55–60.

Wynter, L. E., & Soloman, J. A. (1989, November). A new push to break the glass ceiling. *The Wall Street Journal,* pp. B1–B2.

Yoder, L. (1990). Mentoring: A concept analysis, *Nursing Administration Quarterly, 15*(1), 9–19.

Zuckerman, G. (1977). *Scientific elite: Nobel laureates in the United States.* New York: The Free Press.

CHAPTER 28

From Enabling to Assistive Technology

Highlights

- **Concept of assistive technology**
- **Nurses in need of assistive technology**
- **Exploring new horizons in technology**
- **Assistive technology of relevance to nurse executives**
- **Operationalizing receptivity to assistive technology**

Failure to internalize the learning role as a central feature of the self is a major restraint in the full achievement of human potential (McClusky, 1974). Human learning and problem-solving abilities are therefore important resources in empowering people with the belief that they can control their destiny. Personal goal setting, learning how to learn, and understanding bio-psycho-social-spiritual abilities should replace current procedural patient educational materials that serve as reminders of deficits and do not encourage development of personal control of performance and environment. Self-care and the use of assistive technologies can be learned and can make a tremendous difference in quality of life of people receiving health care and health care professionals delivering care. The purpose of this chapter is to introduce the nurse executive to the abundance of assistive technology available today that can assist activities of daily living for patients and work for nurses. The chapter is also written to stimulate the development of technology by nurses for nursing.

ASSISTIVE TECHNOLOGY

During the past decade, revolutionary changes have involved every aspect of health care in this country. Extensive basic medical research has yielded an expanding array of diagnostic and monitoring equipment. Life-support systems permit surgeons to remove, repair, or replace components of the body as never before in the history of the human race. The manned space programs have yielded a tremendous amount of knowledge related to physiology and communication systems. Major advancements in robotics and the development of assistive technology are dramatically changing patient education and rehabilitation for self-care. As nurses are the principal caregivers in various health care delivery settings, it is essential to take a new look at the nature of the work of nursing and propose innovative models for nursing practice that take into account emerging labor-saving assistive technologies as well as rapidly changing health care needs. In essence, nurses must change the way they do their clinical work and how they spend their time in clinical practice. Moving one's thinking about technology as enabling devices for handicapped people to assistive technology that provides labor savings in time and effort is an important leap in thought.

According to Smith (1988), "The evolving technologies and intelligent clinical information systems will enable health care professionals to extend their therapeutic and protective powers beyond the walls of their offices and hospitals. Systems providing continuous medication and patient monitoring will reduce the need to hospitalize patients, perhaps dramatically. The patients of the 21st century will be connected to their health care providers by webs of telemetry similar to those used in cellular communications; perhaps these communication webs will be coordinated or monitored by computer systems that could trigger responses in advance of crises" (p. 18). Technology will greatly affect the way health care services are organized and delivered in the twenty-first century. The dichotomy between caring and technology in nursing reflects a fear of technology equipment. Nurses must view technology and humanism as complementary in their contribution to human welfare, and nurses must be on the forefront of linking assistive technology with patient empowerment and self-care. Nursing could be considered a late entrant into the field technology-driven services and could offer a highly competitive product in health care delivery.

The Patient Intensity for Nursing Index study, using Division of Nursing definitions, suggests that only one third of nursing time is spent in direct clinical care (Prescott, Phillips, Ryan, & Thompson, 1991). Other work-sampling studies reported by these authors confirmed this finding. The majority of time (over 50 percent) is spent in combined indirect care or unit-management activities. Reducing inefficiencies in information flow and charting routines and reassigning aspects of unit management could save approximately 48 minutes per nurse per shift. Based on their review of selected work sampling studies, Prescott et al. (1991) support *(1)* the redesign of work and work groups through restructuring the role of the registered nurse, *(2)* developing assistive nursing personnel, and *(3)* implementing labor-saving assistive technologies.

NURSES IN NEED OF ASSISTIVE TECHNOLOGY

One of the most disabled groups of people may be nurses who are trying to make do with yesterday's curricula. They lack the physics, engineering, and computer science background that would enable them to become intelligent consumers of rapidly changing technology; nor are current faculty in schools of nursing willing to encourage revolutionary changes in curricula. Many nursing faculties believe that as people get older, they do not need technology, they need good supportive nursing care. What could be more supportive than assistive technologies that could keep persons independent in self-care and in their own homes?

Many tasks in nursing are so demeaning, dehumanizing, boring, tiring, physically exhausting, and even potentially dangerous that to have a robot perform these tasks would be most useful (Haber, 1986). Assistance with personal care activities would free the nursing staff to do those things that only humans can do. The automatic washing machine is a robot that has freed American women to perform other activities. Rarely do nurses have analogous robotics available to them in practice; nor are many nurses emotionally able to deal with introducing robots into nursing care that can conceivably bathe, toilet, feed, and dress people more efficiently and with greater care. Nurses care for a variety of patients who have immobility. Should not there be turning and lifting devices available for those people? Technological support services should be sustained for all disabled citizens and should be available to those seeking prevention of disability (Enders, 1987), including nurses seeking prevention of back injuries.

Record keeping, toileting activities, bedmaking, lifting and moving patients, monitoring wanderers and people with tendencies to fall, feeding patients, collecting specimens, and distributing medications are some of the most time-consuming activities in nursing. Several devices are already on the drawing board in a variety of NASA and rehabilitation engineering studies (NASA Spinoff, 1986). A portable, noninvasive ultrasonic bladder sensor designed to facilitate independence in toileting could potentially have implications for specimen collection.

The potential for computer-assisted communication is phenomenal. The fact that many hospitals do not have computerized information systems probably accounts for much of the lack of computer knowledge among nurses. Furthermore, faculties in even the best schools of nursing are not fully aware of the potential for computer use in record keeping, health education, and direct patient care. Before nursing can take full advantage of large data bases, computerized care plans, and staffing scheduling systems, the computer must become as much a part of the professional nursing skills as the bandage and stethoscopes of yesteryear.

Computers have remarkable potential to enhance the lives of the aging (Gorovitz, 1985). Books, magazines, and a wide variety of courses could be available on terminals in various health care settings, including nursing homes. The size of print and intensity of brightness could be adjusted to the needs of the viewer. Contrary to increased loneliness, the use of modified computer games in some nursing homes for the frail older people, whose average age was 85, suggests that participants show increased vitality, concentration, and greater interaction.

Wandering and propensity for falling frequently require physical or chemical restraints. A variety of restraints such as geri-chairs, beanbag chairs, and tying restraints are commonly used inhuman devices. Surveillance devices could provide wanderers with feedback, which may help them become more oriented in their environment or provide cues that they have entered an unsafe area. Recent work by

Martino-Saltzman, Blasch, Coombs, and McNeal (1987) at the Atlanta VA Medical Center seeks to identify such devices in combination with appropriate training programs.

Review of literature from the National Aeronautics and Space Administration research programs and proceedings of Annual Meetings of the Rehabilitation Engineering Association of North America reveals numerous products that have the potential for influencing the manner in which nursing is practiced. Robotic feeding devices for the disabled population is under development now in research by Seamone and Schmeisser (1985) at the Johns Hopkins University. On the drawing board are programmable, implantable medication systems and sensor-actuated medication systems that can control the availability of medication according to the needs of individual bodies. Czerwinski (1987) in discussing work at the Johnson Space Center noted numerous examples of attending to activities of daily living in a confined space, including showering, oral care, elimination, and menstrual activities. Even in the most modern hospital, nurses must usually work in a confined space in providing personal care. Systems for the odorless disposal of human waste (Jennings & Lewis, 1987) could have tremendous potential for more human care in all settings, especially, in nursing homes.

Nurses need new equipment such as levitation devices, people movers, needleless injection equipment, and range of motion exercisers to do their work now and in the future, as described by Arthur C. Clarke (1986) in his science fiction book about life in the twenty-first century. The significance of the proposed work is that new practice patterns can be designed that will create an environment in which practicing nurses will continue to identify work penetration points at which new technologies and practice patterns can then be tested in practice settings or in newly designed skills labs. It is anticipated that newly designed skills labs could become continuing education centers in which faculty, staff nurses, and even patients and family members could learn how to use new technologies or update practice skills.

EXPLORING NEW HORIZONS IN TECHNOLOGY

Potential applications of technology derived from rehabilitation and bioengineering research could change the nature of nursing work. Libow (1982) suggests that long-term care facilities can become respected places for treating people. He sees nursing homes as major centers of activity in the nation's health care scene and an extension of the university health sciences campus. Although his work has been with older people, his vision for ideal care is appropriate for all groups with special needs. In essence, he believes that a long-term care facility can be a place for education and rehabilitation for self-care, rather than a place to die. Nurses are the principal caregivers in these settings and should have a major role in deciding new ways of delivering services.

Engelhardt and Edwards (1986) describe the work of an applications team formed to investigate potential uses for robots and robotic technologies that could assist the functionally dependent older person. They describe evolving electronic innovations that can contribute to functional rehabilitation such as lifting and transferring robots, daily-living expert systems, voice-technology, smart cards that contain a complete medical history, and other relevant information and emergency alert systems. Goode and Rambaut (1985) discuss the effects of space flight on the human skeleton bearing the results of paralysis or long-term bedrest. The study of skeletal change in space offers a unique opportunity to understand mobility dysfunctions of individuals without disease.

Rushmer (1980) describes the rapidly expanding resources for medical care. Tools developed in basic research have been converted into diagnostic devices, including intrinsic and external energy devices, computerized axial tomography, ultrasound, radioisotopes, thermography, and multiple therapeutic technologies. Diagnoses by satellite using sophisticated satellite communication technology developed in the space program is changing the field of medical diagnosis. There is every reason to believe that these sophisticated technologies will enhance nursing diagnoses and therapies as well.

The cerebrovascular accident (CVA) or stroke patient is an example of a client who requires the full array of nursing skills. An average of 500,000 people suffer from strokes every year, and about 2,000,000 people are still living after a stroke. Stroke is one of the country's leading causes of disability and handicaps and is estimated to account for half the patients hospitalized for acute neurologic disease (Bronstein, Murray, Licata-Gehr, Banko, Kelly-Hayes, Fast, & Kunitz, 1986). Both McCartney (1974) and Dudas (1986) believed that stroke patients would benefit if their early care in the hospital included immediate efforts toward assessment of potential rehabilitation needs. From the moment the stroke patient is admitted, the nurse's efforts must be actively directed toward maintaining both his physical and psychological integrity (McCartney, 1974), and when his medical status stabilizes, the focus of nursing care becomes that of helping the patient to gain independence and function at maximum levels (Dudas, 1986). Thus, the patient begins to relearn skills of daily living or to learn new skills and adaptations to compensate for residual deficits (Dudas, 1986).

In a Swedish comparative study, Hamrin (1982) suggests that an "activation" program of nursing care with special training for the nurses in addition to the usual therapies improved function of the stroke patients in the first month of the stroke. The activation program emphasized psychological activation, verbal communication, prophylaxis against contractures and pressure sores, movement therapy and ambulation, and activities of daily living. Hamrin (1982a) also studied the attitudes of the staff on the wards in which the "activation" program was carried out and those of staff in control wards. There was a significant change in attitudes, judged on a scale constructed of 14 items, among the staff of the experimental wards during a 6-month period. There were also positive changes in individual items, such as attitudes to long-term care. Hamrin concluded that the educational program and also, perhaps, the other activities of the experimental wards seemed to have affected the attitudes of the staff to some extent in a positive direction (Hamrin, 1982a).

An individual who has suffered a CVA or stroke is often devastated by cognitive deficits encompassing a variety of areas (auditory and visual memory, visual perception, logical reasoning and judgment, motivation, calculation, and ability for abstraction). Additionally, the stroke victim may experience an alteration in communication in the form of a speech or language disorder (Pimental, 1986). Mumma (1986) studied the perceived losses of stroke victims and their spouses following a stroke. The top five losses reported were mobility, independence, patient's physical abilities, shared activities, and patient's communication (Mumma, 1986)

The ability to communicate is an important element in life, at any age. Speech and language make humans unique; the diminution of speech and language makes them less human. Human beings have a basic need to communicate and gain much pleasure and mental stimulation from the practice of communication itself (Olson, 1986). When a communication impairment is present, a person loses his ability to interact with others in several spheres from the acute care setting of the hospital to home life, work, and social settings (Kumin & Rysticken, 1985; Ozuna, 1985) and it isolates the person from the main stream of society. Gloag (1986) indicates that in stroke patients, rehabilitation is usually impeded by speech impairment (lack of speech or comprehension). The nurse executive along with other members of the health team should seek to identify alternative methods for the patient to communicate, because people who lose the ability to speak, need not lose the ability to communicate (Kumin & Rysticken, 1985).

Nurse executives are usually in a position to inform patients and staff about possible alternatives and suggest referral to a speech pathologist who specializes in augmentative communication (Kumin & Rysticken, 1985). There is a wide variety of devices that can augment communication, from simple homemade communication boards to computer assistive devices. These devices make things easier for the patient, the family, and the health care professionals by facilitating communication and decreasing the frustrations of the patient's inability to speak.

ASSISTIVE TECHNOLOGY OF RELEVANCE TO NURSE EXECUTIVES

An abundance of innovations and creative uses of a variety of equipment already exist and more are coming. These innovations have a direct application in the nursing practice domain, because their aim is to increase a patient's independence and thereby decrease the workload of their caretakers (Chizeck, 1985). The nursing domains that these innovations may be categorized into are mobility, special senses and communication, maintaining skin integrity, comfort, cognition, elimination, and respiratory areas.

Mobility

Examples of work in this area emanate from the field of robotics, especially in developing prostheses (Engelhardt & Edwards, 1986; Morris, 1986; Peckham, 1987), making modifications on wheelchairs and cars to allow individuals to work effectively at surfaces of varying heights and to facilitate transfers (Kett, Lee, Levine, & Davis, 1987; Levine & Perrint, 1983), and developing devices for assisting in activities of daily living (e.g., grooming, feeding, etc.) (Hedman, Armstrong, Mackesy, Hurd, & Kohlmeyer, 1987) and playing the piano (Koester, Jocz, & Bui, 1985) and other instruments. Functional neuromuscular stimulation is another avenue being explored in the area of mobility and prevention of pressure sores. Chizeck (1985) described the effects of functional stimulation on paraplegics that helped them to lift and release a foot at the right moment as well as helped them to walk some distances, although they needed support when doing so. Also, the idea of closed loop control, which helps the person know the location of his foot and where to place it, was investigated.

Communication

The computer has opened the door of communication to people whose ability to communicate was impaired due to a variety of reasons such as strokes or spinal cord injuries. Even for those patients who, along with their inability to communicate, are unable to operate the computer with their hands, a variety of methods using patients' ability to move their lower extremities or even move their eyelids have been developed (Levine, Gauger, Bowers, & Kahn, 1986; Chesson & Schubert, 1982; Lee, Van Meter, Kett, & Levine, 1986; Bresler, 1987). Not only has the computer helped the person to communicate but also has given him more control in his environment through a variety of devices, for example, to switch the lights on and off.

Besides the computer, on a less complicated level, is the development of telephone communication systems for handicapped individuals. One example of such a system uses operator-assisted dialing, and the individual need only be able to operate two switches that access him to the operator (Levine, Gauger, & Kett, 1984). The development of a self-activated tracheostomy system for quadriplegics is another way that rehabilitation engineering has opened up the world of communication to people. This system allows the person to control the airflow over the vocal cords, thereby facilitating speech, releasing the patient from dependence on others for controlling the air flow (Levine, Koester, & Kett, 1987).

Special Senses

Robotics research is being carried out in the area of touch and tactile sensors. The aim of this research is to provide artificial limbs for the amputee and sensing devices for the paralyzed (Boelter, 1985). These devices will help individuals obtain simple motions of grasp and release using a tactile feedback. Extensive work is being carried out in improving hearing aids to make them more efficient for their users (Levitt & Neuman, 1987; Boothroyd, 1987; Yund, Simon, & Efron, 1987) as well as providing a variety of methods to improve reading abilities of the visually impaired (Hennies, Steele, Goodrich, & McKinley, 1987; Amerson, McNeal, & Ross, 1987).

Skin Integrity

Patients who are confined to bed or a wheelchair for long periods of time have their skin exposed to normal and shear forces that will cause impairment of skin integrity. Studies have been made to describe the changes that occur to impair skin integrity (Kett & Levine, 1987; Sacks & O'Neill, 1987) as well as to test the effect of functional electrical muscle stimulation in the prevention of pressure sores (Levine, Kett, Wilson, Cederna, Gross, & Juri, 1987; Levine, Cederna, Brooks, & Friedman, 1985). In addition, Merbitz, King, Marqui, Carley, Grip, and Morsczek (1987) describe the development of a computer program to improve training in wheelchair pressure-relief lift-offs and leans. Proper performance of these tasks prevents ischial pressure sores among people with spinal cord injury. This program also shows the outcome of teaching interventions so that the effectiveness of teaching can be assessed and, when appropriate, interventions altered. In addition to examining the effects of pressure on skin integrity, other scientists have been looking at the effect of space travel on bone loss in an attempt to find ways to reverse this loss in patients suffering from osteoporosis, especially after menopause and due to the aging process (Goode & Rambaut, 1985).

Comfort

The development of seating systems for disabled individuals is a rapidly growing area of rehabilitation medicine at the University of Michigan (Koester, 1987). A variety of components such as seat cushions, seat backs, trunk supports, pelvic positioners, shoulder positioners, lap trays, etc. can be found that achieve an optimal custom seating system for individual clients. Proper seating and positioning not only affords comfort, it also affords achievement of motor function and participation in self-care, important nursing therapeutic goals.

Elimination

The development of a microenema dispenser to help quadriplegics function independently (Mueller, Miller, & Sherban, 1987) is just one example of the innovations that are being developed to help people with their elimination problems. The National Headquarters of the Association for Retarded Citizens is developing and testing a portable, noninvasive ultrasonic bladder sensor designed to facilitate independence in toileting (Mineo & Cavalier, 1987). This device could apply to the needs of many people who experience urinary neurological dysfunction (e.g., multiple sclerosis, quadriplegia, diabetes, mental retardation, spina bifida, and people of advanced age).

Respiratory Function

Nurses have to continuously suction tracheostomy tubes for accumulated secretions. Balsdon and Hildebrandt (1987) describe the development of a portable suction pump that can be used for the suctioning process. The bioengineers have also designed modifications for wheelchairs to facilitate the carrying of oxygen tanks for those people who need oxygen on a continuous basis.

Cognition

Computers have also been found to be very useful for persons with impaired cognition. Engelhardt and Edwards (1986) describe the potential applications of microprocessor-based technology for increasing independence for those people with declining abilities. Computer programs have been developed to help and guide people through complex tasks as well as correct them during their performance (Levine, Kirsch, Perlman, & Cole, 1984).

OPERATIONALIZING RECEPTIVITY TO ASSISTIVE TECHNOLOGY

One way to introduce the idea of assistive technology equipment is to introduce an innovation such as the bedside terminal, as described in the Appendix under situation J. Another way is to build in self-assessment with the routine health assessment of all clients entering a health care facility. The following self-assessment instrument (Figure 28.1) has been designed to reflect learning needs in the middle and later years. It is important to educate potential users of assistive technology and the addition of self-assessment to current health assessments could encourage a rehabilitation philoso-

HEALTH AND TECHNOLOGY SELF-ASSESSMENT

COPING NEEDS

What are your personal health needs?

What products do you need to assist you in achieving physical well-being? Check all relevant items.

Personal care	—
Mobility	—
Elimination	—
Communication	—
Cognitive function (thinking and remembering)	—
Hearing	—
Vision	—
Other _____	—

What assistive technology do you need to maintain independent living?

What are your strengths?

How can your functional abilities (strengths) be used to balance or offset any dysfunctions?

What would you like to learn about physical, mental, and spiritual fitness?

EXPRESSIVE NEEDS

Would you like to learn how to use a computer? Other technology?

Do you wish to take classes that can prepare you for a new career?

What hobbies and personal interests would you like to develop over the next 5 years?

CONTRIBUTIVE NEEDS

Have you ever considered participating in community activities?

What community activities really make you feel fit?

INFLUENCE NEEDS

Have you ever considered sharing your expertise with others?

Do you think it is important to be active in community/societal events?

What assistance do you need that would help you to carry out desired activities?

TRANSCENDENCE/PERSONAL EMPOWERMENT

What are your learning needs that will allow you to achieve your desired state of well-being?

What goals do you wish to achieve in your life?

Figure 28.1 Example of a health and technology self-assessment questionnaire.

phy for living and development over the life span. When basic coping needs are met, the individual is able to move on, meeting needs at a higher level. A person can begin to think beyond physical needs to contributions to society and even transcendence (McClusky, 1974). A minimum of physical adequacy is needed for survival; more than mere adequacy is needed for health and full function.

This self-assessment schedule can also be introduced as part of regular activities in senior centers. Designed for a paper and pencil format, the guide is easily transferred to computer format. Goal setting has been identified as an extremely important part of continued development over the life span and it is possible, in a later stage of our work, that a modified performance plan will be developed for individual measurement of progress. The challenge for nurse executives is to link meaningful assistive technology with self-care and continuing care and the proposed tool could be one way of proceeding.

Summary

The literature suggests that emerging assistive technology equipment will dramatically change the way nurses work in all settings. Bold new patterns are needed to liberate nurses and clients; patterns that will allow for the introduction of technology into all redesign activities. As medical technology has increased and reimbursement has changed, health care agencies have minimized the role of the patient. To counteract this trend, several initiatives have been introduced that encourage patients to participate in their care. Among these is the Planetree Model Hospital Project (Martin, Hunt, Hughes-Stone, & Conrad, 1990). The Planetree philosophy emphasizes sharing information about illness and teaches skills regarding self-care and healthy behaviors. Patients receive information not only about their specific diseases and treatments, but also about health-promotion activities and independent living. This model provides a cornerstone for the self-care movement in this country and links well with the current emphasis on assistive technology for personal control of one's life and destiny.

References

Amerson, T., McNeal, L., & Ross, D. (1987). Human factors consideration in the design of large print displays for persons with visual impairments. *Rehabilitation Society of North American Proceedings, 10th Annual Conference, San Jose, CA* (pp. 419–421). Washington, DC: RESNA.

Balsdon, G. J., & Hildebrandt, J. R. (1987). A portable suction device for a tracheostomy tube. *Rehabilitation Society of North American Proceedings, 10th Annual Conference, San Jose, CA* (pp. 362–364). Washington, DC: RESNA.

Boelter, S. J. (1985). Restoring touch to the disabled, *Manufacturing Engineering*, February, 74–75.

Boothroyd, A. (1987). Experiments with a two-channel compression-limiting amplification system designed for profoundly deaf subjects. *Rehabilitation Society of North American Proceedings, 10th Annual Conference, San Jose, CA* (pp. 404–405). Washington, DC: RESNA.

Bresler, M. I. (1987). Computer aided construction of non-verbal communication boards. *Rehabilitation Society of North American Proceedings, 10th Annual Conference, San Jose, CA* (pp. 183–185). Washington, DC: RESNA.

Bronstein, K., Murray, P., Licata-Gehr, E., Banko, M., Kelly-Hayes, M., Fast, S., & Kunitz, S. (1986). The stroke data bank project: Implications for nursing research, *Journal of Neuroscience Nursing, 18*(3), 132–134.

Chesson, A., & Schubert, R. (1982). Microprocessors in the hospital-communication for the acutely disabled. *Biomedical Engineering I, Proceedings of the First Southern Biomedical Engineering Conference* (pp. 40–43).

Chizeck, H. J. (1985). Helping paraplegics walk: Looking beyond the media blitz, *Technology Review, 88*(5), 54–63.

Clarke, A. C. (1986). *July 20, 2019 Life in the 21st century.* New York: Macmillan.

Czerwinski, B. (1987, June). Feminine hygiene in space. Sexuality and the menstrual cycle: Clinical and sociocultural implications, *Seventh Conference of the Society for Menstrual Cycle Research*. Ann Arbor, MI: The University of Michigan.

Dudas, S. (1986). Nursing diagnosis and interventions for the rehabilitation of the stroke patient, *Nursing Clinics of North America, 21*(2), 345–357.

Enders, A. (1987). Approaching technological support as a lifelong need: Why rehabilitation technology services need to be sustained in the community. *Rehabilitation Society of North American Proceedings, 10th Annual Conference, San Jose, CA* (pp. 345–347). Washington, DC: RESNA.

Engelhardt, K. G., & Edwards, R. (1986). Increasing independence for the aging, *Byte*, March, 191–196.

Gloag, D. (1985). Rehabilitation after stroke: What is the potential? *British Medical Journal, 290*, 690–701.

Goode, A. W., & Rambaut, P. C. (1985). The skeleton in space, *Nature, 317*(19), 204–205.

Gorovitz, S. (1985). Bringing senior citizens on-line, *Technology Review, 88*(1), 12–13, 76.

Haber, P. A. (1986). Technology in aging, *The Gerontologist, 26*(4), 350–357.

Hamrin, E. (1982). Early activation in stroke: Does it make a difference, *Scandinavian Journal of Rehabilitation Medicine, 14*(3), 101–109.

Hamrin, E. (1982a). Attitudes of nursing staff in general medical wards towards activation of stroke patients, *Journal of Advanced Nursing, 7*(1), 33–42.

Hedman, G. E., Armstrong, W., Mackesy, J., Hund, K., & Kohlmeyer, K. (1987). An adaptive handle for a safety razor. *Rehabilitation Society of North American Proceedings, 10th Annual Conference, San Jose, CA* (pp. 207–209). Washington, DC: RESNA.

Hennies, D., Steele, R., Goodrich, G. L., & McKinley, J. (1987). Development of a portable text communication environment for the visually impaired. *Rehabilitation Society of North American Proceedings, 10th Annual Conference, San Jose, CA* (pp. 431–433). Washington, DC: RESNA.

Jennings, D., & Lewis, T. (1987, May). System for odorless disposal of human waste, *NASA Tech Briefs, 11*(5), 80.

Kett, R. L., Lee, K. J., Levine, S. P., & Davis, D. J. (1987). An adjustable height manual wheelchair for a vocational application. *Rehabilitation Society of North American Proceedings, 10th Annual Conference, San Jose, CA* (pp. 553–555). Washington, DC: RESNA.

Kett, R. L., & Levine, S. P. (1987). A dynamic model of tissue deflection in a seated individual. *Rehabilitation Society of North American Proceedings, 10th Annual Conference, San Jose, CA* (pp. 524–526). Washington, DC: RESNA.

Koester, D. J., Jocz, W. A., & Bui, K. D. (1985). Prosthetic terminal device for playing the piano. *Rehabilitation Society of North American Proceedings, 10th Annual Conference, San Jose, CA* (pp. 260–262). Washington, DC: RESNA.

Koester, D. J. (1987). *An overview of seating and positioning service delivery.* Unpublished manuscript. The University of Michigan Rehabilitation Engineering Program, Ann Arbor.

Kumin, L., & Rysticken, N. (1985). Aids to bridge the communication barrier, *Geriatric Nursing, 6*(6), 348–351.

Lee, K. J., Van Meter, A. M., Kett, R. L., & Levine, S. P. (1986). Communication systems for a severely handicapped individual with visual impairment. *Rehabilitation Society of North American Proceedings, 10th Annual Conference, San Jose, CA* (pp. 416–418). Washington, DC: RESNA.

Levine, S. P., Gauger, J. R., & Kett, R. L. (1984). Telephone communication system for handicapped individuals, *Archives Physical Medicine Rehabilitation, 65*(12), 788–789.

Levine, S. P., Kirsch, N. L., Perlman, O. Z., & Cole, T. M. (1984). Engineering therapy: An approach to treatment of a patient with severe cognitive and physical handicaps, *Archives Physical Medicine Rehabilitation, 65*(11), 737–739.

Levine, S. P., Koester, D. J., & Kett, R. L. (1987). Self-activated talking tracheostomy systems for quadriplegics, *Archives Physical Medicine and Rehabilitation, 68*, 571–573.

Levine, S. P., & Perrint, J. C. S. (1983). Custom powered wheelchair system for a child with lower extremity reduction malformations. *Proceedings Sixth Annual Conference on Rehabilitation Engineering* (pp. 140–141). Washington, DC: RESNA.

Levine, S. P., Gauger, J. R., & Kett, R. L. (1984). Telephone communication system for handicapped individuals, *Archives Physical Medicine Rehabilitation, 65*(12), 788–789.

Levine, S. P., Kirsch, N. L., Perlman, O. Z., & Cole, T. M. (1984). Engineering therapy: An approach to treatment of a patient with severe cognitive and physical handicaps, *Archives Physical Medicine Rehabilitation, 65*(11), 737–739.

Levine, S. P., Koester, D. J., & Kett, R. L. (1987). Self-activated talking tracheostomy systems for quadriplegics, *Archives Physical Medicine and Rehabilitation, 68*, 571–573.

Levine, S. P., & Perrint, J. C. S. (1983). Custom powered wheelchair system for a child with lower extremity reduction malformations. *Proceedings Sixth Annual Conference on Rehabilitation Engineering* (pp. 140–141). Washington, DC: RESNA.

Levitt, H., & Neuman, A. C. (1987). Digital hearing aids. *Rehabilitation Society of North American Proceedings, 10th Annual Conference, San Jose, CA* (pp. 389–391). Washington, DC: RESNA.

Libow, L. S. (1982, April). Geriatric medicine and the nursing home: A mechanism for mutual excellence, *The Gerontologist, 22*(2), 134–141.

Martin, D., Hunt, J. R., Hughes-Stone, M., & Conrad, D. A. (1990). The Planetree model project: An example of the patient as partner, *Hospital & Health Services Administration, 35*(4), 591–601.

Martino-Saltzman, D., Blasch, R., Coombs, F., & McNeal, L. (1987). Wandering behavior of elderly nursing home residents: evaluation and intervention. *Rehabilitation Society of North American Proceedings, 10th Annual Conference, San Jose, CA* (pp. 877–879). Washington, DC: RESNA.

McCartney, V. C. (1974). Rehabilitation and dignity for the stroke patient, *Nursing Clinics of North America, 9*(4), 693–701.

McClusky, H. Y. (1974). Education for aging: The scope of the field and perspectives for the future. In S. M. Grabowski & Mason, W. D. (Eds.). *Education for Aging.* Syracuse, NY: ERIC.

Merbitz, C., King, R., Marqui, H., Carley, D., Grip, J., & Mroczek, L. (1987). Technology for clinicians: Mobile mircocomputer for training pressure sore preventive behavior. *Rehabilitation Society of North American Proceedings, 10th Annual Conference, San Jose, CA* (pp. 333–335). Washington, DC: RESNA.

Mineo, B. A., & Cavalier, A. R. (1987). An ultrasonic bladder sensor for persons with incontinence. *Rehabilitation Society of North American Proceedings, 10th Annual Conference, San Jose, CA* (pp. 232–234). Washington, DC: RESNA.

Morris, H. M. (1986). Controlling multiple robot arms, *Control Engineering*, September, 144–147.

Mueller, L., Miller, J., & Sherban, M. (1987). Micro-enema dispenser for quadriplegics. *Rehabilitation Society of North America Proceedings, 10th Annual Conference, San Jose, CA* (pp. 235–237). Washington, DC: RESNA.

Mumma, C. M. (1986). Perceived losses following stroke, *Rehabilitation Nursing, 11*(3), 19–24.

NASA Spinoff (1986). *Spinoffs in health and medicine* (pp. 60–69). Washington, DC: National Aeronautics and Space Administration.

Olson, D. A. (1986). Communication and the elderly: Overview, *Topics in Geriatric Rehabilitation, 1*(4), 1–4.

Ozuna, D. A. (1985). Alterations in mentation: Nursing assessment and intervention, *Journal of Neurological Nursing, 17*(1), 66–70.

Peckham, P. H. (1987). Functional electrical stimulation: Current status and future prospects of applications to the neuromuscular system in spinal cord injury, *Paraplegia, 25*(3), 279–288.

Pimental, P. A. (1986). Alterations in communication: Biophysiological aspects of aphasia, dysarthria and right hemisphere syndromes in the stroke patient, *Nursing Clinics of North America, 21*(2), 321–337.

Prescott, P. A., Phillips, C. Y., Ryan, J. W., & Thompson, K. O. (1991). Changing how nurses spend their time, *IMAGE: Journal of Nursing Scholarship, 23*(1), 23–28.

Rushmer, R. G. (1980). Technological resources for health. In S. J. Williams & P. R. Torrens (Eds.). *Introduction to Health Services.* New York: John Wiley.

Sacks, A. H., & O'Neill, H. (1987). Skin response to pressure loading by the bent finger technique. *Rehabilitation Society of North American Proceedings, 10th Annual Conference, San Jose, CA* (pp. 302–304). Washington, DC: RESNA.

Seamone, W., & Schmeisser, G. (1985). Early clinical evaluation of a robot arm/worktable system for spinal-cord-injured persons, *Journal of Rehabilitation Research and Development, 22*(1), 38–57.

Smith, G. (1988). The evolution of alternative delivery systems: What will be nursing's role? In *Nursing Practice in the 21st Century.* Kansas City, MO: The American Nurses Foundation.

Yund, E. W., Simon, H. J., & Efron, R. (1987). Speech perception with an eight channel compression hearing aid and conventional aids in a background of speech-band noise. *Rehabilitation Society of North American Proceedings, 10th Annual Conference, San Jose, CA* (pp. 401–403). Washington, DC: RESNA.

CHAPTER 29

Enhancing Productivity Through Computerized Information Systems

Mary L. McHugh

Highlights

- **Productivity concepts**
- **Computer information system applications in nursing**
- **Clinical applications**
- **Efficiency enhancement**
- **Data entry technology**
- **Care scheduling**

Computerized information systems are tools to support information handling activities. They can be used to facilitate nursing documentation. More importantly, they can be used to increase the efficiency and quality of nursing care. That is, they can increase nursing productivity in both clinical and administrative domains. Examples of areas that are now or could be computerized can be found in Figure 29.1.

Clinical Nursing Practice	*Nursing Administration*

1. Reduction in clinical errors
2. Clinical care scheduling
3. Clinical consultation
4. Reducing the volume of documentation
5. Making clinical documents more complete and reliable
6. Increasing clinical records' accuracy, precision & timeliness
7. Quality Management
8. Tracing of clinical outcomes
  • Unexpected Mortality rates
  • Nosocomial Infection rates
  • Functional Status Changes
9. Analysis of the relationship between care protocols and changes in patient status
	1. Staffing and scheduling
	2. Performance evaluation
	3. Project design, scheduling, and evaluation
	4. Management decision support:
	  • System simulation/modeling and analysis of effectiveness/outcomes of management decisions
	  • Forecasting
	  • Trend Analysis
	  • Project evaluation
	5. Financial planning and management
	6. Strategic Planning
	  • Productivity evaluation
	  • Analysis of program costs versus lost opportunity costs for cost comparisons of competing programs
	  • Cost analysis/cost projections

Figure 29.1 Examples of computer applications to enhance nursing productivity.

A framework that organizes a variety of concepts concerned with "productivity" is suggested as a logical structure within which to organize and evaluate concepts and propositions pertaining to computer information systems. This chapter will address the concepts of productivity, quality, and efficiency, and explore the relationships among productivity, efficiency, and quality of care. It will address the role of computer information systems in the management of nursing productivity.

A CONCEPTUAL FRAMEWORK FOR PRODUCTIVITY CONCEPTS

Productivity: A Working Definition

Productivity is conceptually defined as the ratio of inputs to outputs. Inputs include all the human, time, and material resources used to produce a given unit of output. Inputs are usually converted into equivalent dollar costs, including concepts such as the time value of money as well as direct and indirect costs of producing the unit of output. Therefore, "inputs" are often expressed as "costs." Outputs are defined as the number of units of product "of a specific quality." Mathematically, the relationship is expressed as a ratio (McHugh, 1986a) in the following manner:

$$P = I \div O$$

Where *P* is productivity (an expression of the relationship between invested resources and products of work); *I* is inputs (invested resources); and *O* outputs (products of work).

Traditionally, the health care industry has focused on the "number of units" component of the concept "outputs" while sometimes omitting the "quality" component of outputs, simply because service quality is so difficult to quantify. Thus, we have measures of clinical outputs such as "patient days" or "patient visits" and the like. Part of the problem with this approach is that it is insufficient to meet the evolving expectations of consumers and third party payors. Nobody seeks health care to buy "a patient day" or a "service encounter." Patients seek health care for prevention or discovery of health problems, or to achieve a cure of an actual problem, or to abate the negative impact of a health problem on the quality of their lives. Third party payors' interest focuses on ensuring that the money they spend on care for subscribers is used in ways that actually improve health status, not on ineffective or harmful treatments.

The emerging tenor of our clientele (patients and payors) is to demand that we demonstrate (and, of course, document) that patients obtain what they are seeking. In the past, third party payors and health care managers have defined "what patients are seeking" as the services delivered. Services were generally presumed to be effective in producing desired changes in health status. Thus, health services were equated with desired changes in health status. The United States now stands on the verge of a redefinition of the concept, "what patients are seeking." The new approach abandons the assumption that services are effective and defines "what patients are seeking" in terms of changes in the patient's health status or functional status. This change is so radical as to constitute a major paradigm shift in providers' and consumers' view of health care and reimbursement for health care. It will force health care professionals to stop focusing on the quantity of services and to expend more effort in measuring the quality of outputs (defined as patient outcomes).

It may now be useful to redefine a term used in industry that does not fit with the realities of the health care environment. In industry, "throughput" is used to mean a specific quantity of input, "put through" processing in a specific amount of time to produce outputs). This conceptualization fails in health care because patients, on whom health care actions are performed, can never be defined as inputs or outputs per se. Patients are not used or consumed in the process of producing "health care" and therefore are not inputs. Neither are patients created or produced within the health care system, so the patient can not be defined properly as an output.

Health care services ought to act on the patient *in the process of care delivery* in such a way as to produce beneficial changes in the patient's health or functional status. In this sense, the concept of health care services is similar to the concept of throughput. There is not a comparable term to "throughput" in health care. However, such a term may be useful to describe services provided or actions performed on patients. Such a conversion of the term "throughput" may be useful for providing a clear discrimination between inputs (materials and labor), the actions of the supplier (health care providers), which would be called throughput, and the effects of those actions on patients, which would be defined as outcomes of services or care (McHugh, 1989).

Agreement is not yet available on the meaning of the term "outputs" in health care, but clearly differentiating among other, less controversial terms will reduce the amount of confusion about how terms are applied in the health care setting.

In this context, services delivered will be described as throughput. The health care industry has often measured throughput and called it output. For example, nursing outputs have often been defined as counts of services such as "number of intravenous (IV) starts" or "number of dressing changes" and the like. In fact, services are a means to an end, not an end in themselves. This is the crucial problem in defining services as output. The conceptual change now emerging in health care involves redefining services as throughput and patient health/functional status changes as outcomes of care. Eventually, outcomes should constitute one component of the concept "outputs" in health care.

As the concepts "services" and "patient outcomes" change in health care, the concept of "quality" in health care must also change. "Quality of care" has been defined as adherence to standards (written or assumed) defining what services to provide, how to provide them (performance standards), and specifications for documenting those services. In other words, "quality of care" has actually been a measure of quality of throughput. As the health care delivery paradigm shifts to a focus on health/functional status outcomes during the middle 1990s and into the next century, the measures of "quality of care" most familiar to quality assurance (QA) nurses will no longer suffice. "Quality" will be subsumed under measures of productivity. New measures of productivity in the health care industry need to be developed. The new measures need to specify changes in health status as outputs and to clearly differentiate between services and the effects of those services on patients. The implications of this change are at least as significant to the health care industry as was prospective reimbursement. This change will transform quality assessment from a minor irritation—an activity conducted primarily to meet the requirements of accrediting and regulatory bodies—into a critical element in the financial success of the institution.

It is unlikely that the existing paper chart and current work processes in the QA department will be able to support the future requirements of quality measurement and documentation (Oatway, 1987). The volume of data and the content of data required to identify patient outcomes will be such that only a computer-based patient chart will permit the work to be accomplished. Furthermore, the computer chart must be able to be accessed by (or linked to a computer with) programs designed to aggregate data across patients, perform statistical analyses, and facilitate the creation of QA reports. Accordingly, a more detailed consideration of emerging concepts of quality in health care is germane to discussion of the implications of computer information systems for the future of nursing management.

Changing Concepts of Quality in Health Care

Satisfactory measures of productivity are extremely difficult to obtain in nursing and health care (Young & Hayne, 1988), in part because of the difficulty of incorporating quality indicators into productivity measures. Yet, productivity measures that fail to take account of the quality of the output are so seriously flawed as to be nearly barren of meaning. An example from manufacturing may help to illuminate the concept of quality and the contribution of quality to productivity.

In machine tool manufacturing, industrial engineers often develop precise performance specifications for the product. The performance specifications then dictate objective measures of product performance. In this context, quality outcomes may be dichotomized as either "acceptable performance" or "unacceptable performance." The product is "acceptable" only if it meets *all* of the performance specifications. It is "unacceptable" if it fails to meet *even one* specification. A product that fails to meet specifications cannot be sold, and thus counts as zero when the number of outputs are counted. However, inputs necessary to produce a flawed product are usually the same as those used to produce an acceptable product. Therefore, the rate of rejection (quality problems) increases the number of inputs relative to the number of *counted* outputs.

This example illustrates that quality problems are merely one type of productivity problem. Integral to the concept of quality is the concept "performance standards" for the *output*. Performance standards pertaining to throughput refer to aspects of work similar to aspects of care in nursing QA. These must often be done to ensure that degradation of throughput does not produce flawed outputs. But control of quality of throughput is useful only insofar as it improves the quality of outputs.

In nursing, the concept "quality of care" has been interpreted to mean adherence to throughput standards. Output standards (patient care outcomes) have not been measured. In fact, for many patient problems, measures of patient care outcomes do not yet exist. It must be most strongly emphasized that the term "patient care outcomes" has changed significantly. It no longer refers to nursing services. That term now refers to objective, measurable changes in patient condition and/or functional status.

The Concept "Efficiency" and its Relationship to Productivity

Efficiency Defined   Efficiency refers to measures of how fast a particular task or unit of work is accomplished. Efficiency translates into productivity only indirectly. As an example, consider the amount of time an infusion pump can save by eliminating the need to count "drops per minute" when the nurse regulates an IV. If that time saved is spent at the nurses' station in personal conversation with a colleague, no productivity increase is realized. Only if the time saved is used to care for more patients or to deliver better quality care is productivity enhanced (Channon, 1983). The manager must make a conscious effort to use efficiency improvements wisely. Whereas increases in efficiency may or may not be translated into productivity increases, decreased efficiency will almost always damage productivity. This principle can easily be observed by any nurse who must replace an experienced staff nurse with a nurse who is new to the institution. During orientation, the new employee will need to spend significant amounts of time learning where supplies are kept, what numbers to call for lab, pharmacy, dietary, and all the myriad details the experienced nurse will have at her fingertips. Even if the new employee has many years of experience in nursing, the new setting will hamper efficiency for a period of time. That is why most nursing services do not count a new employee as part of the productive staff for a period of time during orientation. Clearly, while increases in efficiency may not be easily translated into productivity improvement, efficiency decreases will almost automatically translate into productivity decreases.

Efficiency, Human Effort, and Productivity   The second component of the productivity formula involves the number of outputs (per unit of input). When one considers productivity enhancement in terms of increasing the number of outputs, the concept of efficiency is critical. Managers with concerns about their department's productivity may try to increase productivity by increasing the efficiency of people's personal work habits. There are two problems with this approach. First, efficiency improvements translate to productivity increases only when the time saved through greater efficiency is reinvested in producing more outputs or into decreasing inputs per unit of output. In nursing, this becomes problematic if increased efficiency produces an extra minute here and three minutes there. It then becomes difficult to reinvest those saved minutes effectively. Second, unsustained productivity improvements represent a zero percent net change. Individual work habits are notoriously difficult to change, and each individual has a personal comfort work pace. The comfortable work pace can be *temporarily* speeded up. Unfortunately, people cannot sustain a work pace that is uncomfortable for long periods of time, and they are *less* efficient for a time after exhaustion is reached. Thus, the productivity gains during the speeded up period are usually lost during recovery from exhaustion.

This author has noticed confusion about the relationships between efficiency improvements and human performance dynamics among many health care managers. All too often managers try to improve productivity through motivational lectures or threats. Sustained productivity increases are *never* achieved in that manner. Sustained productivity improvements are a product of improved work tools.

Improving Productivity

The Strategy of Productivity Enhancement   From these definitions, it is clear that one may increase productivity in two ways. Productivity is enhanced by increasing the number of outputs while holding constant the number of inputs. Alternately, productivity is increased whenever the quality is increased, assuming outputs and inputs are held constant. For sustained productivity improvements to occur, something in the workplace must change to enable the system to produce more or better outputs. History demonstrates that significant, sustained productivity increases have always resulted from application of technological advances in the workplace. Consider the following situation:

A 2-inch-long nail must be driven into a standard 2″ × 4″ piece of lumber. The carpenter has only his bare hand with which to accomplish the work. How long will it take to pound that nail into the board? If the carpenter is provided with a simple hammer, how long will it take? Finally, how many 2-inch nails can the carpenter drive into a house under construction with an electric nail gun?

Clearly, the carpenter will never get a house built without at least a hammer. The carpenter with a hammer might get the house built in a matter of months, whereas with a nail gun, the house may go up in a matter of weeks or, perhaps, even days!

Nurse managers need to avoid unsuccessful strategies and address productivity by seeking out better tools for the work of nurses. In the resource-constrained environment, it is too costly to add Full Time Equivalents (FTEs). Expecting people to work harder is an approach that cannot succeed. Nursing administration needs to take leadership in changing the productivity paradigm now in use in the health care industry. For as long as economic resources for health care delivery are constrained, the old paradigm will be unsuccessful. It cannot succeed because it is founded on a false understanding of the nature of work output and it fails to recognize real, measurable limitations of human performance. What is required of nurse managers is a new look at how nursing work is accomplished — and how that work might be completed more efficiently. The key to productivity lies not in the average nurse's character or work ethic. The key paradigm change involves a view of tools as the key to productivity improvement.

Sources of Productivity Improvement   As nurse managers examine their departments for productivity improvement opportunities, two questions can be used to guide the search. First, "Is the work activity under scrutiny a large enough component of the work of the nurse that a significant efficiency gain in this area can be translated into a meaningful productivity increase?" Second, "Does the technology now exist to achieve a significant efficiency improvement?"

When considering the size of the work activity, time studies may be helpful in determining precisely how much nursing time the activity consumes. If, for example, one can achieve a 90 percent improvement in the efficiency of a nursing activity, but the activity only constitutes 1 percent of the work day, only 4.3 minutes per nurse have been saved per 8-hour shift. On the other hand, if a 20 percent improvement in the efficiency of a nurse can be achieved for an activity that constitutes 40 percent of the nurse's time, 38.4 minutes in an 8-hour shift have been saved. In a unit staffed with five nurses, that savings translates into an extra 3.2 hours available for patient/family teaching, responding to patient requests, or providing care to one additional patient (assuming 9.6 hours of care per patient day).

When considering availability of technology, it is important to focus on what is available here and now. All too often, investigations into productivity enhancement technology are derailed by speculation about the productivity gains that will be achievable when this or that technology advance becomes available. Such conjecture is interesting and valuable when communicating possible directions for product development to vendors. However, it is not productive in the context of current strategic planning. These two questions will serve as a guide to focus attention on realistic planning and budgeting for productivity enhancement technology investments. Once an investment opportunity is identified, determining the value of the investment is necessary.

Justifying Investments in Productivity Enhancement Technology   To justify investment in an item of technology, the manager needs to determine if the investment will produce a net improvement or decrease in productivity. Justifications have more credibility when they focus on a comparative analysis of the cost versus the value of the technology to the institution. "Value" may focus on return on investment, strategic match, competitive advantage, and management information (Parker, Benson & Trainor, 1988). For nurse managers, this may translate into FTE reductions or cost avoidance (avoid the need to add FTEs to accomplish new work required by patient condition or by regulations), improvement in quality of care, improved reimbursement, achievement of strategic goals, etc. For cost justifications the manager often needs to obtain items of information such as:

1. Ability to offer new or expanded services with a good reimbursement profile,
2. Capacity to offer a service or program desired by customers (that may or may not be available from a competitor),
3. The number of nursing hours saved per month or year by the new tool, including both indirect activity hours and direct activity hours,
4. The cost of those nursing hours,
5. A full costing of the labor saving technology. The cost analysis will include yearly maintenance costs, and the cost of any incidentals such as manufacturer provided support, inservice education, new FTEs required to support the technology, etc. The purchase price must also be adjusted for the time value of money to determine the full cost of the labor saving device.

The adjusted cost of the technology should be divided by the cost of the nursing hours saved. The point at which the dollars saved in nursing hours equals the adjusted dollars spent to purchase and support the item is the "break even" point. All useful life of the technology after that point is "profit." Of course, if the useful life of the technology is less than the time necessary to reach the break even point, productivity is decreased by the purchase rather than increased. (This is true because the inputs invested have increased, whereas outputs have remained constant and the organization has suffered a net loss).

Nursing Productivity Enhancement Opportunities   Information handling is the most promising area in nursing for successful productivity enhancement projects. It fits all the criteria previously outlined: it constitutes a large portion of the job, and technology to achieve significant gains now exists. The amount of time nurses spend on communications was measured at 35 to 40 percent during the middle and late 1960s (Jydstrup & Gross, 1966; Richart, 1970). It is obvious that the time spent on information handling has not decreased in the past 20 years. It may have even increased to as much as 45 to 50 percent. As for the technology, there are now a variety of applications that have been developed to support nursing. A careful study of the use of computer information systems in industry reveals that no one industry has information-handling needs like nursing. Nursing has complex and data-intense information-handling problems. Yet, virtually all of the types of information-handling problems found in nursing have computer solutions in at least one other industry. Therefore, the following propositions are offered for the reader's consideration: Significant and material increases in nursing productivity are needed now. These increases in productivity can be achieved with application of existing computer technology to nursing information-handling functions.

COMPUTER INFORMATION SYSTEM APPLICATIONS IN NURSING

Computer information systems can be used to enhance nursing productivity in two ways. First, they can reduce the amount of time required to complete tasks. To the extent that the time saved is invested in accomplishing more work, productivity is enhanced because the number of outputs is increased. Practically, this may be exhibited by doing the same work with fewer people (an FTE reduction is achieved without decreasing number or quality of outputs) or by achieving more work outputs from the people now available. Second, computers can be used to increase quality of outputs. It is important to understand that both clinical and administrative productivity can be enhanced with computer information system technology.

Clinical Applications

Efficiency Enhancement   Today, nurses spend many hours completing flow sheets, care plans, nurses' notes, vital sign graphics, and other records of nursing care. Some of these are in an easy "check-list" or "fill in the blanks" type of flow sheet format. Others continue to require extensive narrative charting. In most care settings, virtually all of this work is done manually. When one considers that performing free-hand narrative charting is very similar to having to write a school term paper or concept paper, it can be appreciated how tedious and time consuming much of this paperwork load has become. The primary goal of putting the clinical chart on computers is to reduce the time required to complete these documents.

Computers can help reduce this burden in several ways. Only a few will be described in this chapter. First, there now exists data entry technology that can greatly streamline the process by which a nurse enters patient care information onto the chart. Second, for some types of data, computers can collect, record, analyze and prepare reports automatically. Third, computers can eliminate or dramatically decrease the work involved in transcribing data (e.g., physician orders) and entering data in several formats (e.g., writing the vital signs and then graphing them). Fourth, computers can help the nurse to organize, prioritize, and schedule the many tasks to be performed each shift.

Data Entry Technology   Writing information on paper in narrative format is the least efficient method of data collection available. Once entered, the use of that narrative information is strictly constrained (Nolan, 1973). Paper-based narrative data cannot be located, retrieved, or analyzed efficiently—even during the care episode that occasioned the narrative note. Costly human time must be invested to convert that narrative information into data that can be aggregated across many patients and analyzed in some fashion. Once stored in medical records, narrative information is effectively lost because of the large amount of time needed to retrieve and search the entire chart for that one note.

Technology exists to permit data to be entered into a computer with minimal or no typing. This technology may consist of application of informatics techniques, or of computer technology (machines and programs) or both. Informatics techniques involve redesigning the chart to permit the majority of data to be entered in numeric format. These formats usually consist of checklists, numbers in a structured format (e.g., vital signs), or graphical data representations.

Checklists may be the most common format for assessment data. Data such as cardiac sounds, lung sounds, skin condition, cardiac rhythms, and the like have a limited number of possible descriptors. These descriptors are presented on the screen as a list and the nurse selects from the list. For example, from normal sinus rhythm to asystole there are 23 commonly described cardiac rhythms. Much time can be saved with a system in which the nurse merely needs to check one of the rhythms instead of writing out a rhythm such as "wandering atrial pacemaker." The checklist format for charting will also help to eliminate the problem of unapproved abbreviations that many health care organizations must address.

Structured number formats and graphical representations of data are informatics methods found in nearly all nursing flow sheets. Structured number formats have proved useful in ICU flow sheets and in other settings where routine care or assessments must be performed and documented in a repetitive manner. Graphics are less commonly applied. Most settings use a vital-signs graphics form, but this is by no means the only application of graphics for representing assessment findings. For example, pupil size is often graphically represented in neurological trauma settings. Some units that specialize in care of the patient with respiratory problems may document adventitious sounds on a drawing of the lungs on the flow sheet. These techniques may be applied to either paper- or computer-based charts, but combined with computerized data entry technology, they offer their greatest power and economy.

A variety of data entry technologies are now available for use in clinical areas. Available today are the light pen, the mouse or track ball, touch screens, and of course, the keyboard and number pad. There are also hand-held terminals, modems for remote access to the computer, and computer networks that permit a direct link to a distant computer.

The equipment most familiar to many nurses is the light pen. Light pens function by either detecting light from the screen or by flashing a light onto a point on the screen. With a checklist or graphic, the nurse places the light pen over the part of the screen to be marked and clicks a button to register "enter." Documenting the average admission assessment with its many checklists and graphics could be made many times faster with light pen entry. With a touch screen the nurse uses a finger to "mark" the correct place on the screen to enter data. A mouse or track ball has a sensor in a movable ball structure. As the mouse or the ball on a track ball is moved, the computer senses the direction change and changes the location of the screen cursor in response. A button on the mouse or track ball serves as an "enter" key.

For data in checklist or graphic format the light pen, mouse, or track ball can be used with a high degree of efficiency. Numeric data can also be selected from a "menu" of numbers with these technologies. However, they require a permanent terminal. Very few settings now have point-of-care clinical computers. Until bedside computers become standard, other data entry methods will be required.

The goal of efficiency is not furthered by increasing the amount of transcribing required in the clinical setting. Paper charts can easily be carried to the bedside. A 70-pound computer cannot. However, it is possible to acquire pocket-sized terminals (similar to a calculator) on which assessment data can be entered. The pocket terminal can be plugged into the main computer for electronic data transfer. In this way, the nurse will not find a need to write down care notes on a piece of scrap paper for later data entry into the computer or paper record. The point here is that there will be problems encountered in converting paper charts to computer information systems. Implementing a computer could be a serious mistake if it forces people to continue their current paperwork load and add computer data entry to the process. It is important to consider tool solutions for these problems rather than FTE solutions when developing a computerized patient record system.

Automatic Data Collection   In some settings, machines are now being used to monitor physical parameters. The monitors in ICUs are now called physiologic monitors instead of heart monitors because they monitor so many different physiologic variables. All of the monitors sold today are based on computer technology, and most (if not all) are designed to permit the monitored data to be stored, trended, and transferred electronically to another computer. Some of the other machines that use computer chips are IV pumps, syringe infusion pumps, ventilators, oximetry, and so forth. Most of these have some capability for transferring data.

These can improve efficiency in two ways. First, they can record the data so that the nurse does not have to enter the data in any format. Second, they can, independently or through data transfer to another computer, perform automatic trending and graphing of the data. In this way, they permit the nurse to avoid some transcribing of data from one part of the record (flowsheet or narrative notes) to another (the graphical record). It may also be that in some cases, they can substitute for manually performed nursing assessment tasks.

For example, if an arterial line is present, the physiologic monitor computer can be programmed to automatically measure and record mean arterial pressure readings and to graph the waveforms. The nurse may not need to take any blood pressure readings but only to validate the accuracy of the machine's measures at the beginning of a shift. For a patient who requires extremely close blood-pressure monitoring (e.g., BP every 5 minutes), this can save the nurse up to 1 and a half hours of work during an 8-hour shift.

Once data are in a computer, programs can be written to perform operations on that data — assuming the computer was designed to permit the data to be used in a variety of ways (Martin, 1976). Computers can be programmed to select a subset of the data for each of many patients. It can store the subset in a new file. Programs can be used to access the data in the new file and perform statistical manipulations and analysis on the data. There are programs that will take raw data or analysis results and format them into a final report. All these activities can be performed manually. Manual data manipulation however, is tedious, error prone, and so time consuming that by the time the report is prepared, it may be obsolete. Properly designed computer systems can be programmed to perform all these tasks in a matter of seconds or minutes.

Efficiencies from Reduction in Transcription Time   Nurses transcribe large amounts of information from one place to another. Part of noting physician orders is usually accompanied by copying the order onto a medication ticket, Kardex, PT schedule, lab requisition, and so forth. People make errors when copying information from one place to another. Children often play the game "telephone" in which one child originates a message and whispers to the next child, who repeats the message to another, and so on until the message at last returns to the originator. As the length and complexity of the "message" increases, the final story is increasingly garbled. Transcribing activities are merely a written and abbreviated form of the telephone game. We ought to expect a certain rate of change with transcribed orders. Yet, nurses always seem surprised when an order is miscopied or omitted entirely. The surprise — not to mention the harsh condemnation of the nurse involved — is inappropriate. A system that relies on human beings to copy large volumes of written materials from one data site to another is a badly designed system.

In industry, there are many examples of computers transcribing important messages to large numbers of different individuals and sites. Computer transmittal is virtually error free. The few errors that do occur in computer data transmission are usually identified by the computer itself as it checks the data for errors. The efficiencies obtained from computer transcription will be augmented by the reduction in time required to complete and investigate incident reports for transcription errors.

Care Scheduling   Nursing care today is more intense, complex, and detailed than at any time in history. Current trends suggest that the situation will worsen. It is also known that the average person usually can retain only about seven items of information in short-term memory. (Most people can remember a number they looked up in the telephone book long enough to dial it. If an area code needs to be added, however, most people need to write the number down. A telephone number without the area code is seven digits). Nurses today have far more than seven items of information to keep in short-term memory. Most have developed their own informal techniques to allow them to function. Yet, many care omissions still happen.

Perhaps a new paradigm is needed. The care system we now have *requires* nurses to function beyond normal human performance limits. Instead of increasing FTEs or, worse, blaming and punishing people for less than super performance, we should redesign the system. The existing manual system offers few memory supports and little or no assistance with scheduling care tasks to the individual nurse. Nurses generally are responsible for a group of patients. The care must be planned so that each patient's requirements are met in a timely fashion. Essentially, nurses schedule care tasks, and scheduling is a cognitive activity.

The cognitive work involved in scheduling is iterative and hierarchical. That is, priorities are determined for each care item and for each patient. Some are bound by time limits such as medications. Others may be scheduled according to unit routine or the nurse's convenience. Once priorities are determined, they are listed on the schedule (whether that be a paper or mental schedule). As higher priority care items are scheduled, lower priority items are left on the unscheduled list. Each review of the unscheduled item list and the partially completed schedule is a cycle or iteration. Computers can iterate rapidly and endlessly. If properly programmed, a computer will produce a work schedule much faster (and thus more efficiently) than a human being could. Furthermore, computers can instantly revise the schedule if a new patient is admitted or new orders written. Preparing or revising a care schedule can be tedious and stressful. That kind of stress often reduces efficiency. A computer scheduler can enhance efficiency by saving time and by reducing the stress factor associated with scheduling tasks.

Clinical Care Quality Improvement   Many of the facilities that promote efficiency can also serve to improve patient outcomes by improving the quality of nursing care. The computer can do this in three ways. First, it can be programmed to reduce or eliminate many errors. Second, it can make expert clinical consultation instantly available to the nurse as care is delivered. Third, it can permit a level of analysis of outcomes of care that is far beyond what can be accomplished with paper charts. Nurses will be able to empirically demonstrate the effects of nursing care on patient health status and functioning. That information will enable nurses to exert more control over changes in practice patterns through the ability to demonstrate the benefits of nursing care protocols.

Performance Limitations and Error Reduction   Previously, it was argued that the current environment requires nurses to function at levels that are beyond normal performance limits. Limits may be absolute or relative. For example, no person can start 500 IVs in an 8-hour shift. Even if the patients were all lined up and all supplies at the ready, a nurse would have to average no more than 57 seconds per IV. That limit is absolute. However, a nurse could start 90 IVs in an 8-hour shift if all the conditions were right, the patients were all lined up, and nobody had difficult-to-access veins. In that case, an average of 5 minutes per IV would be possible. Even under the best conditions, however, nobody could sustain that average forever.

The point is that people can sometimes perform extraordinary feats. Nobody can perform extraordinarily all the time. A system that requires people to function at peak performance at all times is a source of error. The current care environment is so complex and busy and offers so few supports to human memory and cognition that it predisposes to clinical error. Most people do the best they can with the resources they have. Very few nurses are deliberately sloppy or careless. No system can protect against the occasional error. But when we see incident reports averaging more than one or two serious errors a week per unit and notice that even our best nurses are making more errors than expected, we should begin to question the system instead of the quality of the people. Quality cannot be consistently maintained with a seriously flawed care delivery system.

To the extent the computer information system can serve to reduce clinical errors, it will improve quality of care. A medication system provides one example of how a computer can improve care quality. Medication errors can be virtually eliminated by means of a program designed to permit physicians to enter directly their medication orders. It is possible to program the computer to calculate automatically the proper dose range for the patient's body weight and to warn the doctor of a potential dosage error while the order is being entered. Furthermore, incorrect routes or methods of administration can be brought to the physician's attention before a clinical error is made. The computer can be programmed to expect the medication to be charted by a certain time and to warn the nurse about the omission in time to give the drug. If a nurse attempted to enter the wrong dose, the computer could instantly detect and report the error. If an incorrect dose was actually administered, early discovery might permit immediate action to protect the patient from harm. If the error was merely a typographical error, the nurse would have the opportunity to correct the error on the screen before it was permanently recorded in the patient's chart.

Medication errors are only one type of clinical problem that can be alleviated by computer technology. Other situations include activities that require math calculations or need to be performed at specific times. For example, computers can automatically calculate data derived from monitored variables. Therefore, a pulse pressure that is widening in a head trauma patient can be detected and alarmed by a computer attached to the blood pressure monitor. Many errors in documentation could be avoided if computer charts were programmed to recognize the range of correct values and alarm on values that were out of range (e.g., a BP recorded as 60/120). Wrong chart notes would still occur, but would be less frequent if the record itself could detect care not ordered or inconsistent with certain types of expectations. For example, a dressing change charted on a patient who had no wounds or a PAP test recorded on a male patient should not pass unchallenged.

Clinical Consultation The computer can serve to support the clinical knowledge base and decision processes of nurses (Ozbolt, Schultz, Swain, & Abraham, 1985). There are a few systems that have been developed to support the clinical judgement of physicians. These systems work by offering advice or by guiding the thinking and decision processes of the clinician (Brennan & McHugh, 1988). These systems help to improve the quality of clinical judgements by ensuring that all the important information that should be considered is, in fact, taken into account (McHugh, 1986b).

A system that provides a draft care plan derived from the initial nursing assessment is another form of clinical consultation. Ideally, the system should guide and support patient assessment and planning of care (Zielstorff, McHugh, & Clinton, 1988; McHugh, 1989). Although a nurse might overlook or forget a low-priority nursing diagnosis in a multiproblem patient, the computer will not.

Clinical decision support could be of immense value. For the first time in history, a basic level competency in assessment and nursing diagnosis could be defined and maintained. Even very inexperienced nurses would be unlikely to miss important clinical phenomena. The computer would present not only the data, but also a basic level of interpretation of the clinical meaning and importance of the data.

Equally important, the nurse could use the computer as a clinical learning tool. It could be asked to show the nurse the information it used to determine its nursing diagnosis or its care-planning strategy. The computer could be queried by the nurse about its decision process and the decision rules it used to draw its conclusions. Thus, nurses could use the computer to learn new facts and also to improve their own critical thinking and clinical judgement skills.

Improving Clinical Practice Clinical practice is only partially based on evidence of its efficacy. Advancements in the science of nursing are hampered by the expense of research and by the amount of time such research requires. Data collection and preparing data for computer entry usually consumes 70 to 80 percent of all research costs. It is frustrating for a researcher to realize that most of the data needed for a particular study has been collected and stored in the paper chart but, because of the expense, cannot be retrieved. Despite the great expense of collecting data anew, it is often still less expensive than data retrieval from paper charts. Thus, the paper chart often acts as more of an impediment to quality improvement than an asset. A properly designed computer-based patient record could provide enormous opportunity to examine, analyze, and evaluate nursing care protocols and activities across many hundreds or thousands of patients.

If the capacity to evaluate the effects of nursing care on hundreds or thousands of patients were available, changes in practice could be more easily based on sound evidence of the benefits of those changes. Programs could be developed to flag and track unexpected deaths, prolonged lengths of stay, nosocomial infection rates, unusually good patient outcomes, and the like. This information could be linked with the nursing care provided. Commonalities or special differences in these special cases could be evaluated for the need to change practice. If one approach is found to be more highly associated with successful patient outcomes than another, nurses could discover this fact and then change practice to increase success rates. Conversely, care that is ineffective or even deleterious could be identified and abandoned in favor of successful care approaches. The problem now is that we are unable to use the data in our own nursing records to discover and document the effects of our work.

As health care looks more toward changes in patient health status as the most important indicators of care quality, it will become increasingly important for nurses to link nursing practices to patient outcomes. Every blood pressure test, bed bath, dressing change, and patient education session costs money. Some studies have documented the benefits of particular nursing care protocols. However, too much of our care is now based on unit routines or unproven ideas about what will benefit the patient. In the future, we will need to justify nursing care expense with far more credible evidence of the benefits to patients of that care. Until and unless nursing care is documented in a system that permits rapid and inexpensive retrieval, aggregation, and analysis of that data, nursing will be unprepared to respond to the demands of third party payors and regulatory bodies for proof of the quality and effectiveness of our care.

Applications for Nursing Service Administration

In these challenging times, it is increasingly important for nursing care delivery systems to be well managed. All of the principles pertaining to quality, efficiency, and productivity addressed in the context of clinical nursing apply equally to the practice of nursing administration. In some ways, it may be even more important for administrators to examine their practice than for staff. Nursing service administrators must make critical decisions about the fate of their employees and the direction nursing care will take in their institutions. Poor decisions may lead to poor patient care, loss of staff, and ultimately, perhaps, even failure of the entire institution.

Quality of Management Decisions   The body of information needed by nurse managers to make good decisions has increased dramatically in the past 20 years. They have always needed a good foundation in the realities of clinical practice, people management skills, project management skills, and good skills in resource management. None of those skills are obsolete. However, today, managers must also have a good working knowledge of third party payor trends, financial analysis, public relations, requirements of accrediting bodies and regulatory agencies, and a myriad of other facets of the health care industry and its political and social environment.

Increasingly, more pieces of information, more complex information, and the dynamics of interrelationships among disparate items of information need to be understood and analyzed if good management decisions are to be made. Meanwhile, the situation of health care is highly volatile. Almost no one has the time to spend manually collecting, aggregating, and analyzing large volumes of data — even if they have the economic resources to invest in those activities. All too often, these problems force managers to make decisions with faulty and insufficient information. Such decisions may work out well enough if the manager is lucky. Many health care organizations are at risk, however, and poor decisions may threaten their survival.

Computer information systems can be used to improve the quality of management by permitting managers to acquire and *use* more information in their decision-making processes. In this way, they improve the quality of their decisions.

Consider trying to make a decision about choosing between devoting resources to adding four birthing rooms in obstetrics or adding two new operating rooms to surgery. What factors might influence the decision if the only information related to the hospital management team was that both the obstetricians and the surgeons wanted their respective expansions very badly? One suspects that personal relationships with the physicians might influence the decision, or the clinical preference of the decision maker might take precedence. Obviously, the decision has only a 50 percent chance of being the right decision with this paucity of information. Most managers would identify at least five or six more items of information they would need to make a good decision. Critical items of information might include:

1. Information about which program was currently providing the most profit.
2. Community birth rates and the trend upward or downward in births in the service area.
3. The number of women in their childbearing years and population trends in females in the service area.
4. The amount of elective surgery that currently must be delayed due to insufficient operating rooms.
5. Cost projections for each expansion project.
6. Any anticipated loss of surgeons or anesthesiologists because of retirement or relocation and the hospital's potential for replacing those losses.
7. Information about the plans of competing hospitals in the service area.

The answers to any *one* of these questions might have a strong influence on management's decision. If managers have answers to *all* of these questions, they would have a more complete picture of the hospital, its resources, and its environment than any part of the answers could offer. No one aspect of the problem would be likely to create a distorted image of the situation and, thus, have a disproportionate influence on the final choices of the management team. Full information decreases the probability that a wrong choice will be selected.

Unfortunately, the quality of most management decisions can only be evaluated retrospectively. However, some computer-decision support technology exists to permit managers to evaluate in advance the probable outcomes of some types of decisions. These types of applications are called management-decision support systems.

Currently available management-decision support tools include computer simulations, forecasting and trend analysis programs, statistical analysis programs, and financial planning programs. Computer simulations are procedural models. They express dynamic relationships in a system by means of precise symbols and directions about how those symbols remain static or move about in relation to each other. For example, a model of a unit and its access to nursing staff in relation to changing workloads has been developed for the purpose of examining costs and staffing adequacy of a variety of nurse staffing patterns (McHugh, 1988).

Nurse executives must perform financial analysis and make projections about changes in skill mix, clinical specialty requirements, and a host of other problems in which past experience can offer a guide to future performance. Computer programs can be used to support the quality of decisions involving these issues. Specifically, financial planning, forecasting, statistical analysis, and trend analysis programs can be used to improve predictions of changes in the internal and external environment. They can also be used to link these predicted changes to possible outcomes of selected managerial decisions. The computer's predictions of outcomes of decisions can be used as early warning of a need to make adjustments in strategic plans.

Nursing service administrators may want to investigate the value of these types of decision support tools in their own practice. To the extent that nursing service administrators make use of all available resources to support assessment, planning, and evaluation in their management practice, they will be better managers. They will make better quality decisions, and their institutions will have a better chance to survive the stresses of this rapidly changing health care environment.

Efficiency in Nursing Administration   Computer information systems can be used for a wide variety of applications to increase the efficiency of administration. A variety of tasks that must be performed by the nursing service administration require significant amounts of number processing or other data manipulation. Patient classification systems, staffing and scheduling systems, budgeting, and the like are data intensive and data manipulation intensive. Computers can greatly speed up the processing and reduce errors of manual handling.

In this area, conversion from manual processes to computer processing may well permit reduction in FTEs. However, it is more common to find that managers seek computers to avoid increasing secretarial FTEs when their people are simply overwhelmed. On the other hand, they may realize that information that would be extremely useful can be obtained only with the processing power of a computer. Some types of computer programs that have been developed to improve managerial efficiency are patient acuity classification systems, staff scheduling systems, project planning and scheduling applications, budget development and control systems, and programs to support strategic planning efforts. These programs require substantial amounts of information about the current operations of the organization (e.g., average census, workload amount and stability, number of staff, staff mix, among others). These types of programs provide new information by performing analysis on the data about the experience. The value of all of these programs is constrained by the availability of data about the operations of the organization.

Perhaps the greatest danger facing administrators' ability to avail themselves of computer-decision support technology is the dearth and poor quality of information they can retrieve from their own operations. The clinical record contains the source data on the operations of any clinical agency. Few industries would allow their operations data to be lost to illegible, inaccessible paper records. Yet, that is exactly how hospitals treat their clinical operations data. Consider how rapidly your hospital could obtain precise answers to the following questions:

1. How many CCU patients overflowed into SICU last month? Does that number represent our usual experience?
2. How many patients who were at risk for decubitus ulcers actually experienced some degree of skin breakdown?
3. Does the current nursing workload in terms of number and acuity of patients per nursing FTE match the nursing care we had planned to deliver when we prepared the budget?

Many hospitals can quickly answer the third question. Those data are found in an automated patient classification system, if the hospital has such a system. The first question can also be answered fairly quickly. Someone must retrieve the SICU log and make a judgement about every patient listed as to whether or not the patient should have been placed in CCU. A precise answer may never be available, but a good estimate should be obtained in 1 or 2 weeks.

The second question may be a problem. Most hospitals have no practical way to identify patients at risk of complications. Actual complications are usually only available if tracked in a QA study. Yet, answers to the second question relate directly to the effects of the nursing care on patients. The only way that such data can be made available economically is through implementation of the computer-based patient chart. Even then, the desired functionality will be achievable only if the computer-based chart meets the criteria for such systems as described in the ANA Publication, *Computer Design Criteria for Systems that Support the Nursing Process*.

Summary

Computer information systems are primarily useful in the context of productivity enhancement. They help achieve productivity gains by increasing the efficiency or quality of work. In both the clinical and administrative arenas, the amount and complexity of information required for success has grown to such proportions that manual data and information processes no longer suffice. Good decisions are not made in the absence of relevant information. Nurse managers and clinicians need rapid and economical access to an ever-increasing volume and variety of information if their decisions are to lead to clinical and institutional successes. However, computer technology now exists to greatly enhance the power of nurses to improve their performance and the benefits of nursing care. The seeds of future success should be planted now with vendors and other members of the health care delivery team. Vendors must be informed of our needs and the expectations of our computing systems. Other members of the health care delivery team should collaborate with nurses and vendors on the design and implementation of powerful new clinical information systems. The effort will be worthwhile because the benefits of clinical and administrative computing will accrue to all of us — patients, clinicians, and administrators.

References

Brennan, P., & McHugh, M. (1988). Clinical decision-making and computer support, *Applied Nursing Research, 1*(2), 89–93.

Channon, B. (1983). Dispelling productivity myths, *Hospitals, 57*(19), 103–119.

Jydstrup, R. A., & Gross, M. J. (1966). Cost of information handling in hospitals, *Health Services Research, 1*(3), 235–261.

Martin, J. (1976). *Principles of data-base management.* Englewood Cliffs, NJ: Prentice-Hall.

McHugh, M. (1989). Productivity measurement in nursing, *Applied Nursing Research, 2*(2), 99–102.

McHugh, M. (1986a). Increasing productivity through computer communications, *Dimensions of Critical Care Nursing, 5*(5); 284–302.

McHugh, M. (1986b). Information access: A basis for strategic planning and control of operations, *Nursing Administration Quarterly, 10*(1), 10–20.

McHugh, M. (1988, May). Comparison of four hospital nurse staffing patterns for wage costs and staffing adequacy using computer simulation. *Dissertation Abstracts International, 48*(11), 3250-B. B-The Sciences and Engineering. (University Microfilms International Order No. DA8801370)

McHugh, M. (1989). Computer support for the nursing process, *Health Matrix, 7*(1), 57–60.

Nolan, R. (1973). Computer data bases: The future is now, *Harvard Business Review, 51*(5), 98–114.

Oatway, D. (1987). The future of computer applications for nursing quality assurance, *Journal of Nursing Quality Assurance, 1*(4), 61–71.

Ozbolt, J., Schultz, S., Swain, M., & Abraham, I. (1985). A proposed expert system for nursing practice, *Journal of Medical Systems, 9*, 57–68.

Parker, M., Benson, R., & Trainor, H. (1988). *Information economics: Linking business performance to information technology.* Englewood Cliffs, NJ: Prentice-Hall.

Richart, R. (1970). Evaluation of a medical data system, *Computers in Biomedical Research, 3*(5), 415–425.

Young, L., & Hayne, A. (1988). *Nursing administration: From concepts to practice.* Philadelphia: Saunders.

Zielstorff, R., McHugh, M., & Clinton, J. (1988). *Computer design criteria for systems that support the nursing process.* Kansas City, MO: American Nurses Association.

CHAPTER 30

Collective Action— Labor Relations

Richard W. Redman

Highlights

- Concept of collective bargaining
- Nursing and collective bargaining
- Process of union recognition
- Contract negotiation and impasse procedures
- Life with a contract

The purpose of this chapter is to discuss protective legislation for employees and employers as it relates to collective bargaining by nurses. The evolution of collective bargaining in the United States, in general industry and in nursing, is explained briefly. The major legal requirements for collective bargaining are examined and their implications for the nurse executive are discussed.

CONCEPT OF COLLECTIVE BARGAINING

Collective bargaining is often referred to as "bilateral determinism," meaning that two parties, management and a representative group of employees, participate in making decisions that affect the employees in the workplace. This collective or bilateral approach is seen as an alternative to management unilaterally making employee-related decisions. Generally, collective bargaining is viewed as having a close relationship with human resource management. Although they are two distinct programs, they can become related at times; if management does an inadequate job in managing the human resource, they will generally find themselves dealing with a petition by employees to bargain collectively.

The American labor movement has been an important part of U.S. social and economic history. Many feel that American industry owes its present standing in the world marketplace to the labor movement. History supports the fact that prior to the legislated protection of employee rights in the workplace, many employees were exploited and had little say in the workplace issues. Unionism generally has played an integral part in balancing out the relationship between management and staff (O'Rourke & Barton, 1981).

Although the right to bargain collectively is a legislated right, it is often viewed with ambivalence when professional employees are involved. The idea of nurses, physicians, or teachers being involved in collective bargaining activities often evokes strong emotional responses, either pro or con. Those who support collective bargaining for professionals take the position that it is the legal right of all employee groups to seek collective representation over those areas protected by legislation: the mandatory bargaining subjects of wages, hours, and other conditions of employment. Furthermore, it is felt that collective bargaining is the only way to maintain control over professional practice. Those who are against professional employee involvement in collective action generally view unionism as a blue collar activity that promotes strikes, that is, is unprofessional.

In nursing, it presents the additional challenge in that both management and staff generally are professional nurses who are colleagues, yet sitting on different sides of an issue. Also, there are issues related to what type of organization is most appropriate to represent nurses in a bargaining situation, for example, an industrial or trade union or a professional organization that deals with and understands nursing practice issues. These issues notwithstanding, it is the legal right of nurses to bargain collectively just as it is the right of other employee groups to do so. Although management in most organizations would undoubtedly prefer to work directly with employees rather than work with a third party, such as a union, it is also a fact that employees are not always given their due workplace rights and collective action is the only way to ensure that. Many nurses view collective bargaining as the only way to balance their relationship with management and to enhance their professional status (Wilson, Hamilton, & Murphy, 1990). Regardless of personal views, it is essential for the nurse executive to have a thorough understanding of employee and employer rights as they relate to collective action.

MAJOR COLLECTIVE BARGAINING LEGISLATION

Legislation to protect employee rights in the workplace is essentially a twentieth-century phenomenon. The initial legislation focused on railroad employees, but subsequent legislation covered employees in almost all types of industries. Table 30.1 presents a brief chronology of the major federal legislation that defines the rights of employees and employers with regard to collective bargaining.

The National Labor Relations Act (NLRA), passed in 1935, is the major piece of legislation that began to define the rights of employees to organize and bargain

TABLE 30.1 Chronology of Major Federal Labor Legislation in the United States

1898	Erdman Act First federal legislation to deal with collective bargaining; outlawed discrimination by employers against union activities.
1926	Railway Labor Act Established mediation and voluntary arbitration as means to decrease labor/management conflict.
1935	National Labor Relations Act (NLRA) Designed to promote greater self-determination for employees through establishing protected rights to organize and bargain collectively; established the National Labor Relations Board to conduct union elections and provide remedy for unfair labor practices; initially covered all industries, including health care; also known as the Wagner Act.
1947	Taft-Hartley Act Amended the NLRA; quite restrictive of union activities; established the Federal Mediation and Conciliation Service; specifically excluded nonprofit, private, and governmental health care organizations.
1959	Landrum-Griffin Act Directed at the internal affairs of unions.
1962	Executive Order 10988 President Kennedy's order that established employees' right to organize in federal hospitals (such as the VA); prohibits strikes in those facilities.
1974	Taft-Hartley Amendments Amended the NLRA; permitted nonpublic, nonprofit health care facility employees to bargain collectively; established a series of rules specifically for the health care industry (such as required advance notice for strikes).

collectively. It has been amended three times. Initially the NLRA covered all health care employees. The 1947 amendments, however, excluded the nonprofit health care industry from the NLRA, because it viewed nonprofit health care organizations as charitable organizations that were not involved in interstate commerce and thereby exempt (Hirsh, 1990).

The 1947 legislation also excluded federal and nonfederal government-controlled hospitals from collective bargaining. Thus, Veteran's Administration facilities and state and local government-controlled hospitals' employees, as well, could not bargain collectively. This effectively closed off the majority of health care employees from the right to unionize.

Gradually, health care employees were granted rights to organize. In 1962, an executive order established the rights of federal health care employees to organize but prohibited them from striking if an impasse was reached. In 1974, NLRA amendments established the rights of all health care employees in private not-for-profit facilities to bargain collectively.

The legal arena that covers employees' right to organize in a particular type of health care organization is often referred to as the "patchwork quilt of legislation." Federal employees are covered by the EO 10988; employees in the private not-for-profit sector are covered by the 1974 NLRA Amendments. Employees in other types of health care facilities, for example, a state- or city-owned facility, may be covered by "right-to-work" laws if they exist in a particular state. Thus, the right to organize can vary for nurses from one organization to another within the same locale, depending on the type of facility ownership and whether appropriate legislation exists.

The National Labor Relations Board (NLRB), established by the 1935 NLRA, oversees the conduct of the NLRA. The two major activities of the NLRB are *(1)* determination and certification of bargaining units through regulated election procedures and *(2)* prevention and remedy of unfair labor practices (NLRB, 1978). The NLRB also regulates and interprets the NLRA and its amendments through the establishment and promulgation of rules. One important rule that relates to the number of bargaining units permitted in a health care facility has been monitored and challenged over the past 20 years by both nursing groups and hospital management. This rule pertains to the number of bargaining units that can exist in one facility.

The NLRB has ruled that as many as eight bargaining units are appropriate in a given health care facility. The eight bargaining units that may exist in one facility are:

1. nurses
2. physicians
3. other professionals
4. technical employees
5. business office clericals
6. skilled maintenance employees
7. all other nonprofessionals
8. security guards.

This is quite different from an earlier NLRB position that assumed only two bargaining units were appropriate: professional employees (which would include RNs) and nonprofessional employees.

Eligible membership is determined by the "community of interest" doctrine that compares job families in terms of economic concerns, degree to which their work is integrated, and the management structures that apply to them. Nursing groups, such as the American Nurses Association (ANA), have been concerned about RN-only units, taking the position that the "community of interest" of nurses is unique and other job families should not be eligible to participate in a nurses' bargaining unit. Hospital management has been concerned about the number of bargaining units that a facility could potentially have to deal with. Their position has been that bargaining with up to eight units in a facility would be too time consuming and increases the potential for disruption of workflow if negotiations break down with any one group (Gullett & Kroll, 1990).

The NLRB ruling on eight bargaining units was contested in court by the American Hospital Association (AHA). The case was eventually argued before the U.S. Supreme Court, which upheld the NLRB position (AHA vs. NLRB, 1991). Thus, it appears that the potential for eight bargaining units as well as RN-only units will likely remain in any given facility.

NURSING AND COLLECTIVE BARGAINING

Collective bargaining in the health care industry is a relatively new development, with most of the activity taking place in the past 20 years. Most of this activity, especially within nursing, was stimulated by the 1974 NLRA Amendments. Currently, approximately one third of all registered nurses are organized in units that represent 20 percent of all hospitals in the United States (Merker, Blank, & Rhodes, 1990).

Major leadership for collective bargaining in nursing has come from the ANA. The ANA established its commitment to representing the professional and economic interests of nurses when it was established in 1896. In 1946, a national economic security program was developed by ANA. In 1949, the ANA filed with the NLRB as a bargaining agent for nurses. Although the ANA is registered as a national labor organization, it does not directly represent nurses for collective bargaining purposes. That role is filled by the state nurses associations that have economic and general welfare programs. Approximately 70 percent of all unionized nurses are represented by these state associations (Flanagan, 1983). The remainder of organized nurses are represented by other health care unions or general trade and industrial unions that also are involved with health care employees.

Nurses join unions for all the same reasons that any employee group seeks collective bargaining. The major reason is that nurses are dissatisfied with management practices. This dissatisfaction generally relates to inadequate grievance procedures, unsatisfactory wage and fringe benefit packages, inconsistent interpretation of policies by management, and a lack of control over decision making concerning their work and responsibilities. The general levels of dissatisfaction that nurses evidence are generally the type of catalyst that increases interest in what unions can do to address the contributing factors.

Several factors in the contemporary environment have also contributed to an increased interest in collective bargaining by nurses. Many nurses are looking for an increase in autonomy to go along with the increased responsibility they are assuming. Other professionals such as teachers and, to a lesser degree, physicians are increasing their involvement in collective bargaining and this adds legitimacy for nurses who are interested. The impact of the feminist movement has encouraged women to stand up for their rights (Flanagan, 1983). The literature is replete with nurses' growing discontent over general working conditions. Finally, the continuing problems with the economic status of nursing, especially wage compression, remain major issues in nursing (Secretary's Commission on Nursing, 1988).

Although economic factors are often cited as a major factor for unionizing, there are limited data available on the success rate of unions in addressing economic dissatisfaction. Some generalizations about the effect of unions on wages of hospital employees can be made. Overall, wages have increased at a statistically significant level for unionized hospital employees. The effect on nursing salaries has been smaller (about 6 percent) than on nonprofessional salaries (about 10 percent). Another effect to be considered is the "spillover effect," that is, the impact on pay levels in hospitals that are not unionized but compete in the same marketplace for employees with other hospitals that are unionized. Generally, these nonunionized hospitals have to pay higher wages to compete. In addition, the spillover effect can occur within one institution where nonunionized employees benefit from the effects of other employees who are unionized. This effect on wages ranges from 1 to 8 percent (Wilson, 1985).

Critics of unionization often attribute increased costs in health care to union activities. Although limited data exist, it does appear that the impact of unionization on hospital costs has been modest. Less than 10 percent of the increase in hospital costs in the 1970s was attributable to union activity. Furthermore, it has been predicted that the impact during the 1980s and 1990s will be even less (Becker, Sloan, & Steinwald, 1981).

Overall, it appears that the debate over nursing's involvement in collective bargaining is diminishing. Although that does not negate the debate over appropriateness, it does suggest an increased acceptance and recognition of the legal right of nurses to engage in union activities to address both workplace and professional practice issues.

PROCESS OF UNION RECOGNITION

When a group of employees is interested in forming a bargaining unit, stringent requirements, as outlined by the NLRB, must be followed. These legal requirements guide the actions of management, the employees who are potential members of the bargaining unit, and the labor organization that is attempting to represent the employees. Any violation of the legal requirements outlined in the NLRA is designated as an unfair labor practice and punishable by the NLRB, which functions like an administrative court (NLRB, 1978).

The nurse executive must have a good working knowledge of the appropriate legal requirements and must ensure that the entire nursing management team is informed. Generally, when organizing efforts are developing, the senior management team in the facility will work closely with consultants who specialize in responding to union recognition campaigns. These consultants are often referred to as "union busters" by the union representatives (Ballman, 1985). It is important to keep in mind that the employees who are promoting the cause of the union are relying heavily on union staff members and in this regard are working with consultants as well. Several guides exist that offer strategies to both management and the employees interested in forming a bargaining group (see, for example, American Hospital Association, 1991; O'Rourke & Barton, 1981).

The process of union recognition begins with the labor organization filing a petition or a series of union authorization cards signed by a minimum of 30 percent of the employees in the potential bargaining unit. The NLRB then conducts a hearing to determine the appropriate unit membership based on the "community of interest" doctrine. In addition to a determination of which job families are to be included, the NLRB conducts a review of all job titles and the positions they represent to ensure that any title categorized as a supervisor is excluded from the bargaining unit election. Supervisor is defined by the NLRA as someone who has authority to hire, suspend, lay off, promote, discharge, reward, or discipline an employee (Shepard & Doudera, 1981). Generally, employee positions are reviewed on a case-by-case basis and inconsistencies may be found across different health care organizations. For example, assistant head nurses, clinical nurse specialists, and patient care coordinators may be classified as a supervisor in one organization and as a potential union member in another. It is dependent on how an organization defines a particular job title in terms of actual supervisory responsibilities.

After the eligible membership for the proposed bargaining unit has been determined, there is a 30-day period that is referred to as a "laboratory environment." During this time, both management and the union will conduct active campaigns, presenting their views and recommendations to the employee group. Both sides are closely regulated by the NLRB. The NLRA is biased toward the union during this time in that the union can essentially promise the employees all types of gains that will be achieved if the union election is successful. Management, on the other hand, can make no promises about what they will do if the union is not voted in. The intent is that management has had the opportunity for those promises prior to the "laboratory" period and now it is too late for quick fixes. Management can, however, hold informational sessions, called captive audience sessions, in which factual information is presented to employees. Employees are required to attend these sessions if they are scheduled during work time. During this period the union will also be campaigning actively, conducting informational sessions and rallies. Often, other unions in the region will assist with the campaign in support of the labor movement (American Hospital Association, 1991).

At the end of the 30-day period, the NLRB will conduct a secret ballot election. A 51 percent majority of those voting is required to elect the bargaining unit. If successful, the labor organization is then designated as the exclusive bargaining agent for the employees. If not, no additional elections can be held for a period of 12 months (Hirsh, 1990).

In the past 10 years, there has been a general decrease in the number of elections held in health care organizations, although the percentage of those won by unions has increased during that same time. Most predict there will be an increase in election activity, given the impact of prospective payment, the general financial constraints in the health care industry, and the recent Supreme Court ruling that upholds the NLRB position for bargaining units (Merker, Blank, & Rhodes, 1990; Scott & Simpson, 1989).

CONTRACT NEGOTIATION AND IMPASSE PROCEDURES

If the union is recognized by election, then both management and union representatives must bargain in "good faith" to develop a labor contract. The contract covers the mandatory topics outlined in the legislation that applies to that health care facility. The scope of bargaining usually includes wages, hours, and conditions of employment. Any other topic is permissible for bargaining, provided both parties agree to bargain over it.

After the contract is negotiated and agreed to by both parties, the union membership votes to ratify or reject the contract. If ratified, the contract then serves as the legal set of policies that must be adhered to by both parties. Contracts are either 2 or 3 years in length.

Sometimes the negotiation process reaches an impasse where neither side will change its position on a particular contract item. Although a strike is always a potential outcome in impasse situations, generally there are a series of intermediate activities as an attempt to resolve the differences. Some legislation or existing contracts require that unresolvable differences be reported to the Federal Mediation and Conciliation Service (FMCS), which may require mediation before a strike can occur. The FMCS will investigate, conduct hearings in which both sides present their position, and present recommendations that are advisory, not binding. Some contracts may require binding arbitration in which a third party intervenes on unsettled issues. In this situation, an arbitrator holds hearings and makes a binding decision, that is, both parties must accept it.

If an impasse is reached after fact finding and the appropriate legislation permits the union membership to strike, the union generally conducts a vote among its membership. The NLRA requires a 10-day notification of the NLRB before a strike can occur in a health care organization so that necessary arrangements can be made to transfer patients, decrease admissions, and take other appropriate steps to ensure safe patient care.

Two types of strikes are legal: economic strikes and unfair labor practice strikes. An economic strike is called by the union in response to demands made by the employer in terms of wages, hours, or working conditions. In this type of strike, employers cannot discharge workers who are on strike but they can hire either temporary or permanent replacements. The second type of strike is called by the union to protest an unfair labor practice, such as management's bargaining in poor faith. In this type of strike, employees have a legal right to reinstatement and cannot be permanently replaced (Rothman, 1983).

If a strike is to occur, very careful strategic planning is required by the health care facility. The nurse executive assumes a key leadership role in determining patient care management and staffing of those beds that will remain open during the work stoppage. General guidelines are available to assist the facility in planning for a strike (Rothman, 1983).

The overall strike rate in health care facilities is approximately 4 percent, with the majority of work stoppages occurring over first contracts. The major reasons for strikes are not always economic, although management tends to view them as such. Key issues are often related to overtime hours, weekend duty, grievance management, and overall working conditions, such as degree of employee involvement in decision making and general communication patterns between management and employees (Imberman, 1989).

Every attempt is made to encourage settlement of a work stoppage, generally by both parties involved as well as the NLRB. On settlement of a work stoppage, careful consideration must be given to reintegration of the employees as they return to work. This planning should take place during the strike, not after it is settled. Consideration is needed by both employees and management as the organization goes through what is best viewed as a healing process. Blaming and personalizing of issues should be avoided and open communication encouraged. The nurse executive plays an important leadership role for the entire organization by creating an environment where both management and staff can work through their feelings of resentment, anger, and betrayal (Rosenthal, 1990).

LIFE WITH A CONTRACT

After a ratified contract is in place, it becomes important for the organization and its members to accept the reality of the union contract. The existence of the contract will present both advantages and disadvantages to both parties. Most important, it standardizes the treatment of all employees and removes ambiguity from management decision making. The existence of a contract should be viewed as something that will now be used by the organization to move forward and get on with its daily goals.

The contract does not negate the need for a human resource management program. It defines only those areas that have been bargained over and does not address many areas that go beyond the mandatory scope of bargaining. In fact, it would be a mistake for any organization to use the contract as its human resource program.

The nurse executive must ensure that an orientation to the contract is conducted for all members of the nursing management team. It is the management team that will be interpreting the contract on a daily basis through their interaction with bargained-for employees. If they do not have a good understanding of the terms of the contract, they will be generating a lot of grievances for the organization. The managers should also be informed on who to contact if they are not sure how to handle a situation. Periodically, the contract should be reviewed with nurse managers to ensure that they are interpreting the contract with consistency.

Data should be gathered by management throughout the life of the contract in terms of what problems are surfacing that need to be reexamined at contract renewal time. Vague contract language, sources of continual grievances, and areas where the contract is silent all provide important evaluation information for the nurse executive when the next contract is being negotiated.

Living with a negotiated contract does not have to be a difficult experience. Mutual respect and understanding by both parties can provide a solid foundation for collaborative working relationships among management and staff.

Summary

The protective legislation for employers and employees that addresses collective bargaining provides an extremely important body of knowledge for the nurse executive. Often, it is experienced in a crisis situation that is laden with emotions, rather than rational actions. The nurse executive plays a key role in the organization in terms of dealing with employees' concerns and potential collective action. Having a good working knowledge of the rights and responsibilities of both employers and employees in the workplace is essential for the nurse executive. If a collective bargaining contract is in place, it must be integrated into the overall human resource management program that exists within the organization. The nurse executive can assume an important leadership role for the entire organization by creating a working environment wherein the concerns of the employees and the well-being of patients and families are the primary values.

Learning Activities

1. Identify the major pieces of Federal legislation designed to protect the rights of employees and employers in the collective bargaining domain.

2. Describe the prevalence of collective bargaining activities in the health care industry in general and nursing in particular.

3. Discuss the legal requirements that must be followed by employees and employers when collective action is undertaken by employee groups.

4. Discuss the advantages and disadvantages of collective bargaining for employees and employers.

5. Explain the relationship between a collective bargaining contract and a human resources management program.

References

American Hospital Association v. *NLRB*, S. Ct. 90–97 (1991).

American Hospital Association. (1991). *Collective bargaining units in the health care industry.* Office of Legal Regulatory Affairs. Legal Memorandum, No. 16. Chicago.

Ballman, C. S. (1985). Union busters, *American Journal of Nursing, 85*(9), 963–966.

Becker, E. R., Sloan, F. A., & Steinwald, B. (1982). Union activity in hospitals: Past, present, and future, *Health Care Financing Review, 3*(4), 1–13.

Flanagan, L. (1983). *Collective bargaining and the nursing profession.* (Pub. No. D72E IM). Kansas City, MO: American Nurses Association.

Gullett, C. R., & Kroll, M. J. (1990). Rule making and the National Labor Relations Board: Implications for the health care industry, *Health Care Management Review, 15*(2), 61–65.

Hirsh, H. L. (1990). Legal aspects of nursing administration. In J. A. Dienemann (Ed.), *Nursing Administration: Strategic Perspectives and Application* (pp. 29–55). Norwalk, CT: Appleton & Lange.

Imberman, W. (1989). Rx: Strike prevention in hospitals, *Hospital & Health Services Administration, 34*(2), 195–211.

Merker, L. R., Blank, M. A., & Rhodes, R. (1990). *Collective bargaining strategy briefings.* (No. 154902). Chicago: American Hospital Association Center for Nursing.

National Labor Relations Board (1978). *A guide to basic law and procedures under the National Labor Relations Act.* (No. 031-000-00187-1). Washington, DC: U.S. Goverment Printing Office.

O'Rourke, K. A., & Barton, S. R. (1981). *Nurse power: Unions and the law.* Bowie, MD: Robert J. Brady Co.

Rosenthal, E. A. (1990). Good planning alleviates bad effects of stoppages, *Health Care Strategic Management, 8*(12), 13–15.

Rothman, W. A. (1983). *Strikes in health care organizations.* Owings Mills, MD: National Health Publishing.

Scott, C., & Simpson, J. (1989). Union election activity in the hospital industry, *Health Care Management Review, 14*(4), 21–28.

Shepard, I. M., & Doudera, A. E. (Eds.). (1981). *Health care labor law.* Ann Arbor, MI: AUPHA Press.

U.S. Department of Health and Human Services. (1988). *Secretary's commission on nursing.* Final Report. Volume I.

Wilson, C. N. (1985). Unionization in the hospital industry: How are wages affected? *Healthcare Financial Management, 8*, 30–35.

Wilson, C. N., Hamilton, C. L., & Murphy, E. (1990). Union dynamics in nursing, *Journal of Nursing Administration, 20*(2), 35–39.

PART VII

Moving Beyond the Ordinary

CHAPTER 31

Quality in Health Care Environments

Naomi E. Ervin

Highlights

- Structure, process, and outcome relationship
- Quality assurance program for a nursing division
- Interdisciplinary quality assurance program
- Implementation of a quality assurance program
- Fiscal implications

The purpose of this chapter is to discuss the concept of quality of care in health care environments. In this chapter, the definition used for quality of care is that formulated by the Institute of Medicine's Committee to Design a Strategy for Quality Review and Assurance in Medicare. "Quality of care is the degree to which health services for individuals and populations increase the likelihood of desired health outcomes and are consistent with current professional knowledge" (Lohr, 1990, p. 4).

Attempts to assess and improve the quality of care have been made throughout nursing's history. Pressures for quality assurance activities in health care have come from an increasingly informed consumer population, third-party payors, government agencies, accrediting bodies and health care providers themselves. The desire of health care providers to be involved in quality assessment and improvement stems from the responsibility to society for self-regulation. Society gives professions the right to govern themselves. The professions are thus responsible to society for their actions through controlling practice and guaranteeing the quality of services (Phaneuf, 1972). The concept of quality assurance provides a framework that nursing can use to meet this public trust for self-regulation.

In some health care institutions the term quality assurance has been replaced by terms such as quality circles, Total Quality Management, Continuous Quality Improvement, and quality assessment and improvement (see Chapter 19).

Quality assurance is used in this chapter to mean the systematic evaluation of care based on pre-determined standards or criteria, and systematic correction of deficiencies (Zimmer, 1974). The components of quality assurance presented in Chapter 6 were structure, process, and outcome. Structure components are the human, physical, and financial resources needed to provide care. The process components are the activities of health care professionals in the provision of care to patients. The outcomes are the end results of care to the patient (Donabedian, 1969).

As discussed previously, the relationships among structure, process, and outcome are not clear, especially direct relationships of specific processes leading to specific patient outcomes (Given, Given, & Simoni, 1979). Although an analysis of relationships among the quality assurance components is beyond the scope of this text, some of the major areas of lack of agreement will be explored.

STRUCTURE, PROCESS, AND OUTCOME RELATIONSHIPS

Any nurse executive is aware that a particular change does not always culminate in a particular result. Most nurse executives have experienced this first hand when implementing and evaluating changes in such items as nursing practice patterns or information systems. Because of the multitude of variables involved in any such change, many of which are not directly controlled by the nurse executive, the results are frequently not what were predicted or desired. The same is true of structure, process, and outcome relationships.

The factors that contribute to human behavior are, of course, complex and are related to aspects of structure, process, and outcome. Certainly, at this point in the nursing profession's development in quality assurance, we cannot claim that the following relationship exists:

$$\text{structure} \longrightarrow \text{process} \longrightarrow \text{outcome}$$

However, as Donabedian (1980) points out, there is a fundamental relationship among the three elements. For nursing, the influence of structure on process and the influence of process on outcome have not been clearly defined. Such nursing interventions as anticipatory guidance, referral, and teaching have not been tested with a sufficiently large variety of patient populations to enable nursing to posit what interventions are effective with what patient populations under what circumstances.

Quality assurance offers nursing the opportunity to formalize and organize some of our collective experience so that we can share it with each other as practitioners, educators, and researchers. The process of quality assurance can be especially fruitful to nursing if more research efforts are channeled into examining the relationships among structure, process, and outcome.

Nurses experience that all patients do not respond the same to the same nursing intervention; for example, some patients relax when given a back rub, whereas others feel no change or become more tense. This example could be used as an argument for why evaluating outcome is more accurate than evaluating process. Indeed, if the desired outcome is decreased tension in a patient, then the focus of a review of care quality should be the measure of tension experienced by the patient, not the nursing intervention to achieve that outcome. On the aggregate level of patient care, the specific interventions are perhaps less important than the patient's health status — as indicated by outcomes — but if the outcomes are not achieved, the process may be at fault.

However, nursing does not have tested nursing interventions that relate to patients' achieving specific outcomes. In a quality assurance audit, such interventions could be reviewed, and a determination could be made as to which interventions are most successful and, thus, which to use with particular types of patients. Although this type of review is not research, it is a use of the collective experience of a specific nursing service and thus can have validity for a specific nursing care environment. In addition, nurses can assist in formulating research questions related to audit results. The data from audits can provide a rich source of information for clinical research.

An additional complicating factor in the structure-process-outcome relationship is that patients may achieve the desired outcomes without any nursing interventions. For example, some patients learn self-care through the teaching of relatives or a physician. Although the nurse assumes the primary responsibility for teaching patients, the outcome of successful learning cannot be assumed to be the result of only nurse teaching.

Because patient outcomes are products of many processes, nursing cannot be certain that outcomes, as measured, result from nursing interventions. One must also consider the level at which the nursing intervention was directed; that is, how concentrated, intense, skilled, or long was the intervention? For example, implementing a formal teaching plan for a newly diagnosed diabetic should result in more patient learning than a single talk with the patient about diabetes. Similarly, a behavior change is more likely in an adolescent mother who has a series of home visits from a public health nurse, rather than just one visit.

Not achieving specific outcomes is not always due to a lack of proper, adequate, or sufficient process from professional health care providers. Unless process is aimed at achieving the specific outcomes, they will not consistently be achieved unless by chance or other influences. Does this meant that we should abandon the measurement of patient outcomes in favor of measures more demonstrable of nursing care? The question should not be answered with a clear yes or no. Alternative answers follow in the form of two suggested programs: a program for a nursing division and an interdisciplinary program.

Quality Assurance Program for a Nursing Division

In beginning a quality assurance program in a nursing division, a framework is needed for guidance in establishing the organizational structure. In many nursing divisions, a staff position for the quality assurance program is established, and that individual is responsible for developing the program. Because nursing divisions are not always funded for such an approach, the nurse executive frequently plans or delegates to a staff member the development of a quality assurance program.

The structure of a quality assurance program may follow any pattern but may be most useful if it parallels the organizational structure of the nursing division. Such parallel structure offers the advantage of economy of resources, because already existing positions, communication lines, and responsibilities can be built on or modified to incorporate some quality assurance activities. This arrangement should strengthen the philosophy that quality assurance is the responsibility of every nurse and an integral part of each person's functioning. Assuring the quality of nursing care must be the accepted mission of all the staff, not just of a few administrative personnel, if program objectives are to be achieved.

In an inpatient setting, quality assurance organizational structures may be set up to parallel the clinical areas, for example, medical, surgical, pediatric, obstetrical, and newborn nursery. Such a program structure is illustrated in Figure 31.1. Only five nursing clinical areas are illustrated, but as many as are needed could be added to the sub-committee structure. The nursing division quality assurance committee would be composed of a chairperson and the chairperson of each sub-committee. Nurses from the patient care units, clinical specialists, and nursing management personnel would hold membership on the committees, with staff level nurses having the largest number of members.

In a community health nursing setting, an organizational structure could be based on the major subclinical areas of practice or on the major patient populations. In an agency with a focus on primary prevention, such as a health department, the nursing division quality assurance program may be composed of the areas of child health, maternal health, communicable disease, and adult health (see Figure 31.2). In a large agency with many patient populations, more subcommittees could be created, for

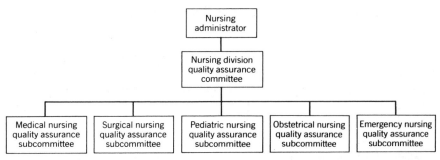

Figure 31.1 Quality assurance program committee structure in an inpatient setting.

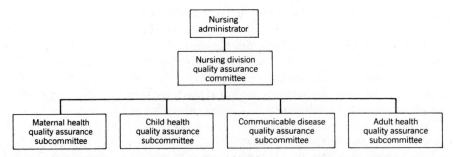

Figure 31.2 Quality assurance program committee structure in a public health nursing setting.

example, infant health, preschool child health, school-age child health, and maternal adolescent health.

After the structure is determined, it is helpful to develop a conceptual framework for implementation of quality assurance program components. Although frameworks in the literature are basically the same, the American Nurses Association (1975) model is comprehensive in its inclusion of structure, process, and outcome components (see Figure 31.3). A total quality assurance program includes all three components — structure, process, and outcome — but all three are not necessarily developed at the same time. Thus, the framework provides the focus for keeping the program development organized and for providing explanation about where specific activities fit into the total program. Nursing staff may especially benefit from an orientation to such a framework so that they can put into perspective what piece of the whole they are involved with and how all the parts may contribute to the assessment and improvement of the quality of care.

The involvement of the nursing staff is crucial to the success of a quality assurance program. Because the single most important objective of a quality assurance program is to improve the quality of nursing care, the people who actually deliver the care must assist in the determinations about what constitutes quality nursing care, how that will be measured, how the care compares with the standards, and what actions should be taken to correct deficiencies.

The nurse executive has several responsibilities in the quality assurance program:

- Appoint committee chairpersons and members.
- Receive and review regular reports from quality assurance committees.
- Meet regularly with the quality assurance committee chairperson to provide guidance, monitor use of resources, and give suggestions for committee direction.
- Monitor audit results.
- Provide resources for or direct implementation of corrective actions aimed at deficiencies found during audits.
- Participate with other agency administrators in the agency quality assurance program.

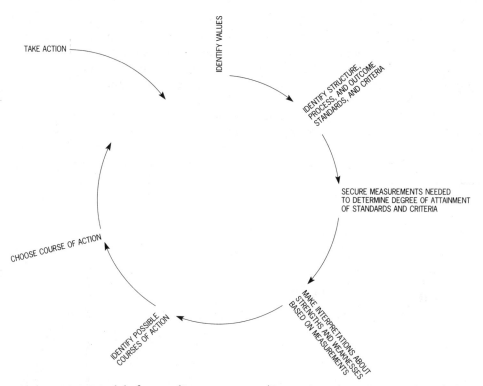

Figure 31.3 Model for quality assurance. (From American Nurses Association. (1975). *A Plan for Implementation of the Standards of Nursing Practice.* Kansas City, MO: Author. Used with permission.)

Interdisciplinary Quality Assurance Program

The final responsibility listed at the end of the previous section—participating with other administrators—is predicated on the assumption that the agency has a quality assurance program. In some instances, nursing may be the only division that has begun quality assurance activities. This is especially prevalent in nonhospital settings because the pressures for quality assurance have not been as great in settings such as health departments, outpatient departments, primary care clinics and nursing centers. In many such agencies, nursing is the primary professional service provided. Thus, an interdisciplinary quality assurance program may have little potential for other discipline participation. In some situations, the agency could use external consultants to provide advice about specified areas of quality assurance, for example, outcome criteria for patients receiving physical therapy at home.

By far the greatest area of need for interdisciplinary quality assurance activities for nursing is with medicine. Nursing and medicine have historically shared responsibilities for patient care. As technology has resulted in more complex diagnostic and treatment plans, medicine and nursing have widened the area of shared responsibilities. Nursing continues to be the recipient of responsibilities handed over to it, temporarily or permanently, by medicine (Bates, 1975). Some of these are shared without conflict, for example, blood pressure measurement by sphygmomanometer. Although other responsibilities may be shared, the sharing is still challenged in some situations by individual physicians or organized medicine; one such responsibility is to provide contraceptive counseling and methods under standing orders or protocols (Selby, 1983).

Because nursing and medicine have common territory of patient care responsibilities, it is to the patient's benefit that the two disciplines collaborate and gain understanding of each other's practice. Quality assurance activities should contribute to the mutual understanding of the interdependence of nursing and medicine in all patient care settings. Quality assurance activities may not clarify all misunderstanding, but a health dialogue may result. Other potential benefits of an interdisciplinary quality assurance program include:

- Increased respect for each other's discipline.
- Changes in patient care that are supported by more than one discipline.
- Increased agreement about distribution of resources.
- Increased joint planning for new projects or programs.

To enjoy these benefits, the other disciplines must support the concept and development of an interdisciplinary quality assurance program. If support is not apparent, the nurse executive would do well to assess the support before making specific recommendations about quality assurance program development. The nurse executive may be able to build support for a quality assurance program by informally educating other division heads or through formal forums. The endorsement of the agency or institution director is a key link in obtaining the support and resources to begin and sustain an interdisciplinary quality assurance program. In some institutions, however, an interdisciplinary quality assurance program may exist in name but have little activity. This situation calls for a reexamination of the quality assurance structure and a revitalization of the program functioning.

If an interdisciplinary quality assurance program does not exist, a structure will need to be developed and implemented. Although the development of the structures should be done by an interdisciplinary committee, the nurse executive would be remiss if not prepared with viable suggestions for committee discussion. A basic interdisciplinary quality assurance program structure that could be adapted to any type of patient care setting is depicted in Figure 31.4. In a health department, the discipline or program committees might be public health nursing, environmental health, health education, and communicable disease. The chairperson of each of these committees would serve on the agency quality assurance committee.

In any setting, the chairperson of the agency quality assurance committee could be appointed by the chief executive or elected by the committee itself from committee membership. If there is a quality assurance coordinator, this individual could serve as chairperson of the committee. Although the chairperson's responsibilities would vary depending on the agency and the number of quality assurance program staff, the basic responsibilities would be to conduct regular quality assurance committee meetings, distribute appropriate materials, provide guidance to quality assurance discipline com-

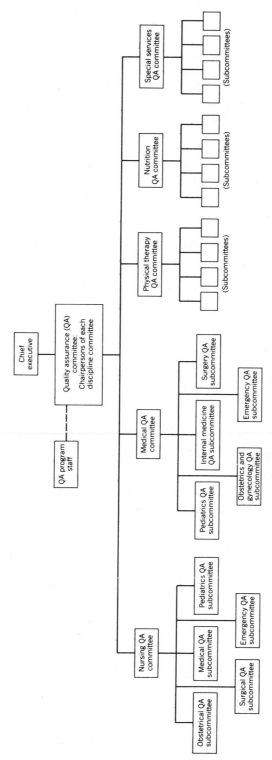

Figure 31.4 Interdisciplinary quality assurance program.

mittee chairpersons, and regularly communicate with the chief executive about committee activities and recommendations.

Components for a quality assurance program should be determined by the chief executive on recommendation from the quality assurance committee, after it has received recommendations from all the discipline committees. Structure, process, and outcome activities should be included in whatever recommendations are adopted. The details about how the committees will interface, how standards and criteria will be ratified, and how interdisciplinary activities will be conducted can be planned to some extent, but many details will need to evolve as the quality assurance program is implemented.

IMPLEMENTATION OF A QUALITY ASSURANCE PROGRAM

After the quality assurance structure and key personnel have been identified and oriented, the quality assurance activities can begin with the first step of the American Nurses Association model (see Figure 31.3) (American Nurses Association, 1975): identifying values based on the institution's philosophy and considering the values of the profession, clients, and society. Specific group exercises are one of the better methods of helping the quality assurance committees deal with this step of identifying values. Part of one meeting could be devoted to one or two group exercises. Once this step is completed, it will not have to be repeated in future cycles of the quality assurance model if the membership of a group remains basically the same.

The second step of the model—identifying structure, process, and outcome standards and criteria—is probably the most time consuming and, thus, most costly for the health care institution. The quality assurance committee or the program coordinator will decide what specific component, tool, and technique will be used as a beginning point. Some examples of structure, process, and outcome tools and techniques are identified in Figure 31.3. If none of these is suitable for the specific setting, a tool can be developed, although this is a costly process.

If structure is chosen as a starting point, a tool could be developed from already existing documents. If other parts of structure are to be examined, the quality assurance committee should inventory what is already in place before other efforts are expended or duplications occur. Because structure is generally broadly measured by external agencies, quality assurance is more frequently directed at process and outcome.

Process is often a practical place to begin in quality assurance for nursing for several reasons:

- Nurses chart in process terms.
- Process criteria may be easier for staff to identify.
- Process criteria may be more available in the literature.
- Process audit tools are available for use with little or no adaptation.

If an already developed tool is used, the committee members will require preparation in using the tool and time to complete the audits or collect data through another method, as shown in step 3 of the quality assurance model.

The fourth step is to make interpretations about strengths and weaknesses of the nursing practice. The degree of correspondence between the previously identified criteria and standards and the current level of nursing practice serves as the data base for these interpretations. Appropriate committees and individuals should be included in the discussions about interpretations of the measurements. Especially nurses who have been directly involved in providing care to the study patient group should have involvement in the discussions. The information that they can contribute to the interpretations will be invaluable in the committees' deliberations.

The fifth step of the model — identifying possible courses of action — should also include nurses who have provided direct nursing care to the patient group. Consideration should be given not only to the degree of attainment of the criteria and standards, but also to the kind and extent of available resources for corrective actions. Examples of types of actions that may be proposed are in-service education, continuing education, system changes, environmental changes, administrative changes, and punitive or reward mechanisms.

After the possible courses of action are identified, the best action or actions should be selected and recommended to the nurse executive if appropriate. If guidelines have not been developed about which actions need administrative approval, the chairperson of the quality assurance committee should have an agreement with the nurse executive so that actions are not begun that are outside the authority of the committee. In addition, the cooperation of the line nursing managers is mandatory if the appropriate long-term changes are to be made. If these managers are not informed or involved in the approval process, they may be less cooperative or resistant to changes aimed at the units for which they are responsible.

The last step is to implement the chosen action or actions. To assure that the action has been implemented completely and as intended, specific individuals need to be assigned specific responsibilities and tasks. No plan of action will be effective unless it is well planned and implemented according to plan. After the plan has been carried through to the satisfaction of those involved, documentation should be maintained for internal records as well as for review by external accrediting groups during site visits. The steps in the model are then repeated after the corrective action has been completed to see if the care has reached the identified criteria and standards (American Nurses Association, 1975).

As an illustration of the use of the model for one specific type of quality assurance mechanism, patient outcome criteria will be used. The quality assurance coordinator, with the overall quality assurance committee, will have already determined the format for the outcome criteria sets. Each subcommittee of the quality assurance committee should start the first work session, after a general orientation to quality assurance, with an exercise that provides for the identification and discussion of values. The type of exercise that is most useful allows the individual nurse to begin to understand how his or her values of patient care compare with those of colleagues.

In a second meeting, each subcommittee would begin to identify outcome criteria for a specific patient population. The patient populations used initially should be the largest groups of the health care agency caseload. For example, the medical nursing subcommittee might choose diabetes as the initial topic for an outcome criteria set. By using the nominal group process (Delbecq & Van de Ven, 1971), a committee can accomplish a great deal of work in a short period of time. Examples of the kind of outcome criteria that may be written by the committee are:

1. Patient or significant other explains that diabetes is a disease in which the body does not produce sufficient insulin.
2. Patient or significant other plans menus for 3 days using the prescribed diet.
3. Patient or significant other administers insulin at prescribed intervals.

The completed outcome set then must be arranged in a way that measurements of each criterion for each patient can be obtained. The most commonly used tool is a retrospective chart audit. A simplistic tool for this is shown in Figure 31.5; other types of forms can be found in the literature (Waltz & Strickland, 1988; Rinke & Wilson, 1987).

After an audit form is completed for each chart, which should have been chosen randomly from those available in the specified time period, composite scores are determined for each criterion. In the example in Figure 31.5, the scores were as follows for 50 audited charts:

Outcome Criteria	Met	Not Met
1	35	15
2	40	10
3	45	5

From analyzing and interpreting these results, the medical nursing subcommittee may determine that more teaching should be done about diabetes as a disease. The actions that seem most appropriate to the committee are a staff development program, development of a patient education booklet, and patient education classes. After discussion, the recommendation is made to the overall nursing quality assurance committee that patient education classes be developed and conducted by nurses and other care providers. Because this recommendation involves hospital resources and other disciplines, the nursing committee would refer it to the nurse executive for approval and implementation.

Criteria	Met	Not Met	Comments
1. Patient or significant other explains that diabetes is a disease in which the body does not produce sufficient insulin.			
2. Patient or significant other plans menus for three days using the prescribed diet.			
3. Patient or significant other administers insulin at prescribed intervals.			

Figure 31.5 Outcome criteria set: diabetes mellitus retrospective chart audit form.

After the implementation of a patient education class on diabetes, an audit would be repeated in 6 to 8 months, a period sufficient for a large enough patient group to have been discharged from the hospital. As mentioned previously, the process does not need to start with the identification of values unless the committee membership has greatly changed. Also, if the committee believes that the criteria are appropriate, they should not be changed, at least until a reaudit is completed. This discussion of the implementation of the American Nurses Association model does not include all the details required for effective implementation. The purpose of the discussion has been to provide the nurse executive with the overview necessary to direct others in implementing the specifics of a quality assurance program.

FISCAL IMPLICATIONS

The implementation of quality assurance mechanisms can be costly. If a quality assurance program is developed and implemented, the initial implementation costs will be a sizable budget item, but the cost of maintaining the system should be much less. Full implementation of a quality assurance program may take 2 years or more in most institutions.

Depending on institutional characteristics, one of two fiscal approaches may be used to plan a quality assurance program: reallocation of current resources or use of newly allocated resources. If fiscal constraints prohibit the allocation of new resources, implementation of the quality assurance program will no doubt require more time. Many nursing divisions have been able to plan and implement quality assurance programs with reallocation of internal resources.

Summary

The American Nurses Association model for quality assurance depicts the steps involved in developing structure, process, and outcome criteria and standards. The model is useful in both nursing division and interdisciplinary quality assurance programs. All levels of registered nurse staff must be included in quality assurance activities for them to have credibility and to increase the likelihood of acceptance and thus success.

The nurse executive should encourage development of an interdisciplinary quality assurance program and should provide leadership in making recommendations and representing nursing at appropriate institutional forums. The quality assurance program structure should incorporate representation for all institution disciplines. The chief executive of the institution has the role of receiving reports and taking action on recommendations.

Whatever terms are used to describe the quality assessment and improvement process, the goal remains the same: to improve the quality of care. The goal of this textbook is to provide the background knowledge for the nurse executive to develop an environment for nursing practice that is designed to deliver quality care with optimal client outcomes. Regardless of our well-intentioned efforts to accomplish this goal, nursing care is not always optimal. Thus, nursing is faced with the ever-present challenge of attempting to do better.

STUDY QUESTIONS

1. What are some benefits of implementing a quality assurance program in a nursing division?

2. If an institution cannot implement a quality assurance program, what five mechanisms should be implemented as a minimum to measure the quality of nursing care?

3. The direct relationship among structure, process, and outcome — that is, structure $\longrightarrow$ process $\longrightarrow$ outcome — is not established. What might the relationship be, other than the one depicted?

4. What are some costs associated with planning and implementing a quality assurance program?

References

American Nurses Association. (1975). *A plan for implementation of the standards of nursing practice.* Kansas City, MO: Author.

Bates, B. (1975). Physician and nurse practitioner: Conflict and reward, *Annals of Internal Medicine, 82*(5), 702–706.

Delbecq, A. L., & Van de Ven, A. H. (1971). A group process model for problem identification and program planning, *Journal of Applied Behavioral Science, 7*(4), 466–492.

Donabedian, A. (1969). *A guide to medical care administration, Vol. 2, Medical care appraisal: Quality and utilization.* New York: American Public Health Association.

Donabedian, A. (1980). *Explorations in quality assessment and monitoring, Vol. 1, The definitions of quality and approaches to its assessment.* Ann Arbor, MI: Health Administration Press.

Given, B., Given, C. W., & Simoni, L. E. (1979). Relationships of process of care to patient outcomes, *Nursing Research, 28*(2), 85–93.

Lohr, K. N. (Ed.). (1990). *Medicare: A strategy for quality assurance,* Vol. I. Washington, DC: National Academy Press.

Phaneuf, M. (1972). *Nursing audit: Profile for excellence.* New York: Appleton-Century-Crofts.

Rinke, L. T., & Wilson, A. A. (Eds.). (1987). *Outcome measures in home care. Vol. II. Service.* New York: National League for Nursing.

Selby, T. L. (1983). NPS appeal unauthorized practice ruling, *The American Nurse, 15*(4), 3, 16.

Waltz, C. F., & Strickland, O. L. (Eds.). (1988). *Measurement of nursing outcomes. Vol. I. Measuring client outcomes.* New York: Springer.

Zimmer, M. J. (1974). Quality assurance for outcomes of patients, *Nursing Clinics of North America. 9*(2), 305–315.

CHAPTER 32

Marketing Nursing and Nursing Services

Sylvia A. Price

Highlights

- **Marketing**
- **Marketing management**
- **Marketing management philosophies**
- **Nursing market arena**
- **Market segmentation**
- **Marketing information and research**

Marketing is a discipline that enables organizations to identify human wants and needs to achieve organizational goals and objectives. Effective marketing is a key factor associated with the survival of health care organizations. An introduction to principles of marketing that will enable nurse executives to integrate these concepts into their nursing administrative practice is the focus of this chapter.

MARKETING

Marketing implies being sensitive to and satisfying individuals' needs and wants through the process of exchange. It involves identifying products that are viewed as capable of satisfying a human want, need, or exchange. Kotler (1988) states that exchange is the core concept of marketing and requires that the following conditions must be satisfied:

1. There must be at least two parties.
2. Each party has something of value to the other party.
3. Each party is capable of communication and delivery.
4. Each party is free to accept or reject the offer.
5. Each party believes it is appropriate or desirable to deal with the other party. (p. 6)

If these conditions prevail, there is potential for exchange. Whether exchange occurs is dependent on whether the exchange will leave both parties better off than before. Exchange is referred to as a value-creating process because the act of exchange brings both parties something of value.

A market is a place of potential exchanges, or trade. Marketing is working within the context of a market to actualize potential exchanges to satisfy human needs and wants. Coping with exchange processes requires considerable deftness. Organizations must demonstrate expertise in managing exchange processes. They must attract resources from specific market arenas, change them into useful products, and trade them in other market arenas.

MARKETING MANAGEMENT

Kotler and Armstrong (1989) define marketing management as the "analysis, planning, implementation, and control of programs designed to create, build, and maintain mutually beneficial exchanges with target markets for the purpose of achieving organizational objectives. It relies on a disciplined analysis of the needs, wants, perceptions, and preferences of target and intermediary markets as the basis for effective product design, pricing, communication, and distribution" (p. 10). Health care marketing management is defined as "the *process* of understanding the needs and wants of a *target market*. Its purpose is to provide a viewpoint from which to *integrate* the analysis, planning, and implementation (or organization) and control of the health care delivery system. The output of the health care marketing process is the development of the means to satisfy or facilitate exchange of values between providers and the target market(s)" (Cooper & Robinson, 1982, pp. 1–2).

Marketing management is essentially demand management. The organization apparently forms an idea of a desired level of transactions with a target market. Kotler and Andreasen (1987) state that "the marketing management's task is to influence the level, timing, and character of demand in a way that will help the organization achieve its objectives" (p. 24). They distinguish eight different states of demand, each presenting a different marketing challenge:

1. *Negative demand.* A market is in a state of negative demand if a major part of it dislikes the product and may even pay a price to afford it. People often have a negative demand for preventive health care (dental services, mammograms). A manager's task is to analyze the reasons the market dislikes the product, if

redesigning a program, lower costs, and more positive promotion can change the market's beliefs and attitudes.

2. *No demand.* Target consumers are disinterested or indifferent to the product. The service may be either unknown or the client is not interested in it. Thus, individuals may not be interested in a well-child clinic, new technology, or surgical procedure. The marketing task is to devise ways to emphasize the benefits of the product with the person's needs and interests.

3. *Latent demand.* Clients may share a strong need that cannot be satisfied by any existing product. Drug treatment centers and crisis rape centers are examples of strong latent demand services that are slowly being used. The marketing task is to determine the size and need of the potential market and develop effective services to satisfy the demand.

4. *Falling demand.* Previous levels of demand are declining. Declining visits to a well-child clinic and referrals to a home health agency are examples of falling demand. The marketing task is to analyze the causes of the decline and attempt to reverse it through creative remarketing of the service.

5. *Irregular demand.* Demand varies and creates inefficiencies in staffing, production, and distribution, such as when hospital operating rooms are overbooked early in the week and underbooked toward the end of the week. The marketing task is to analyze trends in demand and find ways to alter demand through incentives such as price or promotion.

6. *Full demand.* This occurs when the actual demand is congruent with the desired demand. For example, the client is satisfied with the managed health care point-of-service model and is willing to risk inconveniences and still desires it. The marketing task is to maintain the current level of demand, maintain quality, and measure client satisfaction.

7. *Overfull demand.* The demand level is higher than the desired demand. An example would be more patients on a critical care unit than can be safely treated. The marketing task, called demarketing, requires finding ways to reduce the demand by closing nursing units, increasing prices, reducing promotion or service, or referring patients to other units.

8. *Unwholesome demand.* Products are considered undesirable and attract organized efforts to discourage consumption. Alcohol, hand guns, and cigarettes are examples of undesirable products. The marketing task is to encourage consumers to give up these products through advertising campaigns, taxes, and public service announcements.

Marketing challenges health care organizations to be responsive to the motivations of clients or consumers to seek or avoid care: their wants, needs, attitudes, and perceptions of the risks versus the benefits of various services. The influence of such factors as escalating health costs and consumerism have resulted in significant changes in health care delivery. To reduce expenditures, hospitals and community health agencies have responded with incentives to attract more clients. For example, hospitals offer a broad range of services geared to ambulatory care services, whereas home health agencies are expanding their services to meet their clients' needs. Prospective reimbursement based on Diagnosis Related Grouping (DRGs) systems also provides incentives for hospitals to reduce length of stay and procedures and to control expenditures (see Chapter 13).

The advent of wellness and primary care programs is a challenge to hospitals because such programs extend the hospital's traditional role as a provider of inpatient and emergency services. These programs are based on the premise that the consumer or client has a choice as to whether, when, and where to seek health care. In initiating health promotion and primary care programs, hospitals, as well as other community health agencies, must attract clients to the use of such services through the implementation of a marketing approach to health care delivery. Another mechanism to use resources more efficiently is through multihospital systems. These systems have attracted independent hospitals because of the benefit from economies of scale, especially in shared operations such as finance, purchasing, and other services. Greene and Kim (1989) report on a survey by *Modern Health Care* that disclosed that multihospital systems set records in 1988 for revenues, profits, and clients served.

MARKETING MANAGEMENT PHILOSOPHIES

Marketing management is the deliberate effort to achieve outcomes with target markets. It is imperative that organizations formulate philosophies to direct their marketing endeavors. Marketing activities should be administered according to a concept of responsible marketing practices. Three alternative concepts can assist organizations in their marketing activity: the product concept, the selling concept, and the marketing concept.

Product Concept

The product concept is a management orientation that assumes the consumers will desire those products that are good and reasonably priced. Such products require minimal marketing strategies to achieve satisfactory sales and profits. In health care, the physician, as consumer of the product, will respond favorably to good products (or services) and facilities; therefore, minimal marketing strategies are usually required to ensure sufficient use. Nurse executives are also consumers who are seeking new products that will enhance services to clients. Consumers are becoming more knowledgeable about health care through such mechanisms as patient education programs and the media. Federal regulations such as the Patient Self-Determination Act are explained to consumers in the news and lay literature. Readers Digest and Ann Lander's newspaper column are examples of reputable sources of consumer information on health care issues. These mechanisms will enable the consumer to take a more active role in the decision-making process in the health care marketplace. In some cases, consumers actually drive changes in health care practices (e.g., birthing rooms, rooming-in for parents of hospitalized children).

Both profit and not-for-profit organizations can operate according to a product concept. A classic example of the failure of the concept is the demise of the railroad industry, whose management was so convinced it had a superior form of transportation that it underserved its customers. The railroad industry ignored the challenges of the efficient service of the airlines and the trucking industry's capacity to pick up and deliver door to door.

Selling Concept

The selling concept is a management orientation that assumes that users will usually not purchase enough of the organization's products unless they are approached with a considerable selling and promotional venture. The major focus of this concept is obtaining sufficient sales for an organization's products. The concept is based on the assumption that customers will buy again, but even if they do not, a sufficient number of other customers will buy the product. This practice has many disadvantages, particularly when customer satisfaction is secondary to selling the product or service.

Marketing Concept

The marketing concept is a management orientation that accepts the fact that the key task of the organization or system is to ascertain the needs, wants, and values of the target market. The objective is to modify the organization or system so that it delivers the desired level of satisfaction more effectively and efficiently than its competitors.

Drucker (1974) contrasts selling and marketing by emphasizing that "selling and marketing are antithetical rather than synonymous or even complimentary. There will always, one can assume, be need for some selling. But the aim of marketing is to make selling superfluous." He stresses that "the aim of marketing is to know and understand the customer so well that the product or service fits him/her and sells itself. Ideally, marketing should result in a customer who is ready to buy. All that should be needed is to make the product or service available, i.e., logistics rather than salesmanship, and statistical distribution rather than promotion" (pp. 64–65).

To implement a marketing approach, an organization must have a strategic plan of marketing research to determine and attempt to satisfy a defined set of wants of a target group. The enterprise must also recognize that activities related directly or indirectly to the target market must be located under an integrated market control. Cooper and Robinson (1982) note that the success of the health care system in satisfying the client results in repeated usage, support for the system (volunteer services, referrals, positive word-of-mouth publicity), and client loyalty. All of these results contribute to the satisfaction of the system's goals.

Implementing the marketing concept starts with ascertaining existing or potential consumer needs, followed by planning a coordinated set of services and programs to serve those needs and wants. The services and programs are aimed at generating consumer satisfaction as the stimulus to satisfying organizational goals.

The initial step in the implementation process is to identify the market, the individuals who might exchange something they have that the organization desires for something they want that the organization possesses. In this process, important attributes of each party are identified. The next step is to divide the market into homogeneous, distinctive groups to cultivate separate strategies for each one. Specific opportunities and high-probability exchanges with various market segments are then identified. The final step is to decide which of those opportunities to target for specific action and what results are desired.

The marketing concept is particularly significant in nursing because nurse executives must be cognizant of the exchange relationships within the context of the health care organization's external and internal environments. The exchange relationships in nursing practice, whether in the hospital or the community setting, are fundamentally unstable because the value of what is exchanged is constantly changing.

NURSING MARKET ARENA

Within the nursing division, the target market arenas are the members of the organization and the client or service populations. Other internal constituents may include the governing board, employees of other departments, physicians, and volunteers. External environments include clients, community, visitors, suppliers, regulators, supporters, professional associations, and colleagues in other organizations.

These exchange relationships are depicted in the following scenario. The nurse executive represents the organization, such as the hospital, home care agency, long-term care facility, in exchanges with the nursing personnel. The nurse executive is the spokesperson for nursing. The agency exchanges benefits, salary, rewards, and accomplishments for the staff nurse's endeavors, allegiance, and support of the organizational goals, whereas, the consumers exchange money, approval, and satisfaction for technically competent and humane nursing care to improve their health status.

Nurse executives exchange their services for a position of respect, influence, and a desirable place to practice, whereas, the physician exchanges client referrals for a workplace, prestige, influence, and other conveniences. In a hospital setting, physicians are primarily responsible for admitting patients and providing medical care (writing orders for treatment and medications). Nurses perform autonomous nursing activities as well as administer the physician's orders. Client satisfaction is directly related to the attentiveness and competency of the nursing personnel.

MARKET SEGMENTATION

Every market consists of consumers with different needs, preferences, and responses; thus, no one approach will satisfy all consumers. Selecting a target market requires an appraisal of the market opportunities that are available. Each segment of the market requires its own services, marketing strategies, and goals.

For a health care organization, it is imperative to identify whether a distinct group of individuals would or might use a particular service if the need arose. Lovelock (1979) identifies three criteria for the development of meaningful market segments: (1) measurability: it must be possible to obtain information on the specific characteristics of interest; (2) accessibility: management must be able to identify chosen segments within the overall market and effectively focus marketing efforts on those segments; and (3) substantiability: the segments must be large enough or sufficiently important to merit the time and cost of separate attention.

It is difficult to implement market segmentation strategies when the target segment is not clearly identifiable with the population. For example, a health promotion program may be developed to screen potential diabetics, clinics may be established in strategic locations, and a pricing policy determined. However, informing individuals who could benefit from early diagnosis and persuading them to use the services may be difficult.

MARKETING INFORMATION AND RESEARCH

The nurse executive must identify actual and potential markets and institute a two-way flow of communication with all markets to determine the elements that are valued by each segment and what each desires to exchange. Marketing data, such as the needs, wants, and values of the market, must be systematically reviewed and analyzed by the health care organization. When this initial process is completed, strategies are then devised for each segment. To accomplish this, the organization systematically collects and analyzes data from which to make policy regarding consumer preferences in the health care marketplace.

The nurse executive must be intimately involved in forecasting volume and frequency of demands for nursing services, perceptions of clients about the organization and its health care services, and potential demand for new services that are required by the client, physician, and nursing staff. The nurse executive must recognize nursing as a potential revenue-generating service and project the numbers and types of nursing personnel that are needed to meet these demands. Nursing has the potential to be revenue generating with regard to such areas as home care, patient education, midwifery, and rehabilitation.

Marketing Information System

Many health care organizations are analyzing their information needs and developing information systems as a basis for decision making. Kotler and Andreasen (1987) use the term "marketing information system" (MIS) to describe the system for collecting, analyzing, storing, and disseminating marketing information to facilitate decision making regarding planning strategies, execution, and evaluation.

The four MIS subsystems that provide market information are *(1)* internal records, such as patient records, quality assurance reports, patient satisfaction surveys, exit interviews with employees; *(2)* marketing intelligence, which refers to sources and procedures by which marketing managers obtain information about events in the external environment (e.g., nursing journals, newsletters, television, nursing professional organizations); *(3)* marketing research or the systematic design, collection, analysis, and reporting relevant findings to a specific marketing situation or problem; and *(4)* the analytical marketing system, which consists of two sets of advanced tools for analyzing marketing data and problems that include *(a)* a statistical bank or a collection of statistical procedures for analyzing the relationships within a data set and their reliability and *(b)* a model bank or a collection of mathematical models to assist marketers to make better marketing decisions.

Marketing Research Consultants

An important issue is whether an organization should conduct its own research or hire a marketing research consultant. A cost-benefit analysis of using an external consultant versus an organization conducting its own research must be evaluated before a decision is made to hire a consultant. Clarke and Shyavitz (1981) suggest that market research should typically be conducted with the assistance of or by external consultants with expertise in the area of market research. Because such research must be objective, it is important that it be carried out in an unbiased manner. It is difficult for the internal staff of any organization to be objective and unbiased in the way they ask questions of clients; also, confusing market research with promotion activities in an attempt to "sell," or promote, the organization is less likely to occur if market professionals are consulted. These researchers realize that the purpose of market research is for the health care organization to become educated about its market, whereas the purpose of promotion is to educate the market about the health care organization.

Qualitative and Quantitative Research

Market research emphasizes the identification and analysis of information on consumer attitudes, perceptions, opinions, and preferences to devise market strategies. For example, in the health care arena, it is important to analyze consumer reports, post-hospitalization stay, to determine their interest and needs. Qualitative research is a comprehensive analysis of the characteristics and importance of human experience. Qualitative market research emphasizes why consumers like or dislike a product and examines what would change their attitudes and perceptions. Various research techniques are used to identify and evaluate this process. One technique is the focus-group discussion for which a representative group of actual or potential users is brought together. A subject should be introduced by a trained moderator who generates discussion through a few selected "probing" questions. The purpose is to elicit statements regarding the groups' preferences concerning the topics under discussion. These statements are analyzed in an attempt to identify the components of the issues that should be explored with quantitative measures such as a telephone or mail survey.

A second qualitative research technique is the individual depth, or one-to-one, interview. This method is appropriate to use, particularly, when topics may be personal or confidential for the person to discuss in a focus-group situation. This technique may take the form of detailed interviews with an individual conducted by a trained interviewer. The decision making or reasoning of the participants is probed on a one-to-one basis, generally through predominantly open-ended questions. The responses are analyzed to identify and clarify issues rather than to formulate a specific action plan.

Another technique, the nominal group, or Delphi technique, is used when group consensus is desired. A structured format is often used to minimize group interaction and assist the group-reach innovative or judgmental decisions. For example, in a study of nursing shortages, Wandelt, Pierce, and Widdowson (1981) used the nominal group technique at a conference of health care experts. They generated over 150 suggestions for attracting nurses back into the work force.

Quantitative market research, by contrast, refers to systematic statistical sampling of a target market population. Studies are conducted to identify consumer segments in the health care marketplace so that forecasts can be made about their future behavior. The demographic and behavior profiles of the consumers indicate who comprises the market and who provides services to the segments within it. Much of the data needed for these studies can be obtained from secondary sources both internal and external to the organization, such as previous similar research studies and discharge or case-mix records. Data may be collected through survey instruments, such as mailed questionnaires and telephone and personal interviews. The data are then analyzed so that patterns of association or relationship among variables can be determined. In the health care market, quantitative research is conducted in an attempt to control segments so that forecasts predict how the target market will behave (Flexner & Berkowitz, 1979). The information obtained from the qualitative and quantitative phases of the research is used to devise marketing program strategies. Criteria for evaluating these programs are also included. For example, program effectiveness is measured in the health care market by analyses of service utilization, revenues and costs, consumer compliance and satisfaction, and health outcomes.

MARKETING STRATEGIES

In the implementation phase of a marketing plan, the organization should translate marketing research information into strategies and tactics. An important element that must be considered when developing market strategies is planning the marketing mix, represented by the four Ps: product (service), place, promotion, and price. Product, as defined previously, is whatever is offered to a market that is viewed as capable of satisfying a human want, need, or exchange. Place, or distribution, refers to how the product is made available to target segments of the market. Promotion is the activities that make the product available to the consumer. Price refers to the amount of money individuals have to pay for the product. The decision regarding the combination of the various elements—which can be combined in several ways and coordinated in a systematic way to reach targets—is an integral component of marketing strategies. Ireland (1979) emphasizes that success in understanding and applying the marketing mix to a given market "lies in developing a thorough understanding of the people in the market so that the right product can be afforded at the right time in the right place supported by the right promotional effort" (p. 258).

Cost and Pricing

The determination of price in health care organizations is one of the most complex areas of administration. The direct and indirect costs generally related to a specific cost center do not form an accurate indicator of the actual cost of providing and maintaining these services. For example, at a public hospital in the midwest, intravenous solution was marked up from a cost of $0.94 to a charge of $12.00. Clients paid up to $42.00 for the same intravenous solution in the northeast and $4.50 at a private community hospital in the midwest (Traddford & Work, 1983). Pricing practices must be evaluated to make them more equitable and competitive in the marketplace. Health care agencies must develop a pricing structure that reflects the actual cost of providing services. Nurse executives are close to the consumer and capable of evaluating pricing practices. They must be much more involved in determining product costs.

Kotler and Andreasen (1987) note that an organization must decide, in attempting to ascertain a price or pricing policy, the objective that it is trying to achieve. They describe five different pricing policies: surplus maximization, cost recovery, market size maximization, social equity, and market disincentivization. Surplus, or profit, is a situation where the organization will want to determine its price to yield the largest possible surplus. Cost recovery involves setting a price that would help recover a "reasonable" part of the costs. An organization adopts the market size maximization when it seeks to attract the greatest number of customers in the shortest possible time; relatively low prices are set to stimulate the growth of the market or capture a large share of it. Organizations may desire to price their services in a way that contributes to social equity, which implies that public (and by extension, nonprofit) services should not operate to transfer wealth from the poor to the rich. This concept might be achieved by charging users for the service or charging more for services that the wealthier use relatively more often. Last, market disincentivization occurs when pricing is undertaken with the objective of discouraging people from purchasing a particular product or service; for example, the theory behind high government taxes on cigarettes and liquor is to discourage individuals from using those products.

Kotler and Andreasen further state that pricing models applied in practice tend to base prices on factors such as cost, demand, and competition. When an organization is considering a price change—whether a price increase to take advantage of a strong demand or a price reduction to stimulate demand—the action is certain to affect buyers, competitors, distributors, and suppliers. The success of such a change depends on how the parties respond and that their responses are among the most difficult things to predict. Thus, a contemplated price change implies great risks. A market-oriented pricing system that enables health care agencies to more closely match prices and costs is needed.

Promotion

Promotional activities are a strategic part of a marketing campaign. Prospective clients should be knowledgeable regarding the service or product and its desired attributes. The information disseminated must be based on what consumers should know.

Promotion involves advertising, selling, and public relations. In a health care setting, promotional activities usually include identification of services, for example, educational services. Recruitment of nursing staff is also an example of a promotional activity. Recruiters publicize their agency by distributing promotional brochures, participating in professional meetings, and advertising in professional journals. Patton (1991) stresses that a marketing approach to nurse recruitment "promotes your hospital as a competitively superior place of work for satisfying the needs of nurses (and, consequently, the needs of your hospital for competent, motivated, and stable nursing personnel)" (p. 17). Health care agencies are becoming more aggressive in their advertising efforts. Publications and news releases are most effective when designed within the context of a total hospital marketing plan. In the present health care arena, competition is evident for the attraction of consumers in the marketplace.

Competition

In health care, competition is geared toward demand, which restricts the dollars coming into the health system. The assumption is that consumers are involved in making different choices depending on their particular needs. Some spend dollars to have more services. Through control of costs and prices, providers such as physicians compete for clients. There is bargaining with providers over prices by such groups as businesses and labor unions. It is assumed that cost containment results through market forces and consumer choice.

Congress has been involved in several procompetition measures aimed at reducing health care costs. These proposals provide consumers with incentives to decrease unwarranted use of health care and to select the most cost-effective health care plans. The attempt is to reduce the deductions employers can claim for medical benefits, which would encourage them to choose less costly health insurance programs. The proposals also advocate an increase in cost sharing through deductibles and copayments, which would be included in plans for the employed and Medicare and Medicaid recipients. Griffith (1983) stresses "that without direct third-party reimbursement for all licensed professional providers, entry into health care is restricted and true competition is impossible. Physicians and hospitals are the major recipients of direct third-party reimbursement in the current system" (p. 264).

The American Nurses Association has advocated the importance of nursing's interest in developing competition in the health industry. Nursing's interest includes increasing legislative visibility, achieving third-party reimbursement, and interpreting the nurse's role in preventive care, geriatric care, and consumer education.

A preferred provider organization (PPO) has been described as the most powerful marketing tool that providers can use. It is an arrangement or negotiation between a third-party payer and a provider. Panels, providers, or third-party administrators offer a benefit package to employers. PPOs negotiate provider fees and other cost-saving benefits. Characteristics include formation of a panel of providers (hospitals or physicians), negotiated fee schedules that are discounted, a commitment to utilization review methods of quality assurance, and flexibility in the choice of provider with a financial incentive to use the preferred provider.

Models of Managed Care Managed care models can be described by three models: the point-of-service (POS) model, the company-sponsored model, and the Q model. The POS model is a hybrid of the PPOs, Health Maintenance Organizations (HMOs), and traditional indemnity plans. These three health insurance options are integrated to establish a network of providers to meet the company's requirements. The features of the POS model include: point-of-service choice, fee service discounts by providers, utilization management programs, preventive health coverage, provider risk-sharing, and free choice of health care provider. Cost savings in this model are primarily from negotiating lower provider fees and implementing utilization management programs.

In the company-sponsored model, the enterprise sponsors its own health care services such as networks of physicians and hospitals, clinics and pharmacies, or utilization management programs. This model is responsible for all the financial benefits and liabilities.

The Q model philosophy is "total quality principles" that are applied to form a network or system of hospitals and physician group practices. The benefits managers define the company's requirements for purchasing "quality" health care. The suppliers, or health care providers, are expected to achieve these standards. A fundamental principle of this model is that regardless of how it is implemented, a cost-containment

Moving Beyond the Ordinary

assumption is that by pursuing quality, health care costs will stabilize over time (Gray, 1991).

Product-Line Management   Product-line management (PLM) categorizes services or products that have similar functions into multiple strategic business units (SBUs) or product lines. PLM was introduced in 1928 by Procter & Gamble to market their new product, Lava soap™. Several large manufacturing companies adopted this concept to prosper and survive in their competitive environments. The product-line manager is responsible for orchestrating the product or service, from marketing, planning, development, implementation, to evaluation.

MacStravic (1986) defines a product in health services as a "set of activities and experiences that are offered and consumed by an identifiable set of people in ways that are different from other sets . . . or a set of products that when planned, managed, or marketed as a group yields some advantage over being treated as isolated individuals" (p. 35). The PLM approach is currently being implemented to market product lines in a variety of hospital settings. Therefore, PLM is a system of planning, organizing, directing, and evaluating within a product line, such as cardiovascular laboratory services or emergency services, for the purpose of providing comprehensive, high quality, and cost-effective care to clients. It is important to emphasize that product lines represent the hospital's business mission, which is referred to as clear, accurate understanding of the goals and services the hospital desires to represent. Simpson and Clayton (1991) stress that only when this business mission and direction are clear, can a hospital proceed with defining and selecting product lines for profitability management.

Yano-Fong (1988) emphasizes that the implementation of product-line management requires such things as: *(1)* defining the hospital's activities in relation to product lines and services, target markets, and associated costs of services; *(2)* the management of the product lines (managing, organizing, directing, and controlling); and *(3)* targeting specific approaches and treating each service according to the needs of the market population. Product-line managers must consider market needs, health care professional's specialities and competition, and the organization's values, attitudes, and goals.

Newbould (1980) differentiates between programs referred to as "stars" and "cash cows." Stars are programs in high-growth fields in which the institution has market-share dominance in terms of relative numbers of staff. These programs are growing rapidly and typically require extensive resources, such as to add health care personnel, expand the facility, and acquire equipment. If these investments are made and the area proves of enduring interest, the star program will become a cash cow and generate cash in excess of expenses in the future. The cash cows are programs in low-growth fields that attract a high share of the market for such programs. Newbould emphasizes that these programs can be used to support high-growth programs or underwrite those with problems.

Marketing competition is directly affecting the health care industry. As McNerny (1980) eloquently states, "For every force, there will be a countervailing force. Progress will be evolutionary, through competition, voluntary efforts, and regulation."

Summary

Nurse executives must understand marketing principles and techniques and be able to develop marketing strategies to survive in today's economy. Such strategies should be devised to meet competition and increase nursing's influence in the health care sector within the realm of professional nursing practice.

By using a marketing model, the nurse executive can analyze needs, preferences, and perceptions of potential users of nursing service as well as assess the capabilities of the organization to meet the demand for services. Strategies are determined for each market segment, goals and objectives are formulated, and marketing plans are implemented and evaluated. Marketing is a management discipline and must be recognized by the nurse executive to promote high quality, client-centered nursing care within the professional practice of nursing administration.

THOUGHT PROVOKING QUESTIONS

1. What are the similarities between marketing management and health care marketing management?

2. Describe the rationale for using the product and marketing concepts in the health care delivery system?

3. Define marketing management's task. Describe the eight different states of demand and give an example of each that is applicable to the health care marketplace.

4. What are the major differences between marketing information and marketing research?

5. Analyze the impact of issues related to price setting, promotion, and competition within nursing.

6. What are the advantages and disadvantages of product-line management in the health care arena?

References

Clarke, R., & Shyavitz, L. (1981). Marketing information and research: Valuable tools for managers. *Health Care Management Review, 6*(1), 73–77.

Cooper, P., & Robinson, L. (1982). *Health care marketing management: A case approach.* Germantown, MD: Aspen Publications.

Drucker, P. (1974). *Management tasks, responsibilities, and practices.* New York: Harper & Row.

Flexner, W., & Berkowitz, E. (1979). Marketing research in health services planning: A model. *Public Health Reports, 94*(6), 503–513.

Gray, W. (1991). *Implementing managed health care.* New York: The Conference Board Report #968.

Green, J., & Kim, H. (1989). An inward focus: Multi-units providers survey, *Modern Health Care, 19*(5), 27–64.

Griffith, H. (1983). Competition in health care. *Nursing Outlook, 31*(5), 262–265.

Ireland, R. (1979). Marketing: A new opportunity for hospital management. In P. Cooper (Ed.). *Health care marketing issues and trends.* Germantown, MD: Aspen Publications.

Kotler, P. (1988). *Marketing management analysis, planning and control* (6th ed.). Englewood Cliffs, NJ: Prentice-Hall.

Kotler, P., & Andreasen, A. (1987). *Strategic marketing for nonprofit organizations* (3rd ed.). Englewood Cliffs, NJ: Prentice-Hall.

Kotler, P., & Armstrong, G. (1989). *Principles of marketing.* Englewood Cliffs, NJ: Prentice-Hall.

Lovelock, C. (1979). Concepts and strategies for marketers. In P. Cooper (Ed.). *Health care marketing issues and trends.* Germantown, MD: Aspen Publications.

MacStravic, R. (1986). Product-line administration in hospitals. *Health Care Management Review, 11*(35), 35–43.

McNerny, W. (1980). Testimony on S. B. 1968, the Health incentives reform act, to the subcommittee on Health, Committee on Finance, U. S. Senate, March 19, 1980.

Newbould, G. (1980). Product portfolio diagnosis for U. S. universities. *Akron Business and Economic Review,* (2), 44.

Patton, J. (1991). Nurse recruitment: From selling to marketing. *Journal of Nursing Administration, 21*(9), 16–20.

Simpson, R., & Clayton, K. (1991). Automation: The key to successful product-line management. *Nursing Administration Quarterly, 15*(2), 33–38.

Traddford, A., & Work, C. (August 22, 1983). Soaring hospital costs: The brewing revolt. *U. S. News and World Report,* 39–42.

Wandelt, M., Pierce, P., & Widdowson, R. (1981). Why nurses leave nursing and what can be done about it. *American Journal of Nursing, 81*(1), 72–77.

Yano-Fong, D. (1988). Advantages and disadvantages of product-line management. *Nursing Management, 19*(5), 27–31.

CHAPTER 33

Nursing Economics and Politics in a Global Economy

Peter I. Buerhaus

HIGHLIGHTS

- Global economics, health care, and nursing
- Changes in the economics of health care and nursing
- Federal and state regulations to control health care expenditures
- Adopting traditional market forces in health care
- Political effectiveness of nursing

When we think about the economics of nursing and health care, it is sometimes difficult to envision examples of how they are influenced by changes in the world economy. This difficulty arises because the effects of global economic changes on health care are usually indirect and stem from complex economic interactions occurring in the broader U.S. economy that often are not well understood or anticipated, even by economists. Therefore, it is useful to begin this chapter by considering some of the ways that the dynamics of an increasingly global economy exert important effects on the health industry and the nursing profession. Following this, changes in the economic environment, resulting from the use of federal and state regulations, and the emergence of economic competition in health care are examined. The chapter concludes by exploring the political effectiveness of nursing and describing areas of political intervention that will make the profession's economic environment less threatening.

GLOBAL ECONOMICS, HEALTH CARE, AND NURSING

Ten years ago this country experienced a severe economic recession. At the same time, the value of the U.S. dollar strengthened relative to foreign currencies, which resulted in intensifying competition between domestically manufactured products and foreign imports. Both to survive the recession and to be price competitive with imported goods, American business had to lower the cost of producing its products. When seeking ways to reduce its labor-related costs, business realized not only how expensive employees' health insurance premiums had become but discovered that this was the fastest growing part of labor costs. As a result, the business sector initiated a variety of health care reforms aimed at reducing employees' use of costly inpatient facilities. These reforms included incorporating deductible and copayment provisions in health insurance plans; establishing preadmission screening programs; supporting the development of Health Maintenance Organizations (HMOs) and Preferred Provider Organizations (PPOs); starting health care coalitions to monitor the health industry and gather information on providers; offering their own health insurance plans; and pressuring insurers to cover less costly outpatient services and ambulatory surgery. These reforms were so effective that substantial declines in hospital occupancy rates occurred even before the Medicare program's prospective payment system began a few years later and further reduced hospital use (Feldstein, 1986). Had the country not experienced a recession and American firms not found themselves competing with foreign imports in the early 1980s, the business sector might have offset rising health insurance premiums by passing these costs onto consumers in the form of price increases rather than pressuring health insurers and providers to adopt health care reforms.

Although the recession in 1981–1982 slowed the rate of inflation, which had grown significantly during the Carter Administration and eventually reached 10.8 percent in 1983, unfortunately, the recession also created widespread unemployment. However, rising unemployment had two important effects on the health care system and nursing profession. First, it helped end the national shortage of hospital-employed registered nurses (RNs) that had begun in the late 1970s. The shortage ended because, as the spouses of many RNs became unemployed, RNs became the only wage-earner in the family and, consequently, many began to work overtime hours, others switched from part- to full-time employment, and some RNs who were not employed rejoined the labor force. (Increases in real RN wages during this period reinforced the effects of spouse unemployment in stimulating the employment activity of RNs.)[1] Indeed, the

---

[1]Another way that the global economy has influenced nursing and the health industry is the policy of the Philippines to export RNs to the United States. Because students are taught to speak English, nursing education programs are similar to those in this country, and because wages in the United States are higher than in the Philippines, it is worthwhile for hospitals facing shortages of RNs to import RNs from the Philippines. Leaving their country to work in the United States also benefits these RNs because part of their earnings are sent to their families living in the Philippines. By increasing the supply of RNs in this country, however, the importation of RNs from the Philippines and other nations puts downward pressure on the wages paid to American-educated RNs. For these reasons the American Hospital Association has sought changes in Federal regulations that would extend visas for foreign nurses.

overall supply response was so strong that the percentage of employed RNs rose from 76.6 percent in 1980 to 78.4 percent in 1984 (Moses, 1986), and FTE RN hospital vacancy rates fell sharply from a national average of 14 percent in 1979 to 4.4 percent in 1983 (Buerhaus, 1987).[2]

The second way that high unemployment in the early 1980s affected health care was that, even though the unemployment rate declined after 1983, a significant number of people returning to work, and their dependents, did not regain health insurance (Prospective Payment Assessment Commission, 1991). Today, the plight of these nonaged working Americans and millions of others without health insurance has become a major reason for growing interest in adopting a national health insurance program. Moreover, this chain of economic interactions—foreign competition, recession, unemployment, growth in the number of uninsured people, pressure to increase access to health care—illustrates the complexity and often paradoxical nature of economic interactions between domestic and global economic events and health care. Consider, for example, if mandating *employer*-provided health insurance is adopted as a way of partially financing expanded access to health care, then labor-related costs will rise and the ability of American business (especially small firms) to compete with foreign companies will be hampered, and business may raise prices (inflation), lay off workers (unemployment), lower wages, or apply greater pressure on providers and insurers to lower health care costs.

But perhaps the most dramatic example of how global economics influences health care in this country is illustrated by examining the impact of the nation's federal deficit. Despite public calls for smaller government and a balanced federal budget, federal spending under the Reagan and Bush administrations has greatly exceeded revenues. Year after year, the excess federal spending was financed in large part by foreign countries (namely, Japan). Had other nations not been in strong economic positions or their government's not willing to lend the United States needed capital, federal spending would probably have been constrained and yearly deficits would not have grown to the point where, now, fully 14 percent of federal spending is used to pay the *interest* on the national debt! The consequence of accumulating huge annual deficits is that the country has become a debtor nation, and essentially all domestic policy decisions, including health care, are made on the basis of how they effect the federal budget deficit.

Over the past several years, the brunt of federal budgetary policy has been felt by U.S. hospitals who have received Medicare payments less than the costs of providing services for the program's beneficiaries. Today, most hospitals have negative Medicare operating margins and their overall financial positions have become so vulnerable that managers face extraordinary challenges. Nursing is especially pressured because the costs of labor account for a large portion of hospitals' expenses. Thus, as long as huge annual budget deficits continue and other nations are willing and able to finance them, then the financial pressure on hospitals and the nursing

---

[2]It is ironic that the economic conditions of the 1990s reflect some of the same characteristics of the 1980s: the country is experiencing a recession, although it is not as severe as the one in the early 1980s; unemployment has increased; and hospital-employed RN vacancy rates have fallen to 10.96 percent in 1990 from 12.6 percent in 1989 (American Hospital Association, 1990).

profession will intensify and last indefinitely (Federal support for nursing education and research budgets will continue to be affected as well). Finally, when contemplating how global economic developments might affect the country's health care system in the future, if the administration and Congress respond favorably to the billions of dollars in economic assistance requested by the Soviet Union and Eastern Europe to help finance their transition to a market economy, it is not difficult to imagine how future federal budget deficits will be affected or that the dollars saved by further reducing federal spending on health care will be transferred overseas.

CHANGES IN THE ECONOMICS OF HEALTH CARE AND NURSING

Beyond global economic developments, which work their way through the U.S. economy and eventually influence the health industry, other changes are occurring that more directly influence the economic environment of health care and nursing. For the most part, these changes are the result of public and private policies aimed at reducing health care expenditures. The two major strategies that have been used to carry out these policies involve a regulatory approach used by Federal and state governments and the adoption of economic competition to guide decisions concerning the production and consumption of personal health care services. Examining these strategies and their effects on the health industry will reveal how the economic environment is changing and provide clues concerning what nursing can expect in the future.

FEDERAL AND STATE REGULATIONS TO CONTROL HEALTH CARE EXPENDITURES

Federal Regulations

To understand the federal government's primary motivation for using regulations to control health spending, it is necessary to appreciate the budgetary perspective of the administrations that have occupied the White House during the 1980s: They have witnessed government health expenditures increasing so fast (reaching $215 billion in 1989) that the annual rate of increase was surpassed only by the annual growth rate of the national debt (Prospective Payment Assessment Commission, 1991). Because the administration has responsibility for preparing the federal budget and overseeing Federal agencies, it has a political interest to limit spending and reduce the size of budget deficits. But given the political difficulty associated with cutting spending on entitlement programs (namely, social security) or substantially decreasing defense spending, the Reagan and Bush administrations (and Congress) have had little choice but to target health care spending as a primary area for achieving significant budget savings. Despite their publicly voiced disdain of government intervention and regulations, both administrations have directed health agencies, especially the Health Care Financing Administration (HCFA), which administers the Medicare and Medicaid programs, to promulgate regulations aimed at reducing payments to health care providers.

Given the federal government's perspective, it is not surprising that the cost-based retrospective reimbursement system used by Medicare to pay hospitals was replaced by a prospective payment system (PPS) based on Diagnostic Related Groups (DRGs). Indeed, Medicare's PPS has slowed the annual growth rate in Medicare hospital payments to between 4 and 6 percent in the beginning years of the system and in subsequent years held increases below double-digit levels in all but 1989. Moreover, Medicare's PPS has prevented the bankruptcy of the Medicare Hospital Trust Fund. But despite these impressive results, Medicare outlays to hospitals are projected to increase an average 8.9 percent per year between 1990 and 1996 (Prospective Payment Assessment Commission, 1991). Thus, federal budget policy-makers want the Medicare program to make DRGs payments more inclusive so that these expenditures can be constrained.

The two areas that HCFA intends to incorporate into Medicare DRG payments are hospitals' capital-related costs and services provided to Medicare beneficiaries in hospital outpatient settings. Including capital-related costs in DRGs would further reduce Medicare payments to hospitals (nationally, capital as a percentage of hospitals' total operating costs averages about 7 percent), and could jeopardize nursing's acquisition of capital items at a time when there is an acute need to obtain information technology and other equipment to make the provision of nursing care more efficient. With regard to including outpatient services in hospital DRG payments, this policy decision came about because hospitals reacted to shrinking inpatient revenues by shifting more care to the outpatient setting where payments were relatively higher. This shift resulted in a substantial increase in federal expenditures, which HCFA believes can be better controlled if a DRG-like system is used to pay for them. When outpatient (and eventually ambulatory) DRGs are implemented, nurses and other professionals can anticipate fewer resources and will have to make adjustments similar to what was required when DRGs were implemented in the inpatient setting.

Beyond extending the coverage of DRGs and continuously fine-tuning the prospective payment system, the administration wants HCFA to sharply reduce Medicare payments to teaching hospitals for graduate medical education (GME). The Administration believes that Medicare is not in the business of financing the education of physicians and that teaching hospitals have been overpaid for operating these programs. Although teaching hospitals have been successful in avoiding large cuts in Medicare GME payments during the past decade, in light of mounting pressures to decrease the size of the budget deficit, it is unlikely that current GME payment levels will continue much longer. If teaching hospitals respond to eventual payment decreases by reducing the number of interns and residents in their education programs, then nurses employed in teaching hospitals can anticipate that they will probably be used as substitutes for physicians and the provision of more *medical* care will be shifted onto them.

In addition to these regulatory approaches, HCFA is carrying out a variety of other initiatives aimed at limiting Medicare outlays to hospitals and pressuring them to lower costs. These include restructuring and strengthening its peer review system by focusing on patterns of care for individual beneficiaries and improving the performance of Peer Review Organizations (PROs); issuing increasingly tough regulations requiring that the cost effectiveness of new procedures and technology be demonstrated before Medicare will pay for them; increasing the enrollment of Medicare beneficiaries (currently 1.5 million) in HMOs as a means to further decrease hospital use; and, applying strong pressure on insurance companies to improve their claims review functions. Additionally, the Agency for Health Care Policy and Research (AHCPR) has begun an ambitious agenda involving the development of new practice guidelines for treating various medical conditions. These guidelines will be disseminated to physicians and hospitals and eventually used in Medicare quality assurance programs. Thus, in the years ahead, nurse executives can expect more inclusive and restrictive Federal regulations influencing more and more of nursing's management and clinical decisions. Perhaps one of the most significant ways that the environment of nurses will change is when physicians begin to experience the effects of Medicare's new physician payment system.

Medicare Payments to Physicians

Annual increases in Medicare physician spending ranged between 13 and 18 percent during the 1970s to mid-1980s, fell to between 8 and 10 percent in the mid-1980s due to congressionally imposed fee freezes, and are projected to be 9.9 percent from 1990 to 1996 (Prospective Payment Assessment Commission, 1991). Bolstered by the success of DRGs in reducing Medicare's spending on hospitals, and because 75 percent of Medicare dollars to pay for physicians is funded by *tax revenues*, in 1989 the administration and Congress developed the political fortitude to target physician expenditures as a source to achieve additional budget savings and enacted legislation to develop a new physician fee schedule known as Resource Based Relative Value Scales (RBRVS).

The RBRVS methodology (its development was partially funded by the American Medical Association) has begun a 4-year phased implementation starting in January 1992. Although the methodology is too complicated to describe here, at least two consequences are already apparent: there will be sharply limited growth in Medicare spending on physicians; and specialists (namely anesthesiologist, pathologist, radiologists, and surgeons) can expect fee reductions as high as 35 percent, whereas internists and family physicians will see fee increases as high as 15 percent. Not surprisingly, physicians have bitterly renounced physician payment reform, and they may succeed in using their political influence to modify the RBRVS method or delay its date of implementation. Nevertheless, it is important that nurse executives recognize, even if physicians do not, that the era of excessive government payments to physician is coming to an end. More important, executives should anticipate how payment reforms may affect nurse-physician relationships. For example, it is not inconceivable that some physicians may become so upset by declining incomes that their anger is occasionally vented on unsuspecting and undeserving nurses. Unit managers and staff nurses will be better able to deal with these potential outbursts if they understand what will be happening to physicians in the years ahead.

State Regulatory Initiatives

During the past decade most regulatory efforts at the state level have centered on reducing Medicaid spending. The proportion of state budgets allocated to Medicaid has risen from 4 percent in 1970 to 14 percent in 1990, and Medicaid spending now accounts for 25 percent of total government health spending and 10 percent of all U.S.

health expenditures (Prospective Payment Assessment Commission, 1991). In fact, since the mid-1980s, federal expenditures for Medicaid have increased more rapidly than for Medicare, and the National Association of State Budget Offices (cited in Prospective Payment Assessment Commission, 1991) reports that state spending has almost doubled from $18.5 billion in 1985 to $32.6 billion in 1990. However, despite these spending increases, only 42 percent of those below the federal poverty level are covered by Medicaid (Prospective Payment Assessment Commission, 1991). This low percentage is explained by eligibility restrictions mandated by the Omnibus Reconciliation Budget Act (OBRA) of 1981 and because the percentage of the population under the poverty level has increased in the past 10 years, whereas the percentage that Medicaid covers has not changed. OBRA (1981) also permitted states to experiment with various payment systems, and about 30 states have developed some form of Medicaid PPS for paying hospitals (many states face legal action by state hospital associations alleging that payments are too low). Additionally, states have begun to negotiate prices with providers, selectively contract with HMOs and PPOs, and develop their own managed care programs.

By far the most dramatic regulatory initiative to control Medicaid expenditures is the State of Oregon's proposed rationing plan. The state has determined that everyone eligible for Medicaid should receive a basic set of health care benefits, but to finance them, certain high-cost procedures such as organ transplants will not be covered. The rationing proposal has been debated in public forums throughout the state, and citizens have been integrally involved in selecting the services that should and should not be included in Medicaid's benefits package. If Oregon's plan turns out to be politically and financially successful, other states will undoubtedly embrace similar approaches.

ADOPTING TRADITIONAL MARKET FORCES IN HEALTH CARE

In addition to federal and state regulations aimed at reducing *payments* to providers, traditional market forces that are based on principles of economic competition have emerged in the 1980s. By introducing incentives to promote efficiency in both the production and consumption of personal health services, economic competition is expected to slow the rate of cost increases and help lower overall spending. However, because competition and regulation are contrasting ways to govern the economic activity of a market, it is somewhat perplexing that the competitive approach emerged at the same time that there was intensifying use of strong federal price regulations via DRGs (and now RBRVS) and a variety of state level regulations. This contradiction can be explained by recalling the relatively weak form of regulations (with the exception of Nixon's 1971–1974 economic stabilization programs, which affected the entire economy) that were used in the 1970s (e.g., Certificate of Need, Voluntary and State Health Systems Planning, Professional Standards Peer Review, hospital rate setting, etc.). Rather than accomplishing their intended objective of reducing health care expenditures and improving quality, regulatory agencies were so manipulated and controlled by hospitals, insurers, and health professionals (namely physicians) that these groups were able to use the regulatory process to monopolize "their" respective health submarkets. As monopolists, they charged high prices, earned above normal incomes, stifled the development of lower-cost innovations such as HMOs and ambu-latory surgery facilities,[3] and prevented competition from other providers.[4] Conse-quently, the output of the health industry was less than optimal, resources were not used efficiently, prices and total expenditures grew rapidly, and too many decisions were made on the basis of how hospitals' and physicians' economic interests were advanced as opposed to satisfying consumers.

During the early 1980s, however, a number of events and economic forces con-verged such that the emergence of competition could no longer be restrained. Among them were growing doubts about the effectiveness of regulations, several court rulings effectively removing legal issues clouding the application of competition in health care, a growing supply of physicians, an excess number of hospital beds, and pressure by business to control health insurance premium increases and reduce hospital use (Feldstein, 1986). Given these developments and the failure of the 1970s approach to regulating health care, competition in health care began to develop, even though there was a concurrent revitalization of regulatory activity by federal and state governments.

Economic Competition In Health Care

When thinking about competition, it is important to realize that although there may be many hospitals or professionals existing in an area, this does not mean that they compete on the basis of *price*. In economics, competition means price competi-tion, whereas in health care, people usually refer to competition in the sense of non-price competition, as when hospitals compete for physicians by offering them the latest equipment, modern facilities, etc. Enthoven (1990) explains the true meaning of competition:

Price competition is present only if alternative suppliers are offering their goods or services to purchasers who really care about price because they are using their own money and must give up something else of value if they choose to pay a higher price. In other words, for there to be price competition, the purchasers must be seeking value for their money. (p. 368)

For competition (in the economic or "true" sense of the word) to exist in health care, suppliers (hospitals, HMOs, among others) must feel economic pressure to compete on price exerted by demanders (employers, unions, consumers, and so forth), or otherwise they will use non-price competition as a way to increase their market share. Although more competition is developing in health care, most remains non-price in nature.

Enthoven (1990) and McClure (cited in Iglehart, 1988) believe that competition (price) has been slow to develop in health care because large employers (demanders)

---

[3]For example, because they would reduce hospital use, hospitals obtained regulatory barriers that slowed the growth of HMOs, and hospitals prevented insurers from covering out-patient surgery because this would have decreased hospital revenues.

[4]Physicians have obtained regulatory protection from nurse practitioners, nurse midwives, and nurse anesthetists who have sought to expand their practice privileges, gain hospital admitting privileges, or receive fee-for-service payments directly from insurers and the government.

have failed to exert appropriate pressures on suppliers. For example, employers do not allow employees to keep any savings that result from choosing a less costly health care plan. This weakens employees' incentive to choose such plans and thereby removes some of the economic pressure on plans to compete on the basis of price. Additionally, many employers do not even offer their employees the opportunity to choose more economical HMO or PPO plans but restrict their choices to expensive fee-for-service providers. Also, employers rarely insist that health care plans provide good information, describing the quality of their services or conveying it in a way that indicators of quality can be compared with other plans. Finally, current tax policies give employers an incentive to purchase more costly and comprehensive health care plans, which makes it hard for employers to insist that employees and their unions adopt a cost-conscious approach to selecting health care insurance plans (Enthoven, 1990).

It will take time before these barriers to the development of price competition break down, but when they do, nurse executives can expect hospitals and competitive medical plans to have even stronger economic incentives to minimize production costs so that they can price their products and services competitively. Formal barriers, such as regulations, or informal ones that rely on traditional ways of doing things, will be broken down, if management believes they are keeping production costs higher than necessary and if their removal will not exert an important negative effect on quality. For example, employers may seek to remove restrictions preventing Licensed Practical Nurses (LPNs) from giving medications or performing procedures currently done by RNs, or employers might lift restrictions preventing nurse aids or nonnurses (e.g., pharmacist technicians) from doing nursing functions. To counter the development of these actions, nurse executives should examine their institution's traditional barriers and involve hospital senior management to work with them in cases where they cause nursing costs to be higher than necessary. Furthermore, to survive in a competitive environment, providers will have to constantly improve their reputations for high quality patient care, which means that they will truly have to become concerned with satisfying consumers. For nursing to gain, it must visibly demonstrate its unique contribution to increasing consumer satisfaction and anticipate their evolving expectations. Finally, as price competition develops in health care, providers will use more promotional initiatives to inform purchasers on the *price* and *quality* of their services and products. Advantages can be obtained if nurse executives are involved in these initiatives so that nurses' contributions to patient outcomes are highlighted and become the means to favorably distinguish the parent organization's reputation (i.e., non-price competition) from its competitors.

POLITICAL EFFECTIVENESS OF NURSING

The extraordinary changes that occurred in health care during the 1980s helped national nursing organizations become more effective in representing the interests of the nursing profession. Recognizing that nurses would be excluded from the public policy-making process unless they became more politically sophisticated, national nursing organizations strengthened their lobbying capability, improved the ability to conduct timely policy analysis, expanded information networks, and diminished some of the rivalry existing among different organizations. These changes were assisted by two nurses in Washington, Sheila Burke, who was Senator Robert Dole's chief of staff (Dole was Senate Majority Leader in the mid-1980s), and Carolyne Davis, who was the administrator of HCFA when DRGs were being implemented. Both nurses helped nursing's political leaders gain better access to influential political leaders, enrich their networks, and educated countless politicians and federal bureaucrats on the value of nurses' contributions to the health care system. As a result, one can argue that today, the nursing profession's political effectiveness at the national level has never been better.

Unfortunately, it is impossible to make such a claim when considering the political effectiveness of nursing at the state level. The following quotation from a member of the House Public Health Committee in the State of Michigan poignantly reflects the political situation in many states:

Nurses are rarely heard from, they are rarely seen, they are seldom included in the consensus-building process. If the nurses association has a representative, I don't know who it is. (Zimmerman, 1990, p. 96)

For several reasons the political effectiveness of nursing at the state level will become an especially important area of vulnerability. First, as the federal government attempts to shift more of the responsibility for providing health care onto the states as a way to decrease federal spending and reduce budget deficits, the states will increasingly exercise more control over the allocation of health resources. If nursing's political leadership continues to be invisible at the state level, then the profession will risk being shut out of an expected increase in the number of important health policy-making decisions that will affect the profession. (The state of Oregon's rationing proposal illustrates the type of policy making that will be taking place in more states in the future.) Second, a recent Supreme Court ruling concerning collective bargaining in the health field will increase the chances of unions being more successful in organizing RNs than they have been in the past. Thus, it can be expected that state nursing association bargaining units, which currently represent the majority of RNs, will become increasingly focused on dealing with the competitive threats of other unions trying to attract RNs. As important as this issue is, nevertheless, it may prevent nursing's state political leaders from paying adequate attention to other health policy developments that also effect the interests of RNs. This may result in missed opportunities to advance the interests of the nursing profession. The third reason that the political effectiveness of nursing at the state level will become an especially important area of vulnerability is due to the economic pressure that competition will exert on traditional health care providers. As the survival of hospitals and HMOs becomes more dependent on their ability to minimize production costs, they can be expected to invest the time and political resources to attempt removing or weakening state regulations and nursing practice acts that prevent tasks and procedures traditionally done by RNs from being performed by lower cost personnel. Because such changes will likely be perceived as enhancing the economic positions of LPNs, aides, physician assistants, and pharmacy, laboratory, and respiratory technicians, groups representing these health personnel will support the political efforts of large employers of RNs. To defeat such a formidable coalition and maintain RNs' present political and economic advantages vis-à-vis these rivals, the nursing profession's state political leadership will have to become far more visible and effective than it is today. The profession's political leaders have much to do before they can successfully handle these and other future challenges.

Summary

The nursing profession faces significant challenges arising from global economic developments, federal and state regulations, and from strengthening price competition among providers of personal health care services. To be sure, it will take a great deal of insight and conviction on the part of nurse executives to direct their nursing departments through such a dynamic economic environment. Their chance of succeeding will be affected by how well nursing's political leaders understand these changing economic conditions and anticipate their political implications. Because a great number of the challenges that lie ahead can be influenced by political intervention, especially at the state level, it is in the interest of nurse executives to avoid directing all of their energy to solving internal matters but use some of it to develop and implement strategies that promote the political effectiveness of organizations representing professional nurses.

References

American Hospital Association, Center for Nursing. (1991). *Nursing Roundup 1990 Hospital Nursing Personnel Survey Executive Summary.* Chicago: Author.

Buerhaus, P. I. (1987). Not just another nursing shortage, *Nursing Economic$, 5*(6), 267–279.

Enthoven, A. C. (1990). Multiple choice health insurance: The lessons and challenges to employers, *Inquiry, 27*(4), 368–373.

Feldstein, P. J. (1986). The changing health care delivery system, *Trustee, 39*(2), 15–17, 21.

Iglehart, J. K. (1988). Competition and the pursuit of quality: A conversation with Walter McClure, *Health Affairs, 7*(1), 79–90.

Moses, E. (1986). The registered nurse population: Findings from the national sample survey of registered nurses, November 1984. Rockville, MD: Health Resources Services Administration, Bureau of Health Professions, NTIS #HRP-0906938.

Prospective Payment Assessment Commission. (1991). *Medicare and the American health care system. Report to Congress.* Washington, DC: Author.

Zimmerman, J. B. (1990). *Setting the agenda in health care: Politics and processes in the Michigan legislature.* Unpublished doctoral dissertation, University of Michigan, Ann Arbor.

CHAPTER 34

Humor in Administration/ The Comedy of Management

Marjorie M. Jackson

Highlights

- State of the comic art
- The nature of comedy
- Comic research
- The gender gap in comedy
- Managing creativity and humor

The purpose of this chapter is to call attention to an unnoticed relationship between comedy and management. Examination of the relationship will not make you laugh, but a comic outcome may be achieved: a restructuring of your perception of comedy and management. This chapter develops the thesis that the qualities inherent in good management are similar to those of good comedy.

During the past two decades, there has been a virtual explosion of information in the field of management, ranging from the popular and brief *One Minute Manager* by

Kenneth Blanchard (1982) to Robert L. Veninga's (1982) *The Human Side of Health Administration* to the scholarly conceptualizations of *The Definition of Quality and Approaches to its Assessment* by Avedis Donabedian (1980). These same decades have seen a parallel emergence of comedy in literature, theater, research, and the information media. Current conferences on humor and laughter are playing to full houses across the country, just as conferences on management thrive and proliferate. However disparate the two arenas appear, they share a basic theme: how people behave, both as individuals and as members of organizations. Managers and comedians have much in common. Managers focus on the survival of the organization, namely, on improving productivity, ensuring quality, and reducing costs through people. Comedians focus on the survival of people and their attitudes and values for dealing with the content and context of their environments.

Humor can be used constructively to influence human behavior in health service organizations. In particular, nurse executives like comedians, can be bearers of a special kind of wisdom and grace: the wisdom to see humor as a rich and versatile source of new knowledge and the grace to create the comic vision. Appreciating humor, even recognizing it, requires human skills of the highest order, as does managing enterprises of human service.

STATE OF THE COMIC ART

There was widespread ignorance among scientists and professionals of our humor heritage and the potential for the positive use of the comic tradition. Interest in the serious study of humor by scholars, educators, scientists, and therapists is a fairly new phenomenon that has only recently captured popular attention. Cummings (1979) notes that the pioneers in developing constructive use of humor in therapy in the treatment of retarded children, alcoholics, and drug addicts have been greeted by a majority of their professional colleagues with a lack of enthusiasm not dissimilar to that demonstrated by many members of the medical profession when innovators in that field insisted that nutrition be recognized as an important factor in physical and emotional well-being.

Recently, innovations in the teaching field have intentionally demonstrated the use of humor in textbooks to enhance learning; not a new idea, as the Talmud instructs its readers to "begin a lesson with humorous illustrations." Vera M. Robinson (1977) was the first nurse to legitimize humor as a fruitful concept and tool in communication and intervention with clients in *Humor and the Health Professional*. Norman Cousins' article "Anatomy of an Illness" in *The New England Journal of Medicine* (1976) stirred immediate and persistent controversy in the medical world. The publication of his book by the same title became popular literature, with its message that human beings possess remarkable powers of self-healing both of the body and mind. Cousins' use of humor to enhance his self-healing has become a modern legend.

Comedy has two essential ingredients: incongruity and surprise. Surprise and incongruity are exemplified in the unlikely perspectives of two students of comedy: Conrad Hyers and John Allen Paulos. Conrad Hyers (1981) presents an engaging interpretation of the religious dimensions of laughter, humor, and comedy in *Comic Vision and the Christian Faith*. John Allen Paulos (1980) has comprehensively studied the formal properties of humor by mathematical analyses in *Mathematics and Humor*. The ubiquity of humor is seen in the diversity of studies currently under the umbrella of the Workshop Library on World Humor, a nonprofit organization headquartered in Washington, D.C., which serves as a clearinghouse for the humor movement. Among topics under study are psychological theories of humor, the shaping power of comic strips, stand-up comedy, the holy fool, construction and implications of ethnic and disparagement humor, children's humor, and the comedy styles of humorists such as Rabelais, Chaplin, and Robin Williams.

All of these examples illustrate the range and depth of the humor revolution. The promise of the comic viewpoint in the affairs of people and their organizations is a sudden insight, a fresh and accommodating change in viewpoint, an ability to see things in a new way, as Thoreau would say, to affect the "quality of the day." Beyond each day, "the importance of the comic vision in our time is amplified by the unparalleled knowledge and technological power available to us for dehumanizing and destroying as well as benefiting one another" (Hyers, 1981).

THE NATURE OF COMEDY

The plea for the comic vision begins with understanding the nature of comedy and an appreciation of the comedic rules. Finding a universal definition of comedy is as difficult as finding a universal definition of nursing. Our authorities on comedy speak from a heritage accumulated over the past several thousand years. No one of the following observations tells the whole story; neither do all of them together; none of them, you will observe, is good for much of a laugh:

- Plato first noted that the genius of comedy and tragedy were the same: a true artist in tragedy was also an artist in comedy.
- Aristotle reflected the attitude of the classical writers who considered comedy base and ignoble. Comic heroes were smaller than life. Audiences looked up to tragic heroes and looked down on comic heroes.
- In Roman comedy, the characters who are comic are from real life, are common people. The emphasis is on the physical, on social problems, and on the community setting of the city. Roman comedy established that catastrophe in comedy is never permanent. There are those whom we laugh at and those whom we laugh with.
- Satire results from moral indignation. It seeks to reform or at least expose vice and stupidity by attacking with sarcasm, wit, irony, or ridicule. It is not always fun or funny. There are basically two categories: Horatian and Juvenalian. The satire of Horace presents folly and lets it be its own worst enemy through accurate reproduction, only subtly exaggerated. The satire of Juvenal attacks folly full tilt; its contempt and anger are undisguised and overt.
- Moliere's play *Tartuffe* was banned as immoral and blasphemous when he attacked the vices of the age by depicting them in ridiculous guises.
- Schiller, poet and dramatist, declared that high comedy is the greatest of literary forms. The more comedy tends to be physical, the lower it is; the more it tends to be intellectual, verbal, concerned with the play of ideas, the higher it is.

George S. Kaufman once defined high comedy as "a show that closed last Saturday."

- Meredith (1918) instructed us that true comedy is not contempt as is satire, but seeks thoughtful laughter.

- Kronenberger (1952) compared tragedy and comedy: both comedy and tragedy are about human limitations and human failure. Tragedy is idealistic and says, "The pity of it." Comedy is skeptical and says, "The absurdity of it." Tragedy laments the flaws of humanity; comedy looks for them. In tragedy, humans aspire for more than they can achieve; in comedy, they pretend to it. Comedy is criticism. It does not deny idealism but shows how far human beings fall short of it.

- Bergson (1911) observed that comedy is based on our sense of the full, rich, spontaneous variety of human nature. When the human becomes nonhuman and acts mechanical, we laugh. Comedy is social.

- Freud (1961) proposed that laughter is the surplus energy released when fear is appeased. Jokes release the anger or fear resulting from stress. All jokes release bottled-up anger or fear by presenting them in disguise so that we can laugh at stress; the disguise protects us from direct personal pain. We laugh for two reasons: *(1)* the catharsis of relief ("thank God this has not happened to me") and *(2)* the warding off of suppressed anxiety ("by God, this might happen to me").

- Grotjahn (1966) refined the concept of comic distance. A joke is funny according to the efficiency of its disguise. The better the disguise, the better the joke. The disguise gives the audience the safety of comic distance or protecting objectivity.

- Frye (1956, 1958) speaks of mature comedy and comic grace. Comedy is designed, not to condemn evil, but to ridicule a lack of self-knowledge. "The essential comic resolution . . . is an individual release which is also a social reconciliation. The normal individual is freed from the bonds of . . . society, and a normal society is freed from the bonds imposed on it by . . . individuals." Comic grace is the grace of acceptance. A fundamental principle of comedy is to include rather than exclude, to soften and reduce distance between people.

- A cartoonist is a sit-down comic. The cartoonist Al Capp (1950) has observed that we laugh when we feel superior to the comic figure. The more secure one feels, the more ready one is to laugh. So Charlie Chaplin, the instant he appeared, gave us all a feeling of security. Certainly, none of us, no matter how bad off we were, were as bad off as this bundle of rags.

- Webster's Dictionary (1968) defines humor as the mental faculty of discovery, expressing or appreciating ludicrous or absurdly incongruous elements in ideas, situations, happenings, or acts. Many other definitions litter the comic landscape, each trying to capture essential elements of the humor experience.

- Arthur Koestler (1964) links creativity and comedy on the principle of connectivity. A good joke connects two unrelated things in an unexpected surprise.

Koestler cites humor as one of the most basic forms of "bisociative" thinking—two different frames of reference collide to produce the surprising result.

- Pollio's study (Pollio & Talley, 1991) of the language of comedy suggests that whenever there is comedy, there is originality, spontaneity, superiority, and social significance. The comic event is best considered as a coherent gestalt—it does not seem reducible to any single principle.
- The stand-up comedians of our time still serve the basic function that court jesters did in times of yore. We expect, as did kings, that comedians be in touch with the chaotic forces in the universe, to protect and assure us that all will turn out all right, eventually.

From the abundance of these random observations on the nature of comedy over time, one can readily see that comedy is a wide roof under which every man and woman can find shelter. The brotherhood of comedy and tragedy is significant and clear. Comedy is serious business. It is also clear that comedy is relative, a matter of opinion.

Vera Robinson (1977) provides us with a generic definition. She views humor as any "communication which is perceived by any of the parties as humorous and leads to laughing, smiling, or a feeling of amusement." Robinson notes that within health care settings, most of the humor is spontaneous or situational in nature, unlike the formal humor of literary work or the planned inclusion of jokes in speeches or lectures. Humor as a communication that results in certain observable behavior is an operational definition that serves the researcher's need for measurement. To the humor researcher, measurement is the riddle to be solved. Humor depends on so many emotional, social, and intellectual facets of human beings that it appears immune to quantitative analysis.

COMIC RESEARCH

Researchers who have confronted the complexities and the inherent ambiguity of the humor response have in the main produced descriptive studies, typologies, and functional analyses. Three primary foci of study have been *(1)* how funny a joke or situation is rated, *(2)* how jokes might be classified into different types of humor, and *(3)* how humor can be described in terms of its social, psychological, psychodynamic, and physiologic functions (Linn & Demalleo, 1983). Coser (1959) observed the joking relationship as a status phenomenon in her study of humor in hospital settings. Others have tried comic principles on for fit. Jackson (1980) uses the analogy of nurses as clowns, and Paulos (1980) applies mathematical logic and laws to understand and model the structure of jokes.

Research on the relationship between humor and healing has not produced the hard experimental evidence required to convince the scientific and medical community. Attempts to connect laughter to the production of endorphins or to the activation of the immunological system are under way by cheerful medical researchers. Dr. William Fry (1984), a psychiatrist and researcher at Stanford University, is currently conducting experiments that seek to prove a definite physiological relationship between laughter and the production of catecholamines by demonstrating laughter's effects on the circulatory system.

The requirements of reliability and validity and use of human subjects in experimental research are immediate obstacles. Linn and Demalleo (1983) have developed an instrument to identify and measure the communication skills used by providers with their patients. Their instrument is the *Communication Preference Inventory*, in which the willingness of a person to send or receive humorous responses when given other carefully defined choices is measured. The researcher claims to have developed a "moderately reliable, face valid, self-report measure of the degree to which consumers or physicians value the use of humor in physician-patient communication." Mindess (1984) has developed a *Sense of Humor Inventory* similar to an IQ test. The instrument assesses the type of humor one likes and the role it plays in one's personality. Mindess' premise is that if we understand who will laugh at what and why, we can learn more about our important differences.

Gender differences in the response to and appreciation of humor have been discussed and studied by scholars ever since Eve handed Adam the apple and, particularly, since Freud. Apte (1985) reports that women's humor generally lacks the aggressive and hostile quality of men's humor. The use of humor to compete and to belittle others seems generally absent among women. Institutionalized forms of humor are rarely reported for women, but in the private domain in which there is an all-female audience, women are actively humorous. The results of numerous studies of late are inconsistent and contradictory. Prerost (1982) suggests that humor preferences based on gender seem to be narrowing. Taboos against female humor and sex-role stereotypes are being demolished as women use humor as a change strategy. In the academic community, humor is now respectable, producing theoretically minded researchers. Most recent theories on humor have used cognitive and linguistic mechanisms to explain aspects of humor such as Victor Raskin's (1987) script based semantic approach.

A current center of scholarly attention is the creation of a general taxonomy as a shared tool for researchers and a means for scientific rigor. The paradoxical nature of humor designates it as a realm of cognitive chaos. A taxonomy would be useful to humor researchers attempting to resolve apparently contradictory findings.

Research on humor is wide and varied, cutting across academic disciplines and engaging diverse and unlikely schools of thought. All disciplines, however enthusiastic, face challenging methodological and measurement tasks. Students of humor have a lifelong career of imaginative inquiry.

A COMIC HISTORY

We have seen that comedy defies definition, resists measurement, is a matter of opinion, is an ancient art enjoying a modern lifestyle. Humor may be a contemporary phenomenon of inquiry, but it has a natural history that is instructive. The ancient conception of comedy was narrower than ours, confined to farce, burlesque, and slapstick. This conception persisted until 1651, when the English philosopher Thomas Hobbes introduced a theory of laughter referred to as the superiority or disparagement theory. A sense of satisfied superiority and self-satisfaction are factors in many kinds of humor and play a prominent role in sick and ethnic jokes. Superiority is the primitive base on which humor theory was developed.

In 1776, James Beattie identified incongruity as a comic principle. Incongruity as oddness, or inappropriateness, was further developed in the eighteenth and nineteenth centuries by the philosophers Schopenhauer and Kant. Schopenhauer was so funny that countless adherents to his pessimistic philosophy committed suicide. Kant in 1790 called attention to the element of surprise, the unexpectedness of incongruity: "laughter is an affection arising from a sudden deflation of a strained expectation into nothing" (Paulos, 1980). Herbert Spencer and Charles Darwin observed the physiological bases of laughter, laughter as a release of energy, an observation that influenced later theorists, in particular, Freud.

In the early twentieth century, the critic George Meredith (1918) emphasized a different aspect of humor: the social regulatory function. He wrote that the comic spirit is a sort of social corrective and springs into action whenever men wax out of proportion — whether they are planning short-sightedly or plotting dementedly. Meredith noted that humor, societal health, and the social equality of men and women were closely related.

The French writer Henri Bergson crafted a celebrated phrase in 1911 when he attributed laughter to the mechanical encrusted on something living. In other words, when humans become rigid, machinelike, and repetitive, they become comic, because the essence of humanity is its flexibility of spirit.

A well-known theory was developed by Freud in 1905. Through jokes and witticisms, a person vents his or her aggression or sexual anxieties in a disguised or playful manner. Max Eastman (1936) emphasized the relationship of humor and play as well as the requirement of an objective disengagement to appreciate humor. Eastman developed the derailment theory of humor. Humor is context dependent; that is, normal events are derailed by the situation. Humorous events are not incongruous per se but become incongruous given their situation. Perhaps this theoretical insight is the origin of the popular situation comedies rampant in the television media.

In 1964, Arthur Koestler compared the continuity of creative insights in humor with the creative insights of science and poetry: the logical pattern of the creative process is the same in all three fields: creativity consists of the discovery of hidden similarities, but the emotional climate is different . . . the comic smile has a touch of aggressiveness, the scientist's reasoning by analogy is emotionally detached, that is, neutral; the poetic image is sympathetic or admiring, inspired by a positive kind of emotion. Koestler's principle is that creative insight in all fields share the same logical patterns. Koestler's theory synthesized incongruity theory with the psychological theory of humor. Laughter is the discharge of emotional energy resulting from the "biociation" of two incompatible frames of reference. Koestler has a disciple in John Allen Paulos (1980).

Paulos explores the operations and structures common to humor and in the formal sciences of logic, mathematics, and linguistics. He develops a mathematical model of jokes using the mathematical theory of "catastrophe." Paulos exemplifies the universality of humor across disciplines and promises a humorous continuity in the age of information and its computer technology.

This chronology is admittedly incomplete, but the common ingredients of humor emerge despite the different approaches of theorists of humor. An essential ingredient of humor is the juxtaposition of two or more incongruous ways of viewing events, ideas, people, and their roles. For something to be funny, some unusual, inappropriate or odd aspect of it must be perceived and compared with the norm. Another essential ingredient of humor is the proper psychological and emotional climate. The proper emotional climate is both subjective and objective and, in the current understanding of comedy theory, an undefined conjecture.

THE GENDER GAP IN COMEDY

When we review the historical development of comedy, the maleness of comedy hits us like a pie in the face. Comedy as the domain of males is evidenced in their numbers, in attitudes expressed, and in determining the way comic routines are done and who does them. Traditionally, women have been the objects of the put-down; wife and mother-in-law jokes are the stock and trade of disparagement humor. Women have been seen as a community of fools. Jokes that degrade women (and men) seem to correlate with one of the personality characteristics called "tough poise" in Mindess' (1985) typologies. Such people tend to be aloof and to believe that stereotypes of the opposite sex are true. A cartoon depicting a woman jacking up the wrong end of a car to fix a flat tire is funny only if you really believe women are stupid.

Comedy has been a field dominated by male thought and male themes in much the same manner as the field of management. Both arenas are at last welcoming women. Women are proving that they can be bright, assertive, attractive, and funny. The phenomenon of women going for laughs and recognition in all aspects of comedy — writing, cartooning, producing, and performing in movies and on stage — is no longer novel. Collier and Beckett (1980) have examined the experiences of 17 women humorists in a series of interviews to see how they live, to hear how they think, and to listen to their personal stories. The barriers comediennes face are familiar barriers to women in management: image problems (the difficulty of retaining their femininity while being funny); accepting attention (a nice girl does not draw attention to herself); and overcoming the socialized fear of taking the spotlight away from men.

Again, equity is a common issue. Women humorists feel that they are forced into being better than men. Vocabulary and understanding present elusive barriers. There is a women's culture that men just do not know about, a repetitive lament of nursing. The essence of comedy is familiarity and surprise. One cannot laugh unless one knows what one is laughing about. Male comedians do not ask, "Do you understand this?" they seldom inquire, "Do you know what a carburetor is?"

Women humorists, once confined to a small and limited role, are now creating the structure of humor and its content as well as performing it. The maturing of comedy by women is more significantly evidenced in the increased number of comediennes doing humor on issues, in the prevalence of message comedy, and in working toward a cohesion of attitude in setting up a point of view intelligible to both men and women. Collier and Beckett (1980) noted that this is a good time for women's humor and a hard time for men's humor.

An illustration is Rita Rudner, who won accolades as the best female stand-up comic in 1990. Her style is bemused, wide-eyed, and soft-spoken. Her witticism is playful yet shrewd, based on startling contrasts and a wide range of topics. Rudner recalled her decision to explore comedy in a 1991 *Ann Arbor News* interview with Whitley Setrakian, a *News* special writer. "I found I loved the science of comedy: figuring it out, listening to the comedians I loved. And I loved creating a style all my own. I realized that there is a whole area of comedy for women." Nancy Walker's (1988) recognition that women humorists "tend to be storytellers rather than joke tellers" is an important insight that Rudner demonstrates. Rudner is excited about writing a book. "It's essays on life. When you do jokes everything is immediate, but with writing you can expand, turn a phrase, go off on a tangent."

Blumenfeld and Alpern (1986) suggest "the real power of using humor is not controlling other people but for gaining their trust and approval which in turn makes them more receptive to your ideas." The power of laughter for women is to build relationships, to share self-knowledge, and to encourage joining in common purposes. Thoughtful use of humor by women appears to side-step the historically aggressive, competitive characteristics of humor by men.

The expressive direction of comedy by women is a dramatic shift since Coser (1960) wrote that the use of humor is rarely initiated by women. Today, women humorists are creating humor on their own terms and turf. Notably, there are others who recognize the (past) gender gap and the significance of women's contribution to the literature of comedy. Two influential voices are Ken Hope of the MacArthur Fellowship and Justin Kaplan, editor of the latest revision of *Bartlett's Familiar Quotations.* Ken Hope (Hoopes, 1991) acknowledges that in the 13 years of the MacArthur Foundation "there are too few minority people and women selected. The figures are appallingly low. Fewer than 20 percent of the fellowships have been awarded to women. The Foundation is trying to improve on that."

Justin Kaplan (Grave, 1991) has just completed a full-scale revision of Bartlett's book of quotations—its 16th revision since 1855. He addressed this cultural task with a far richer sense of humor than former editors. In Kaplan's view "humor is tragically underrated. People tend not to take it seriously enough." Kaplan has cut 300 authors, but added Erica Jong. In efforts to include women, he invited Gloria Steinem and her sister feminists Betty Friedan and Barbara Ehrenrich to suggest quotes from their own writings or to nominate the work of other authors involved in the women's movement. To his astonishment, he reports, none responded to his invitation.

It is the author's hope that Kaplan's search for women's voices includes the freshly minted phrases of Felicia Lamport, a poet and verse satirist. From the Nixon era to that of Bush, Lamport has displayed her remarkable talent as witty political commentator and brilliant versifier in a series of syndicated columns entitled "The Muse of the Week in Review." Richter (1990) describes Lamport as employing a variety of humorous literary devices from parody and burlesque to *reductio ad absurdum*. She has created a gallery of lively and memorable comic portraits of America's chief executives and their cohorts through political wit unequaled since satire's heyday in eighteenth-century England. Richter's accolades of Lamport include "insights may be gained into her ability to achieve lasting rather than merely ephemeral impressions of character and episode by examining her idiosyncratic comic imagination, her extraordinary mastery of language, and the unique perspective of her gender." Richter confers upon her full and unrestrained honor. She is a national treasure. Her satire is "truth dancing."

The role of women in the comic tradition of the theater has been reconstructed by Susan Carlson, professor of English at Iowa State University. In the first comprehensive study of its kind, Carlson (1991) explores the contradictory connection between women and dramatic comedy. The work shows how a genre that has been used historically to restrict women's behavior is being reconfigured to express women's triumphs. It thus redefines the assumption with which both traditional comedy and contemporary comedy and contemporary women's plays are read and reviewed.

Instead of an imitation of male comedy, humor by women is becoming the comedy of friendship, or reacting with one another as colleagues about aspirations and anxieties and shared experiences. All comedians talk (and write) about things they know well. Nurse executives know the world of nursing, its culture, and its vocabulary. Nurse executives know the structure of care, the significance of an atmosphere of trust. Being or thinking funny has so much to do with trust, confidence, and intelligence that nurse executives are in a fortunate time and space not only to humanize but to humorize the practice of management.

HOW TO BE A COMEDIAN

To humorize management in constructive and productive ways requires awareness, accumulation of comic knowledge, and the progressive mastery of comic skills. A generous appreciation of comedy, its relative nature, and its rules is developed in individuals and in organizations by the same process of developing and using new knowledge and new technology from other relevant fields. Currently, nurse executives are addressing the business of nursing, establishing the economic rationality of practice, and integrating complex information technology into their professional practice. The arguments for an economic framework for nursing practice, whether clinical or administrative practice, carries the urgency of survival. Similarly, if no other argument can be made that will convince nurse executives of the value of the comic perspective, humor as a conferment of survival skills, is the most compelling.

Vera Robinson has developed guidelines for increasing a humor conscience, identifying appropriate uses, and establishing a knowledge base for comedy and comic techniques for the health professional. Another survival manual for administrators is Carolyn L. Vash's book, *The Burnt-out Administrator*, which is written with insight and humor (1980). Assuming an informed student of the comic tradition, what possibilities are at hand for the nurse executive and his or her staff to step outside themselves and their bureaucratic systems, to see themselves and their organizations from a comic perspective? Just as humor and jokes have at least two levels of meaning, organizational theory has two levels of conceptualization, normative and descriptive, what ought to be and what actually is. The organizational chart and job description are two handy hooks with which to begin practicing humor. What insights might emerge if a humorist designed an organizational chart that truly reflected organizational decision making, actual power centers, and patterns of information flow? Is there a department of applied humor, a committee on utilization of humor, or a consultant on comedy? Is there a locus for maintaining an organizational sense of humor? What would a job description reveal about the reality of nursing, if actual work performed were described instead of work expected? Would a recognition program change if humor or the ability to create laughter were among the criteria of achievement? How would a humor break affect the work of committees? Would instruction or policy be followed more willingly if formulated in a comic vocabulary? Would the graffiti of disenchantment that peppers the walls of a unit or department in crisis or under threat change from rage to more accommodating slogans? If humor were legitimized, what would happen to the relationship between management and labor? Would communication failures persist if subject to comic analysis?

The folklore of an organization and the ambiguous context of organizational reality is a dazzling lode for the comedian. Humor ranges in a continuum from healthy to unhealthy. It is healthy when it deals with immediate issues and helps the individual or the organization handle reality. It is dysfunctional or unhealthy when it denies reality.

In an entirely different context from that of the inherent absurdities of organizational endeavors, humor has the potential for enriching nursing diagnostic and therapeutic practice. The American Nurses Association's Social Policy Statement defines nursing as "the diagnosis and treatment of human responses to actual or potential health problems" (1980). The document includes a partial list of human responses that call for nursing intervention, such as self-care limitations, impaired functioning, and pain and discomfort. Laughter is a human response, inherent in humanness. It is also a functional ability amenable to nursing assessment and nursing treatment. Inability to laugh or to respond appropriately to the comic is a health problem. Recent research on the relationship of the right and left sides of the brain promises diagnostic criteria in brain-damaged patients such as in stroke. "Only when the brain's two hemispheres are working together can we appreciate the moral of a story, the meaning of metaphor, words describing emotion, and the punch lines of jokes" (Gardner, 1981).

Using the sense of the ridiculous has also been posited as a memory enhancing device; the more ridiculous the image created in terms of association, the more likely the name, place, or event will be remembered. Laughter presupposes a system of shared values and beliefs. Laughing with someone enfolds him or her in a system of support and care. The therapeutic use of humor treats the people in pain, not the pain in people. Recognizing laughter as evidence of a positive patient care outcome expands opportunity to collaborate with patients in their own self-regulation.

MANAGING CREATIVITY AND HUMOR

Within the economic dynamics of the 1990s, nursing service organizations that purposefully and persistently manage the generation and development of new ideas will have a significant competitive edge in the future marketplace. Dennis D. Pointer (1985), senior research fellow at the Rand Corporation, prophesied "organizational creativity and innovation will become 'the high ground' of the health care industry." To varying degrees all organizations resist creativity, innovation, and change, particularly large scale organizations and those dependent on complex routines such as hospitals. "An organization's climate and culture are among the most important barriers to or facilitators of creativity and innovation," declares Pointer.

It is within the climate and the culture of an organization that a friendly sense of humor, the comic vision, and healthy laughter play constructive roles. Humor experiences such as having humor consultants or workshops that entertain, even energize, the participants are temporary in effect if there are no sustaining or organizational values that integrate humor into the daily grind of work. Humor in the workplace connects our shared experiences of organizational life. It connects things in a way we never suspected. Most of us operate from only one frame of reference at a time. A new frame of reference gives a new center of gravity. Discovery of surprising relationships among the ordinary and mundane startles our imagination out of habit and cliché. The catapult of humor is an effective yet frequently neglected pathway to creative and innovative behavior. Many corporations are beginning to take serious interest in humor to be used in training, employee relations, and other day-to-day activities.

The manager's use of humor is purposeful—to help pace, lighten, and highlight the content and context of work. Humor brightens the corner where you are. The manager is not an entertainer, but a role model and facilitator who seeks and empowers a natural and healthy sense of organizational humor. For instance, Ben and Jerry's Ice Cream in Vermont has a joy committee. The concept of a sense of humor residing in an organization humanizes the organization and allows a fresh orientation from which to see how to make conflict manageable and goals clear. Given the popular advocation of humor in management evident in current literature (Ross, 1989, Paulson, 1989, Kushner, 1990), humor is acknowledged as one of the easiest and most accessible and most effective ways to stimulate new ideas and new approaches to old problems. The spontaneity of humor frees us to step outside one's own discipline and traditional behavior to seek new sources of knowledge to serve the organization. In particular, humor demands originality and creativity in thought and action.

Both humor and creativity are boundary free and have a natural connection. They are kissing cousins. Both are nonlinear phenomena characterized by divergent thinking through which many solutions to address problems become possible. Both share wide ranging knowledge sources and a repertoire of language and conceptual skills. Howard Gardiner's (1982) psychological research on various types of intelligence has shown that the best predictor of creativity is an active sense of humor, not intelligence as currently measured. Koestler (1964) in the first chapter titled "The Jester" in his book *Act of Creation,* makes a convincing argument for the basic nature of creativity as expressed in the process of humor. For Koestler, the studies of creativity and humor are inseparable—sharing a common cognitive pathway. The commonality is the same process of appreciating a joke, for solving a problem and for having an artistic, high experience.

Alice M. Isen's (1987) research on creativity and states of mind or mood found that 70 percent of students put into a cheerful mood by a comedy film correctly solved problems; on the other hand, only 20 percent of those who watched a math film came up with a correct answer. Isen speculates that positive mood influences creativity by changing the way cognitive material is organized—being in a happy mood may cue you into a cognitive context that could significantly affect your creativity. An aspect of

Isen's work is the implication that creativity can be manipulated, can be fostered, can be enticed by laughter — therefore, learned.

The author of *Uncommon Genius*, Denise Shekerjian (1990), believes creativity can be learned but not through a formula or recipe slavishly followed. "The phenomenon of the creative spark is larger than any of my findings can suggest. But I do firmly believe that if we cultivate a consciousness about the way we think and work and behave, improvement in our creative abilities is possible — and improvement is not something to be taken lightly." Her computer search in preparation for her book produced six thousand, eight hundred and twenty-one "hits" on creativity in print from 1967 to date — and those are just the ones in English. Shekerjian interviewed 40 winners of the MacArthur Foundation Fellowships to write her guide to creativity. She blends her conversations with the 40 awardees with theory and literature and life and shows us how to nurture creativity in our lives.

Researcher David Perkins of Harvard University is codirector of Project Zero, a project studying cognitive skills of scientists and artists. Perkins (McAleer, 1989) contends "there is no justification for assigning abilities such as math or music or general faculties like intuition and rationality to the left or right hemispheres of the brain. The two hemispheres interact and cooperate in a variety of complex ways not yet fully understood." According to Stanford University neurologist, Karl Pribrim (McAleer, 1989) the frontal lobe is more verbal on the left and more visual on the right. "If there is an important simple anatomical way of dividing the brain in relation to creativity it's a front/back, not a right/left division."

Not since the post-Sputnik years has there been such a surge of creative research about creativity and innovation. As creativity and innovation shape the template of the twenty-first century, nurse executives have a profound and joyful resource in humor.

THE PUNCH LINE

At this time in this routine, a disquieting question should be raised and resolved. Is there a comedy of management or a management of comedy? Is there a distinction here that makes a difference? A Soviet diplomat was asked what in his mind was the difference between capitalism and communism. With a straight face he responded that in capitalism, humans exploit humans and in communism, it is the other way around. The alignment of management and comedy demonstrates two key characteristics of humor: opposition and relational reversal. Opposition is the articulation of contrasts: expectation vs. surprise, the mechanical vs. the spiritual, superiority vs. incompetence, balance vs. exaggeration. Reversal is cognitive restructuring that produces a change in perspective. It is the setting up of a premise, an expectation or a process that suddenly shifts direction and meaning (for example, "that is not dirt in your soup; it is earth"). Like a relational reversal, a pun forces one to perceive in quick succession two incongruities or unlikely sides of an idea.

The comedy of management resides in the response to the dynamics of unruly oppositions common in administrative practice: predictability vs. surprise, control vs. freedom, stability vs. chaos, full knowledge vs. inevitable ignorance. Comedy of management is keeping the people who dislike you from the people who are undecided.

The management of comedy is exemplified in the dynamics of relational reversal, in securing a new way of looking at the mundane to find the marvelous or beyond the marvelous to find the mundane. Through the management of comedy, human resources of imagination and creativity are liberated for invention and experimentation. Responding to events is the comedy of management, whereas shaping events is the management of comedy.

Summary

Humor is a distinct universe of discourse with its own logic and its own reason. Constructive humor integrates, combines into one view or framework, the best of two worlds: nursing and management. Humor makes possible new connections between two dissimilar theory and practice universes. Good management is the constructive and creative use of human resources. Good comedy enlightens and informs us about our self-concept and our organizational concept. A comic perspective leads an organization toward greater awareness of its strength and weaknesses and allows an organization to respond to one of the most powerful human drives: the urge to try something new. When you have a hammer in hand, you look for nails. When you have a comic perspective, you look for new ways to respond and express creativity.

STUDY QUESTIONS

1. What value does humor have in your personal and professional life? Examine what makes you laugh. Do you initiate and create humor?

2. What do you mean when you say someone has a sense of humor? Can you specify or qualify your definition of a sense of humor?

3. Select an organization with which you are familiar and analyze it according to a comic perspective. What kind of humor is characteristically expressed? What patterns of joking relationships characterize the organization? How does the organization utilize comic framework and techniques to accomplish organizational work or goals? How much fun or playfulness is tolerated or sanctioned by the organization?

References

American Nurses Association. (1980). *Nursing: A social policy statement* (p. 9). Kansas City, MO: Author.

Apte, M. (1985). *Humor and laughter: An anthological approach* (pp. 70–76). Ithaca: Cornell University Press.

Bergson, H. (1911). *Laughter: An essay on the meaning of the comic.* New York: Macmillan.

Blanchard, K. (1982). *The one minute manager.* New York: Berkley.

Blumenfeld, E., & Alpern, L. (1986). *The smile connection.* Englewood Cliffs, NJ: Prentice-Hall.

Capp, A. (1950, February). The comedy of Charlie Chaplin. *Atlantic Monthly.*

Carlson, S. (1991). *Women and comedy: Rewriting the British theatrical tradition.* Ann Arbor: University of Michigan Press.

Collier, D., & Beckett, K. (1980). *Spare ribs: Women in the humor biz.* New York: St. Martin's.

Coser, R. (1959). Some social functions of laughter: A study of humor in the hospital setting. *Human Relations, 12*(2), 171–182.

Coser, R. (1960). Laughter among colleagues: A study of the social functions of humor among staff at a mental hospital. *Psychiatry, 23,* 81–85.

Cousins, N. (1976). Anatomy of an illness. *New England Journal of Medicine, 295*(26), 1458–1463.

Cummings, H. (1979). *The importance of not being ernest in the arts, sciences and professions.* Address presented at the Second International Conference on Humor. Los Angeles.

Donabedian, A. (1980). *The definition of quality and approaches to its assessment.* Ann Arbor: Health Administration Press.

Eastman, M. (1936). *Enjoyment of laughter.* New York: Simon & Schuster.

Freud, S. (1961). Jokes and their relation to the unconscious. In J. Strachey (Ed.), *The complete psychological works of Sigmund Freud* (p. 8). London: Hogarth Press.

Fry, W. (1984). *Laughter and health in Encyclopedia Britannica, Medical and Health Annuals: Special report* (pp. 259–262). USA: Encyclopedia Britannica, Inc.

Frye, N. (1956). *The anatomy of criticism.* Princeton: Princeton University Press.

Frye, N. (1958). The structure of comedy. In S. Barnett (Ed.), *Eight great comedies.* New York: New American Library.

Gardner, H. (1982). *Art, mind and brain: A cognitive approach to creativity.* New York: Basic Books.

Gardner, H. (1981). How the split brain gets a joke. *Psychology Today, 15*(2), 74.

Grave, R. (1991). The "Pope" who is revising our Bible of sayings. *Smithsonian, 22*(3), 69–77.

Grotjahn, M. (1966). *Beyond laughter: A psychoanalytical approach to humor.* New York: McGraw-Hill.

Hoopes, R. (1991). Virtue rewarded. *Modern Maturity, 34*(2), 62–67.

Hyers, C. (1981). *The comic vision and the Christian faith.* New York: Pilgrim Press.

Isen, A. (1987). A creative muse. *Journal of Personality and Social Psychology, 52,* 1122–1131.

Jackson, M. (1980). The nurse as clown: The comic spirit in nursing. *Michigan Nurse, 53*(4), 12–14.

Koestler, A. (1964). *The act of creation.* London: Hutchinson.

Kronenberger, L. (1952). *The thread of laughter.* New York: Knopf.

Kushner, M. (1990). *The light touch: How to use humor for business success.* New York: Simon & Schuster.

Linn, L., & DeMalleo, M. (1983). Humor and other communication preferences in physician-patient encounters. *Medical Care, 21*(12), 1224–1230.

McAleer, N. (1989). On creativity. *Omni, 11*(7), 42–44.

Meredith, G. (1918). *An essay on comedy.* New York: Scribner's.

Mindess, H. (1985). *The Antioch humor test: Making sense of humor.* New York: Avon Books.

Paulos, J. (1980). *Mathematics and humor.* Chicago: University of Chicago Press.

Paulson, T. (1989). *Making humor work: Take your job seriously and yourself lightly.* Menlo Park, CA: Crisp Publications.

Pointer, D. (1985). Responding to the challenges of the new health care marketplace: Organizing creativity and innovation. *Hospital and Health Services Administration, 30*(6), 10–23.

Pollio, H., & Talley, J. (1991). The concepts and language of comic art. *Humor, 4*(1), 1–20.

Prerost, F. J. (1982). *A decade of change in humor appreciation among males and females: A relaxation of social and sex role restraints.* Paper presented at the Third International Conference on Humor. Montgomery College, Washington, D.C.

Raskin, V. (1987). *Semantic mechanisms of humor.* Boston: Reidel.

Richter, P. (1990). *The mocking of presidents continue: A solitary American Bard, Felicia Lamport.* Paper presented at the Eighth International Conference on Humor. Sheffield University, Sheffield, England.

Robinson, V. (1977). *Humor and the health profession.* New Jersey: Slack.

Ross, B. (1989). *Laugh, lead and profit: Building productive workplaces with humor.* New York: William Morrow.

Shekerjian, D. (1990). *Uncommon genius.* New York: Viking Penguin.

Vash, C. (1980). *The burnt-out administrator.* New York: Springer.

Veninga, R. (1982). *The human side of health administration.* Englewood Cliffs, NJ: Prentice-Hall.

Walker, N. (1988). *A very serious thing: Women's humor and American culture.* Minneapolis: University of Minnesota Press.

Webster's Third New International Dictionary. (1968). Springfield: Merriam.

CHAPTER 35

The Nursing Administration Imperative: Integrating Practice, Education, and Research

---

Highlights

- **A historical perspective**
- **Need for integration of service and education**
- **Models of integration**
- **Collaborative practice within nursing**
- **An approach to interdisciplinary collaborative practice**

The purpose of this chapter is to summarize the major concepts of professional nursing administration within a framework of integration and collaboration. Nursing service and nursing education can no longer exist separately. Together, they blend and build on quality research to bring harmony in the practice setting. Nurse executives hold the key to professional integration and must be the leaders in this effort.

The relationship between nursing service and nursing education has moved full cycle and is now back on a trajectory of integration within a conceptual framework of "nursing community." The concept of nursing community develops from the highest order of collaboration within nursing, a collaboration such that the separate terminologies of practice and education are no longer meaningful. Within this conception, professional nurses assume key leadership positions and practice clinically, administratively, or both as well as teach. This arrangement negates the guest or visitor faculty role in practice settings and the lack of nursing service involvement in the teaching of students.

Nurse executives in service and education play a unique role in developing this concept and creating the environment in which professional practice can occur and endure. To function in this unique leadership role, nurse executives must have a better understanding of integrated models and collaboration within and beyond nursing. There must also be a better understanding of the unfortunate separation of nursing education and services over the late nineteenth and early twentieth centuries.

A HISTORICAL PERSPECTIVE

The idea of integration of education and practice has existed since the development of nursing schools in 1873 (Bullough and Bullough, 1969; Gelinas, 1946). Early schools of nursing were hospital based, and nurses were trained through apprenticeship, with little emphasis on formal education. Nearly all schools of nursing were owned and controlled by the hospitals they served. Students were used for service to maintain low costs. Early schools were designed to function in much the same way as religious orders, with the hospital being the training center for educational and practice activities (Goodnow, 1942). There was much confusion as to their purpose: service or education. Differences in the roles of the nursing student and of the graduate nurse were not clearly defined.

By 1923, the need for self-directed, independent schools of nursing was identified. The Goldmark report stressed the need to establish university-based schools of nursing (Goldmark, 1923). The dual role of the hospital school of providing education and service was viewed as detrimental to the needs of patients and students. Furthermore, the training of nurses was considered a serious educational business that required direction by those who were committed to quality nursing education.

Throughout the next four decades, a gradual transition occurred from hospital-based to university- and college-based schools of nursing. Concomitant with this change was a dramatic decrease in faculty involvement in direct service in hospitals. Although the primary purposes of universities are teaching, research, and service, the service component became deemphasized. As faculty moved away from practice, nursing service personnel moved away from education. In the process of developing the strong research focus so important in quality nursing education, many faculty drifted away from problems related to direct care.

In the early 1960s, some nursing leaders began to seriously question the separation and began to devise approaches for reintegrating nursing practice and education.

Noted initiatives are the programs at the University of Florida, Case Western Reserve University, University of Rochester, and Rush-Presbyterian-St. Luke's Medical Center (Powers, 1976).

These programs have shown great promise, but several persistent difficulties hinder implementation in some settings. Doctorally prepared faculty hesitate to assume leadership roles in practice. Lack of agreement about academic preparation for nurses interferes with professional integrated models. Nationwide, the deficit of nurses prepared for leadership roles interferes with selection of nursing practice patterns appropriate for specific integrated models. Integrated models are not accepted by all nurses, and, indeed, crises are brewing in nursing that demand the most creative thinking by nursing leaders.

NEED FOR INTEGRATION OF SERVICE AND EDUCATION

Professional nursing practice emphasizes interdependence and collegial relationships between schools of nursing and clinical practice settings. The distinction between faculty and nursing service personnel in this relationship becomes diminished because all are participating in multiple aspects of practice. Practitioners in educational and clinical practice settings must be active participants at all levels of policy formulation and implementation in both the educational and clinical settings. Such professional accountability for all aspects of practice by all participants is essential.

In addition to professional accountability, mature professional practice requires the acceptance of the following assumptions:

- Clinical nursing is central to all other aspects of the profession of nursing, thus forming the unifying base for administration, education, research, and practice.
- Professional nursing is practiced in all settings, including acute, long-term, ambulatory, and home care settings.
- In these various settings, nursing care is based on the most advanced nursing knowledge.
- Nursing is responsible for nursing administration, education, practice, and research.
- The relationship between a school of nursing and a practice setting fosters a mutually productive environment that enhances the tripartite missions: education, practice, and research.
- The organizational and decision-making structures of the practice settings have direct effects on the extent to which educational missions can be achieved.
- Excellence in nursing practice in health care settings facilitates nursing education.

These assumptions, although necessary for professional practice, also form the basis for developing organizational models that allow for and foster the integration of nursing education and service. Although a variety of models can provide this, the ultimate goal is quality nursing care through an integration of administration, education, research, and clinical practice.

Though marriages of service and academia are coming into vogue in the form of born-again models (20 to 30 years ago, deans were directors of nursing), the criteria are similar. The following conceptual framework adapted from Christman's work on centers of excellence in nursing suggests potential criteria for integrated models (Christman, 1979a; Christman, 1979b).

Criteria for Integrated Models

Complete Opportunity for Practice   Educators are practitioners, practitioners are educators, and a variety of opportunities exist for joint appointments. Shared responsibilities are assumed, and research, both individual and interdisciplinary, is an expected behavior. Administration is recognized as a legitimate component of professional nursing.

Appropriateness for Size of Institution and School of Nursing   In some settings, the dean of the school of nursing may be the director of nursing. In other settings, it may be appropriate to have an associate dean for clinical practice. Top-level administrative responsibilities in practice and education are assumed by the best and most appropriately prepared nurses.

Open Communication Between Nursing Service and Education   Open communication is maintained through joint appointments and shared committee or task force responsibilities. Joint positions are crucial to maintaining open communication, and nurses in these positions are the viable linkage. For example, curriculum and research review committees, formerly considered the total prerogative of schools of nursing, have nursing service and faculty members, for they are one and the same in an integrated model.

Ability to Be Realized in a Variety of Health Care Settings   Because of the close involvement with the delivery of patient care, faculties with joint appointments can be more realistic in assignment of patients for student experience. All models portray the teacher as a participant in care rather than as a visitor to a patient care setting.

Participation in Policy Making at the Executive Level   The size and type of institution dictate the nature of governance; however, successful implementation of any model requires the participation of the dean or director at the executive level. This includes but is not limited to voting membership on the institution and school of nursing executive boards. In academic centers, nursing bylaws are shared across education and service.

Comparable Rewards for Education, Practice, and Research   Because of the tripartite mission of most teaching hospitals, some nursing homes, and community health nursing agencies, the successful integrated model allows for comparable rewards for education, practice, and research activities. These include promotion, merit increases, and public recognition.

Promotion of Interdisciplinary Collaboration   The success of any integrated model depends heavily on the acceptance and support of other health professionals.

Nurses, physicians, and hospital administrators must collaboratively define and implement an integrated model appropriate for each particular institution.

MODELS OF INTEGRATION

The mid-1970s signaled the beginning of a time of revolutionary change in the organization and operations of departments of nursing and their relationships with schools of nursing. To grasp the magnitude and scope of these changes, one has only to recognize two concurrent yet contrasting trends. At one extreme is the organizational model, characterized by the absorption of autonomous schools of nursing and departments of nursing into the medically dominated systems. An opposite trend is characterized by the integration of schools of nursing and nursing services into a unified structure for the provision of nursing care and nursing education. Between these two extremes are multiple other organizational structures in which nursing provides clinical care, education, and management of services. Whatever organizational context prevails, nursing contends with multiple authority systems and issues related to the direction and scope of practice.

Variations for models of integration exist in the real world and on the drawing board. As indicated previously, Case Western Reserve University, Rush-Presbyterian-St. Luke's Medical Center, and the University of Rochester present established unification models. Grace (1980) presented a taxonomy for integrated models at the Fall Conference of the Midwest Alliance for Nursing in September 1980. This taxonomy represents a progression of development:

1. Nightingale model: historical hospital training model with no organized external education.
2. Medical model: current state of the art; structures in nursing match the medical organization.
3. Collaborative model: characterized by consultative arrangements in selected roles and at selected levels of institutions; institution specific.
4. Affiliative model: based on the "associated with" concept; found in shared services and multihospital systems.
5. Independent faculty practice model: a specific mutant of the field on the edge of the movement with realignment of roles and current fiscal issues.
6. Transition model: undefined conceptually and operationally; the conversational model of integration without firm commitment by any of the involved members; goal clear, but process for achievement unclear.

Other model variations could potentially be established around:

1. Contract for nursing services by clinically expert faculty (for example, gerontological or pediatric specialists).
2. Unreimbursed adjunct appointments in the practice setting.
3. Research facilitation by nurse executives.
4. Collaborative research involving participants from practice and education.
5. Collaborative scholarly efforts among researchers, clinicians, and educators.

6. Shared teaching by faculty and clinical practitioners.
7. Integration of hospital nursing services with nursing home and home care services.
8. Alternating appointments by term in nursing practice and education.
9. Shared nursing consultation within and across multihospital systems.
10. Combination of the above in a newly designed transformation model.

The extent to which integration occurs depends primarily on the creativity, flexibility, and autonomy of nurse executives in both education and service. Sharing common mission, philosophy, and goal statements is the first step in collaboration within nursing and the development of a nursing community within a geographic area. Differentiating nursing practice can then provide a transitional step to achievement of a dynamic integrated practice/education model.

COLLABORATIVE PRACTICE WITHIN NURSING

In the final analysis, it is unreasonable to talk about joint or collaborative practice with physicians if there is no collaboration within nursing. The integrated models proposed by Grace (1980) essentially are designed for academic centers. However, integration (internal collaboration) can and should occur in any setting where professional nursing is practiced. All nursing divisions have, at a minimum, practice and quality assurance committees or councils. Is this not the first level of integration? Is this not an opportunity for faculty involvement? All schools of nursing have curriculum committees. Are these not opportunities for service involvement? The education of students should be a high priority for nurse executives, and opportunities for clinical practice and research should be available for nursing students. Figure 35.1 depicts a collaborative nursing model, freestanding from medical structure, that could optimize communication between and among educators and practitioners.

The collaborative model could be modified to meet the needs of any practice setting in acute, home, or long-term care. It builds on trust, mutual respect, and pride in professional nursing. Although the same person could be in the designated positions, this is not necessary. In a collaborative approach, two or more nurses can work together to achieve common goals related to excellence in practice, education, and research.

AN APPROACH TO INTERDISCIPLINARY COLLABORATIVE PRACTICE

Not long ago, the relationship between physicians and nurses was clear-cut. Nurses understood their place in the world, and physicians were captains of the health care team. The team consisted of two people: the physician and the nurse. Today, the relationship has changed dramatically as care has become more complex and there is strong support for multidisciplinary patient-centered care.

In today's world, there seems to be a lack of opportunity for interpersonal understanding. Many more nurses are ready to do battle over real or perceived nonrecognition. Where once the alliance of medicine and nursing was strong, there is increasing evidence of a bonding between administration and medicine, much to the dissatisfac-

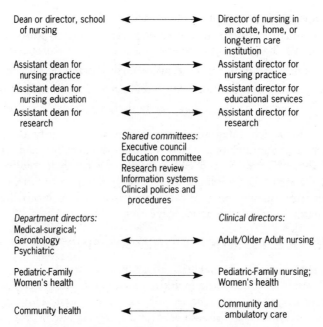

Figure 35.1 Collaborative nursing model.

tion and concern of nurses. Small irritations become major incidents, and it is not unusual for nursing strikes to occur. Interpersonal relationships are important, and much more attention is devoted to joint or collaborative practice in most health care settings.

Between 1978 and 1981, the National Joint Practice Commission (1981) offered four different but typical hospitals the opportunity to demonstrate how to successfully alter the physician-nurse relationship with resulting benefits to patients, nurses, physicians, and the hospital from establishing joint practice. The commission was supported by the American Medical Association, the American Nurses Association, and the W. K. Kellogg Foundation, and it established guidelines for nurses and physicians to use in collaborating as colleagues in providing patient care.

The emphasis on joint practice can be attributed to reasons related to changing times and changing professional goals:

1. Emergence of professional nursing.
2. Upgrading of education for nurses.
3. Increased interest in patient-centered care.
4. Conflict in images of nursing projected by nursing service and nursing education.
5. Breakdown in communications among health professionals.

Emergence of Professional Nursing

Over the past decade, nurses in this country have sought to become recognized as health professionals. This has not been easy, as society awards professional status only to those groups that are recognized as professionals by virtue of advanced preparation and a body of knowledge that is the unique basis for practice. Nurses seek an independent as well as interdependent role as they make a strong plea for an increased voice in decision making in health care delivery settings.

Education for Nurses

Although associate degree programs continue to flourish in community colleges and diploma programs have not ceased to exist, it is increasingly apparent that graduate education for nurses is here to stay. New master's and doctoral degree programs continue to develop. Baccalaureate education is considered by many schools of nursing to be the entry point to professional practice. In addition, the American Nurses Association proclaimed 1984 as the implementation date for requiring the B.S.N. for entry into professional practice. Although the proclamation was not widely accepted by the hospital industry, the very existence of the statement gave credence to the belief that advanced education in nursing is important. More recently, differentiating practice has become the focus of redefining technical and professional nursing roles (American Academy of Nursing, 1991; Malloch, Milton, & Jobes, 1990).

Quality Patient Care

Direct patient care has been largely the provision of services by institutions and physicians. With the advent of interest in quality patient care and patient-centered care, nurses are expected to play an ever-increasing part in monitoring and evaluating quality of care. Emphasis on care outcomes demands a look beyond chart audits and encourages collegial interaction from admission to discharge. Concern about continuity of care further supports joint planning.

Conflicts in Images of Nursing

Historically, medicine and nursing have always been allied around care of the sick and helpless patient. As the needs of humanity have changed, the scope of nursing has broadened beyond the care of the sick. In the past decade, nursing has been reconceptualized as legitimately being involved in wellness and illness. Health is no longer considered as being the mere absence of disease but, rather, as optimum biopsychosocial functioning and the ability to cope with problems of daily living. This emphasis on wellness care in many schools of nursing has created many problems for health care institutions where patients are getting older and sicker. As might be expected, baccalaureate-prepared nurses may feel unprepared to provide acute care. On the other hand, clinical specialists may feel well prepared for their positions and may lack opportunity for full use of skills.

Breakdown in Communications

There have been dramatic advances in medical knowledge and new techniques. The advent of antibiotics has helped to rout infectious disease, and many people are living longer and reaching the age in which chronic disease is more prevalent. Highly sophisticated diagnostic and monitoring techniques, coupled with intensive surgical treatments at any age, have created an environment of machines such that human interaction can be avoided or misused. The purchase of new equipment is ever a bone of contention as arguments go on over how scarce funds will be allocated. The very complexity of the environment interferes with both the time and place of normal conversation.

The Joint Practice Commission Model

Five factors have contributed to divergent goals on the part of physicians and nurses, such that in the 1980s, it has again become necessary to emphasize cooperation and collaboration in decision making. The collaborative model developed by the Joint Practice Commission (1981) is dependent on the following steps:

- Establishing a centralized joint practice committee representing practicing nurses and physicians, supported by administration
- Introducing primary nursing, with registered nurses individually responsible for nursing care within a collegial relationship with physicians
- Encouraging nurses' individual clinical decision making within the scope of nursing practice as defined by the hospital
- Integrating the patient record in a manner that reflects both nurse and physician assessment and action
- Conducting joint nurse-physician patient care record reviews.

Advantages of the Joint Practice Model

Many advantages are cited in the literature as being atttributable to joint practice. Mamana (1981) discusses joint practice as a new concept with promise and problems. Bates (1982) emphasizes the importance of level of preparation for an expanded role such as the clinical nurse specialist. Adelson and Werner (1981) also emphasize the importance of professionalism and competence for the role.

In general, the following advantages are described (Nayer, 1980):

1. One primary nurse caregiver: no nursing care is given by nonprofessionals. Clinical nursing functions are carried out by registered nurses, with minimal or no delegation of nursing tasks to others.

2. Increased job satisfaction: contributions of the registered nurse are recognizable. There is improved accountability and less blurring of the lines around who delivered what care to whom. This promotes individual recognition.

3. Improved recruitment and retention: although hard data are not available, a joint practice emphasis is thought to be related to an improvement in recruitment and retention.

4. Recognition of nursing: joint practice legitimizes nursing inputs and emphasizes the importance of optimal physician-nurse relationships. Furthermore, it promotes the integration of medical cure and nursing care philosophies.

5. Professional nursing competence: it is the expectation in joint practice that the primary nurse is knowledgeable, competent, and supportive of 24-hour responsibility.

6. Ongoing evaluation: in a sense, joint practice is an ongoing form of evaluation of care. The integrated record provides a readily available data source for reviewing observations, treatments, and actions. Joint discussion of care problems and goals further enhances the quality of care.

7. Communication, competency, and trust: these three elements are repeatedly cited as essentials for and advantages of joint practice.

The goal of joint practice is to improve health care, not to protect or preserve professional prerogatives. Interdependent relationships and willingness to reformulate roles are facilitated when practitioners are mature, experienced, and comfortable in their own role. The extent to which collaboration takes place between physicians, nurses, and administrators depends on the support of professional autonomy and the sharing of care activities between and across participating disciplines.

Multidisciplinary collaborative practice needs to be conceptualized, planned, supported, and evaluated, taking into account the specific characteristics of the organization and the individual patient care situation. In determining either the need for or planning the evaluation of selected models, one might well raise the question: How does one know if collaborative practice exists in a institution? Its existence can be recognized by the following criteria: *(1)* effective communication patterns, verbal and written, between and among physicians, nurses, and administrators; *(2)* the rewarding of improved patient care and units in which it is practiced; and *(3)* established efficient and effective support services. If these criteria are not met, collaborative practice does not really exist.

Summary

Integration of nursing service and education and multidisciplinary practice are of importance for nurse executives. The phenomena resemble religion, and proponents of integration are like born-again believers, flag bearers for the truth. The concepts of integration and collaboration are not new. They are developing patterns of professional organization in health care settings in which nursing administration, practice, education, and research are integrated and consolidated into a professional entity recognized by other health professionals.

Resurgence of interest in intra- and interdisciplinary integration is most likely due to the maturing of the profession and the recognition by professional nurses that clinical practice without research is not recognized in the professional world. Research is basic to administration, practice, and education, and good research comes out of collaboration between nursing service and education as well as across disciplines.

Nursing is a clinical practice discipline. To teach effective nursing practice, faculty members must be involved in clinical settings in some way to have credibility and to have access to research environments. Nurses in clinical practice lose credibility if they do not maintain expertise through continued education and research utilization.

Throughout the 1990s and into the twenty-first century, there will be an increased emphasis on research that has relevance for both nursing practice and education. Faculty members will be increasingly criticized for their lack of practice-based research and their rusty clinical skills. On the other hand, nursing service personnel will be expected to provide sophisticated, cost-effective patient care based on research. Research is the primary means of documenting effectiveness and efficiency of nursing education and practice, and nurses in the near future will be expected to provide data to justify nursing's portion of education and health care costs.

This book attempts to reach the heart and soul of the practicing nurse executive. At no time in the history of nursing has there been a better opportunity for the profession to move from adolescence to full maturity. The major studies of the decade carried out by non-nursing groups support the mandate for leadership within nursing. Although leadership must be present in education, research, and clinical practice, it is in administration that leadership is most likely to make the significant difference in bringing the profession to maturity.

By virtue of personal skills as well as clinical and administrative knowledge, the practicing nurse executive has the opportunity to create a professional practice environment that optimizes the development of staff to the fullest potential and enhances quality care delivery. This we believe. We also believe that the results of effective leadership in nursing administration can be measured in terms of:

- Recognized professional nursing image throughout the institution.
- Ongoing credible nursing research conducted by doctorally prepared nurses.
- Scholarly nursing publications by nurse executives and staff members.
- High level of staff satisfaction and work excitement.
- Quality patient care.
- Projects that demonstrate attention to changing trends (for example, special concern for the aged; drug abuse; AIDS).
- Cost-effective practice patterns.
- Clinical and administrative ladders.
- Upgrading of entire nursing division programs by increase in master's prepared nurses in middle management roles and B.S.N.s in primary nurse roles.
- Demonstrated collaboration with other health professionals (for example, interdisciplinary research).
- Integrated practice-education model in place.
- Decreased number of voluntary leavers.
- Demonstrated ability to attract, recruit, and retain excellent nurses at all levels.

- **Master's prepared nurses in newly designed clinical positions with care coordination responsibilities across settings.**

In the house with effective nursing leadership, people know each other, talk to each other, and are enthusiastic about common goals. They are working in concert on a regular basis, not trying to make ends meet through occasional, casual encounters.

The time for procrastination is over. As Styles (1983) states so vigorously, "Our future is now." It is time to realize that universal access to health care means access to all care providers as well as recipients and we must integrate our clinical and management skills. Just as Florence Nightingale decried the terrible conditions contributing to the death of British soldiers in the Crimea, so, too, can we in nursing administration say "No more!" It is time for nurses to assume the mantle of professional behavior, with all its inherent privileges and responsibilities, and it is time for nurse executives in all settings to assume the leadership for professional nursing.

STUDY QUESTIONS

1. Review Chapter 20, "Nursing Research in a Professional Practice Climate." Then describe three potential research projects that could use the expertise of educators and practitioners.

2. Visualize your setting for administrative practice. Describe a collaborative nursing model that links service and a related educational setting.

3. In the same setting, identify the key factors essential for collegial relationships with physicians and administration.

4. Identify the forces in your setting that interfere with the development of collegial relationships within nursing. With other disciplines.

5. To what extent should your nursing practice environment change to establish a climate for research-based decisions? Consider current and projected needs for substantive data.

6. How could staff nursing positions in your setting be redesigned to bring in doctorally prepared nurses with both clinical and teaching responsibilities?

References

Adelson, B., & Werner, J. (1981). Fostering collaborative relationships. *The Hospital Medical Staff, 10*(3), 5–11.

American Academy of Nursing (1991). Differentiating Practice. Kansas City, MO: American Academy of Nursing.

Bates, B. (1982). Doctor and nurse: Changing roles and relations. *New England Journal of Medicine, 783*(3), 129–134.

Bullough, V. L., & Bullough, B. (1969). *The emergence of modern nursing* (2d ed.). London: Macmillan.

Christman, L. (1979a, October). *The center of excellence in nursing: The conceptual model.* Paper presented at the Third Annual Nurse Educator Conference. Detroit.

Christman, L. (1979b). On the scene: Uniting service and education at Rush-Presbyterian-St. Luke's Medical Center. *Nursing Administration Quarterly, 3*(3), 7–40.

Gelinas, A. (1946). *Nursing and nursing education.* New York: The Commonwealth Fund, E. L. Hildreth and Co.

Goldmark, J. (1923). *Nursing and nursing education in the United States, committee for the study of nursing education.* New York: Macmillan.

Goodnow, M. (1942). *Nursing history.* Philadelphia: Saunders.

Grace, H. (1980, September). *Taxonomy of unification models.* Paper presented at the Fall Conference of the Midwest Alliance for Nursing on Designs for Collaboration: Nursing Service and Nursing Education. Rapid City, SD.

Malloch, K. M., Milton, D. A., & Jobes, M. O. (1990). A model for differentiated nursing practice. *Journal of Nursing Administration, 20*(2), 20–26.

Mamana, J. P. (1981). New concept has promise and problems. *The Hospital Medical Staff, 10*(3), 2–5.

The National Joint Practice Commission. (1981). *Guidelines for establishing joint or collaborative practice in hospitals.* Chicago: Neely Printing Co.

Nayer, D. D. (1980). Unification: Bringing nursing service and nursing education together. *American Journal of Nursing, 28*(6), 1110–1114.

Powers, M. J. (1976). The unification model in nursing. *Nursing Outlook, 24*(8), 482–487.

Styles, M. M. (1983, October). *Our future is now. Keynote address.* American Society for Nursing Service Administration. Minneapolis.

Bibliography

Baggs, J. G., & Schmitt, M. H. (1988). Collaboration between nurses and physicians. *Image, 20*(3), 145–149.

Davidson, R. A., Fletcher, R. H., & Earp, J. A. (1981). Role disagreement in primary care practice. *Journal of Community Health, 7*(2), 93–102.

DeRose, J. (1981). Implementing the basic elements of collaborative practice. *The Hospital Medical Staff, 10*(3), 19–25.

Ehrat, K. S. (1979). Service and education together: A working model. *Nursing Administration Quarterly, 3*(3), 1–5.

Huckabay, L. M. (1979). Point of view: Nursing service and education—is there a chasm? *Nursing Administration Quarterly, 3*(3), 51–54.

Joint Practice Committee of the State Medical Society of Wisconsin. (1980). Guidelines for implementation of joint practice of physicians and nurses. *Wisconsin Medical Journal, 79*(6), 30–33.

Koerner, B. L., Cohen, J. R., & Armstrong, D. M. (1986). Professional behavior in collaborative practice. *Journal of Nursing Administration, 16*(10), 39–43.

Mailick, M. D., & Jordan, P. A. (1977). A multimodel approach to collaborative practice in health settings. *Social Work Health Care, 2*(4), 445–454.

Simms, L. M., Dalston, J. W., & Roberts, P. W. (1984). Collaborative practice: Myth or reality. *Hospital and Health Services Administration, 29*(6), 36–48.

Steel, J. E. (1981). Putting joint practice into practice. *American Journal of Nursing, 81*(5), 964–967.

Steenson, C. B., & Sullivan, A. R. (1980). Support services in the school setting: The nursing model. *Journal of School Health, 50*(5), 248–249.

Weil, T. P. (1992). A universal access plan: A step toward national health insurance? *Hospital and Health Services Administration, 37*(1), 37–51.

Appendix

Situations for case study

A — Implementation of a change process
B — Gainsharing as an innovative approach
    Deborah Hooser
C — Problem-oriented recording
D — Community/rural hospital nursing system
E — Urban hospital nursing system
F — Sharing of services as a cost-effective measure
G — Operationalizing professional nursing
H — Introducing quality assurance in a nursing home
I — Marketing a product line
    Betty Sue Cox
J — Introduction of bedside terminals
    Kathryn Barnoud

SITUATION A

Describe a situation requiring implementation of a change process in a health care agency with which you are familiar. Recommend a change model and describe the desired outcomes or resultant situation. Identify the forces resistant to the change and the methods you would use to minimize stress and resistance.

SITUATION B

Gainsharing as an Innovative Approach
    Deborah Hooser
Read the description of the case situation below and answer the questions that follow it:

Gainsharing, an innovative approach, is a bonus and involvement system to reward performance and productivity. It is a responsive way to enhance the wages of employees for the improved performance of their unit and/or the total organization. The philosophy includes rewarding employees for improved productivity, cost reduction, or quality improvement in the form of cash bonuses.

This concept is coming of age in increasing numbers of health care agencies. It is a profit-sharing concept in several not-for-profit hospitals. The objective of gainsharing in a nursing division is to reward employees individually for efficient and effective resource management in their pursuit of quality and excellence in client-centered nursing care.

Clark Community Hospital is an 800-bed urban facility in the mid-south. Ten nursing administrators (nurse executive and directors of the clinical areas), a financial planner, and the risk manager met to consider the feasibility of using gainsharing as an incentive for rewarding employees within the nursing division. Current literature regarding this concept was reviewed. The administrative council initially endorsed the gainsharing plan. The nursing administrators explained the concept to each of their respective nurse managers and their staff. A survey instrument was used to assess the acceptance by the employees of the process of gainsharing. The majority of the staff indicated an interest in participating in the plan.

Educational and organizational change strategies were then developed to facilitate positive outcomes of the gainsharing plan. Before implementing the plan, the administrative council decided that the staff must be responsible and accountable for decision making at the nursing unit level (budgetary and personnel decisions were a centralized function). After 6 months the majority of the nursing units reported progress in this empowerment process.

The administrative council then formed subcommittees to examine critically the philosophy and goals of the gainsharing plan and how it is designed to benefit the organization, the staff, and the client. One subcommittee was charged with determining whether the legal aspects and personnel policies were congruent with the reward structure of the proposed gainsharing plan. An example of the application of gainsharing in a nursing unit is when staff are committed to conserve resources and use other innovative methods so that they are below or within their allocated budget. When this goal is achieved, all the employees will receive cash bonuses or shares. A formula for determining the bonuses and how they will be paid to staff is included in the plan. Also built into the plan is a structure that reflects staff input. Their ideas are crucial to the successful implementation of gainsharing, an innovative approach for rewarding nurse performance and productivity.

Questions

1. Who should be eligible to participate in this gainsharing plan? Why?
2. How should unit shares be distributed?
3. What happens to a share if the employee transfers, becomes disabled, or is deceased?
4. Should there be a penalty if there is a monetary deficiency, for example, due to a high rate of absenteeism in a nursing unit? If yes, what would you suggest the penalty should be?
5. If your nursing division wanted to operationalize a gainsharing plan to reward nurse performance and productivity, describe the steps that should be included to implement the plan.
6. Describe how this case situation would be applicable to Rogers' diffusion of innovation decision model.

Situation C

Read the description of the situation below and answer the questions that follow it:

North Community Hospital recently hired a master's-prepared nurse executive with no previous administrative experience except as a student and one summer as a night supervisor in a medium-sized hospital. Mary Turner is enthusiastic about her new position at this 150-bed community hospital. She has plans to implement primary nursing with the current staff and believes that this can be done within 6 months. Approximately three of the registered nurses are baccalaureate prepared. These three nurses are not head nurses. Another priority that Turner has identified is to revise the charting format. She has seen problem-oriented recording work successfully in other hospitals and is eager to have it implemented at North Community.

Questions

1. Would your priorities for the environment for nursing practice be the same as Turner's?
   a. If yes, why?
   b. If not, what would they be?
2. What additional data would you need to identify other priorities?
3. What specific outcomes might a nurse executive want to achieve by implementing primary nursing?
4. Are there other means by which the outcomes might be achieved?

Situation D

Read the description of the situation below and answer the questions that follow it:

James Community Hospital was opened in 1956 with a licensed bed capacity of 126 general medical-surgical, pediatric, and obstetrical beds to serve the town of Jamesville, population 3,100, and the surrounding county. Since the original opening of the hospital, 22 beds have been added, 10 of them for intensive care patients. The hospital has an emergency room as well as a labor-delivery area and a newborn nursery.

The department of nursing is headed by Joan Miller, a nurse with a baccalaureate degree in nursing. Miller works with an assistant director of nursing, who reports to her. The 10 nurse managers for the patient care units report to Miller. They are responsible for care 24 hours a day, but each has an assistant nurse manager who works evenings and a team leader RN, who works nights.

Three nursing supervisors report to the assistant director of nursing. Each supervisor works a specific shift and has other assigned responsibilities. For example, the day supervisor is responsible for coordinating the quality assurance activities, and the evening supervisor coordinates development and revision of the policy and procedure manuals. One of the problems encountered by the supervisors is their lack of communication with each other when decisions need to be made.

The nursing administrative staff, along with the RNs, agreed to implement primary nursing on all units. However, because of the difficulty of recruiting sufficient numbers of RNs, each unit has a modified primary nursing patient assignment pattern.

James Community Hospital provides care for acutely ill patients but refers complex patients to the nearest larger hospital, 25 miles away. Because the hospital serves a rural community, farm accident victims are commonly brought to the emergency room in spring and summer.

Questions

1. What purposes does the department of nursing serve in this community hospital?
2. Develop a philosophy and objectives for the James Community Hospital department of nursing. Indicate aspects of an organizational plan that would facilitate the implementation of the philosophy and objectives.
3. Design a system or flow of communication among the supervisors to expedite decision making.
4. Assess the current reporting relationships. What would you suggest for proposed changes?

Situation E

Read the description of the situation below and answer the questions that follow it:

Hospital X is a 900-bed university hospital located in a large metropolitan area. The hospital serves as a community facility for a population of 100,000 people in the surrounding communities and also as a referral center for a region comprising the entire state and portions of three contiguous states. The nursing division employs a staff of 800 registered nurses, 150 licensed practical nurses, and 100 nursing assistants.

The original pattern of nursing care was a combination of team and functional nursing. The nurse coordinator for quality management presented to the nursing staff a proposal to adopt primary nursing. This proposed change in the pattern of nursing care received mixed reactions among the staff of all units. However, staff members of the medical nursing unit decided to initiate the case-managed model.

The medical nursing unit assumed the following organization. A clinical nursing director is responsible for nursing services rendered in 7 patient care units (4 of them intensive care units) comprising 220 beds, 8 head nurses, 5 clinical nursing specialists, and 200 staff personnel, including registered nurses, licensed practical nurses, and nursing assistants. The clinical nursing director is responsible directly to the associate director for nursing, who is responsible for maintaining collaborative and consultative relationships with hospital administrative and medical staff. The staff registered nurses are accountable for the design and implementation of nursing care plans for their patients. Staff nurses report directly to the nurse managers of their unit, and the nurse managers report to the clinical nursing director. A clinical nursing specialist who had experience with such a system at a similar hospital agreed to provide consultation to the staff. She reports directly to the clinical nursing director in a position of functional responsibility.

Continuing support was pledged by nursing and hospital administration. The differentiation of clinical and nonclinical activities facilitated decisions concerning operation of support services. The satisfaction nurses have experienced with case management has supplied a motivating force. The positive response expressed by patients has fed the intrinsic reward system for nursing, and as this unit has become more adept in the use of the model, motivation to emulate it has been manifested by staff in other units.

Questions

1. Discuss the major factors to consider when designing an organizational structure for the division of nursing.
2. Prepare an organizational chart depicting the line, staff, and functional relationships. Indicate communication patterns and authority relationships.
3. Does the organizational chart reflect a wide or narrow span of control? State the rationale for your answer.
4. Does the organizational structure of the division of nursing influence nursing assignment patterns? If so, how? If not, why?

Situation F

Read the description of the situation below and answer the questions that follow it:

Ridgewood Hospital, a 500-bed hospital, is located in a large metropolitan area. It is a member of a five-hospital cooperative association that has the objectives of providing quality patient care and minimizing the costs to its members. The administrators (hospital, nursing, and physician) of the five hospitals constitute the association's executive committee, which meets bimonthly. A recent agenda item concerned the sharing of services as a cost-effective measure.

The administrators from the Ridgewood Hospital have advocated that there should be a formal program of ambulatory surgery. Hospitals throughout the country have developed ambulatory surgery, in which, for selected procedures, patients can be discharged the same day they are admitted. The hospital administrator from Ridgewood proposed to the association executive committee that, of the 10,000 surgical procedures per year performed at the hospital, as many as 1,000 could be done on a same-day basis. The hospital's occupancy rate is 87 percent, and an ambulatory surgery program would be likely to reduce occupancy.

In each of the member hospitals, the organizational structure within the nursing department is very similar. The units within the nursing department are functionally oriented (OB, medical-surgical, psychiatric, community health).

Decision-making authority is vested in the top administrative hierarchy, with limited staff input. Planning and mandating changes of direction or programs for the organization are functions of the top management. The medical staff maintain an autonomous position in relationship to the hospital and resist controls on their activities.

The nurse executive, the associate clinical directors, and the hospital administrator, in collaboration with the chiefs of medical services, are proposing that each member hospital have a separate program in ambulatory surgery. Three of the hospitals employ clinical nurse specialists in ambulatory care. The proposal is that these three specialists would function as a team in a staff relationship with the hospitals to coordinate planning activities for the establishment of the ambulatory surgery program. The hospital administrator will represent the proposal to the governing board of the hospital cooperative association for their approval.

Questions

1. Identify the type of organizational structure depicted in this situation and explain the advantages and disadvantages of this structure.

2. If the proposed program is approved, what type of organizational structure would be most advantageous for the implementation of this program? Support your answer.

3. Should a center operated by the five hospitals with an emphasis on ambulatory surgery be developed? Or should none or all of the hospitals establish such a program of their own, so that outpatients would be merged with inpatients?

4. What impact will the proposal have on costs, quality of care, and hospital personnel?

5. Utilize the proposed design, discuss the implications for nursing practice, the empowerment of nurses, and greater staff input.

Situation G
Read the description of the situation below and answer the questions that follow:

As the new nurse executive in a 250-bed community hospital, you have assessed that two major problems exist in the division of nursing: high turnover of the registered nurse staff and lack of communication from nursing administration to the nursing staff. Although the reasons for these problems are not known with certainty, several key nursing staff have stated that they agree that these are the major problems. Reasons given for the problem of high nurse turnover include low salary, no opportunity for advancement, and lack of recognition as professionals. Lack of communication from nursing administration to the nursing staff has been attributed to an autocratic previous nurse executive, and a centralized organizational structure of the nursing division.

The hospital administration has expressed support for the nursing division and offered to work on decreasing the turnover rate. The hospital medical staff have expressed a desire for improvement in the nursing care and agreed to work with the new nurse executive.

Over the next 3 years, this hospital has plans to begin a hospital-based home care program and to explore the feasibility of a hospice program. Although the hospital has always been community oriented, in the past few years some of the community programs have been discontinued because of fiscal problems.

Questions

1. If you, as the nurse executive, wanted to operationalize professional nursing in this hospital, what prerequisites should be present? Which seem to already be in place?
2. How would you go about determining the reasons for high nurse turnover and lack of communication from nursing administration?
3. What theories or conceptual frameworks may be applicable in this situation to the nurse turnover problem? To the communication problem?
4. Choose one theory or conceptual framework for each problem and develop the derived constructs that may lead to the operationalized results that you specify.

Situation H
Read the description of the situation below and answer the questions that follow it:

Restful Nursing Home is planning to implement an interdisciplinary quality assurance program soon. The facility has 100 beds, 25 of them skilled beds. The director of nursing has been designated the coordinator of the quality assurance program, with the responsibility of developing the structure and chairing the quality assurance committee. In addition to 16.8 FTE (full-time equivalent) registered nurses, the nursing home has a staff of a full-time physical therapist, a part-time occupational therapist, and a full-time dietition as well as consultation from a social worker and a family practice physician. The chief executive of the nursing home is concerned that the quality assurance activities are aimed at meeting regulatory requirements for documentation and quality control.

Questions

1. What quality assurance committee structure might be put in place in Restful Nursing Home?
2. What do you see as three possible specific priority areas for quality assurance activities, for example, monitoring medications, auditing patient outcomes?
3. What role should the discipline of medicine have in the quality assurance program?
4. What costs will be incurred for the nursing home to implement this program?

Situation I
Marketing a Product Line
    Betty Sue Cox
Read the description of the case situation below and answer the questions that follow it:

Williams Hospital is a 1000-bed, tertiary, not-for-profit hospital in the southeastern United States. It offers a full range of medical services, including neurology, cardiovascular, orthopedics, and oncology. Referrals originate primarily from a four-state area covering approximately a 200-mile radius. There are also two other hospitals in the locality offering similar services that rely on referrals from the same geographic area.

Over the past 3 years, Williams Hospital has maintained status quo with its cardiovascular services, despite the analysis of marketing research predications of a 20 percent increase in cardiovascular-related conditions in the region. One of the local hospitals has begun an aggressive, regional advertising campaign promoting their cardiovascular services. Another has initiated a specialized chest pain emergency department to attract local consumers experiencing symptoms related to cardiovascular disease. As cardiovascular services contribute 40 percent of Williams Hospital's annual revenue, hospital and nursing administration formulated strategies to strengthen their cardiovascular presence in the region and gain new market share.

Market Analysis

Market analysis was conducted by a consulting firm specializing in market research. Data revealed areas where Williams Hospital had gained, remained the same, or lost cardiovascular market share locally or in the region. The patient demographics and payer mix of the region were also analyzed as to their current and future impact on the hospital.

Results of patient-satisfaction surveys were trended for areas of concern specific to cardiovascular patients. Comments revealed concern for the lack of teamwork among nursing units, delays in test scheduling and results, and unmet specific needs of the cardiovascular patient. The next step was to focus on another key customer, the medical staff. Needs and expectations of the physicians were solicited as well as their suggestions for improvement in cardiovascular services. The marketing research consultants interviewed physicians on the staff and regional physicians referring their patients to Williams Hospital. The purpose was to compile information for strategic planning related to cardiovascular services.

Results indicated useful suggestions for strategic planning. The medical staff of Williams Hospital expressed frustration over the levels of "bureaucracy" and the lengthy time it took to obtain decisions or follow-up on issues of concern. There was also discontent regarding both the varying standards of care and inadequate nursing staffing on the patient care units. Some physicians felt that continuity of care did not occur between these units. The regional physicians expressed concern over referral of patients to the "big Williams Hospital" and oftentimes not receiving feedback regarding the care their patients received. Once referrals were initiated, patients would continue to receive care from Williams Hospital, a "loss" to the referral physician.

Reorganization

One of the strategies implemented to improve the cardiovascular service at Williams Hospital was to reorganize the existing cardiovascular-related departments into one department that emphasized the care of the patient with cardiovascular disease. The traditional functional organization of the institution was reorganized into a matrix model, aligning all services for cardiovascular patients into one strategic business unit (SBU). A vice-president became responsible for all areas related to cardiovascular services: cardiac patient care units, transplant services, cardiac rehabilitation, cardiac catherization laboratory, noninvasive cardiac laboratories, and the emergency departments. Responsibilities of the position included marketing, planning, development, implementation, and evaluation of all cardiovascular-related services at Williams Hospital.

An advisory board was established for the cardiovascular product line. Members included physicians, nurse managers and directors, cardiac laboratory director, marketing services, and administration. Ancillary support services such as radiology, clinical laboratory, and pharmacy were included as needed. The advisory board analyzed the data provided from the market research analysis and internal data related to financial performance and patient satisfaction surveys. The purpose was to develop strategies aimed at improving the current cardiovascular service and market share.

Strategies

The advisory board then implemented strategies that would target the following three basic goals: improve quality of patient care, maximize revenues, and reduce costs. The market analysis and the physicians' surveys indicated that one of the strategies for maintaining a high-quality reputation for cardiology in the designated market areas was state-of-the-art equipment and facilities. The next step was the renovation and expansion of patient care units and the cardiac laboratories. Telemetry was expanded and updated on all of the cardiac patient units. Innovative nurse recruitment efforts were initiated to address the inadequate staffing on the cardiology areas. The cardiac catheterization laboratories were upgraded with digital equipment. Research in cardiovascular disease was supported monetarily for the medical and nursing staff. New procedures such as coronary athrectomy and transesophageal echocardiography were initiated.

The emergency department was renovated to provide a specialized cardiac area. Patients with symptoms related to cardiovascular disease were triaged to this area for immediate treatment. Cardiac patients referred for admission from regional physicians were also evaluated in this area. The cardiologist then consulted with the regional physician regarding the patient's plan of care before the patient left the admission cardiac area.

The cardiologists and cardiovascular surgeons established a speakers bureau, which was available to regional hospitals and their medical staff. Topics ranged from technological advances to clinical case studies. The regional physicians also received invitations to continuing medical educational seminars offered by Williams Hospital. The enthusiasm expressed by the physicians from the regional hospitals prompted the nursing department to initiate a similar speakers bureau and continuing education seminars with the regional nursing staff.

The market analysis also indicated a significantly higher percentage of repeat cardiac admissions from patients who were enrolled in the hospital's cardiac rehabilitation program. This program was assessed by the medical and nursing staff as a mechanism to improve the quality of patient care as well as generating a sense of loyalty of the cardiac patients. Changes implemented were *(1)* hours were extended to improve patient access; *(2)* new educational classes were offered that were taught by staff such as cardiologists and cardiovascular clinical nurse specialists; *(3)* former patients received "VIP" invitations to public seminars, as well as being recruited for the hospital volunteer program for the cardiac service areas.

Market advertising focused on the excellent quality of the cardiac care and the full range of cardiac services available at Williams Hospital. Emphasis was on television and newspaper advertisements that promoted this comprehensive, state-of-the-art cardiac care. A "hot-line" was established for patients to call for information related to cardiovascular disease.

Analyses of data specific to cardiovascular-related DRGs revealed opportunities for cost reduction associated with length of stay (LOS) and resource utilization. Case management using the clinical pathways approach was implemented. The clinical pathways were developed with physician, nursing, and ancillary services input emphasizing quality of care, LOS, and resource utilization. The attempt was to standardize physician practice patterns and to assist with the planning of care for patients and their families. Several systems within the hospital were reorganized to become more "patient focused" rather than "hospital focused." For example, rather than a centralized electrocardiogram (ECG) department that employed technicians to perform ECGs, staff on the units were cross-trained to do the procedure. Not only did this eliminate another staff member entering the patient's room that they did not know, it reduced costs and improved service delivery time.

After cost-reduction activities were implemented, package pricing of all related services, including physician charges for a particular episode of care, was started at the hospital. Third party payers were interested in the cardiovascular speciality as an area to concentrate on package pricing because an episode of care is fairly predictable (such as coronary artery bypass and angioplasty).

Summary

Williams Hospital has demonstrated major commitments to the cardiovascular consumer population that it serves. Through working together as a service line team, the hospital's goals of improving quality of care, maximizing revenues, and reducing costs are continuing to be realized.

Questions

1. What should be the qualifications and desirable characteristics of the vice-president leading a major product line? Should the leadership for a product line be promoted from within or should it be someone from outside the organization?
2. Describe the role of nursing in a matrix organization focused on one service line.
3. What strategies would you use to influence those departments and/or individuals who did not support a matrix organization for a service line?
4. How would you market a unit's or department's service to patients, physicians, and other customers? What is your staff role?
5. What are the goals of your organization related to your speciality area? How are you currently supporting those goals?

Situation J

Introduction of Bedside Terminals

Kathryn Barnoud

The oldest hospital in Tennessee, The Regional Medical Center at Memphis (The MED) is a private, not-for-profit hospital with a public mission, which includes providing health care services to the indigent citizens of Shelby County. The hospital's mission statement: "BY THE MID 1990s WE WILL BECOME THE MOST RESPECTED HEALTH CARE ORGANIZATION IN THE REGION KNOWN FOR PASSION FOR MEDICAL AND MANAGERIAL EXCELLENCE COMPASSION FOR ALL INDIVIDUALS"; is supported by these corporate values: customer responsiveness, empowerment, leadership excellence, innovation, and systems measurement. These values aid The MED in challenging the boundaries of existing MED systems in the journey to operate as efficiently and effectively as possible.

In the summer of 1988, the Medical-Surgical Nursing Department of The MED embarked on a project to improve the quality of patient care. The Vice-President of Patient Care Services contracted a joint appointment with The University of Tennessee College of Nursing for a project coordinator to develop nursing protocols for the most prevalent medical diagnoses. These standardized nursing care plans could be individualized for patients, ensure that standards of care were met, and eliminate redundant creation of similar care plans. A medical-surgical pilot unit was chosen for the purpose of creating teams to develop the care plans.

In the fall, the project coordinator invited a graduate student in nursing administration interested in automation of the protocols to join the project. They approached the Medical-Surgical Director of Nursing (DON) with the idea of automating the care plans and nurse's charting. The student shared information about new, available technology that would enable nurses to do this at the bedside. The DON was intrigued and wanted to pursue the idea, so the student began to design a plan for an automation phase of the project.

The team consisting of the project coordinator, the student, the DON and the pilot unit nurse manager made a presentation to the executive leadership that introduced the concept of bedside automation as "phase II" of the protocols project. Responses were varied. The Director of Hospital Information Systems (HIS) took the position that this new technology was not "market-proven." However, the Vice-President of Patient Care Services stated that she was not afraid to be a "pioneer" in the field and the Chief Executive Officer (CEO) said to give the project team whatever they needed.

In the spring (1989), the DON hired the student part-time to develop phase II. Through literature review, attending conferences, and making site visits to vendor locations and hospitals using the technologies, the student researched information regarding bedside terminals and presented it to the project team and Vice-President of Patient Care Services for review. Potential vendors were identified and invited on site to demonstrate their systems to nursing, HIS and other key hospital staff, as well as outside "experts" from the University's College of Nursing and its Bio-Medical Information Center. Surveys were completed to measure staff reactions to the systems they reviewed. When the selection was narrowed, profiles were drawn to analyze the history and financial stability of the vendors of choice.

All of this information was compiled in a proposal to pilot the system of choice and presented in August 1989 to the Chief Operating Officer (COO) and Vice-President of Patient Care Services. In addition, the proposal included an identification of the need for the system, an outline of the benefits to be gained, a timeline for the pilot project and expansion (if successful), expected Return on Investment (ROI), and proposed criteria for the evaluation, which would be completed by the project team. The COO gave her approval with added evaluation requirements. A contract for the pilot unit was negotiated with the vendor and signed by the CEO in February 1990.

The project team was aware that the implementation would be a dramatic event for the nursing staff. It required total relearning of ingrained daily work habits. The technology was "scary" and intimidating to many. To prepare the nursing staff for the implementation, several key unit staff members were chosen to work for a day with nurses in a hospital where the system had been successfully implemented. This experience helped to persuade the doubtful and encourage those already enthusiastic.

In March, the student moved into another full-time position and a Bedside Terminal Coordinator was hired to coordinate the installation and implementation of the pilot unit. The terminals were installed during the month of April and after much staff training and preparation, the unit "went live" on the system in May.

Eight months after implementation of the system, the "pilot" was evaluated on the preestablished parameters.

A work sampling, consisting of over 18,000 observations, was used to measure the impact of the terminals on nursing care time and charting time. There was an overall positive trend for increasing the direct nursing care time and decreasing indirect care time for all categories of workers. LPNs, the group of workers doing the largest amount of charting prior to implementation, were saving an average of 21 minutes per shift. Also, in part because of the change in location of charting, there was an average time gain of 23 minutes per caregiver (all nursing unit personnel) spent at the bedside.

Patients on the nursing unit were interviewed by an objective outside party. The results showed that the patients were pleased with the system, saw it as enhancing nursing care, and felt they had increased access to their nurses. Increasing time that caregivers are accessible to patients was used to demonstrate that the system was supporting the corporate value, "customer responsiveness."

Monitors were developed to look at 18 specific criteria about the quality of charting before and after implementation. A dramatic improvement in the quality of documentation in terms of completeness was seen. For example, in intravenous (IV) management documentation: whether an IV solution was charted went from 79 to 98 percent compliance, whether an infusion rate was charted went from 47 to 98 percent compliance, and charting of needle sites went from 70 to 98 percent compliance. Also, whether intake and output was charted went from 7 to 100 percent compliance. In addition, the appearance, legibility, accessibility, and timeliness of charting was also enhanced.

Several methods were used in an attempt to quantify financial impact of the bedside system. An analysis of overtime was made, looking for overall trends in overtime reduction. An average of 1 hour and 15 minutes savings per week for the unit was identified. One of the greatest areas of financial impact was seen in capturing lost charges for purposes of third party reimbursement. This criteria was evaluated by conducting "mock" chart audits. The areas with the most significant changes were pharmacy intravenous fluids, 22 percent decrease in lost charges, and supply cart exchange, 28 percent decrease in lost charges.

Although implementation of the system required a complete reorganization of the daily work habits of personnel on the nursing unit, staff surveys revealed that they were very pleased with the system and prefered not to return to the old system of manual charting. This was confirmed during the December holidays when the unit was temporarily closed due to low census and staff were reassigned. Returning to manual charting on the other units met with strong resistance and complaint!

Being the only hospital in the region to have implemented the bedside technology, The MED soon began hosting interested visitors from all aspects of health care, information systems, and education. Local nursing schools began competing for clinical time for their students on the unit. This by-product of the project provided an avenue to demonstrate the values of innovation and leadership excellence.

In December 1990, these evaluated criteria were compiled in a report and presented to the executive staff by the project team. In the report, the "pilot" experience and evaluation outcomes were demonstrated as having exercised the corporate value system and supporting the mission statement. The project was determined to be successful and approved for expansion to other medical-surgical units.

Questions

1. Describe the key ingredients involved in this change process.
2. Explain how the corporate value system supported the innovation.
3. Identify Rogers' five-step process to the diffusion of innovation in this case study.
4. Are you able to identify change agents in the case study?
5. Describe a change or innovation that you have experienced in your health care setting and identify the change agents and the process that occurred.
6. Describe a change or innovation that was proposed but unsuccessfully implemented. Identify the change agents and the process that occurred. Identify ingredients or strategies that may have altered the outcome.

Index _____

Page numbers followed by the letter t refer to information in tables.

Accounting
  assets in, 175–176
  expenses in, 176–177
  financial, 175
  fiscal year in, 177
  liabilities in, 176
  managerial, 175
  revenues in, 176
Accounting accrual, 178
Accrual accounting, 178
Action research
  action learning through,
    242–244
  group learning through,
    236–238
Administration
  clinical, human side of, 49–52
  concept of, 30–31
  excellence in, leadership styles
    and, 68–70
  historical perspective on,
    477–478
  humor in, 460–473
  nursing, 476–487
    integration of service and
      education in, 478–480
  nursing service
    computerized information
      systems in, 406–409
    efficiency of, computerized
      information systems and,
      408–409
Administrative support to institute
  change, 85
Aging, secondary, frail older
  people and, 210–211
American Nurses Association
  model for quality
    assurance program, 427,
    430–433
Anger
  in communicating with self,
    353, 355
  process of, 356
Assets, 175–176
Assistive technology, 379–388
  for cognitive disorders, 386
  for comfort issues, 386
  concept of, 380

  for elimination problems, 386
  exploring new horizons in,
    382–384
  for mobility problems, 384
  nurses in need of, 380–382
  operationalizing receptivity to,
    386–387
  relevant to nurse executives,
    384–386
  for respiratory function
    disorders, 386
  for skin integrity problems,
    385–386
  for special senses deficits, 385
Authority
  to approve nursing practice
    components in instituting
    change, 85
  chain of command and, 96–97
  delegation of, 97
  functional, 96
  line and staff, 96
  of nurse executive, 84–85
Authority relationships, 95–97
Autocratic-democratic continuum
  of leadership, 70
Autocratic leader, traits of, 68
Avoidance in conflict resolution,
  193–194

Behavior
  changing, in developing human
    potential, 163–164
  networking, men and women
    and, 374–375
Behavioral science approach to
  management, 36–37
Boundaries, managing, 57–58
Budgetary control to institute
  change, 85
Budgeting in managing fiscal
  resources, 180–183
Bureaucratic model of
  management, 35–36
Business skills, nurse executives
  and, 147

Care
  health. See also Health care
  patient, quality of, in

    interdisciplinary
      collaborative practice, 483
  quality of, ethics and, 223
  scheduling of, computer
    information systems in,
    403
Change. See also Innovation
  innovation theories/models and,
    105–110
  resistance to, 116–117
  stages of, 113–114
  strategies for, 114–116
Climate of organization, 81
Clinical administration, human side
  of, 49–52
Clinical practice, blending
  organizational design
  with, 90–102
Closed system organizations,
  38, 39t
Coercive power as source of
  conflict, 189, 190
Cognition, assistive technology
  innovations for, 386
Collaboration in conflict
  resolution, 197–199
Collaborative nursing research,
  273–274
Collective bargaining, 411–416
  concept of, 411–412
  in conflict resolution, 199–200
  legislation on, 412–414
  nursing and, 414–416
Comedian, how to be a, 469–470
Comedy
  gender gap in, 467–469
  ingredients of, 461–462
  of management, 460–473
  nature of, 462–464
  punch line in, 472–473
Comfort, assistive technology
  innovations for, 386
Comic art, state of, 461–462
Comic history, 465–467
Comic research, 464–465
Committees, nature of,
  organizational design and,
  93–94
Communication, 351–420

assistive technology and, 379–388
innovations in, 385
breakdown in, in interdisciplinary collaborative practice, 483–484
computer technology in, 361–362
effective, 352–363
formal and informal groups in, 360–361
group, 357–359
in interview, 357
mentorship and, 365–377
networking and, 365–377
nonverbal, 360
one-to-one, 355, 357
by public speaking, 362–363
with self, 353–357
    anger in, 353, 355
    revitalization of self in, 355
verbal, 359–360
Company-sponsored model of managed care, 445
Competency, 285–286
Competition
as marketing strategy, 444–446
in strategic planning, 252
Computer as communication aid, 385
Computerization, quality management and, 267
Computerized information systems applications of
    in nursing, 400–409
    for nursing service administration, 406–409
    for enhancing productivity, 392–410
Conceptual model(s) for nursing
Levine's, 25–27
theories of nursing practice and, 16–27
Conflict
characteristics of, 187–188
functional and dysfunctional, assessment of, 191–193, *194, 195*
intergroup, 189
interorganizational, 189
interpersonal, 188
intrapersonal, 188
sources of, 189–190
types of, 188–189
Conflict management, 185–201
in building effective work groups, 328
historical background of, 186–187
philosophical background of, 186–187
Conflict resolution
avoidance in, 193–194
collaboration in, 197–199
collective bargaining in, 199–200
confrontation in, 196
containment in, 195–196

defusion in, 194
lose-lose, 196
negotiation in, 197
strategies for, 193–200
techniques of, 197–200
win-lose, 196
win-win, 197
Confrontation in conflict resolution, 196
Conservation principles, 25–27
Construction in facility planning, 307–308
Containment in conflict resolution, 195–196
Contingency management movement, 40–41
Continuity of care, emerging practice settings in, 155–156
Contract, union, life with, 418–419
Contract negotiation, 417–418
Conviction in successful nurse executive, 72
Coordinating in building effective work groups, 328
Corporate culture, relationship of, to subgroup cultures, 124–125
Correctional systems, opportunities in, 148
Cost centers, 177
Costs in marketing strategies, 443–444
Courage in successful nurse executive, 71–72
Creativity
managing, humor and, 470–472
in successful nurse executive, 72–73
Cultural anthropologist's perspective on organizational culture, 121
Culture, organizational, 120–133. *See also* Organizational culture

Data
collection of, automatic, in enhancing efficiency, 402
entry of, technology for, in enhancing efficiency, 400–402
Debate in group communication, 359
Deci's theory of motivation, 165–166
Decision making
ethical, 222–229. *See also* Ethics
models for
    descriptive, 225
    ethical, 225–226
    generic, 224–225
    prescriptive, 225
Deductive theory construction, 14
Delegation in building effective work groups, 328
Demand states in marketing management, 436–437

Descriptive model for decision making, 225
Design process, facility planning and, 298–307
Developmental psychology in developing human potential, 167–168
Disease prevention, health promotion and, emerging practice settings in, 153–155
Diversification in hospitals, emerging practice settings and, 149–150

Economic competition in health care, 456–457
Economic factors in strategic planning, 250
Economic issues involving emerging practice settings, 149–151
Economics, 449–457
global, health care and nursing and, 450–452
of health care and nursing, changes in, 452
Education
for nurses in interdisciplinary collaborative practice, 483
power of, human potential and, 162–163
and service, integration of models of, 480–481
need for, 478–480
Educational needs, McClusky's, 65–67
Effective unit workplace, 331–333
Efficiency
definition of, 396–397
enhancement of, computer information systems in, 400–403
productivity related to, 397
Elimination, assistive technology innovations for, 386
Empirical-rational strategies of change, 114–115
Empowerment, 231–246
definition of, 232–233
effective practice and, 241–242
job satisfaction and, 239
perceptions of work and, 238–239
visioning and, 234–235
work excitement and, 239–241
Entrepreneurship, nurse executives in, 147
Environment
changes in, fiscal implications of, 87–88
concept of, 82–84
definition of, 80
health care
    quality in, 422–434
    structure-process-outcome relationships in, 423–425
internal, 80–81

nurse executive and, 81–85
for professional practice,
creating, 80–88
Error reduction, computer
information systems in,
404–405
Ethical decision making
moral judgments and, 222–229.
See also Ethics
in nursing administration,
224–226
Ethical dilemmas, dealing with,
157–158
Ethics
applied benefits and, 224
content of, ethical decision
making and, 226
current practice and, 223–224
definition of, 223
nurse executive and, 156–157
nursing, quality management
and, 266–267
professional practice of nursing
administration and,
227–229
quality of care and, 223
related to organizational culture,
133
theories of, ethical decision
making and, 226
Ethos, unit, in building effective
work groups, 335–336
Executive, nurse, 61–76. *See also*
Nurse executive
Expectancy theory of motivation,
165
Expenses, 176–177
Expert power as source of conflict,
189

Facility planning, 295–309
bid-award process in, 307–308
block plan drawings in, 302–305
construction documents in,
307–308
construction in, 307–308
design development in, 306–307
design process and, 298–307
functional evaluation in, 298, 300
master program phase of,
300–302
mission in, 298
nursing in, 296–298
physical evaluation in, 298, 300
postoccupancy evaluation in, 308
role study in, 298
schematic drawings in, 305–306
space program in, 302, 303*t*
Factor-isolating theories, 15
Fayol, Henri, management
principles of, 33–35
Federal funding, emerging practice
settings and, 149
Federal regulations to control
health care expenditures,
452–454
Fiedler model of leadership, 70

Financial accounting, 175
Fiscal implications
of environmental change, 87–88
of operationalizing professional
nursing, 143–144
of quality assurance program, 433
Fiscal resources
budgeting in, 180–183
managing, 173–183
operating cycle in, 174–178
reimbursement methods in,
178–179
monitoring results in, 180–183
Fiscal year, 177
Flexible work group, 292–293
Followers, developing, 168–171

General systems theory, 38–40
Geriatric population, 203–218. *See
also* Older people
Global economics, health care and
nursing and, 450–452
Global system, emerging practice
settings in, 151–152
"Great man" leader, traits of, 68
Group communication, 357–359
Group learning through action
research, 236–238

Health, promotion of, nursing in,
4–5
Health care
economic competition in,
456–457
economics of, changes in, 452
expenditures on
federal regulations to control,
452–454
Medicare payments to
physicians and, 454
state regulatory initiatives on,
454–455
global economics and, 450–452
market forces in, adopting
traditional, 455–457
for older people, standards of,
208–210
quality movement in, 259–260
quality of, changing concepts of,
395–396
reform of, nursing agenda for,
quality management and,
267
Health care agency boards, nurses
on, 147
Health care environment
quality in, 422–434
structure-process-outcome
relationships in, 423–425
Health Care Financing
Administration (HCFA),
452–454
Health organization-environment
model, 82, *84*
using, 85–87
Health promotion, disease
prevention and, emerging

practice settings in,
153–155
Home health care, opportunities
in, 150
Hospital context in building
effective work groups,
328–330
Hospital image in strategic
planning, 252
Human relations approach to
management, 36–37
Human resources frame,
organizations viewed
from, 47
Humor
in administration, 460–473
managing creativity and,
470–472

Iceberg phenomenon, conflict and,
187
Inductive theory construction,
14–15
Infection control in integrated
quality management, 263
Innovation. *See also* Change
organization development model
of, 108–110
organizational behavior model
of, 110–112
participatory action research and,
110
receptivity to, 104–118
resistance to, 116–117
theories of
Lewin's force field, 105–106
Lippitt's, 106–107
Rogers' diffusion of, 107–108
Inpatient practice settings, 147–148
Instrumental leader, traits of, 68
Integrated professional nursing
administration,
components of, 10–11
Integrated quality management,
257–268
components of, 261–264
strategies for, 264–265
Interdisciplinary collaborative
practice, approach to,
480–485
Interdisciplinary quality assurance
program, 427–430
Intergroup conflict, 189
Internal environment, 80–81
Interorganizational conflict, 189
Interpersonal conflict, 188
Interview, communication in, 357
Intrapersonal conflict, 188

Job satisfaction, empowerment and,
239
Joint Practice Commission model,
484
Joint practice model, advantages
of, 484–485

King's general systems theory,
23–25

Labor relations, 411–420
 collective bargaining in, 411–
  416. *See also* Collective
  bargaining
 contract negotiation in, 417–418
 impasse procedures in, 417–418
Laissez-faire leader, traits of, 68
Leader(s)
 developing, 168–171
 nurse executive as, 63–64
Leadership
 in care of older people, 203–218
 styles of, 68–70
Learning
 action
  participatory action planning
   from, 245
  through action research,
   242–244
 group, through action research,
  236–238
 worker, 53–55
Learning organizations, nurse
  executive role in, 55–57
Learning window, 53–55
Legislation, collective bargaining,
  412–414
Legitimate power as source of
  conflict, 189, 190
Levine's conceptual model for
  nursing, 25–27
Lewin's force field theory of
  innovation, 105–106
Liabilities, 176
Lifestyle trends in strategic
  planning, 251
Lippitt's theory of innovation,
  106–107
Load in McClusky's theory of
  margin, 65
Lose-lose in conflict resolution, 196

Managed care models, 445–446
Management
 behavioral science approach to,
  36–37
 bureaucratic model of, 35–36
 comedy of, 460–473
 concept of, 31
 contingency approach to, 40–41
 creativity in, humor and,
  470–472
 human relations approach to,
  36–37
 management science approaches
  to, 37–38
 product-line, 446
 of resources, 279–350. *See also*
  Resources, management of
 span of control of, 95
 theories of
  classical, 31–35
  contingency, 40–41
  evolving, 30–45
  F, 43
  X, 41–42
  Y, 42
  Z, 42–43

Management decisions, quality of,
  computerized information
  systems and, 406–408
Management science approaches to
  management, 37–38
Management theorist's perspective
  on organizational culture,
  121–122
Managerial accounting, 175
Manpower in strategic planning,
  252
Margin, McClusky's theory of, 65
Market segmentation, 440
Market trends in strategic planning,
  251
Marketing, 435–447
 quality management and, 267
 strategies for, 443–446
Marketing concept in marketing
  management, 439–440
Marketing information system,
  441
Marketing management, 436–438
 philosophies of, 438–440
Marketing research consultants,
  441–443
Maslow's hierarchy of needs, nurse
  executive and, 64, *65*
Maslow's theory of motivation,
  nurse executive and, 64
Master planning, 249
Matrix organizations, 99–102
McClusky, Howard, nurse
  executive and, 65–68
Mentor(s)
 becoming, 372
 benefits of mentoring for, 371
 characteristics of, 367–368
 definition of, 366–367
 role of, 366
 women and, 368–369
Mentor relationships, characteristics
  of, 367–368
Mentoring
 attitudes and behavior for,
  372–374
 benefits of, 370–371
 cross-gender, 368
 of nurses, 369
 same-gender, 370
Mentorship, 365–377
 choosing, 371–372
Mission, business-centered,
  defining, in strategic
  planning, 253–254
Mobility, assistive technology
  innovations in, 384
Mobility devices for older people,
  212
Model(s)
 of management, bureaucratic,
  35–36
 of nursing, 16
  conceptual, Levine's 25–27
  implications of, for nursing
   administrative practice, 27
  Roy adaptation, 21–23
Moral judgments, ethical decision

making and, 222–229.
  See also Ethics
Motivation
 in developing human potential,
  164–167
 Maslow's theory of, nurse
  executive and, 64

Nadler-Tushman transformation
  model, 111–112
National Labor Relations Act
  (NLRA), collective
  bargaining and, 412–414
Navy Nurse Corps, opportunities
  in, 147
Needs, educational, McClusky's,
  65–67
Negotiation in conflict resolution,
  197
Networking, 365–377
 professional, 375–376
 theory of, 374
Networking behavior, men and
  women and, 374–375
Nightingale, Florence, as nurse
  executive, 3
Normative reeducative strategies of
  change, 115
Nurse(s)
 auxiliary personnel and, ethical
  problems between, nurse
  executives in resolving,
  227–228
 education for, in interdisciplinary
  collaborative practice, 483
 mentoring, 369
 in need of assistive technology,
  380–382
 nurse executives and, ethical
  problems between,
  resolving, 228–229
 physicians and, ethical problems
  between, nurse executives
  in resolving, 228
 shortage of, perceived, 283–285
Nurse executive
 in advancing nursing research,
  271–272
 assistive technology relevant to,
  384–386
 authority of, 84–85
 barriers to, 369
 chance and, 75
 conviction in, 72
 courage in, 71–72
 creativity in, 72–73
 in dealing with ethical
  dilemmas, 157–158
 developing, 67
 emergence of, 3–5
 energizing responsibilities of,
  345–348
  nursing's contribution in, 347
  performance planning in,
   347–348
  technical/professional roles in,
   346–347
 environment and, 81–85

ethics and, 156–157
as leader, 63–64
leadership styles of, 68–70
in learning organizations, 55–57
Maslow and, 64, *65*
McClusky and, 65–68
nurses and, ethical problems
    between, resolving,
    228–229
person in role of, 61–76
personal support systems for,
    74
successful, personal attributes of,
    70–73
time management and, 74–75
Nurse staffing, 310–324. *See also*
    Staffing
Nursing
collaborative practice within, 481
collective bargaining and,
    414–416
economics of, changes in, 452
in facility planning, 296–298
global economics and, 450–452
in health promotion, 4–5
images of, conflicts in, in
    interdisciplinary
    collaborative practice, 483
nature of, 7
political effectiveness of,
    457–459
professional
    emergence of, in
        interdisciplinary
        collaborative practice, 483
    operationalizing, 137–144. *See
        also* Operationalizing
        professional nursing
    vocational nursing
        differentiated from, 7
vocational, professional nursing
    differentiated from, 7
Nursing administration
efficiency of, computerized
    information systems and,
    408–409
ethical decision making in,
    224–226
model of, 138–139
professional practice of, ethics
    and, 227–229
in strategic planning, 254–255
Nursing administrative practice,
    implications of theories
    and models for, 27
Nursing division, quality assurance
    program for, 425–426
Nursing homes, opportunities in,
    147
Nursing market arena, 440
Nursing model for ethical decision
    making, 226
Nursing practice, 7–8
interactive model of, 8–9
Nursing service administration,
    computerized information
    systems in, 406–409
Nursing staff, ethical dilemmas

within, nurse executives
    in resolving, 227

Older people
demographics of, 203–208
emphasis on, obstacles to,
    215–216
female, special needs of, 216–217
frail, secondary aging and,
    210–211
leadership in care of, 203–218
    assuming, 213–215
not-so-frail, 211–213
standards of health care for,
    208–210
Open system organizations, 38–39
Operating cycle in managing fiscal
    resources, 174–178
Operationalizing professional
    nursing, 137–144
fiscal implications of, 143–144
model for, 140–141
    use of, 141–143
prerequisites for, 139–140
Orem's self-care theory, 16–20
Organization(s)
boundaries in, managing, 57–58
climate of, 81
clinical, windows on, *48–49, 50*
making sense of, 46–59
matrix, 99–102
perspectives on, 47–48, *48–49*
philosophy of, organizational
    design and, 91–92
process of, in strategic planning,
    253
purpose of, organizational design
    and, 92
structure of, 94–95
    centralized, 99
    decentralized, 98–99
    models of, 98–102
    in strategic planning, 253
Organization development (OD)
    model of innovation,
    108–110
Organizational behavior model for
    innovation, 110–112
Organizational culture, 120–133
assessing, 131–133
changing, possibility of, 128–130
corporate and subgroup,
    relationship between,
    124–125
definitions of, 123–124
ethics related to, 133
perspectives on, 121–123
sources of, 125–127
understanding, value of, 127–128
Organizational design
authority relationships and,
    95–97
blending clinical practice with,
    90–102
of care delivery systems, impact
    on, 53
context for practice and, fit
    between, 91

nature of committees and, 93–94
participatory approaches to,
    52–53
purpose and philosophy of
    organization and, 91–92
shared governance in, 92–93
span of control in, 95
Organizational practitioner's
    perspective on
    organizational culture, 122
Organizational theorist's
    perspective on
    organizational culture,
    121–122
Organizational universe model of
    environment, 82, *83*

Participative leader, traits of, 68
Participatory action planning from
    action learning, 245
Participatory action research, 110
group learning through,
    236–238
Participatory approaches to
    organizational design,
    52–53
Path-goal theory of nursing
    leadership, 70
Patient classification
as component of nurse staffing
    systems, 312–313
tools for, 313–316
Performance planning in
    energizing responsibilities
    of nurse executive,
    347–348
Personal support systems of nurse
    executive, 74
Persuasion in group
    communication, 358–359
Philosophy of organization,
    organizational design and,
    91–92
Physicians, nurses and, ethical
    problems between, nurse
    executives in resolving,
    228
Planning
in building effective work
    groups, 327–328
facilities, 295–309. *See also*
    Facility planning
master, 249
participatory action, from action
    learning, 245
performance, in energizing
    responsibilities of nurse
    executive, 347–348
strategic, 248–256. *See also*
    Strategic planning
Point-of-service (POS) model of
    managed care, 445
Political effectiveness of nursing,
    457–459
Political frame, organizations
    viewed from, 47
Political issues

involving emerging practice
settings, 152–153
in strategic planning, 251
Potential, human, developing,
162–171
changing behavior and, 163–164
developmental psychology in,
167–168
for leaders and followers,
168–171
meeting needs and, 171
motivation in, 164–167
power of education in, 162–163
Power
in McClusky's theory of margin,
65
non-zero-sum model of, 233
nursing, 235–236
personal and group, 235–236
as source of conflict, 189–190
zero-sum conception of, 232–233
Power-coercive change strategies,
115–116
Practice
collaborative, interdisciplinary,
approach to, 480–485
current, ethics and, 223–224
effective, empowerment and,
241–242
nursing research applications in,
275–276
patterns of
redesigning, new approach to,
287–292
conceptual framework in,
288–292
traditional, 286–287
Practice settings, emerging,
147–148
in continuity of care, 155–156
economic issues involving,
149–151
in global system, 151–152
in health promotion and disease
prevention, 153–155
political issues involving,
152–153
Prescriptive model for decision
making, 225
Pricing as marketing strategy,
443–444
Product concept in marketing
management, 438
Product-line management (PLM),
446
Productivity, 339–348
concepts of, conceptual
framework for, 393–399
definition of, 341
efficiency related to, 396–397
energizing responsibilities of
nurse executive and,
345–348
enhancing, through
computerized information
systems, 392–410. *See
also* Computerized
information systems

high, characteristics of systems
with, 341
human effort and, 397
improving, 397–399
low, 343–345
measuring, methods of, 343
units of production and, 342–343
working definition of, 393–395
Profession, criteria essential for, 5–6
Professional associations, 57
Professional networking, 375–376
Professional nursing, 139
emergence of, in interdisciplinary
collaborative practice, 483
operationalizing, 137–144. *See
also* Operationalizing
professional nursing
vocational nursing differentiated
from, 7
Professional practice
environment for, creating, 80–88
of nursing administration, ethics
and, 227–229
Professional practice disciplines,
8–11
Professionalism, definition of, 5
Promotion as marketing strategy,
444
Protégé, benefits of mentoring for,
370–371
Psychology, developmental, in
developing human
potential, 167–168
Public speaking, 362–363

Q model of managed care, 445–446
Quality
assessment and improvement of,
in integrated quality
management, 261–263
of care, ethics and, 223
of clinical care, improvement in,
computer information
systems in, 404–406
definition of, 260
of health care, changing
concepts of, 395–396
in health care environments,
422–434
of management decisions,
computerized information
systems and, 406–408
Quality assurance model of
environment, 82
Quality assurance program
fiscal implications of, 433
implementation of, 430–433
interdisciplinary, 427–430
for nursing division, 425–426
Quality control, industrial model
for, 258–259
Quality management, 260
computerization and, 267
goals of, 264
integrated, 257–268
marketing and, 267
nursing agenda for health care
reform and, 267

nursing ethics and, 266–267
nursing research and, 265–266
trends in, 265–267
Quality movement in health care,
259–260
Quality patient care in
interdisciplinary
collaborative practice, 483
"Queen bee" syndrome, 370

Rational-legal authority in
bureaucratic model of
management, 35
Recession, health care and,
450–452
Recruitment, 281
Referent power as source of
conflict, 189, 190
Regulatory factors in strategic
planning, 251–252
Reimbursement
methods of, in managing fiscal
resources, 178–179
third-party, for nursing services,
150–151
Relicensure, 285–286
Research
action
action learning through,
242–244
group learning through,
236–238
marketing, 441–443
qualitative and quantitative,
442–443
nursing
advancing
nurse executive in, 271–272
in professional practice
climate, 270–277
applications of, to practice,
275–276
collaborative, 273–274
developing emphasis for, 275
quality management and,
265–266
researchable nursing problems
for, 272–273
utilization of, 276–277
participatory action, 110
Resources
existing, mobilizing, 280–291
competency in, 285–286
flexible work group in,
292–293
recruitment, retention, and
turnover in, 281–283
relicensure in, 285–286
management of, 279–350
mobilizing existing resources
in, 280–293
Respiratory function, assistive
technology innovations
for, 386
Retention, 281–282
Revenue, 176
Revenue centers, 177

Reward power as source of conflict, 189, 190
Risk management in integrated quality management, 264
Robots to assist functional dependent older persons, 382
Rogers' diffusion of innovation theory, 107–108
Roy adaptation model of nursing practice, 21–23

Safety management in integrated quality management, 264
Scheduling
  of care, computer technology for, 403
  workweek patterns for nursing personnel and, 320–322
Self
  communicating with, 353–357
    anger in, 353, 355
    revitalization of self in, 355
    revitalization of, 355
Self-assessment and personal empowerment, 235
Self-care
  development, 18
  health-deviation, 18–19
  universal, 17–18
Selling concept in marketing management, 439
Senses, special, assistive technology innovations for, 385
Service and education, integration of
  models of, 480–481
  need for, 478–480
Shared governance in organizational design, 92–93
Situation-depicting theories, 15
Situation-producing theories, 15–16
Situation-relating theories, 15
Skin integrity, assistive technology innovations for, 385–386
Skinner's theory of motivation, 166
Social trends in strategic planning, 251
Specialized devices for older people, 213
Sponsor, role of, 366
Staffing, 310–324
  patient classification tools and, 313–316
  systems for
    current, overview of, 316–317
    evolution of, 311–312
    next generation of, 322–323
    patient classification as component of, 312–313
    work measurement in, 317–319
State regulatory initiatives to control health care expenditures, 454–455
Strategic planning, 248–256

competition/hospital image in, 252
concept of, 248–249
critical issue examination in, 253
defining business-centered mission in, 253–254
economic factors in, 250
of facilities, 295–309. *See also* Facility planning
internal assessment in, 252–253
manpower in, 252
market trends in, 251
nursing administration in, 254–255
organizational structure and process in, 253
plan development in, 254
political issues in, 251
process of, 249–252
regulatory factors in, 251–252
social/lifestyle trends in, 251
technology trends in, 251
Stroke patient, assistive technology for, 383–384
Structural frame, organizations viewed from, 47
Subgroup cultures, relationship of, to corporate culture, 124–125
Symbolic frame, organizations viewed from, 47–48
Systematic abstraction, definition of, 14

Taylor, Frederick W., scientific management and, 32–33
Teacher-learner leader, traits of, 68
Technology
  assistive, 379–388. *See also* Assistive technology
  data entry, for enhancing efficiency, 400–402
  productivity enhancement, justifying investments in, 398–399
  trends of, in strategic planning, 251
Theory(ies)
  construction of, 14–15
  factor-isolating, 15
  general systems, 38–40
  implications of, for nursing administrative practice, 27
  King's general systems, 23–25
  of management, evolving, 30–45. *See also* Management, theories of
  nursing, 13–16
  Orem's self-care, 16–20
  situation-depicting, 15
  situation-producing, 15–16
  situation-relating, 15
Therapeutic self-care demand, 19
Third-party reimbursement for nursing services, 150–151
Time management by nurse executive, 74–75

Transcription time, efficiencies from reduction in, 402–403
Transformation, 231–232
Turnover, 281–283
  implication of nursing practice pattern for, 291–292

Unions
  nurses and, 415–416
  recognition of, process of, 416–417
Unit ethos in building effective work groups, 335–336
Unit nursing work, 333–334
Unit work context in building effective work groups, 330–331
Utilization management in integrated quality management, 263–264

Verbal communication, 359–360
Visioning, empowerment and, 234–235
Vocational nursing, professional nursing differentiated from, 7

Wald, Lillian, as nurse executive, 4
Weber, Max, bureaucratic model of management of, 35–36
Win-lose in conflict resolution, 196
Win-win in conflict resolution, 197
Women, older, special needs of, 216–217
Work
  context of, in building effective work groups, 328
  perceptions of, empowerment and, 238–239
  unit nursing, 333–334
Work excitement, empowerment and, 239–241
Work excitement, model for, 239–240
Work groups
  effective, building, 327–337
    effective unit workplace in, 331–333
    hospital context in, 328–330
    unit ethos in, 335–336
    unit nursing work in, 333–334
    unit work context in, 330–331
    work context in, 328
  flexible, 292–293
Work measurement in nursing, staffing and, 317–319
Work penetration points, identification of, from unit data, 244–245
Worker learning, 53–55
Workplace, effective unit, 331–333
Workweek patterns for nursing personnel, scheduling and, 320–322